ANATOMY TO COLOR AND STUDY

2nd edition

Ray Poritsky, Ph.D. Emeritus

Department of Anatomy
Case Western University School of Medicine
Cleveland, Ohio

ISBN: 978-0-9835784-2-0

Digitally Reproduced by:
CONVERPAGE
23 Acorn Street
Scituate, MA 02066
www.converpage.com

CONTENTS

Part III: Pelvis and Perineum

Part IV: The Upper Limb

Part V: Back

Part VI: The Lower Limb

Part VII: Head and Neck

PREFACE to Second Edition

This book allows the reader to learn human anatomy in a simple and direct manner by coloring and labeling key anatomical structures. It is intended to augment and reinforce the student's anatomical knowledge. Many students will be engaged in anatomical dissection in the gross anatomy laboratory (the word *anatomy* comes from the Greek "to cut"). In addition to dissection, the study of human anatomy involves reading anatomy textbooks, and studying formal anatomical atlases, both artistic and photographic. A careful coloring and labeling of the figures in this book can serve as either an introduction to or as a review of one's knowledge of anatomy.

The book is arranged in regional order to follow the method used in most courses in anatomy. In this edition the number of plates to color and label has been expanded from 265 to 415. These plates cover the seven regions of the body. The use of the book should be fairly intuitive. The traditional color scheme of anatomy textbooks and atlases is red for arteries, blue for veins, yellow for nerves, pink to reddish brown for muscles, and white or light tan for bones. The reader will find that good quality sharp color pencils work quite well. The student may wish to keep these colored and labeled plates as useful references in the future, as aids when explaining anatomy to their patients.

There is very little explanatory text. In a few places, short paragraphs have been added that impart important aspects of applied anatomy, but this book is not intended to serve as an anatomy textbook. Etymological cartoons are interspersed throughout for a brief change and convey some information about Latin and Greek roots.

Color pencils ready… go!

Ray Poritsky, Ph.D.

ACKNOWLEDGMENTS

The majority of the illustrations were drawn by the author, who has had formal training in anatomy and medical illustration. Additional drawings were done by Helen Williams, Susan Weil, Cheryl Owens, and James Bille. The author used the following texts as source materials: Spalteholz and Spanner: *Atlas of Human Anatomy, 16th ed.*, Philadelphia, F.A. Davis, 1961; Wolf-Heidegger: *Atlas of Systematic Human Anatomy*, New York, Hafner, 1962; Hollinshead and Rosse: *Textbook of Anatomy, 4th ed.*, Philadelphia, Harper and Row, 1985; Netter: *The Ciba Collection of Medical Illustrations*, Summit, NJ, Ciba Pharmaceutical Company, 1959, 1962; Clemente: *Anatomy: A Regional Atlas of the Human Body, 3rd ed.*, Baltimore and Munich, Urban & Schwarzenberg, 1987; Rohen and Yokochi: *Color Atlas of Anatomy: A Photographic Study of the Human Body*, New York and Tokyo, Igaku-Shoin, 1984; Moore: *Clinically Oriented Anatomy*, Baltimore, Williams & Wilkins, 1982; Clemente: *Anatomy of the Human Body, 13th ed.*, Philadelphia, Lea & Febiger, 1985; Williams and Warwick: *Gray's Anatomy, 36th British ed.*, Edinburgh, Churchill Livingstone, 1980; Anson: *Morris' Human Anatomy: A Complete Systematic Treatise, 12th ed.*, New York, McGraw-Hill, 1966; Pernkopf: *Atlas of Topographical and Applied Human Anatomy*, Munich, Urban & Schwarzenberg, 1980. I also found certain Somso anatomical models most helpful for several of the drawings.

I also acknowledge Dr. Thomas Oelrich for his generous help relating to his work on pelvic anatomy and the medical students at Case Western Reserve University School of Medicine for their suggestions, criticism, and encouragement.

The following sources were employed for the section on The Upper Limb and The Lower Limb and are gratefully acknowledged. Several figures were drawn by Cheryl Owens and Wayne Timmerman. Illustrations are reworked and updated figures from Eycleshymer and Jones: *Hand Atlas of Clinical Anatomy*, Lea & Febiger, 1925. Other atlases and texts consulted include: Wolf-Heidegger: *Atlas of Systemic Human Anatomy*, Hafner, 1962; Spalteholz and Spanner: *Atlas of Human Anatomy, 16th ed.*, F.A. Davis, 1961; Hollinshead and Rosse: *Textbook of Anatomy, 4th ed.*, Harper and Row, 1985; Clemente: *A Regional Atlas of the Human Body, 3rd ed.*, Urban & Schwarzenberg, 1987; Töndury: *Angewandte und Topographische Anatomie*, Fretz & Wasmuth, 1949; Williams (ed): *Gray's Anatomy, 38th British ed.*, Churchill Livingstone, 1995; Netter: *The Ciba Collection of Medical Illustrations*, Ciba Pharmaceutical Company, 1959.

I thank and warmly dedicate this book to my wife Connie.

Part I: Introduction and Thorax

The Four "Birds" of the Thorax (A Shameless Pun)

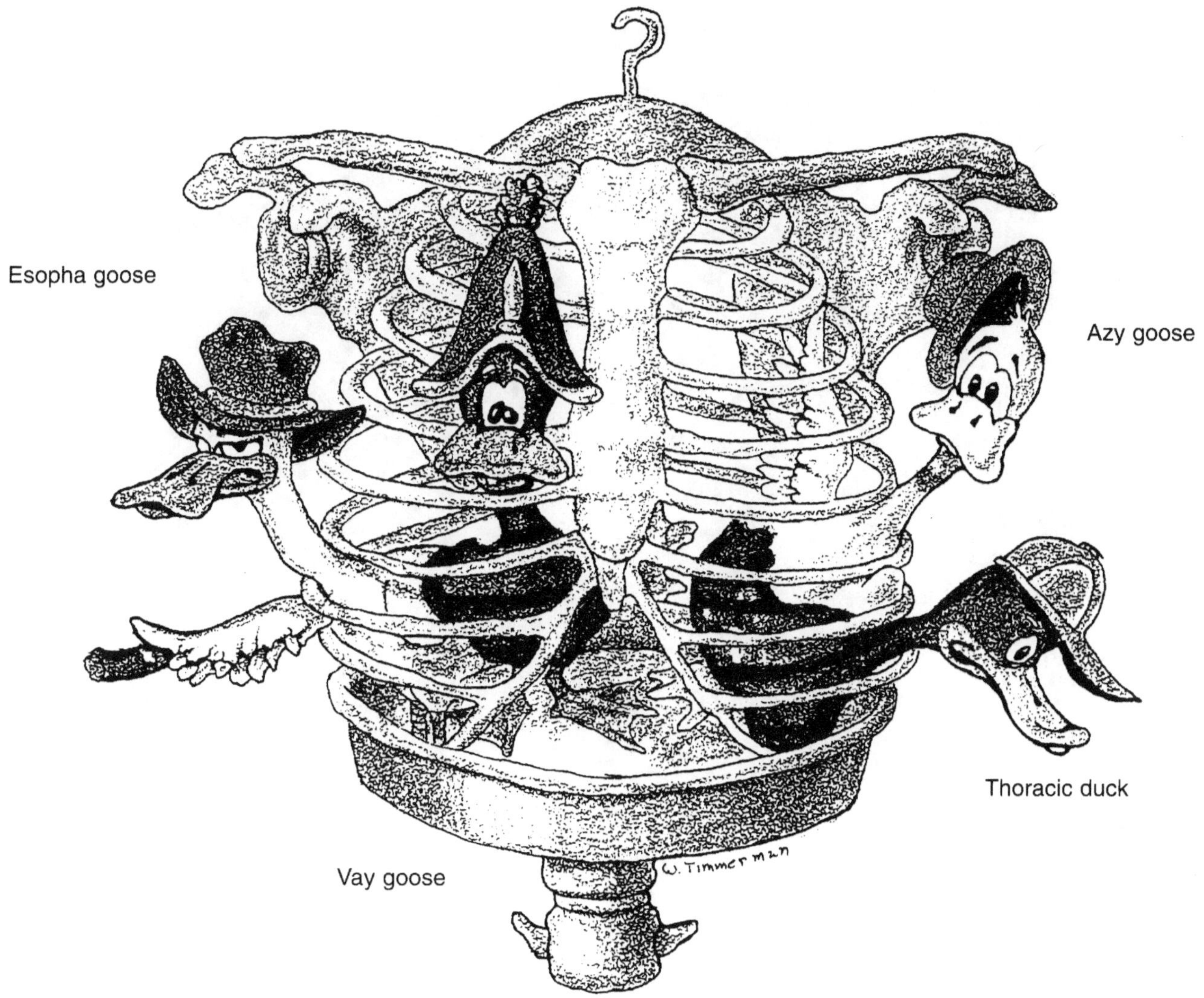

The "Esopha goose" is the esophagus

The "Azy goose" is the azygos vein

The "Vay goose" is the vagus nerve

The "Thoracic duck" is the thoracic duct
(the largest lymph vessel in the body)

Th-1 Planes of the Body

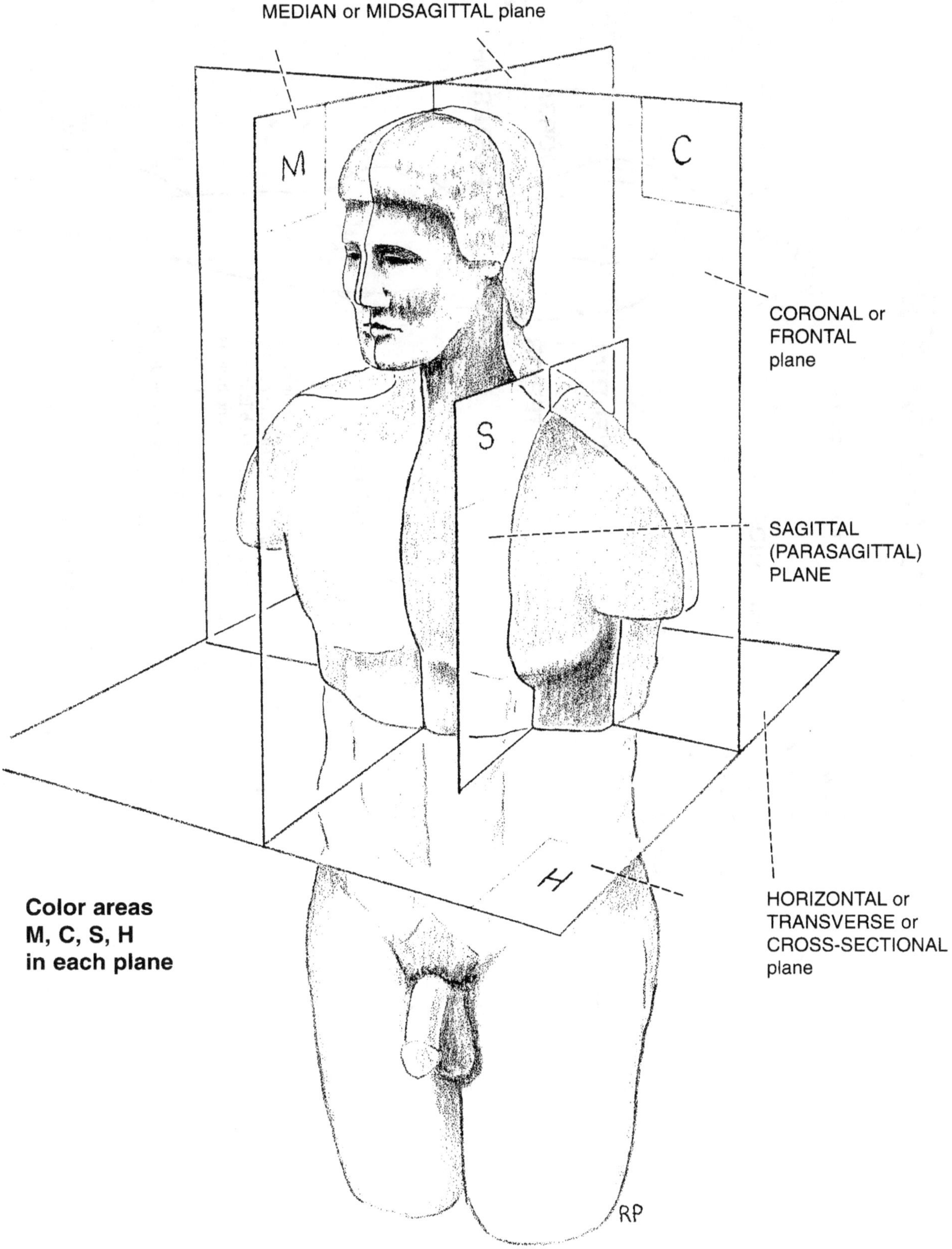

Color areas M, C, S, H in each plane

Th-2 Anatomic position

Color each arrow

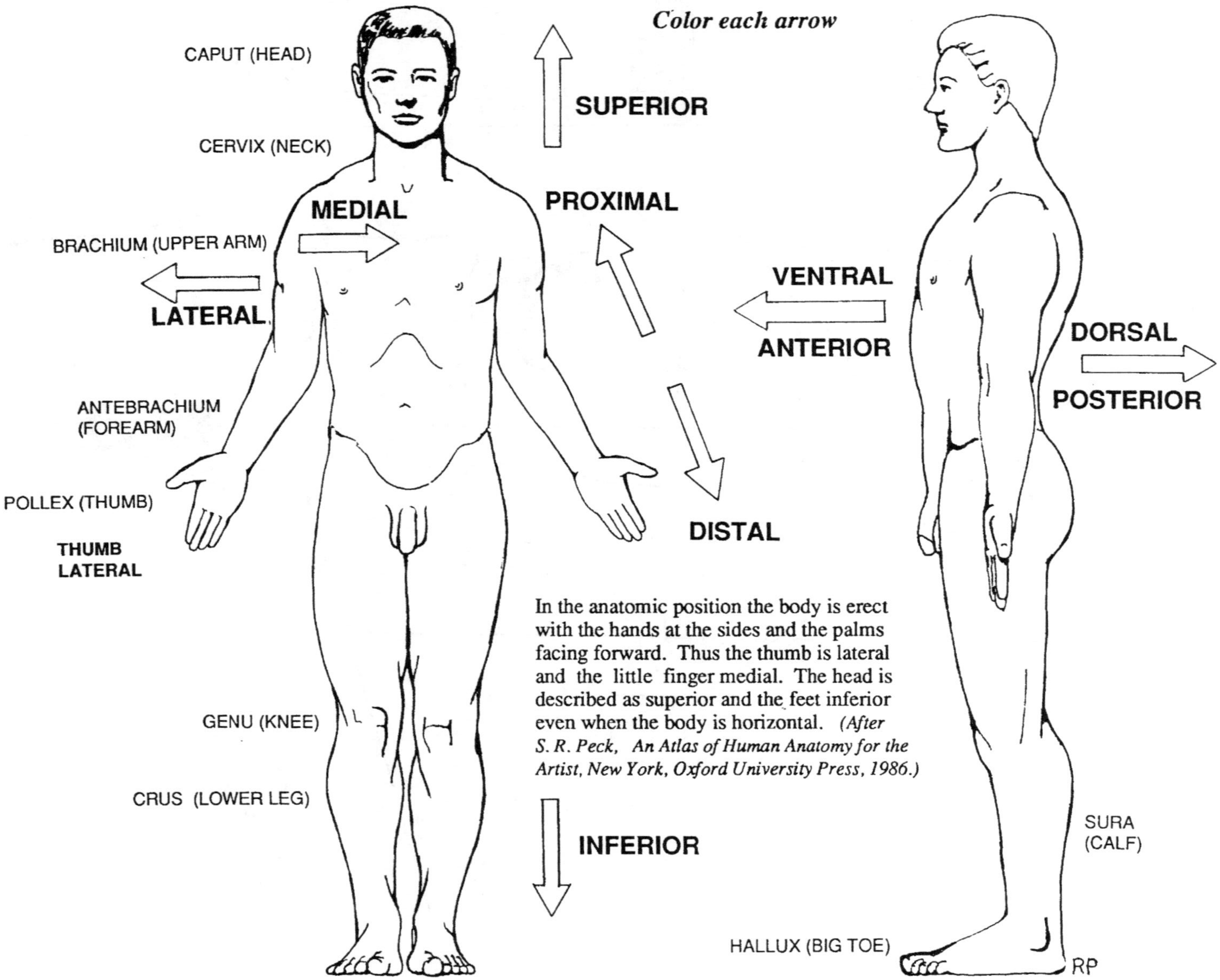

In the anatomic position the body is erect with the hands at the sides and the palms facing forward. Thus the thumb is lateral and the little finger medial. The head is described as superior and the feet inferior even when the body is horizontal. *(After S. R. Peck, An Atlas of Human Anatomy for the Artist, New York, Oxford University Press, 1986.)*

Th-3 Some common movements

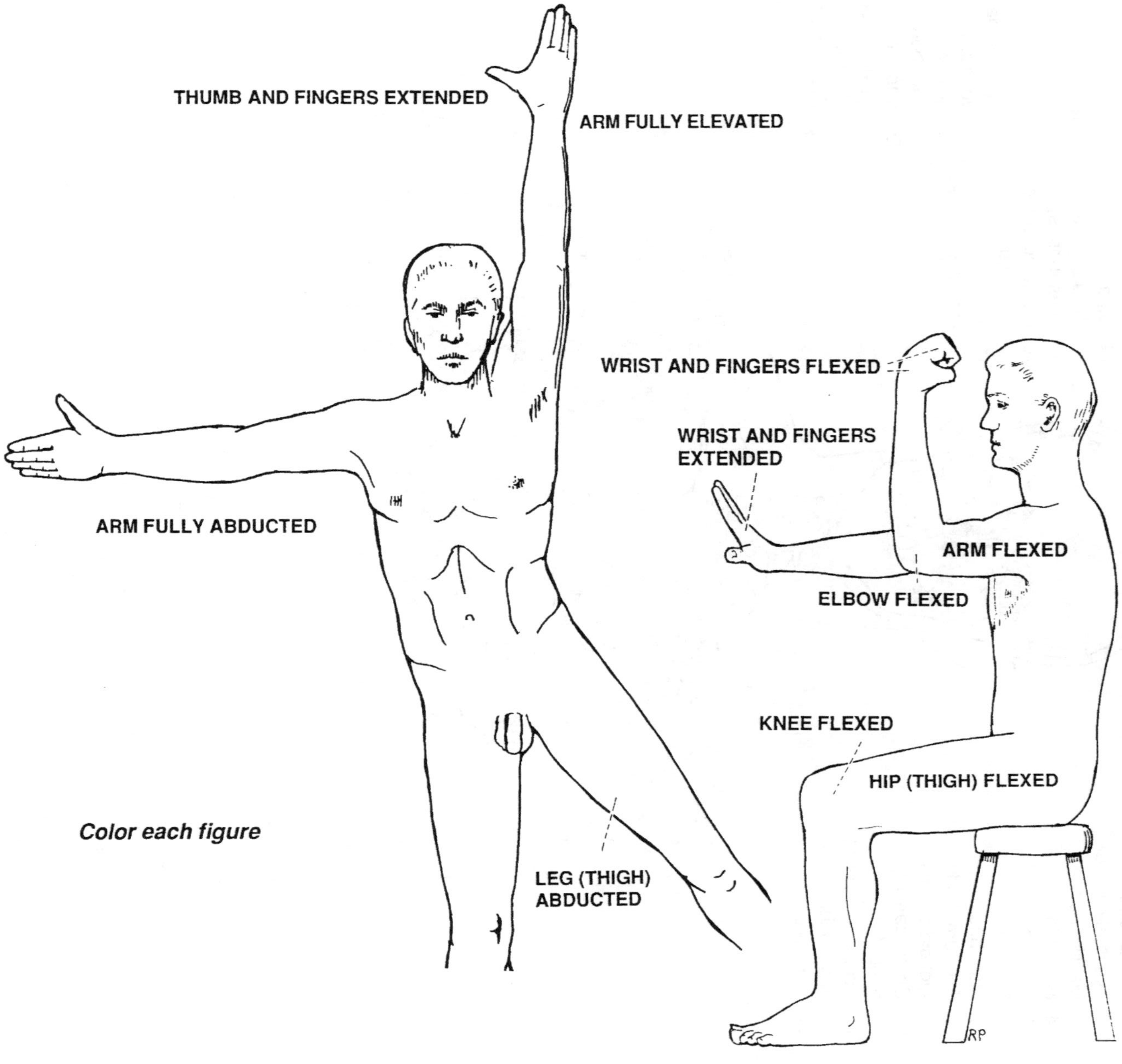

Color each figure

Th-4 Skeletal landmarks

(upper anterior view)

Color and label

1 Frontal bone
2 Zygomatic bone
3 Maxillary bone
4 Mandible
5 Clavicle
6 First rib
7 Manubrium
8 Sternum (body)
9 Xiphoid process
10 Costal cartilage of rib 7
11 Acromion process of scapula
12 Humerus
13 Radius
14 Ulna
15 Carpal bones (wrist bones)
16 Coracoid process of scapula
17 Scapula (shoulder blade)
18 Fifth lumbar vertebra
19 Ilium of coxal (hip) bone
20 Sacrum
21 Greater trochanter of femur
22 Pubic symphysis

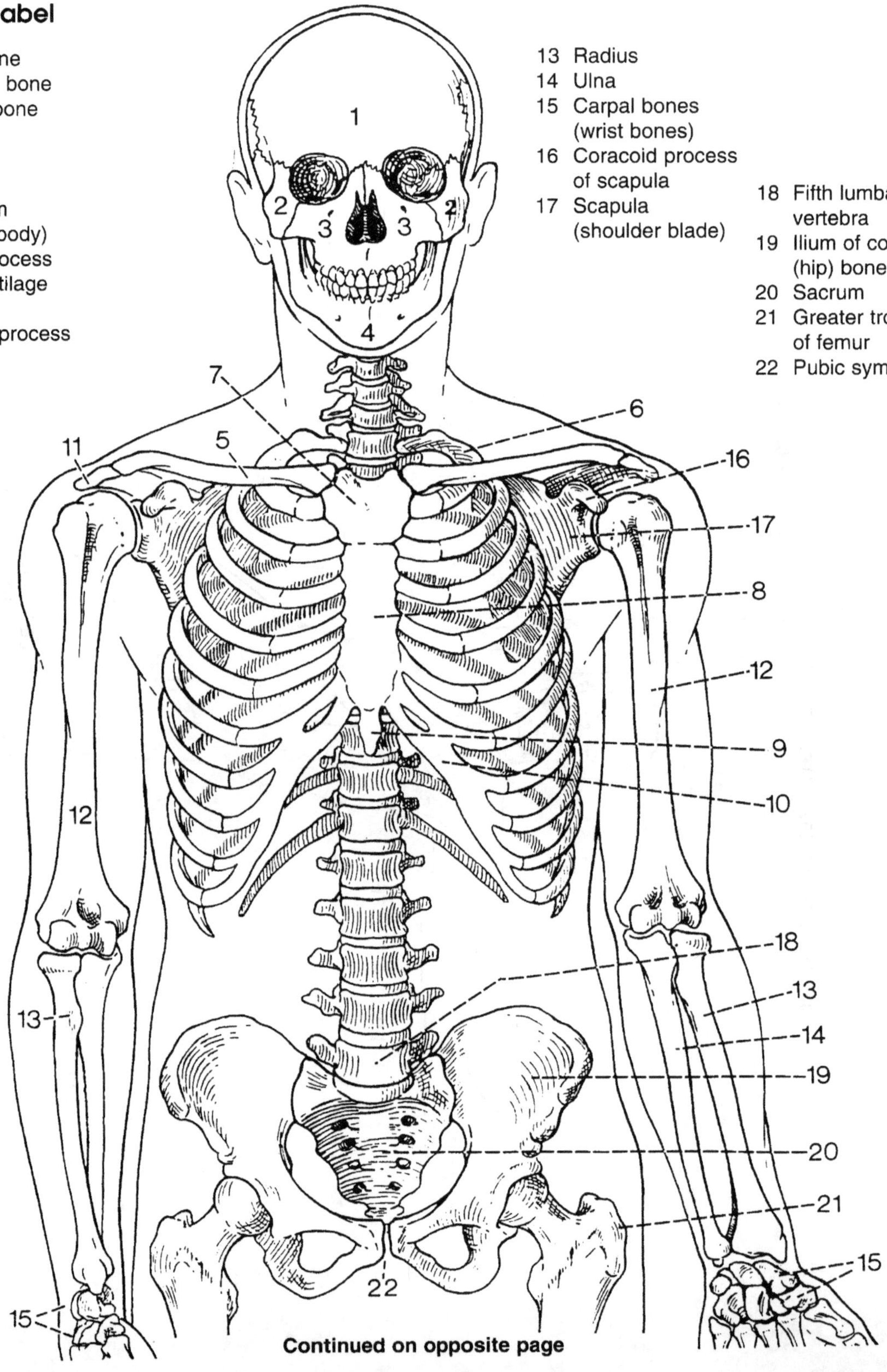

Continued on opposite page

Th-5 Bones of the skeleton

(lower anterior view)

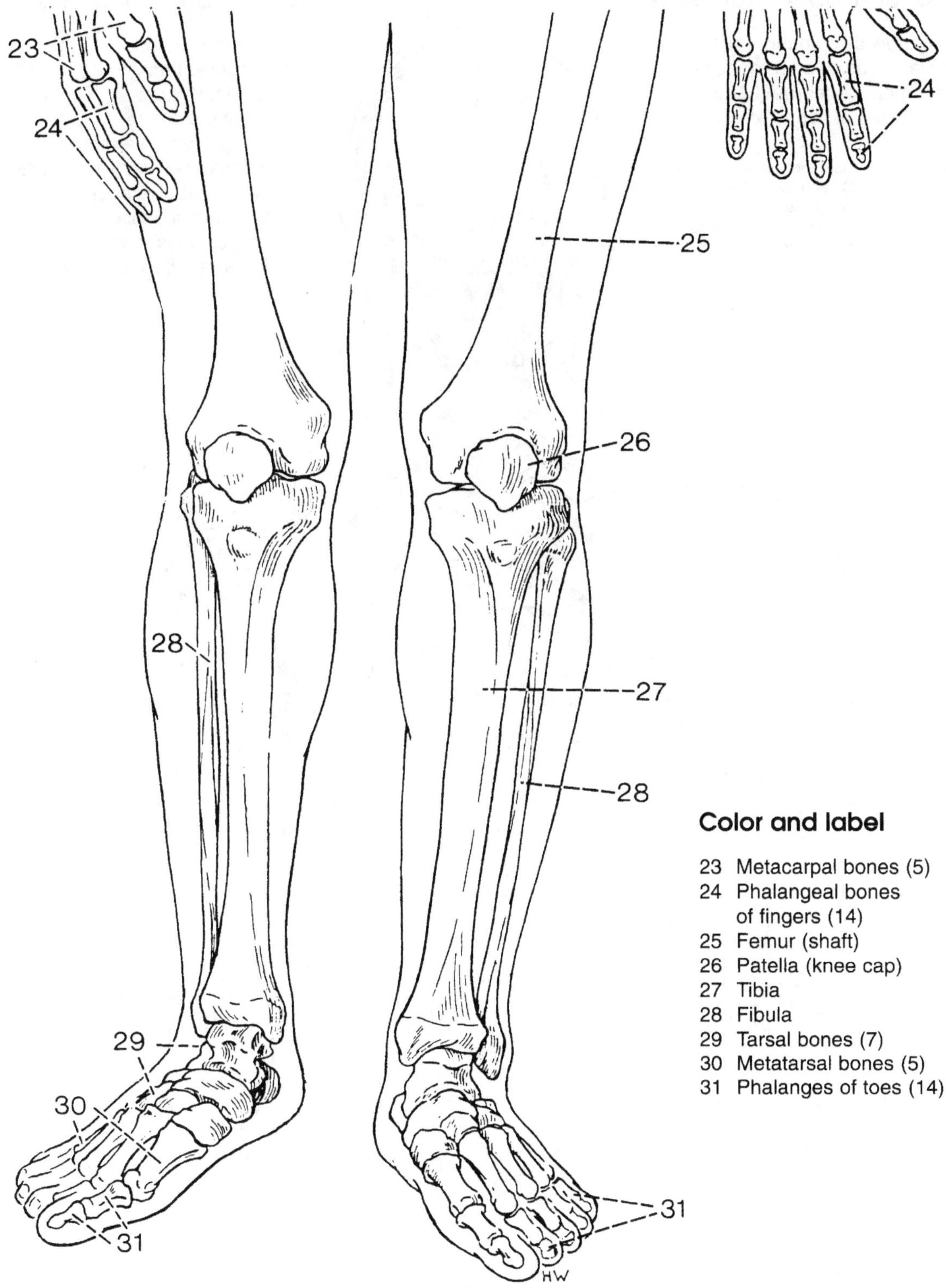

Color and label

23 Metacarpal bones (5)
24 Phalangeal bones of fingers (14)
25 Femur (shaft)
26 Patella (knee cap)
27 Tibia
28 Fibula
29 Tarsal bones (7)
30 Metatarsal bones (5)
31 Phalanges of toes (14)

Th-6 Skeletal landmarks

(upper posterior view)

Color and label these bones

Seven cervical vertebrae (C1-C7)
Twelve thoracic vertebrae (T1-T12)
Five lumbar vertebrae (L1-L5)
Twelve pairs of ribs
Scapula
Humerus
Ulna
Radius

Note that cervical vertabrae C1 and C2, unlike the other 25 vertebrae, have their own names, **atlas** and **axis** respectively.

Label these landmarks

1 Parietal bones
2 Occipital bone
3 Sagittal suture
4 Lamboid suture
5 First cervical vertebra (atlas)
6 Second cervical vertebra (axis)
7 Acromion of scapula
8 Spine of scapula
9 Infraspinous fossa
10 Greater tubercle of humerus

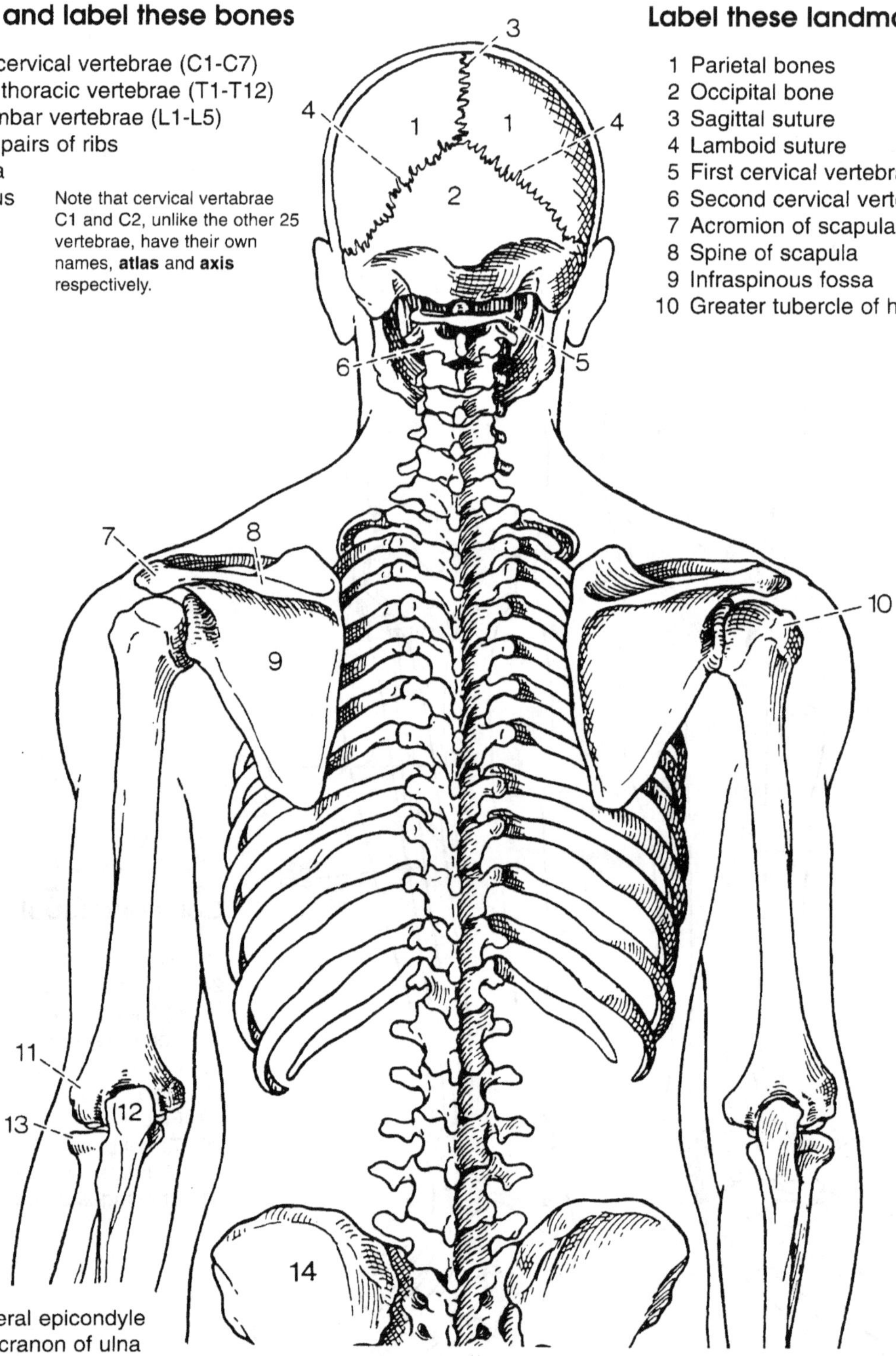

11 Lateral epicondyle
12 Olecranon of ulna
13 Head of radius
14 Ilium of coxal bone

Continued on opposite page

Th-7 Skeletal landmarks

(lower posterior view)

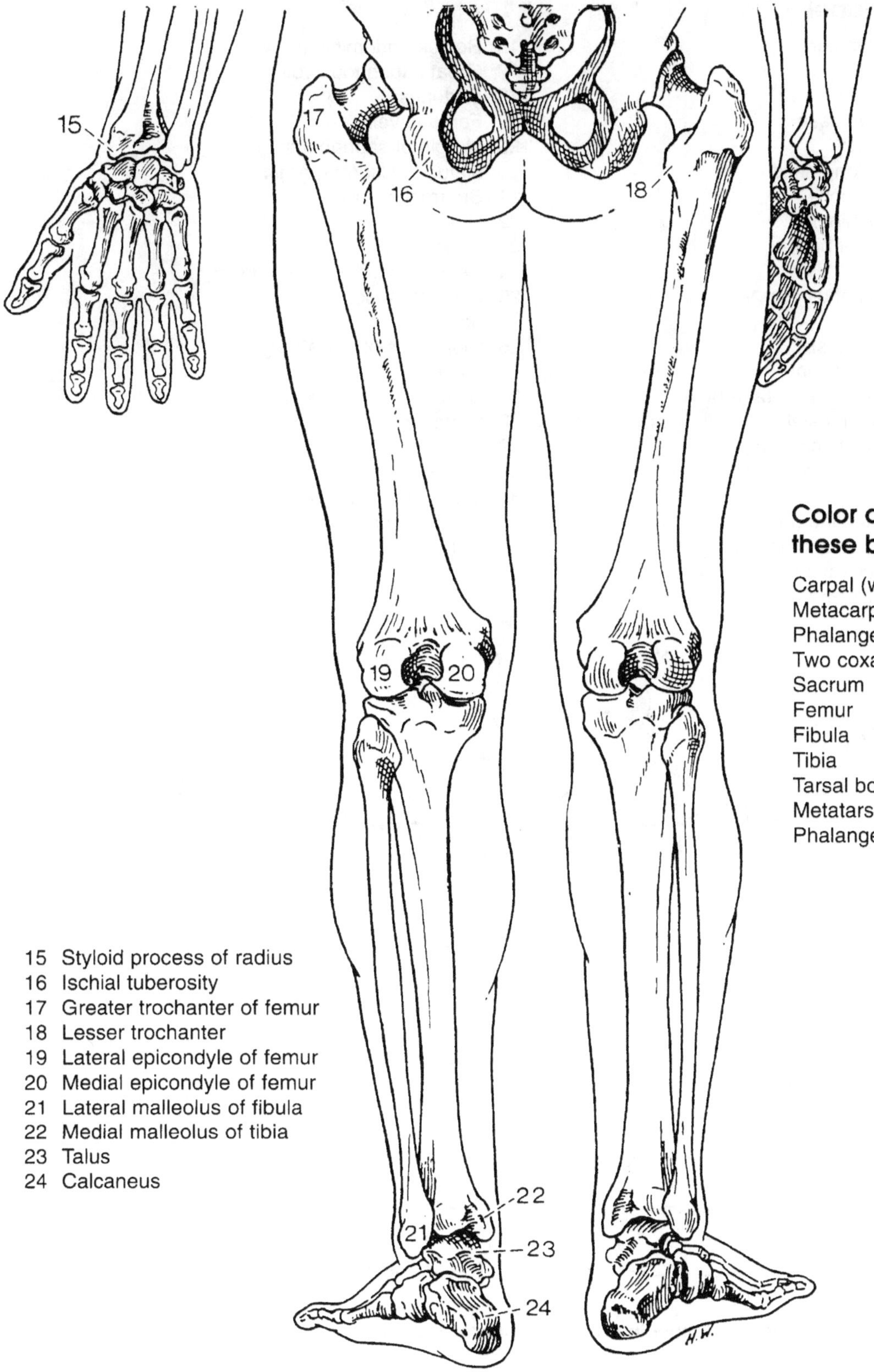

Color and label these bones

Carpal (wrist) bones
Metacarpal bones
Phalanges of fingers
Two coxal (hip) bones
Sacrum
Femur
Fibula
Tibia
Tarsal bones
Metatarsal bones
Phalanges of toes

15 Styloid process of radius
16 Ischial tuberosity
17 Greater trochanter of femur
18 Lesser trochanter
19 Lateral epicondyle of femur
20 Medial epicondyle of femur
21 Lateral malleolus of fibula
22 Medial malleolus of tibia
23 Talus
24 Calcaneus

Th-8 Muscles of the anterior trunk

(opposite page)

Color and label

1 Pectoralis major
2 Subclavius
3 Trapezius
4 Coracoid process
5 Deltoid (cut)
6 Tendon of long head of biceps brachii
7 Pectoralis minor
8 Long head of biceps brachii
9 Short head of biceps brachii
10 Latissimus dorsi
11 Internal intercostal seen beneath membrane of external intercostal
12 Rectus abdominis (cut)
13 Rectus sheath (posterior layer)
14 Semicircular line (lower border of posterior layer)
15 Internal abdominal oblique
16 Rectus abdominis (cut)
17 Great saphenous vein
18 Sartorius
19 Femoral vein
20 Margin of saphenous hiatus (falciform margin)
21 Spermatic cord
22 Umbilicus
23 Linea alba
24 Rectus sheath (anterior layer)
25 External abdominal oblique
26 Digitations of serratus anterior
27 Deltoid
28 Sternum
29 Clavicle
30 Trapezius
31 Sternocleidomastoid
32 Sternocleidomastoid sternal clavicular origins (cut)

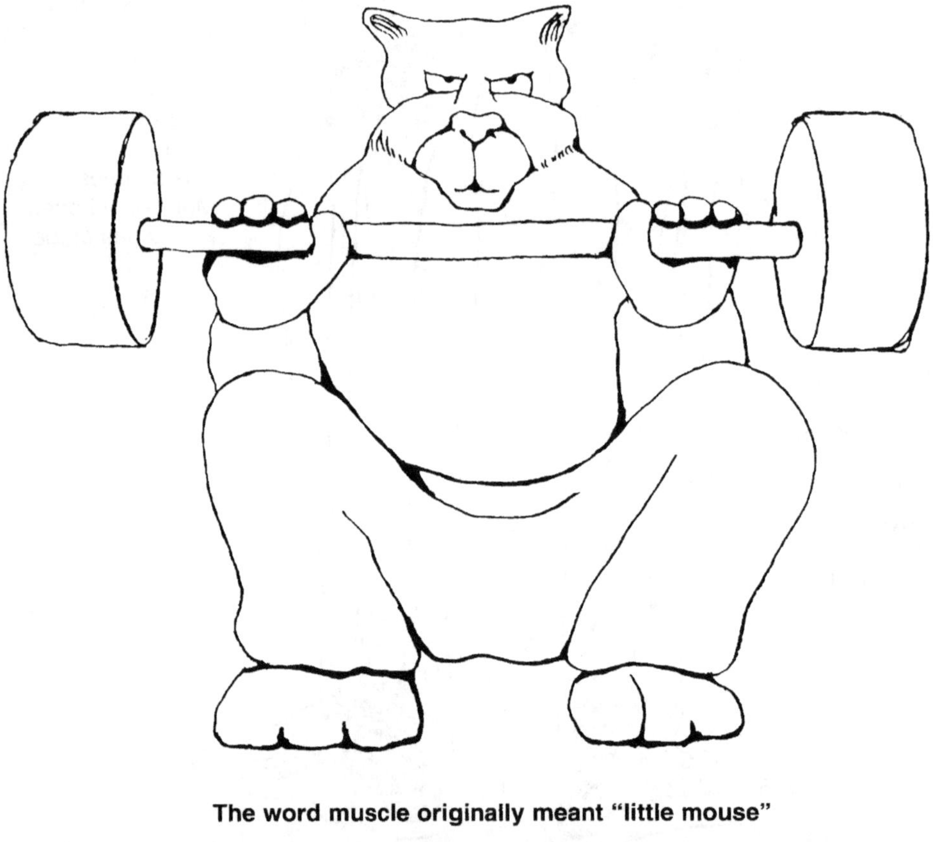

The word muscle originally meant "little mouse"

Th-8 Muscles of anterior trunk

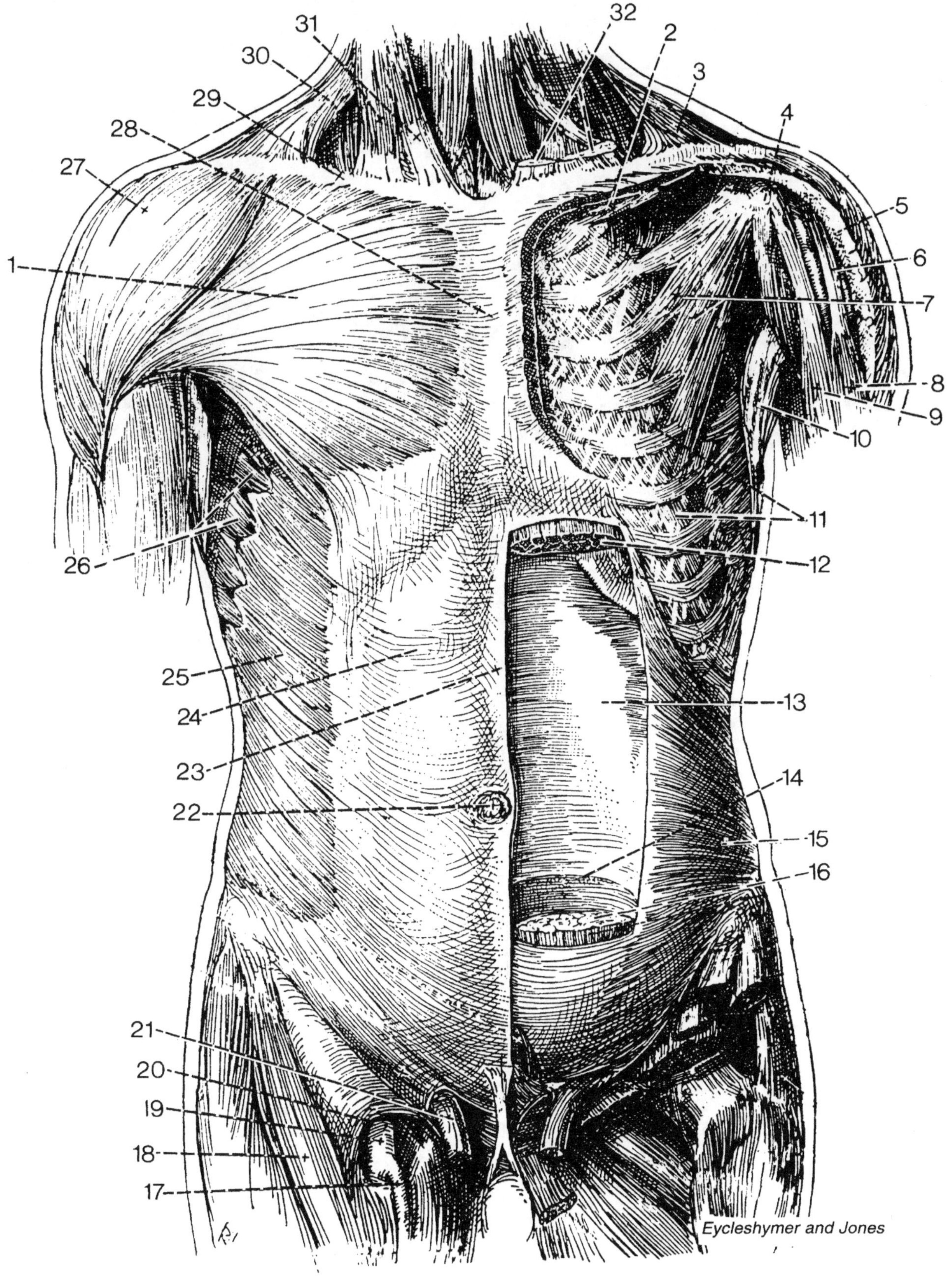

Th-9 Muscles of anterior thorax and abdomen

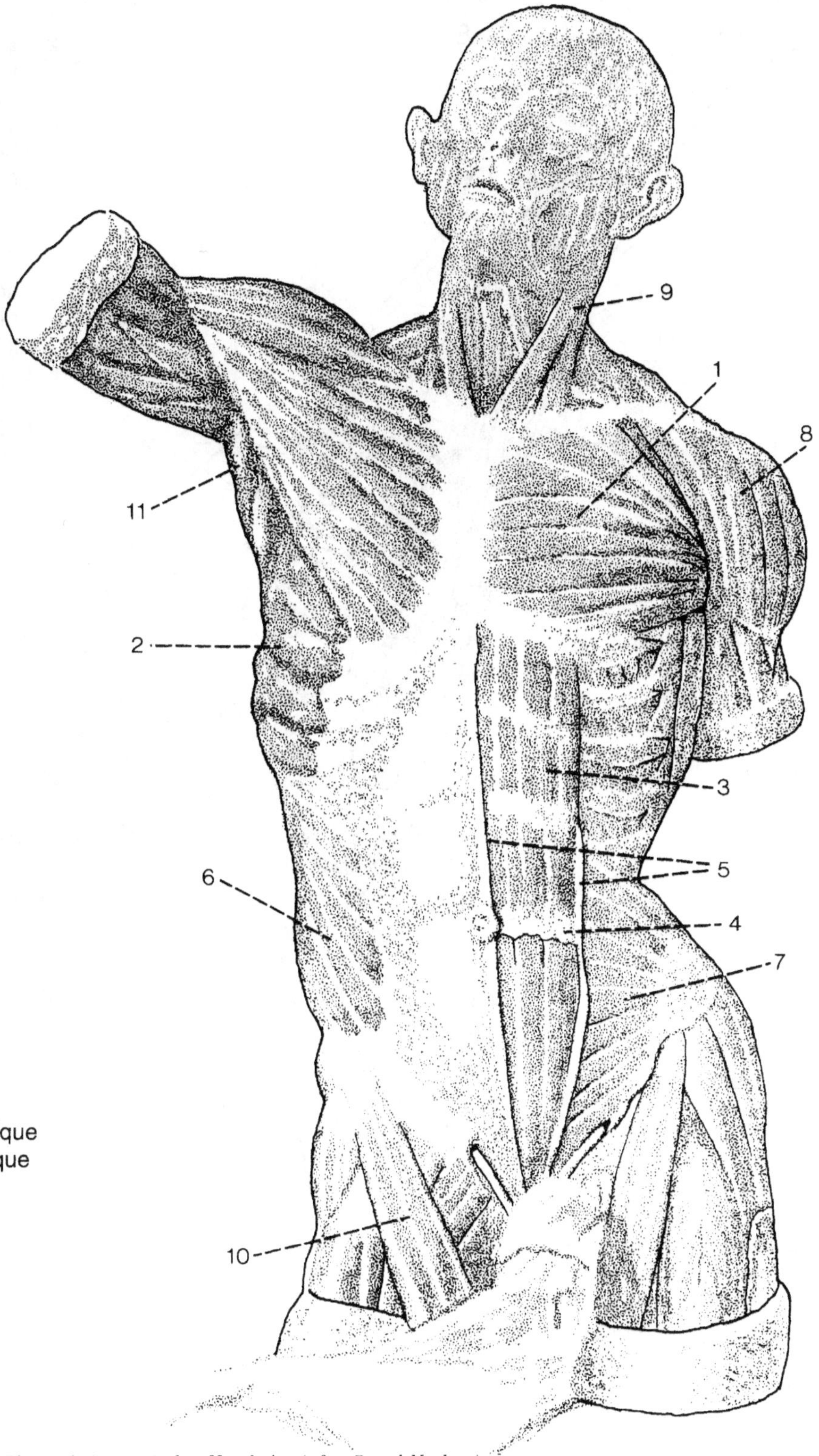

Color and label

1 Pectoralis major
2 Serratus anterior
3 Rectus abdominis
4 Tendinous intersection
5 Rectus sheath (cut)
6 External abdominal oblique
7 Internal abdominal oblique
8 Deltoid
9 Sternocleidomastoid
10 Sartorius
11 Latissimus dorsi

After E. A. Seeman, Fritz Schiders Plastisch-Anatomischer Handatlas (after Duval-Neelsen). Leipzig, M. Averbach and Franz V. Stuck Verlag, 1929.

Th-10 Section through lactating breast

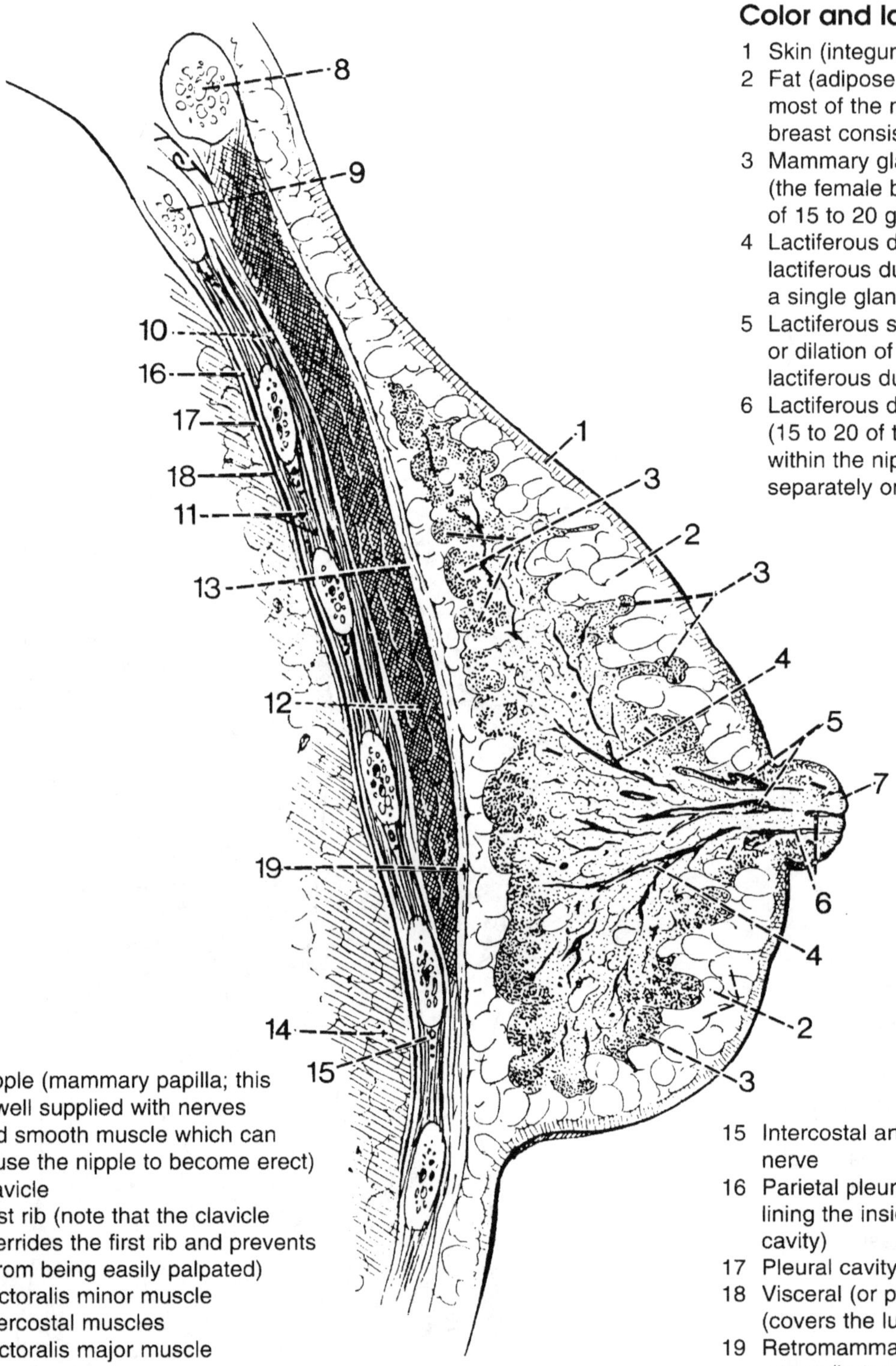

Modified from Eycleshymer and Jones

Color and label

1 Skin (integument)
2 Fat (adipose tissue; most of the non-lactating breast consists of fat)
3 Mammary gland lobes (the female breast consists of 15 to 20 glandular lobes)
4 Lactiferous ducts (each lactiferous duct arises from a single glandular lobe)
5 Lactiferous sinus (swelling or dilation of the lactiferous duct)
6 Lactiferous ducts in nipple (15 to 20 of these converge within the nipple and open separately on the tip of the nipple)
7 Nipple (mammary papilla; this is well supplied with nerves and smooth muscle which can cause the nipple to become erect)
8 Clavicle
9 First rib (note that the clavicle overrides the first rib and prevents it from being easily palpated)
10 Pectoralis minor muscle
11 Intercostal muscles
12 Pectoralis major muscle
13 Deep fascia
14 Lung
15 Intercostal artery, vein, and nerve
16 Parietal pleura (a thin membrane lining the inside of the pleural cavity)
17 Pleural cavity (a potential space)
18 Visceral (or pulmonary) pleura (covers the lung)
19 Retromammary (or submammary) space (between breast and deep fascia; allows some movement of the breast on the deep fascia)

Th-11 Fibrous supporting membranes in the breast

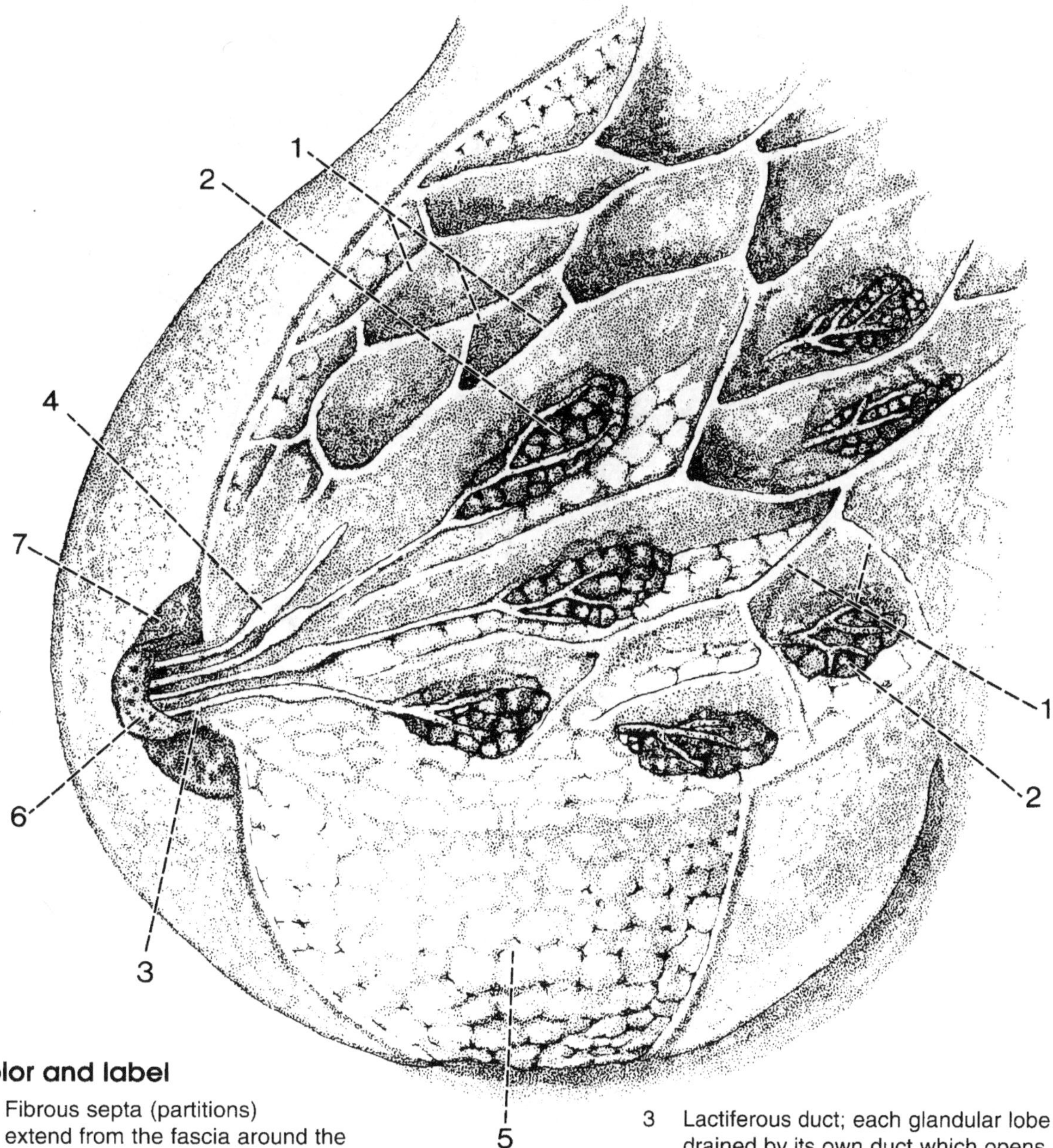

Color and label

1 Fibrous septa (partitions) extend from the fascia around the mammary gland lobes to the skin; they are most prominent in the upper part of the breast where they were once called the suspensory ligaments of Cooper.

2 Mammary gland lobes 15 to 20 in number; these are roughly pyramidal in shape with their apices pointed towards the nipple. Most, but not all, enlarge during lactation and secrete milk.

3 Lactiferous duct; each glandular lobe is drained by its own duct which opens separately as one of 15-20 tiny orifices on the nipple.

4 Lactiferous sinus; swellings in the ducts which accumulate milk during lactation

5 Fat (adipose tissue)

6 Nipple (Latin, *papilla*); note that the nipple is traversed by 15-20 lactiferous ducts.

7 Areola; pigmented area of skin that surrounds the nipple; during pregnancy and lactation, small areolar glands secrete a protective oily substance.

Th-12 Lactating breast

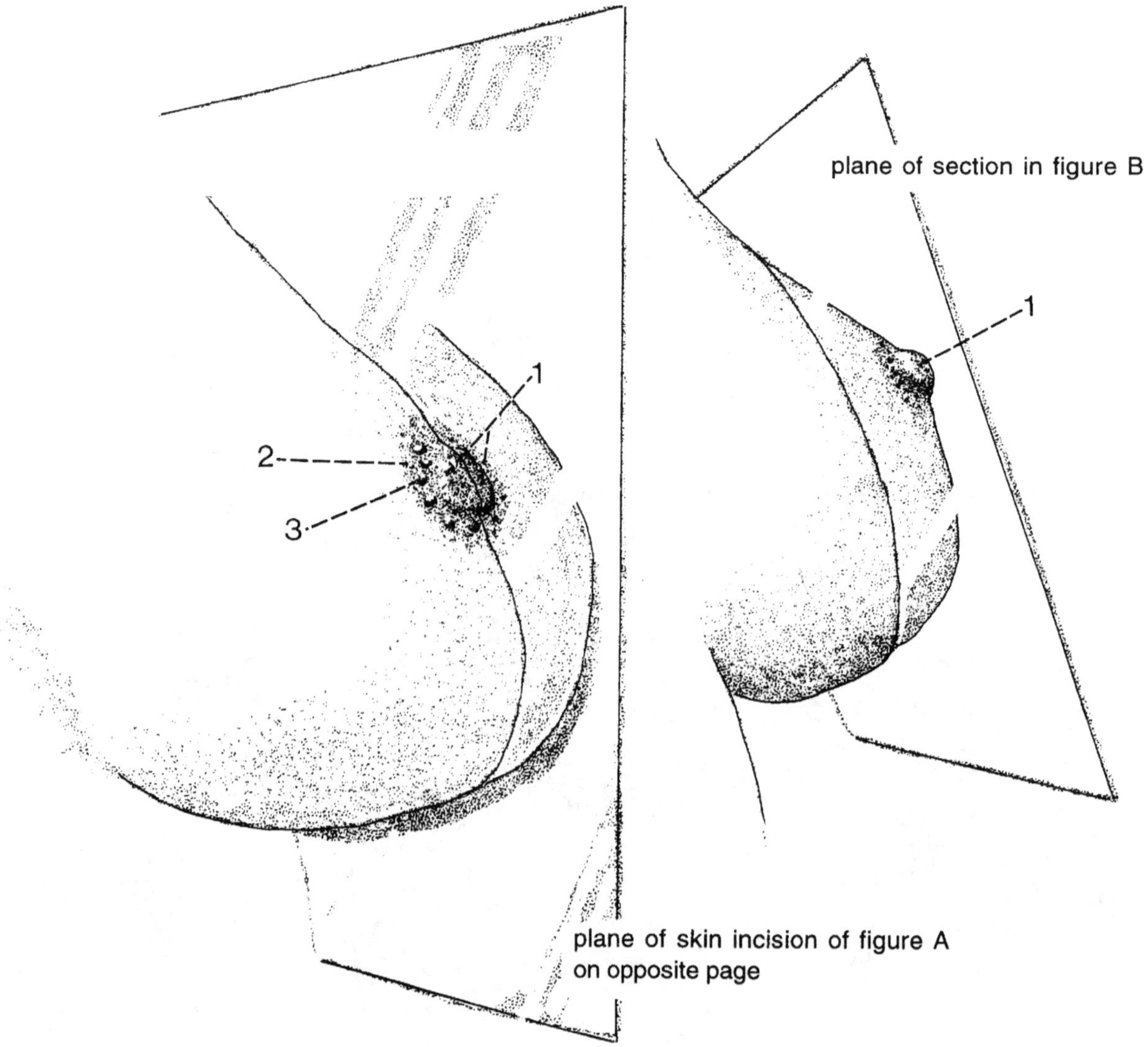

Color and label

1 Nipple (papilla)
2 Areola
3 Areolar glands
4 Nipple with 15 to 20 openings (orifices) of main lactiferous ducts
5 Main lactiferous duct (each drains a single glandular lobe)
6 Mammary gland lobes (15 to 20 in number; note their pyramidal shape with their apices directed forward towards the nipple; these are greatly enlarged during lactation)
7 Lactiferous ampulla (sinus or dilation of the lactiferous duct)
8 Fat (fills the spaces between the glandular lobes and smooths out the contour of the breast; fat is metabolically consumed during lactation)
9 Fibrous membranes or septa (these extend from the glandular lobes to the skin; they are most prominent in the upper part of the breast where they are called the suspensory ligaments of Cooper; the fibrous septa also form pockets which hold the fat)

Th-12 Lactating breast

A

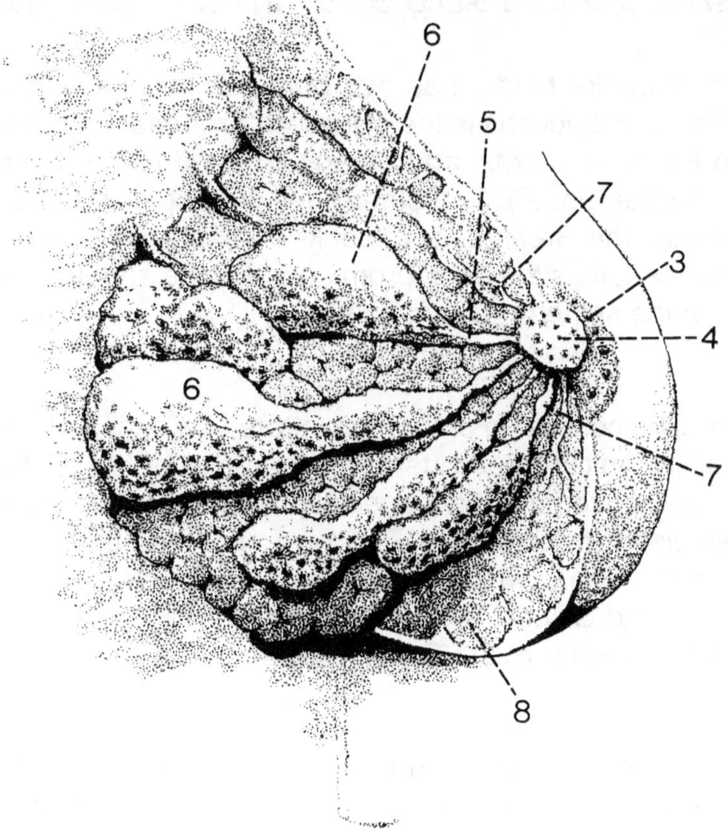

B

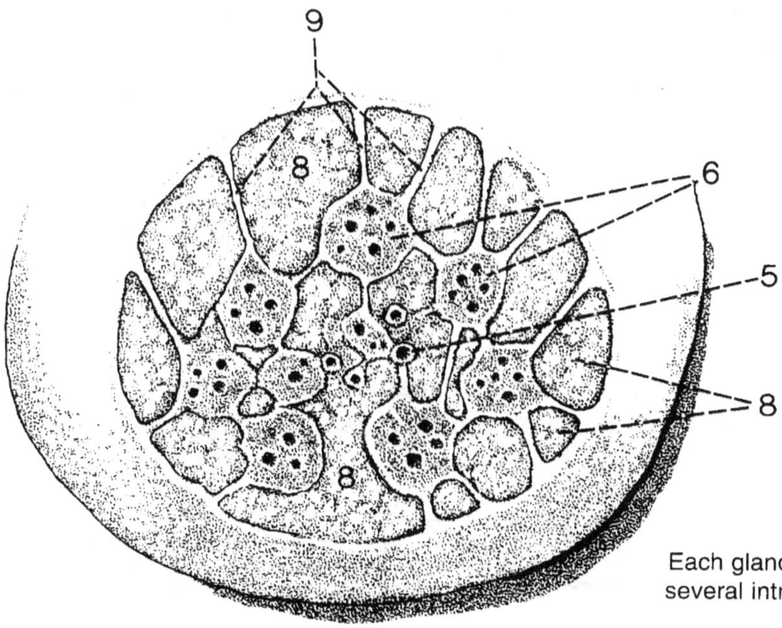

Each glandular lobe shows several intraglandular ducts

Coracoid Process and Acromion

The **scapula**, or shoulder blade, has two bony projections with rather interesting names. One of these projections is the **coracoid process**. Its name is derived from the Greek word for raven, *korax*, and means "shaped like a raven's beak" (*korax*, "raven" + *eidos*, "appearance"). The other bony projection is the **acromion**, and its name is derived from the Greek *akron*, "peak" or "extremity", and *omos*, "shoulder". The acromion can be felt as the bony prominence of the shoulder where it forms the expanded apex of the spine of the scapula.

An *acronym* is a word consisting of the first letters of a series of words. It is derived from *akron*, "first" or "initial" (used here in the sense of the *first* or *initial letter*) + *onyma*, "name". The government is especially adept at alphabetizing the names of government agencies with acronyms. The very early and famous acronym *ichthus* or *ichthys*, Greek for "fish", was used by early Christians as a symbol for "Jesus Christ, Son of God and Savior". The X in Xmas is from the Greek letter *X*, or chi, and stands for the first letter of the Greek word for Christ.

Rostrum means "beak" or "snout". In anatomy *rostrally* means "toward the nose". *Rostrum* also means a "ship's prow". The Roman Forum was ornamented with prows of ships captured from their enemies. These prows were used by orators to make speeches; thus, the word *rostrum* came to mean a stand for a speaker.

Scapula meant shoulder blade in Roman times, as it does today. A winged shoulder blade or scapula results from damage to the serratus anterior muscle often caused by the shoulder rest of a crutch repeatedly rubbing against the long thoracic nerve, which supplies the serratus anterior muscle.

Calcar avis ("bird's spur"; *calcar*, "spur" + *avis*, "bird") is a bump on the medial wall of the posterior horn in both lateral ventricles of the brain.

Pinna, or ***penna***, means feather. Muscles are sometimes described as *bipennate* (like a feather with a central tendon) or *unipennate* (all the fibers obliquely attached to a tendon on one side).

Coracoid process and acromion

An etymological cartoon

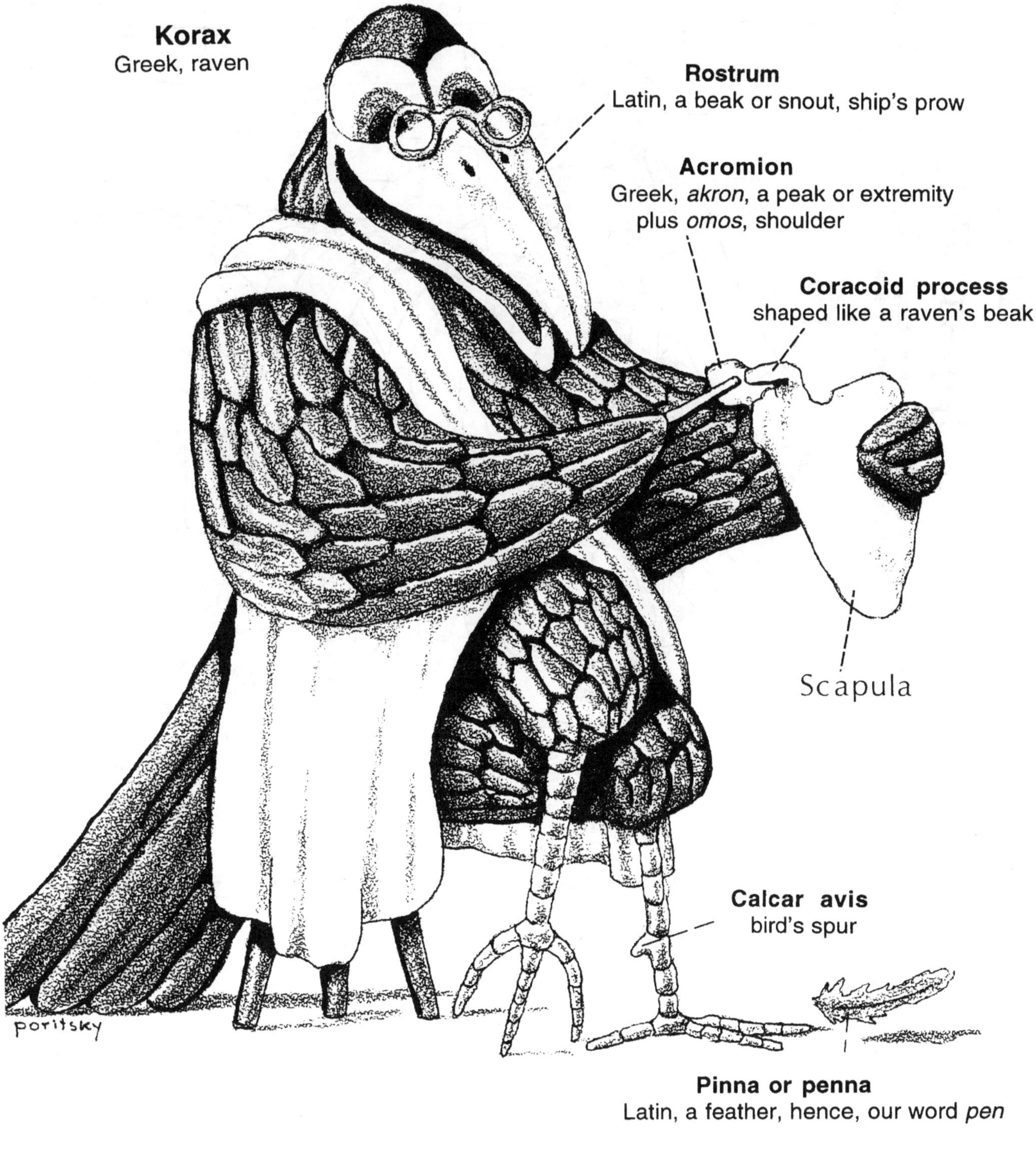

Th-13 Skeletal landmarks (thorax and upper arm)

Color the skeleton and label each of these landmarks

1 Greater tubercle of humerus
2 Lesser tubercle of humerus
3 Intertubercular groove
4 Head of humerus
5 Glenoid fossa of scapula
6 Coracoid process
7 Deltoid tuberosity

The bony thorax consists of the sternum (manubrium, body, xiphoid process), the 12 pairs of ribs on each side, and the 12 thoracic vertebrae.

8 Clavicle
9 Jugular notch
10 Sternoclavicular joint
11 Acromion of scapula
12 Sternal angle
13 Rib 7; the first 7 ribs are "true ribs" because their costal cartilages attach directly to the sternum.

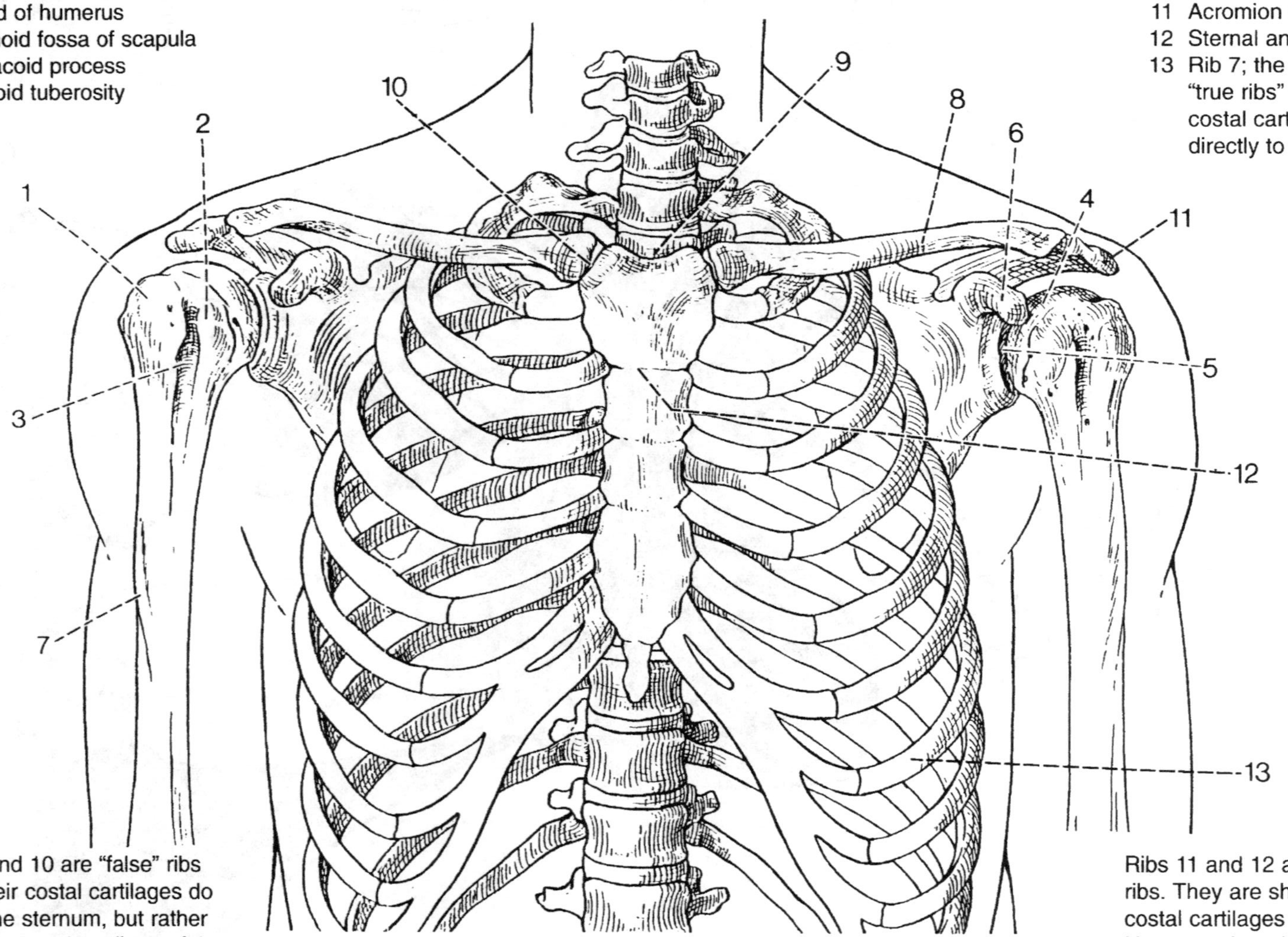

Ribs 8, 9, and 10 are "false" ribs because their costal cartilages do not reach the sternum, but rather attach to the costal cartilage of the rib above.

Ribs 11 and 12 are the "floating" ribs. They are short with very short costal cartilages that end freely. However, they do not float, since they articulate with thoracic vertebrae 11 and 12.

Continued on opposite page

Th-14 Skeletal landmarks (pelvis and hip)

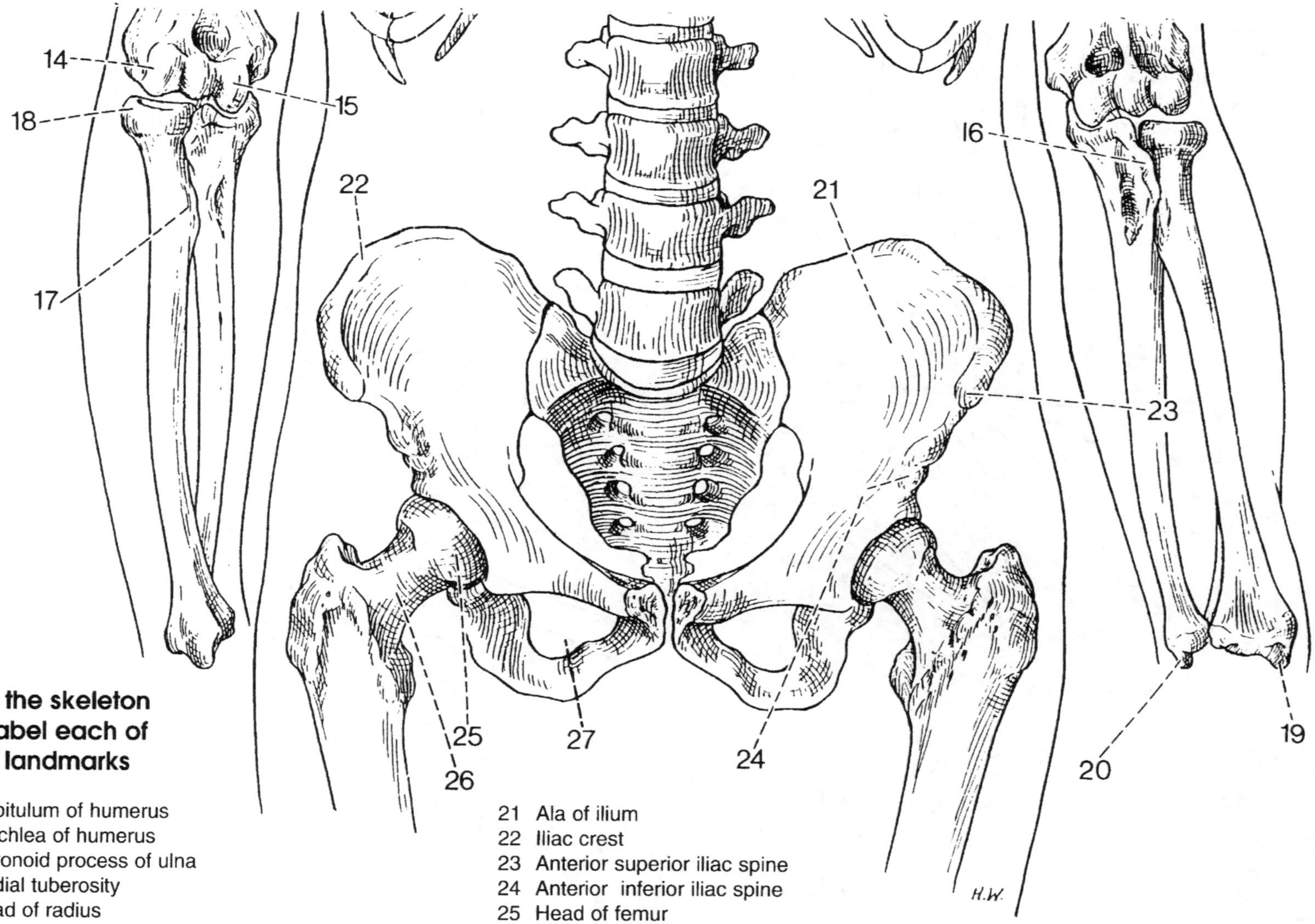

Color the skeleton and label each of these landmarks

14 Capitulum of humerus
15 Trochlea of humerus
16 Coronoid process of ulna
17 Radial tuberosity
18 Head of radius
19 Styloid process of radius
20 Styloid process of ulna

21 Ala of ilium
22 Iliac crest
23 Anterior superior iliac spine
24 Anterior inferior iliac spine
25 Head of femur
26 Neck of femur
27 Obturator foramen

Th-15 Anterior thoracic muscles

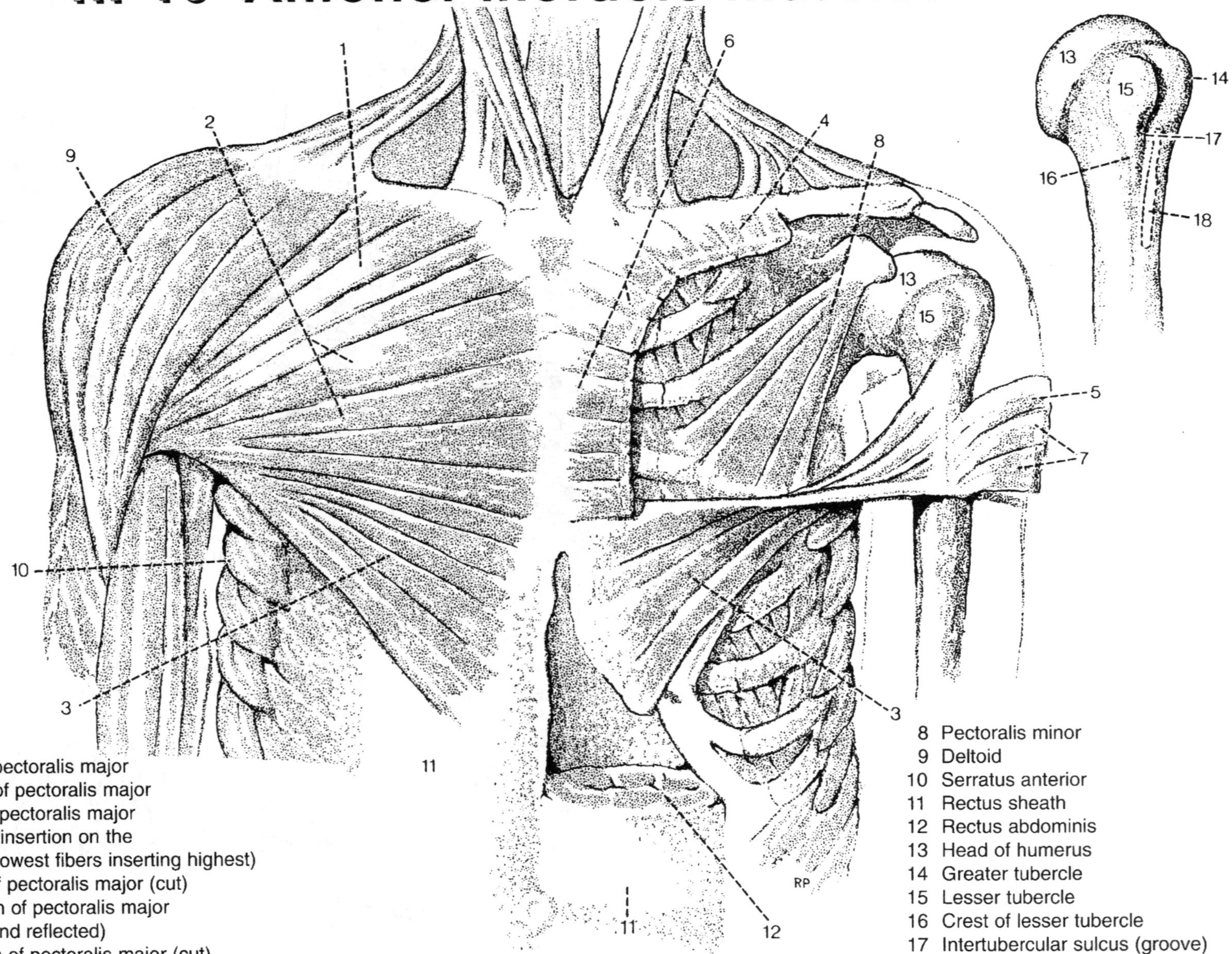

Color and label

1 Clavicular part of pectoralis major
2 Sternocostal part of pectoralis major
3 Abdominal part of pectoralis major (notice its twisting insertion on the humerus with the lowest fibers inserting highest)
4 Clavicular origin of pectoralis major (cut)
5 Clavicular insertion of pectoralis major on humerus (cut and reflected)
6 Sternocostal origin of pectoralis major (cut)
7 Sternocostal insertion of pectoralis major (note the bilaminar insertion of the pectoralis major tendon with abdominal part inserting deeper and the sternocostal and clavicular parts inserting more superficial)
8 Pectoralis minor
9 Deltoid
10 Serratus anterior
11 Rectus sheath
12 Rectus abdominis
13 Head of humerus
14 Greater tubercle
15 Lesser tubercle
16 Crest of lesser tubercle
17 Intertubercular sulcus (groove)
18 Insertion of pectoralis major on crest of greater tubercle

Th-16 Muscle attachments of the anterior thorax

Color and label the muscle origins (O) red and insertions (I) blue

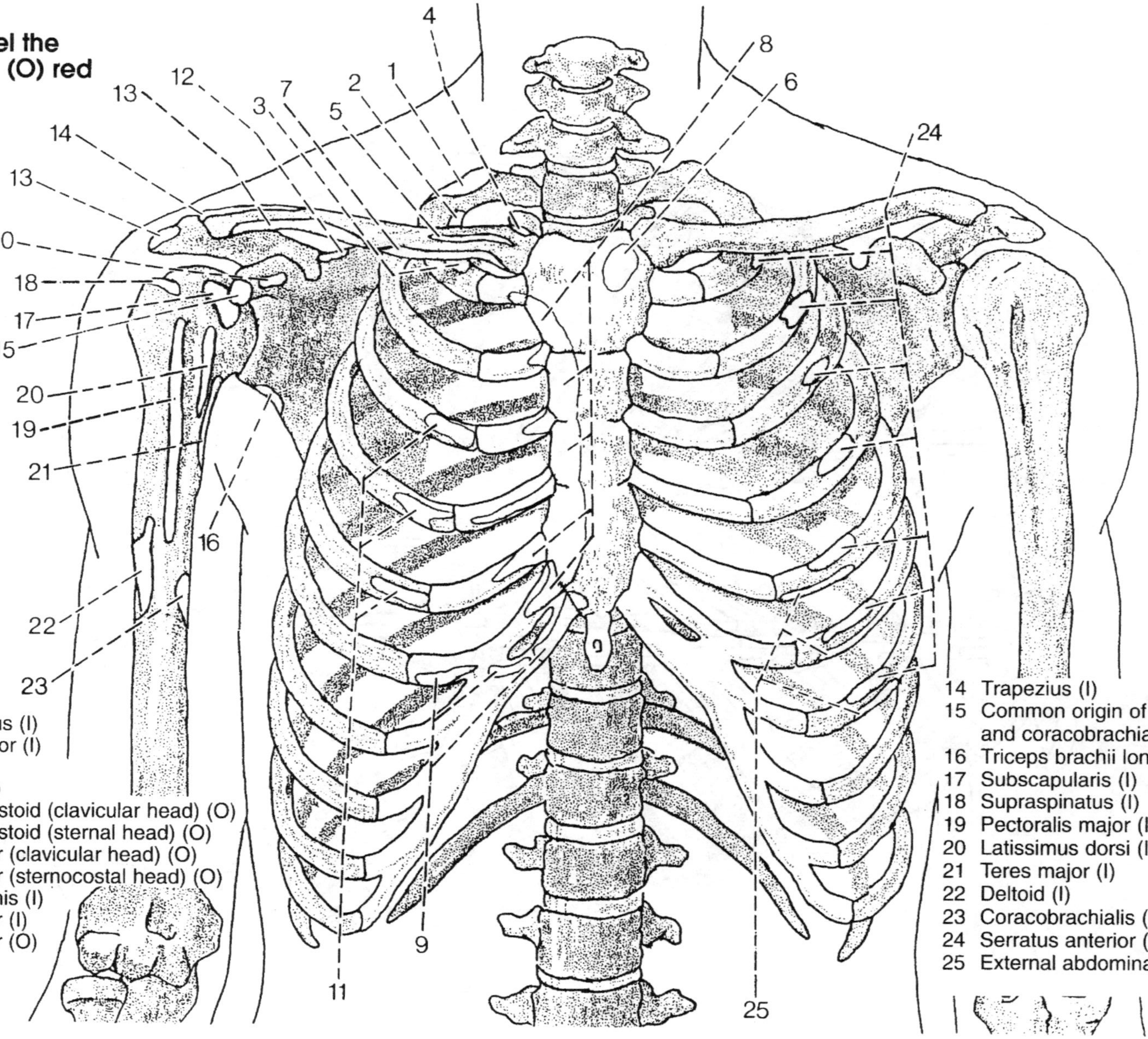

1 Scalenus medius (I)
2 Scalenus anterior (I)
3 Subclavius (O)
4 Sternohyoid (O)
5 Sternocleidomastoid (clavicular head) (O)
6 Sternocleidomastoid (sternal head) (O)
7 Pectoralis major (clavicular head) (O)
8 Pectoralis major (sternocostal head) (O)
9 Rectus abdominis (I)
10 Pectoralis minor (I)
11 Pectoralis minor (O)
12 Omohyoid (I)
13 Deltoid (O)
14 Trapezius (I)
15 Common origin of biceps brachii and coracobrachialis (O)
16 Triceps brachii long head (O)
17 Subscapularis (I)
18 Supraspinatus (I)
19 Pectoralis major (I)
20 Latissimus dorsi (I)
21 Teres major (I)
22 Deltoid (I)
23 Coracobrachialis (I)
24 Serratus anterior (O)
25 External abdominal oblique (O)

Th-17 Anterior thoracic wall seen from inside

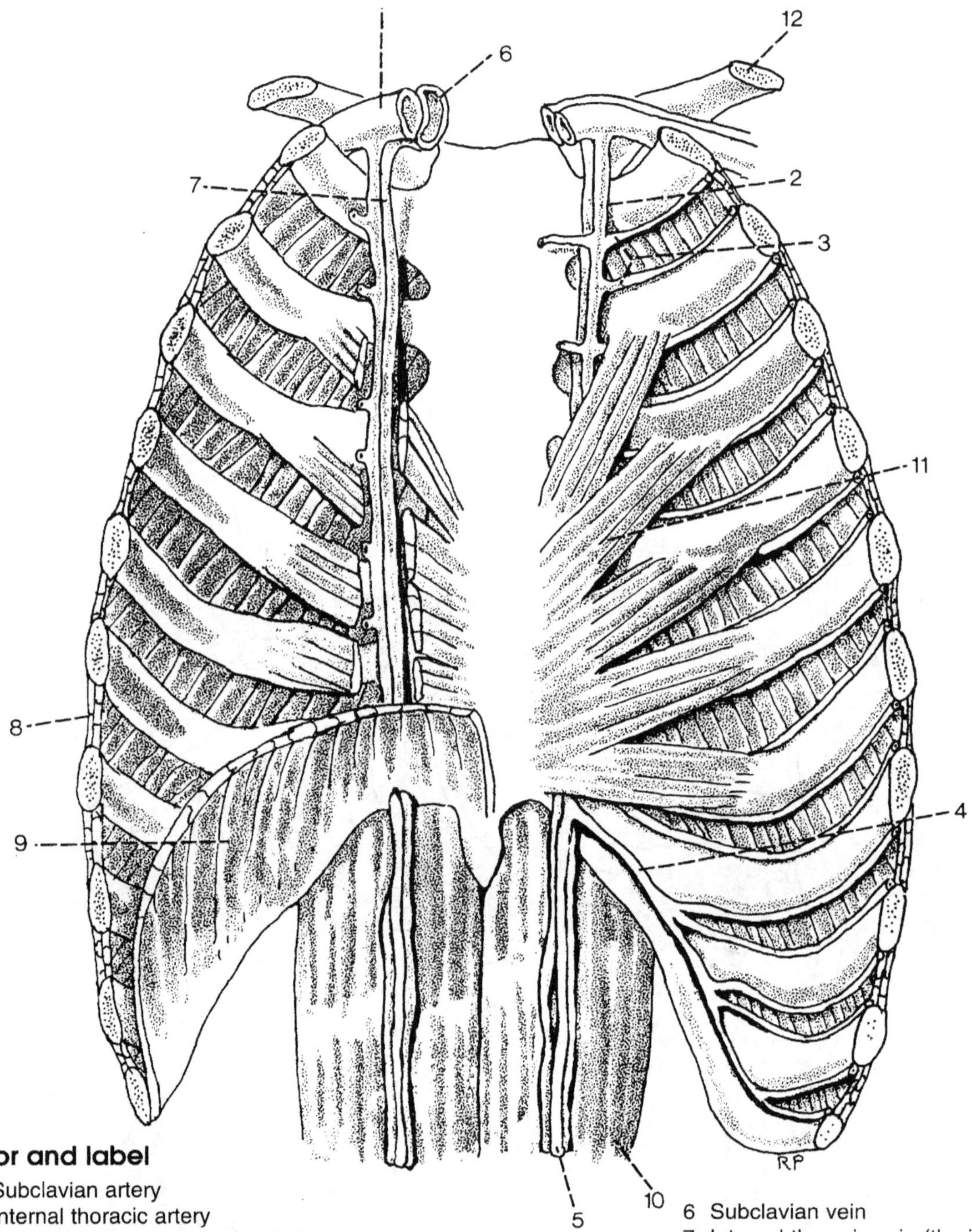

Color and label

1 Subclavian artery
2 Internal thoracic artery (old name, internal mammary artery)
3 Anterior intercostal arteries
4 Musculophrenic artery (phren refers to the diaphragm, which it helps supply)
5 Superior epigastric artery (the internal thoracic artery ends by dividing into the musculophrenic artery and the superior epigastric artery, which supplies the rectus abdominis muscle)
6 Subclavian vein
7 Internal thoracic vein (the internal thoracic vein is often doubled, resulting in two veins and one artery)
8 Intercostal muscles
9 Diaphragm
10 Rectus abdominis muscle
11 Transversus thoracis muscle
12 Clavicle (cut)

Th-18 Contents of thorax with anterior wall removed

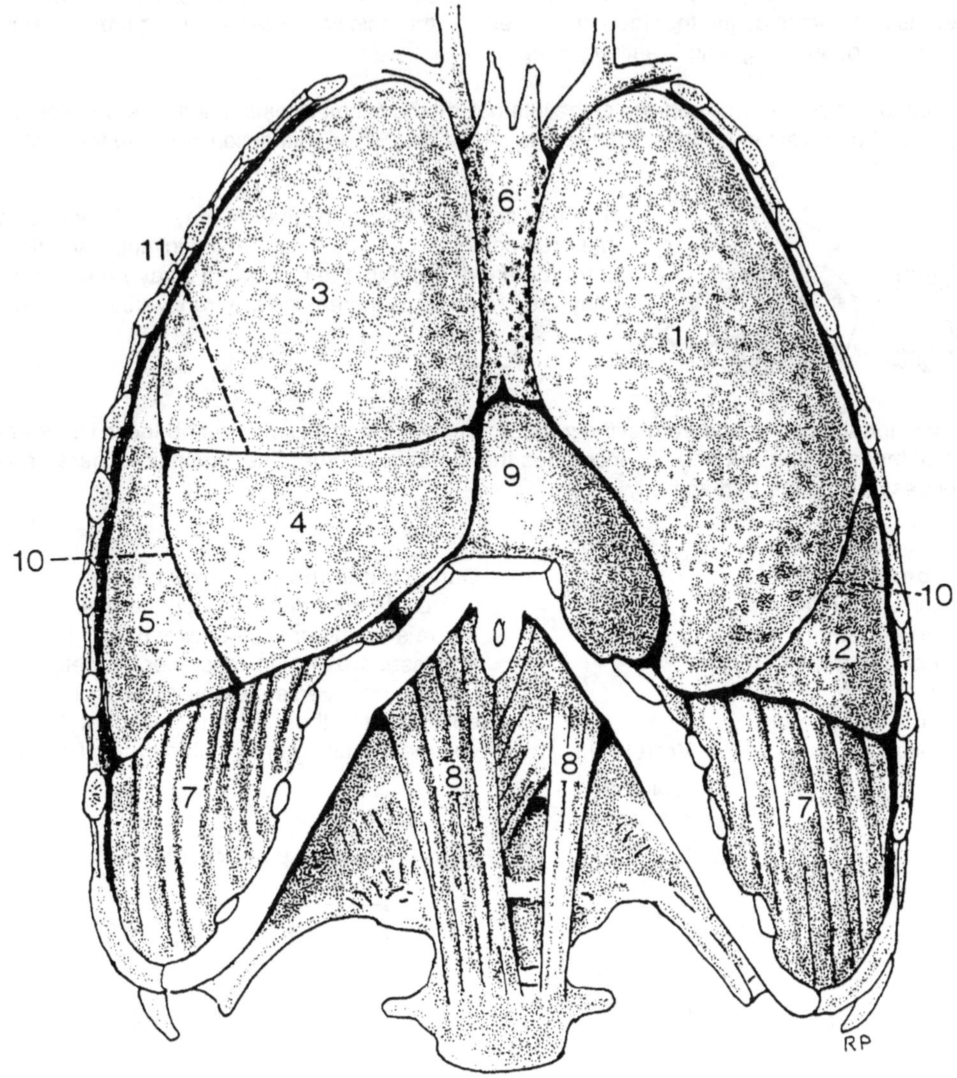

Color and label

1 Superior lobe of left lung
2 Inferior lobe of left lung
3 Superior lobe of right lung
4 Middle lobe of right lung
5 Inferior lobe of right lung
6 Thymus (remains)
7 Diaphragm
8 Crura of diaphragm
9 Pericardium
10 Oblique fissures (present in both lungs)
11 Horizontal fissure (present in right lung only)

Note that the right lung has three lobes, whereas the left lung has only two. However, the fissures separating the lobes are not always present so that an isolated right lung with an obliterated horizontal fissure may appear to have only two lobes and be mistaken for the left lung.

Th-19 Intercostal muscles

The external intercostal muscles along with the parasternal (intercartilaginous) portions* of the internal intercostal muscles are active during inspiration. They raise the ribs, thus drawing air into the lungs. The remainder of the internal intercostal mucles depresses the ribs. In quiet breathing the elastic recoil of the costal cartilages and the elasticity of the lungs play the major role in depressing the ribs and pulling the thoracic wall inward. Both the external intercostal and internal intercostal muscles acting together strenghten the thoracic wall against strong internal and external pressure as occurs in singing, shouting, and breathing deeply.

*Note that the incline of the parasternal portions of the internal intercostal muscles bears the same geometric relation to the costal cartilages as that of the external intercostal muscles to the ribs. Their contraction will raise the costal cartilages.

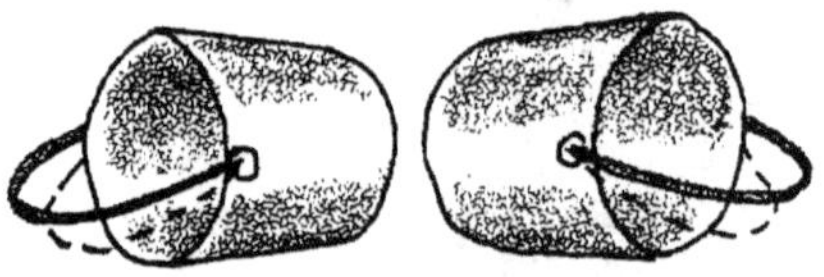

The movement of ribs in respiration may be likened to that of the handle on a pail or bucket. Just as the semicircular handle swings away from the rim of the pail, the ribs swing away from the midline when they are raised, thus increasing the transverse diameter of the thorax.

A simple two-dimensional model made from stiff cardboard or popsicle sticks and thumb tacks illustrates how the external intercostal muscle by raising the ribs increases the thoracic volume. The dimensions here apply only to the model and not necessarily to the human body.

During **expiration:** the external intercostal muscles are relaxed; the incline (slant) of ribs from back to front and from the midline to each side is greater; the spaces between the ribs are smaller.

During **inspiration:** the external intercostal muscles contract; the ribs are raised; the spaces between the ribs increase; the anterior-posterior diameter and the transverse diameter both increase, thus enlarging the thoracic (and pulmonary) volume, resulting in air being drawn into the lungs.

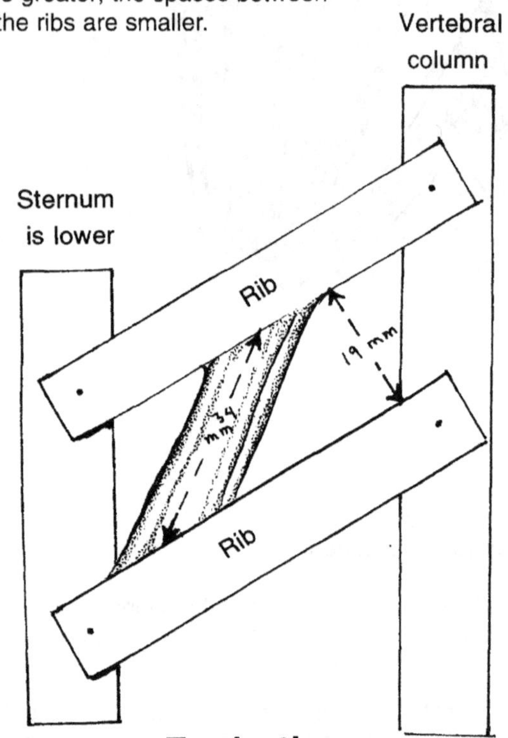

Expiration

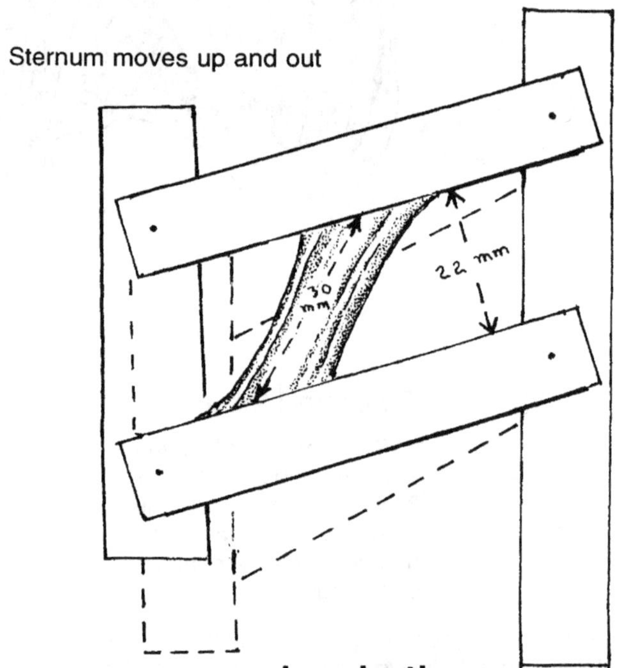

Inspiration

Th-20 Intercostal muscles

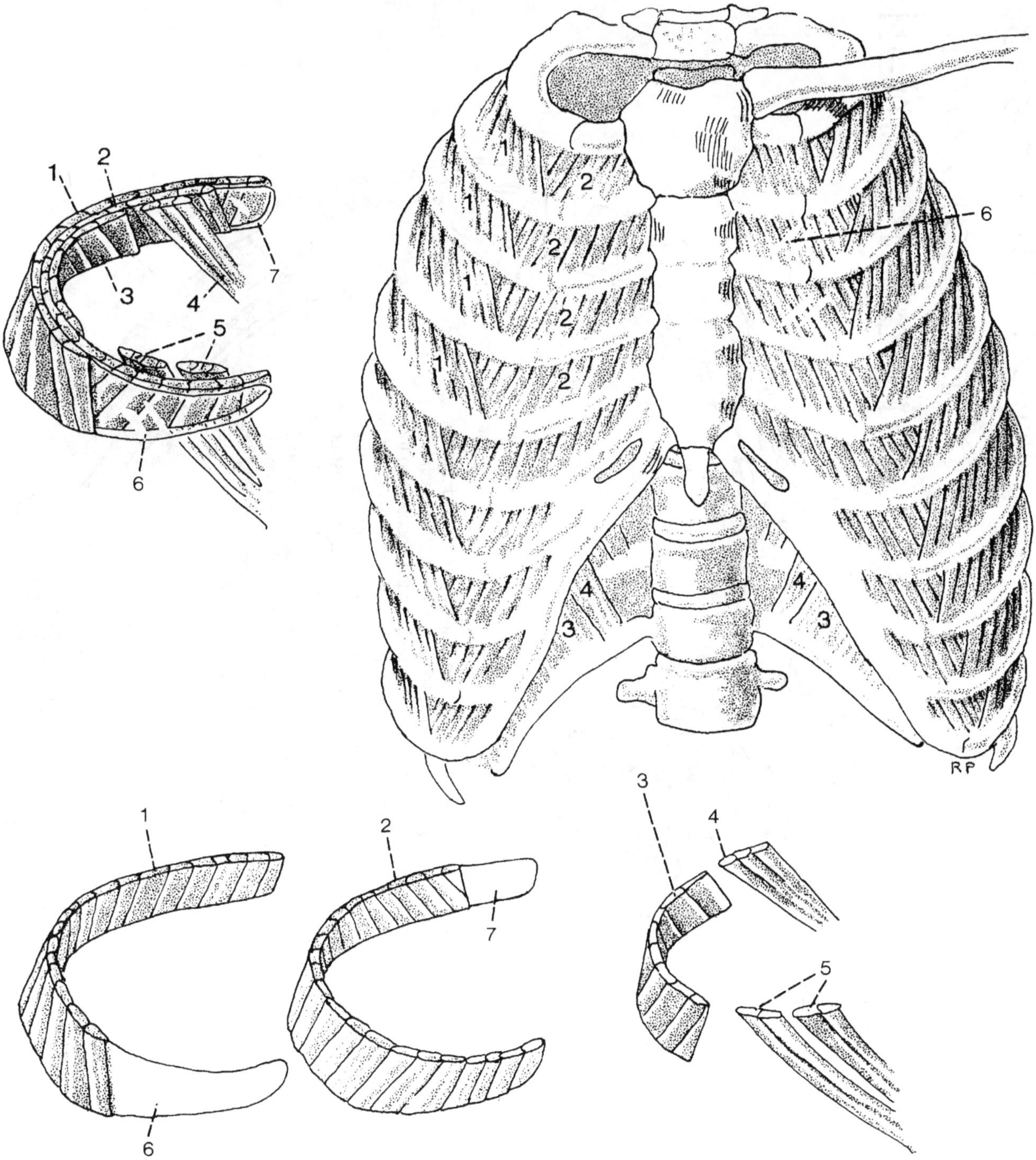

Color and label

1 External intercostal
2 Internal intercostal
3 Innermost intercostal
4 Subcostal
5 Transversus thoracis
6 External intercostal membrane
7 Internal intercostal membrane

Notice the direction of fibers in each layer. Also notice that neither the external intercostal nor the internal intercostal muscles completely fill in the intercostal spaces; rather each has a membranous portion that fills in its missing muscular portion. The parasternal (intercartilaginous) portions of the internal intercostal muscles (2) are visible beneath the membranes of the external intercostal muscles (6).

Th-21 Cross section of thoracic wall with intercostal arteries

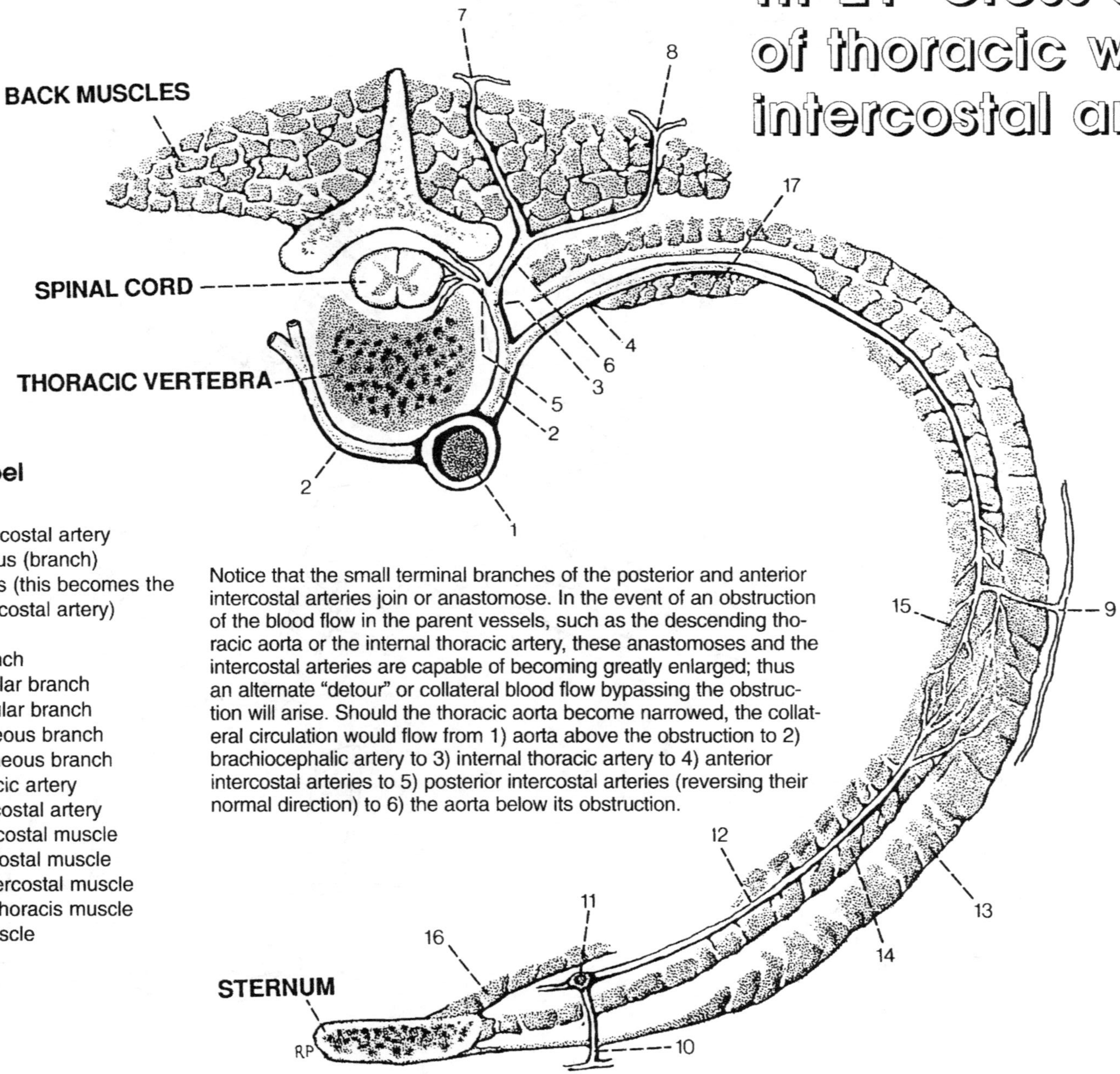

Notice that the small terminal branches of the posterior and anterior intercostal arteries join or anastomose. In the event of an obstruction of the blood flow in the parent vessels, such as the descending thoracic aorta or the internal thoracic artery, these anastomoses and the intercostal arteries are capable of becoming greatly enlarged; thus an alternate "detour" or collateral blood flow bypassing the obstruction will arise. Should the thoracic aorta become narrowed, the collateral circulation would flow from 1) aorta above the obstruction to 2) brachiocephalic artery to 3) internal thoracic artery to 4) anterior intercostal arteries to 5) posterior intercostal arteries (reversing their normal direction) to 6) the aorta below its obstruction.

Color and label

1 Aorta
2 Posterior intercostal artery
3 Posterior ramus (branch)
4 Anterior ramus (this becomes the posterior intercostal artery)
5 Spinal branch
6 Muscular branch
7 Medial muscular branch
8 Lateral muscular branch
9 Lateral cutaneous branch
10 Anterior cutaneous branch
11 Internal thoracic artery
12 Anterior intercostal artery
13 External intercostal muscle
14 Internal intercostal muscle
15 Innermost intercostal muscle
16 Transversus thoracis muscle
17 Subcostal muscle

Th-22 Section of thoracic wall with intercostal arteries

Color and label

1 Aorta
2 Posterior intercostal arteries
3 Collateral branch
4 Internal thoracic artery
5 Anterior intercostal arteries
6 Thoracic vertebra
7 Sternum
8 Internal intercostal muscle
9 Innermost intercostal muscle

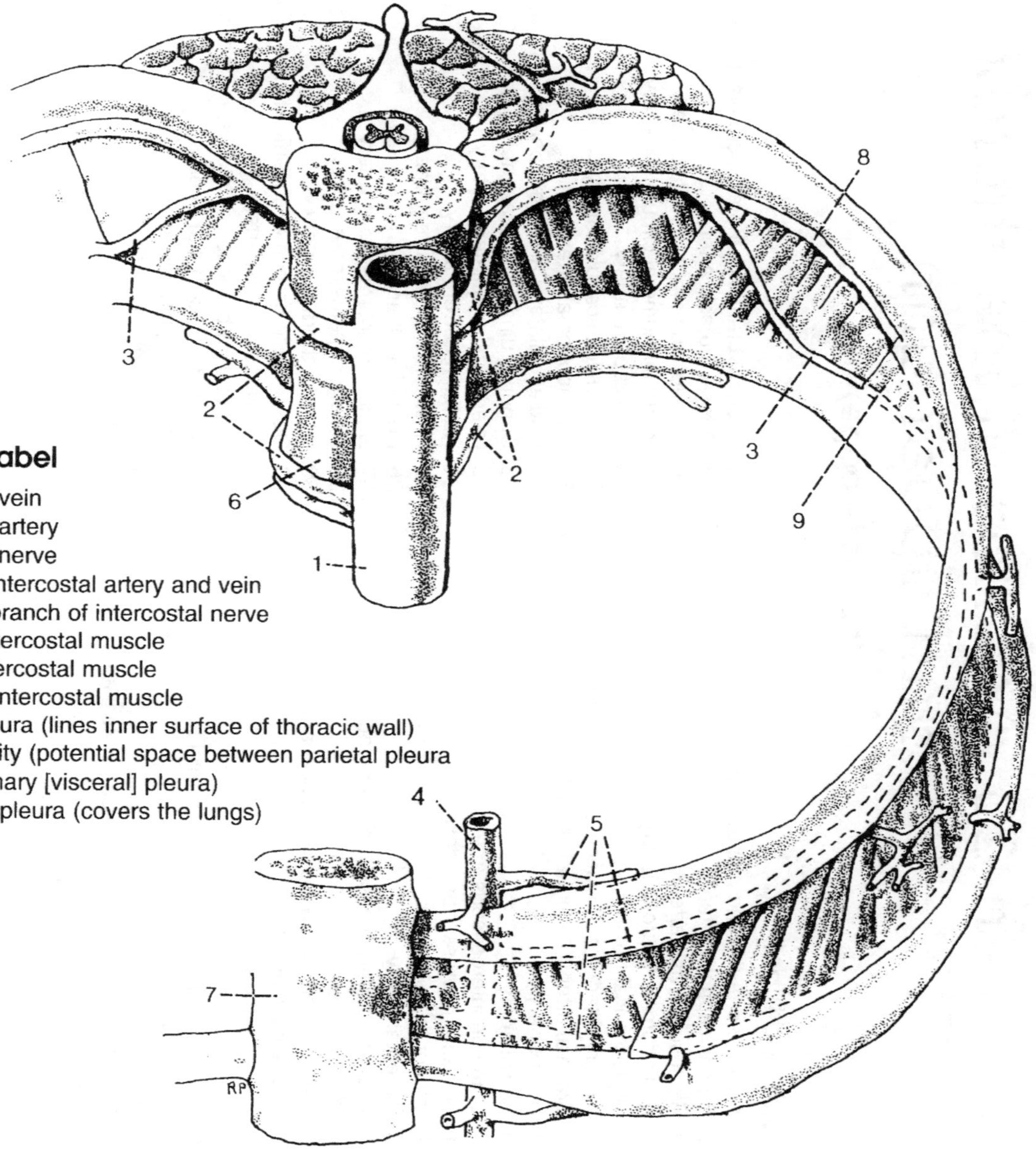

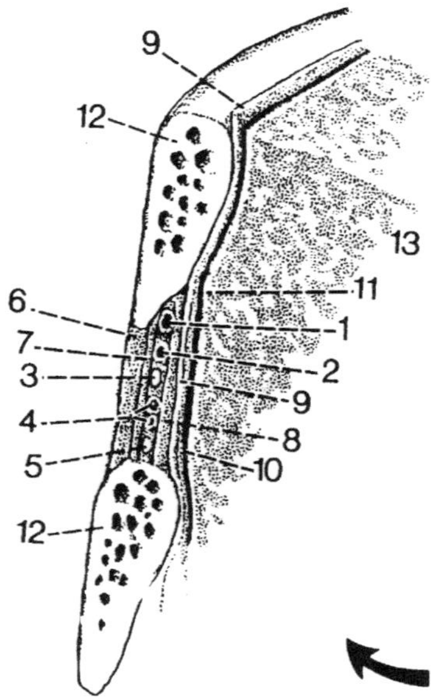

Color and label

1 Intercostal vein
2 Intercostal artery
3 Intercostal nerve
4 Collateral intercostal artery and vein
5 Collateral branch of intercostal nerve
6 External intercostal muscle
7 Internal intercostal muscle
8 Innermost intercostal muscle
9 Parietal pleura (lines inner surface of thoracic wall)
10 Pleural cavity (potential space between parietal pleura and pulmonary [visceral] pleura)
11 Pulmonary pleura (covers the lungs)
12 Ribs
13 Lung

Th-23 Arteries of the thorax and upper arm

(opposite page)

Color and label

1 Arch of aorta (behind manubrium)
2 Brachiocephalic artery
3 Right subclavian artery
4 Right common carotid artery
5 Thyrocervical trunk
6 Axillary artery (continuation of subclavian artery)
7 Brachial artery (continuation of axillary artery)
8 Ulnar artery
9 Radial artery
10 Common interosseous artery
11 Posterior interosseous artery
12 Inferior thyroid artery
13 Vertebral artery
14 Ascending branch of superficial branch of transverse cervical artery
15 Deep branch of transverse cervical artery
16 Suprascapular artery
17 Supreme thoracic artery
18 Thoracoacromial trunk
19 Acromial branch of thoracoacromial trunk
20 Clavicular branch
21 Deltoid branch
22 Superficial branch of transverse cervical artery
23 Transverse cervical artery
24 Pectoral branch of thoracoacromial trunk
25 Lateral thoracic artery
26 Anterior humeral circumflex artery
27 Posterior humeral circumflex artery
28 Subscapular artery
29 Circumflex scapular artery
30 Thoracodorsal artery
31 Radial collateral artery of deep brachial artery
32 Superior ulnar collateral artery
33 Inferior ulnar collateral artery
34 Radial recurrent artery
35 Anterior ulnar recurrent artery
36 Posterior ulnar recurrent artery
37 Recurrent interosseous artery
38 Anterior interosseous artery
39 Internal thoracic artery
40 Descending branch of superficial branch of tranverse cervical artery
41 Perforating branches of internal thoracic artery
42 Anterior intercostal arteries
43 Superior epigastric artery
44 Musculophrenic artery
45 Xiphoid process
46 Deep (profunda) brachial artery (behind humerus)

Th-23 Arteries of the thorax and upper arm

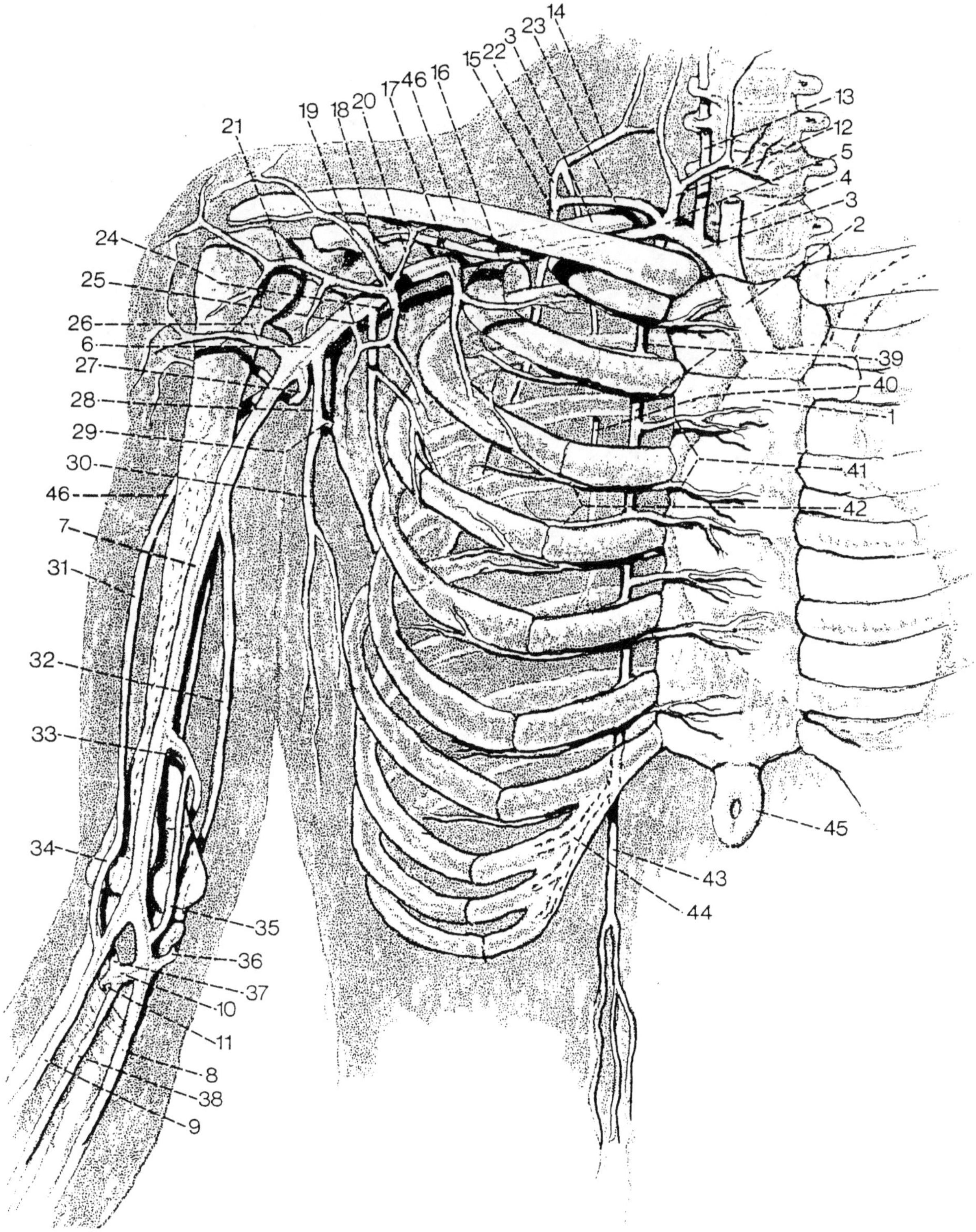

Th-24 Thoracic spinal nerve

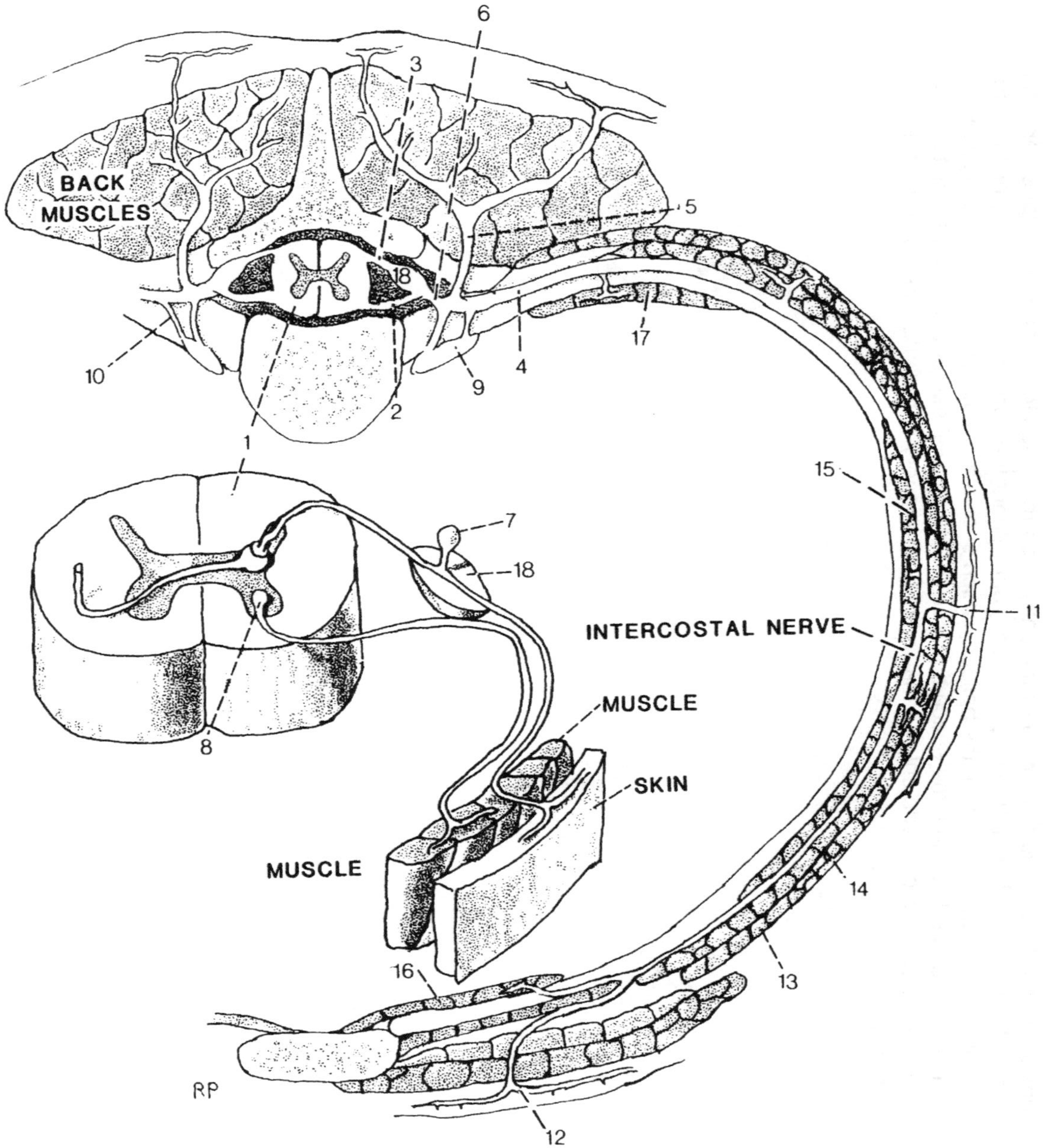

Color and label

1 Spinal cord
2 Ventral root of spinal nerve; contains out-going (efferent**) motor fibers; a nerve fiber is an axon.
3 Dorsal root of spinal nerve; contains in-coming (afferent**) sensory fibers.
4 Ventral ramus; the ventral and dorsal rami contain both motor fibers and sensory fibers.
5 Dorsal ramus
6 Spinal nerve; note that each spinal nerve arises from two roots, a ventral root and a dorsal root; it then divides into two rami, a ventral ramus and a dorsal ramus; the ventral ramus becomes the intercostal nerve; in fact all the nerves in our arms and legs are continuations of ventral rami; the dorsal rami innervate the large back muscles and supply sensation to the skin in the middle of the back.
7 Cell body of sensory neuron; all the sensory spinal nerve fibers have their cell bodies in the dorsal root ganglia.
8 Motor neuron cell body; these large alpha motor neurons innervate striated muscle, such as the intercostals.
9 Sympathetic ganglion*; these neurons give rise to fibers that supply blood vessels, sweat glands, and arrector pili (hair erector) muscles in hair follicles.
10 Communicating rami
11 Lateral cutaneous branch
12 Anterior cutaneous branch
13 External intercostal muscle
14 Internal intercostal muscle
15 Innermost intercostal muscle
16 Transversus thoracis muscle
17 Subcostal muscle; note that the intercostal nerve courses between the innermost intercostal muscle and the internal intercostal muscle.
18 Dorsal root gangion* (or spinal ganglion)

* A ganglion is a collection of nerve cell bodies outside the brain and spinal cord. The brain and spinal cord comprise the central nervous system (CNS).
**Efferent and afferent simply mean "going away from" and "coming toward", respectively.

Th-25 The pericardium

(opposite page)

The pericardium, or pericardial sac, is a tough fibrous membrane that surrounds the heart. It consists of two fused membranes: a strong outer fibrous membrane, the fibrous pericardium, and an inner thin serous membrane, the serous pericardium. The inner serous pericardium both lines the inside of the pericardial sac (parietal part) and is reflected over the proximal parts of the eight great vessels and onto the heart where it forms the outer layer of the heart, the epicardium (visceral part of the pericardium). The pericardial sac is strong and not capable of expansion, so that if blood leaks into the pericardial space, the heart may be compressed to the degree that there is insufficient atrial capacity for blood to return and hence insufficient arterial outflow. This condition is called **tamponade** and can be life-threatening.

The relationship between the heart and the surrounding serous pericardium may be likened to a fist (the heart) being pushed into a soft balloon (the serous pericardium; top figures A and B). The part of the balloon that covers the fist corresponds to the visceral serous pericardium or epicardium, whereas the remainder of the balloon corresponds to the parietal serous pericardium that lines the inside of the pericardial sac, but without the surrounding fibrous pericardium. However, unlike the diagram of the balloon, which shows a considerable amount of space inside the indented balloon, the space between the pericardial sac and the heart is actually a potential space and contains only a small amount of slippery serous fluid secreted by the serous pericardium.

Th-25 The pericardium

Label the cut edge of the balloon

1 "Parietal" layer
2 "Visceral" layer

A

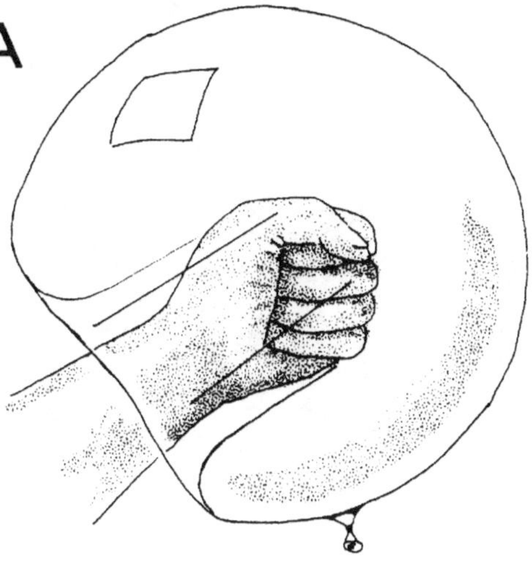

B

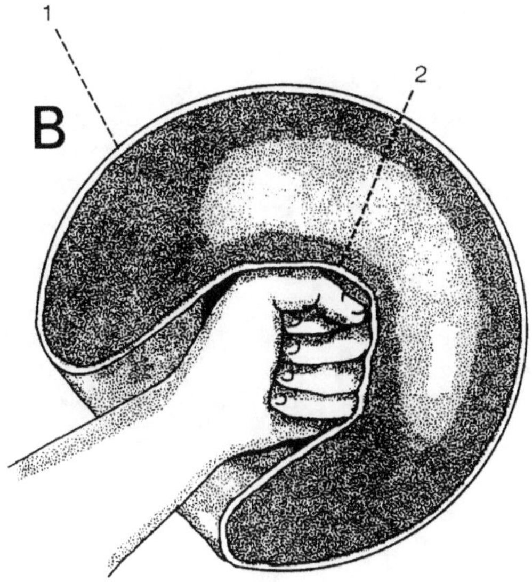

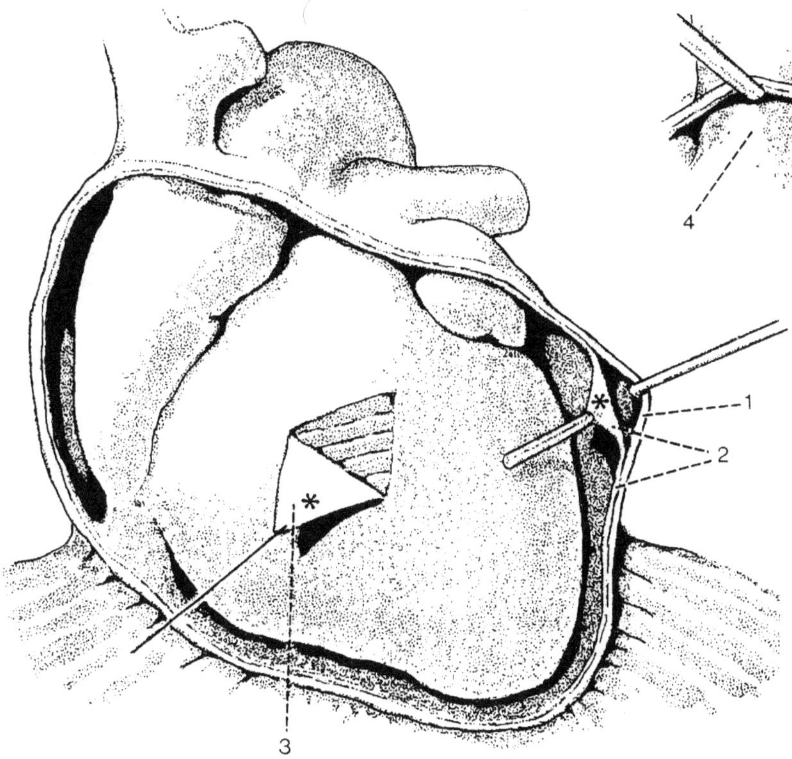

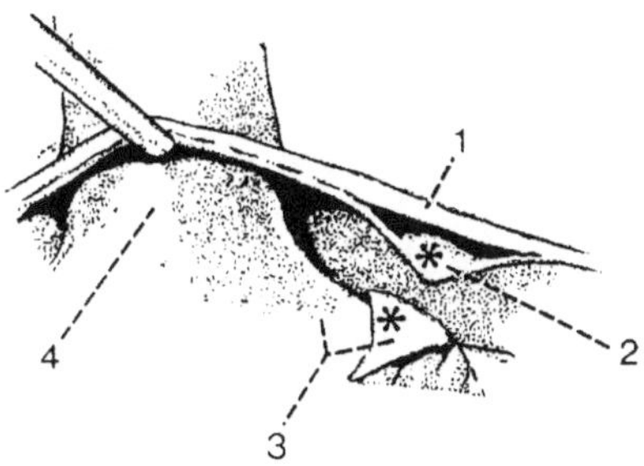

Color and label

1 Fibrous pericardium (forms the outer strong layer)
2 Parietal part of serous pericardium* (thin and delicate layer; lines inside of fibrous pericardium)
3 Visceral part of serous pericardium* (covers outside of heart; also called epicardium)
4 Great vessels such as the aorta penetrate pericardial sac and are covered by the serous pericardium inside the pericardial sac.

*Serous pericardium peeled off at asterisk

Th-26 The interior of the posterior pericardial sac with the heart removed and the great vessels cut

Viewed from the front

The serous pericardium forms two infolding covers of the great vessels which divide the area in back of the heart into the two pericardial sinuses, the straight sinus and the oblique sinus. One infolding of serous pericardium surrounds the intrapericardial parts of the aorta (5) and the pulmonary trunk (6); the other "tube" surrounds the intrapericardial portions of the remaining six great vessels.

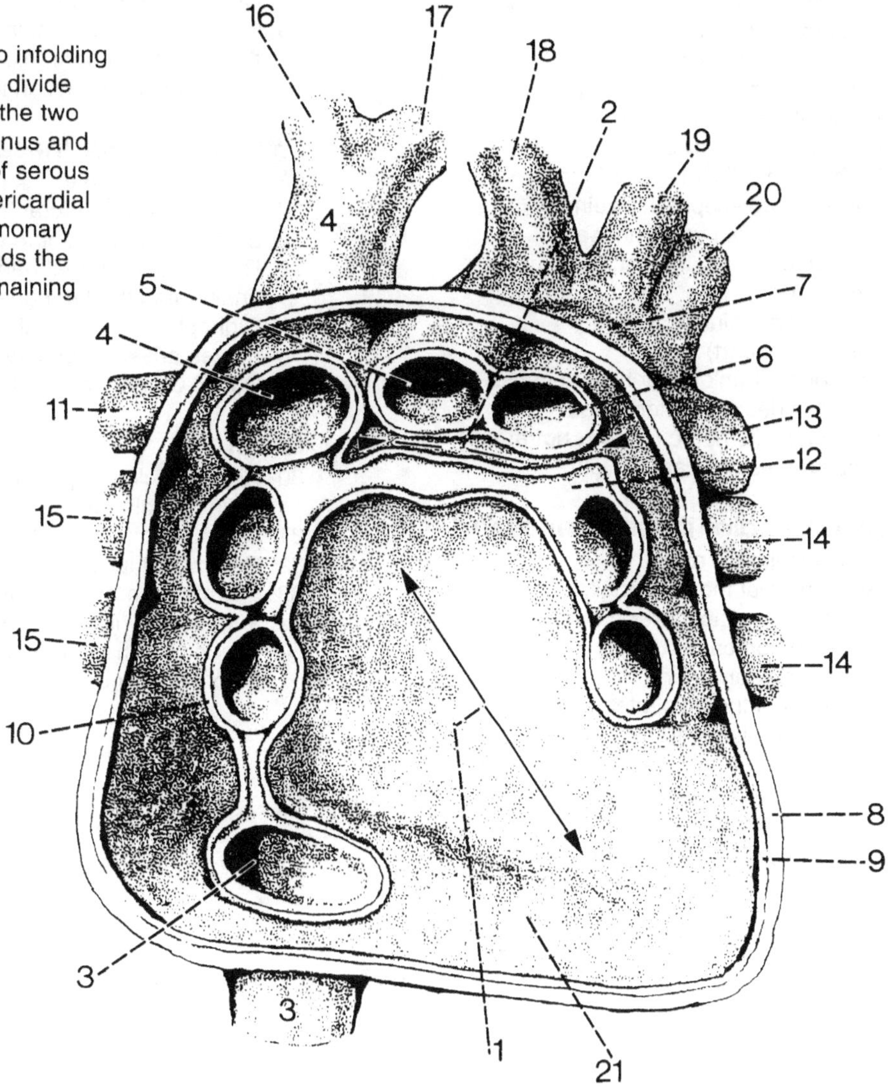

Color and label

1 Oblique pericardial sinus (occupied by back of left atrium)
2 Transverse pericardial sinus (between arrowheads; immediately in front of right pulmonary artery)
3 Inferior vena cava
4 Superior vena cava
5 Aorta
6 Pulmonary trunk
7 Arch of aorta
8 Fibrous pericardium (its thickness somewhat exaggerated)
9 Serous pericardium (parietal layer; lines inside of fibrous pericardium)
10 Serous pericardium covering intrapericardial parts of great vessels
11 Right pulmonary artery
12 Bare area of fibrous pericardium (not lined with serous pericardium)
13 Left pulmonary artery
14 Left pulmonary veins
15 Right pulmonary veins
16 Right brachiocephalic vein
17 Left brachiocephalic vein
18 Brachiocephalic artery
19 Left common carotid artery
20 Left subclavian artery
21 Base of pericardium (fused inferiorly to central tendon of diaphragm)

Th-27 Exterior of the heart

(opposite page)

Label and color these veins blue

1 Right brachiocephalic vein
2 Left brachiocephalic vein
3 Superior vena cava
4 Inferior vena cava
5 Right internal thoracic vein
6 Left internal thoracic vein
7 Right pericardiacophrenic vein
8 Left pericardiacophrenic vein
9 Anterior cardiac veins (these drain directly into the right atrium)
10 Great cardiac vein* (this becomes the coronary sinus on inferior surface of heart)
11 Pulmonary trunk (color blue because it carries deoxygenated blood; remember, its name is trunk, not artery)
12 Small (or lesser) cardiac vein

Label and color these arteries red

13 Brachiocephalic artery
14 Right internal thoracic artery
15 Right pericardiacophrenic artery
16 Left common carotid artery
17 Left subclavian artery
18 Left internal thoracic artery
19 Left pericardiacophrenic artery
20 Right coronary artery*
21 Right marginal branch
22 Anterior interventricular artery* (branch of left coronary artery; also called left anterior descending)
23 Ascending aorta

Label the serous membranes

24 Cut edge of parietal pleura
25 Cut edge of pericardium; the phrenic nerve and the pericardiacophrenic artery and vein are "sandwiched" between these two membranes

Label and color these nerves yellow

26 Left phrenic nerve
27 Left vagus nerve (cranial nerve X; supplies parasympathetic fibers to the heart)
28 Recurrent laryngeal nerve (innervates the laryngeal muscles)
29 Right phrenic nerve (the two phrenic nerves arises from cervical nerves C3,C4,C5 and innervate the diaphragm)

Label

30 Right auricle (outpouching of right atrium; *auricula*, Latin for little ear)
31 Left auricle (outpouching of left atrium)
32 Root of left lung
33 Ligamentum arteriosum (remnant of fetal ductus arteriosus which diverted oxygenated blood headed for the nonfunctional lungs to be shunted from the pulmonary trunk directly to the aorta)

*Coronary vessels lie under fat which must be removed for the vessels to be seen.

Th-27 Exterior of the heart

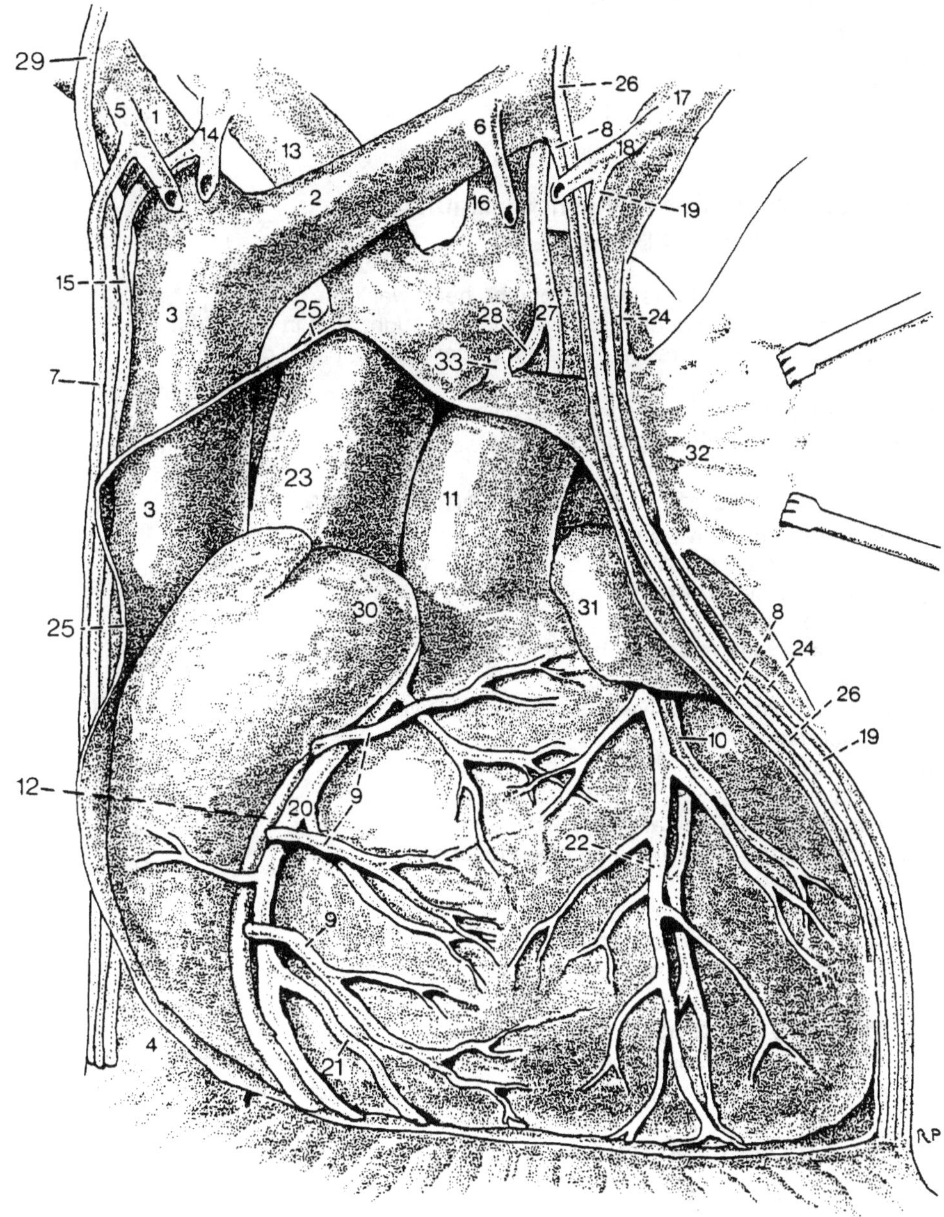

Th-28 Interior of the heart somewhat schematic

(opposite page)

Label and color these veins blue

1 Right brachiocephalic vein
2 Left brachiocephalic vein
3 Superior vena cava
4 Azygos vein
5 Inferior vena cava

Label and color the interior of the right atrium blue

6 Ostium (opening) of superior vena cava
7 Ostium of inferior vena cava
8 Ostium of coronary sinus (returns blood from the heart wall)
9 Fossa ovalis (remains of the opening between left and right atria in the fetus)
10 Musculi pectinati (comb-like strands of heart muscle; *pecten*, Latin, comb)
11 Crista terminalis
12 Sinoatrial node (pacemaker; here somewhat dissected out)
13 Right auricle (ear-like outpouching of right atrium)

Label and color the interior of the right ventricle blue

14 Anterior cusp of tricuspid valve (leave white)
15 Chordae tendineae (leave white)
16 Anterior papillary muscle (pink)
17 Trabeculae carneae (pink)
18 Septomarginal trabecula (moderator band) (pink)
19 Conus arteriosus
20 Anterior valvule of pulmonary valve (no muscles in valves; leave white)
21 Myocardium (heart muscle; pink)
22 Endocardium (leave white)
23 Epicardium (leave white)
24 Interventricular septum (muscular part; pink)
25 Pulmonary trunk (carries deoxygenated blood to lungs)
26 Right pulmonary artery
27 Left pulmonary artery
28 Superior branch of right pulmonary artery
29 Inferior branch of right pulmonary artery

Label and color the left atrium red

30 Ostia (openings of right pulmonary veins; these carry oxygenated blood from right lung back to heart)
31 Left pulmonary veins (carry oxygenated blood from left lung back to heart)

Label and color the left ventricle

32 Anterior cusp of mitral valve (leave white)
33 Posterior cusp of mitral valve (leave white)
34 Chordae tendineae (leave white)
35 Anterior papillary muscle (pink)
36 Left valvule of aortic valve (leave white)
37 Ostium of left coronary artery (coronary arteries supplies blood to the heart)
38 Aortic arch (aorta carries oxygenated blood to the whole body)
39 Brachiocephalic artery carries blood to right arm and right side of neck and head)
40 Left common carotid artery (carries blood to left side of neck and head)
41 Left subclavian artery (carries blood to left arm)

Th-28 Interior of the heart

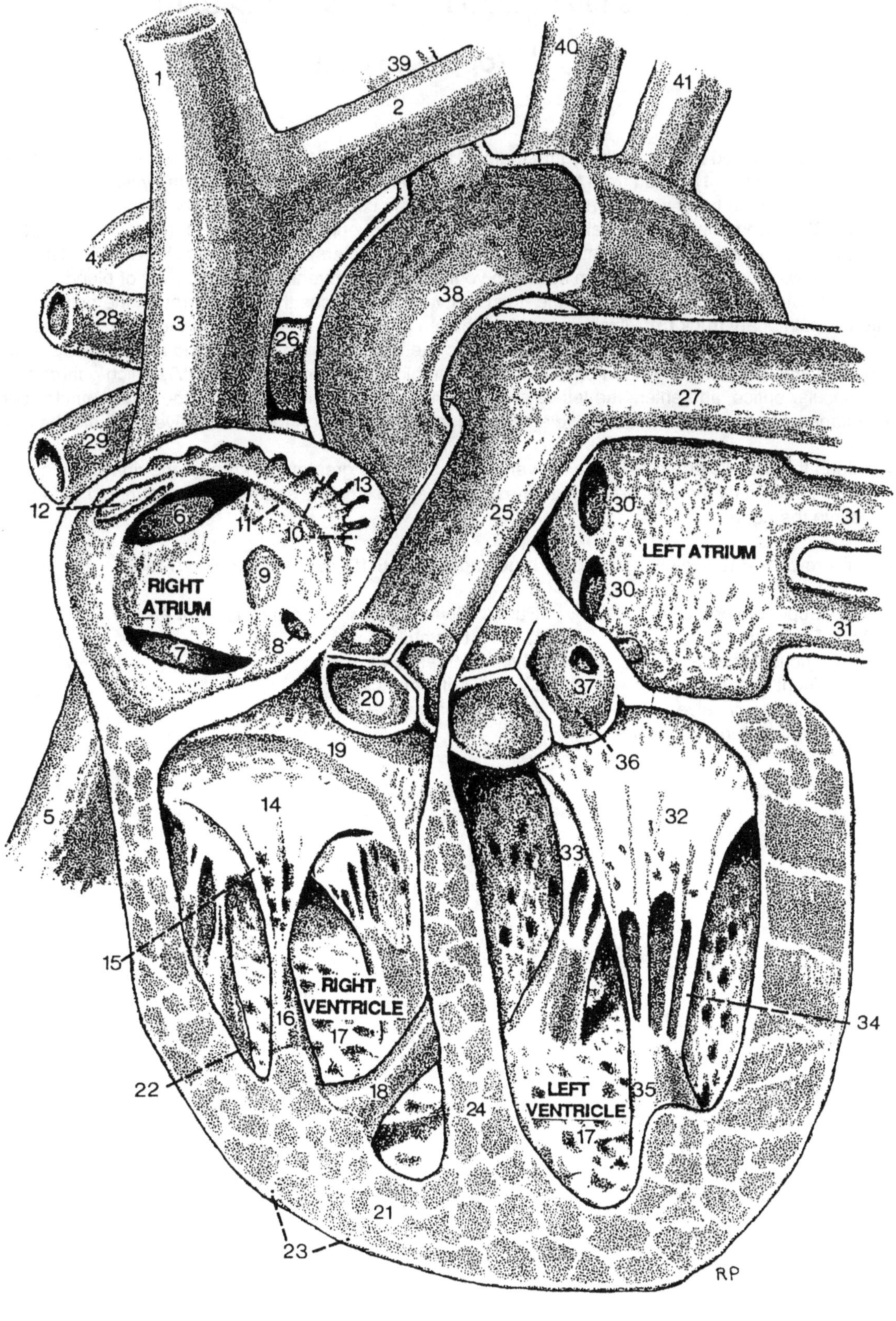

Th-29 Trace the course of blood through the heart

(opposite page)

Deoxygenated blood returns to the right atrium (R At) of the heart from the head, arms, and thorax by way of the superior vena cava **(1)**. Blood from the legs and abdomen reaches the right atrium by way of the inferior vena **(2)**. Blood from the heart wall returns mainly by way of the coronary sinus **(3),** which also empties into the right atrium. Blood from the thoracic wall drains into the superior vena cava by way of the azygos vein. Blood leaves the right atrium through the right atrioventricular orifice and enters the right ventricle (RV) **(4)**. The tricuspid valve (TCV) allows blood to flow only from atrium to ventricle, thus preventing any backflow of blood from ventricle to atrium. Ventricular contraction closes the tricuspid valve and forces the blood through the pulmonary valve (PV) into the pulmonary trunk **(5),** which divides into the left pulmonary artery **(6)** and the right pulmonary artery **(7)**. Oxygenated blood from the lungs is carried back to the the left atrium (L At) of the heart by way of four pulmonary veins **(8)**. The blood then passes through the bicuspid or mitral valve (MV), which guards the left atrioventricular orifice, and enters the left ventricle (LV) **(9)**. Ventricular contraction (the two ventricles contract simultaneously) closes the mitral valve and forces the blood through the aortic valve (AV) into the aorta **(10).**

Although the systolic pressure in the left ventricle is six times greater than that in the right ventricle, the amount of blood pumped by the right ventricle to the lungs is approximately equal to the amount pumped by the left ventricle into the aorta.

Color arrows **1- 6** (deoxygenated blood) **blue** and arrows **6-10** (oxygenated blood) **red**

SVC Superior vena cava
R At Right atrium
TCV Tricuspid valve
RV Right ventricle
PV Pulmonary valve
LA Ligamentum arteriosum
Pul Tr Pulmonary trunk (note, *trunk*; not artery)
L At Left atrium
MV Mitral valve
LV Left ventricle
AV Aortic valve

Th-29 Trace the course of blood through the heart

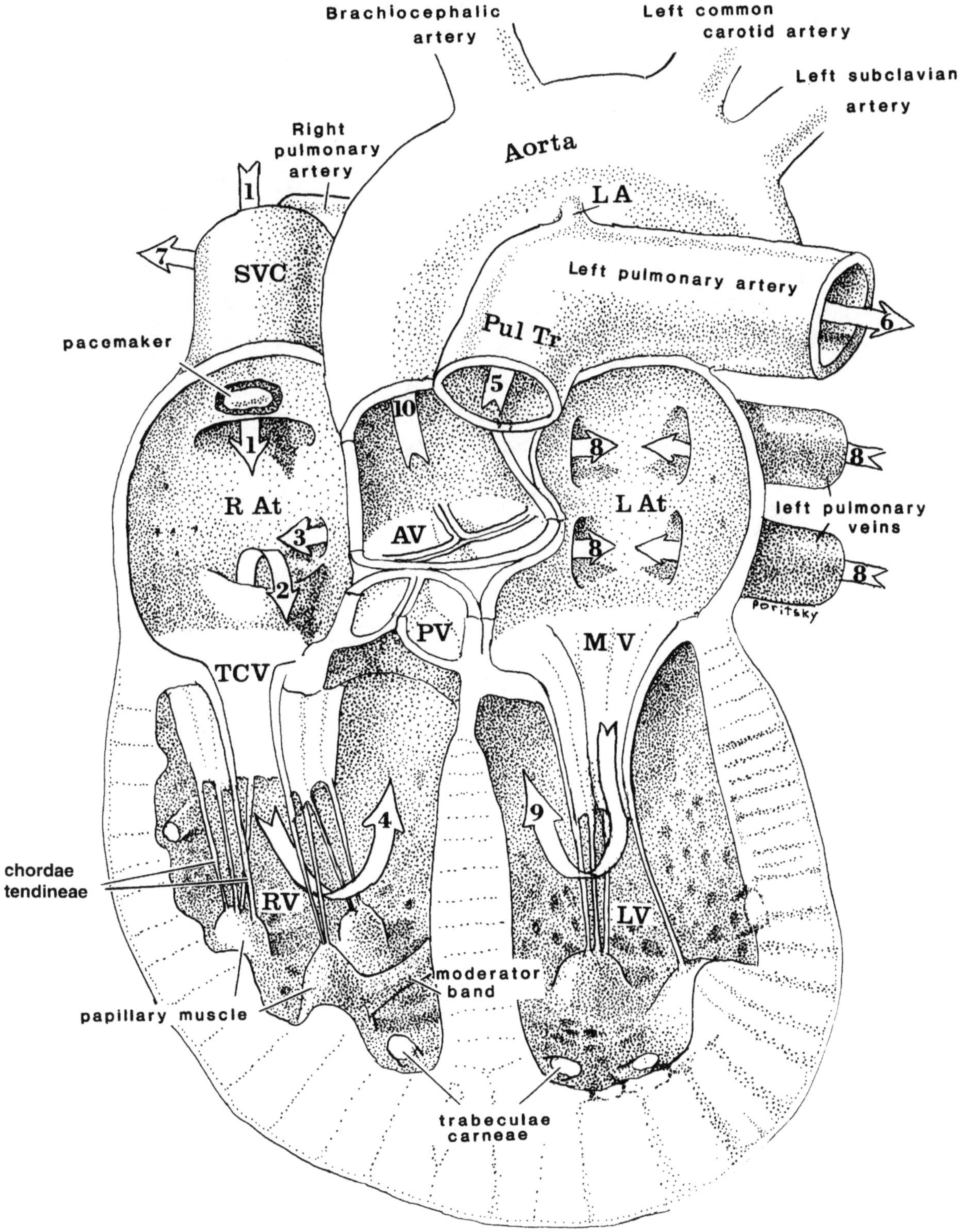

Th-30 The heart. Ventricles exposed

Much of the anterior wall has been removed to reveal the interior of the ventricles

Color and label

1 Arch of aorta
2 Pulmonary trunk
3 Anterior interventricular artery
4 Superior branch of left pulmonary artery
5 Inferior branch of left pulmonary artery
6 Left auricle
7 Left superior pulmonary vein
8 Left inferior pulmonary vein
9 Pulmonary valve
10 Anterior cusp (leaflet) of mitral valve
11 Chordae tendineae
12 Trabeculae carneae in wall of left ventricle
13 Anterior papillary muscle in left ventricle
14 Anterior interventricular artery
15 Great cardiac vein
16 Trabeculae carneae in wall of right ventricle
17 Right marginal artery
18 Inferior vena cava
19 Papillary muscle
20 Chordae tendineae and septal leaflet of tricuspid valve
21 Right coronary artery
22 Small cardiac vein
23 Right auricle
24 Infundibulum (conus arteriosus) of right ventricle
25 Superior vena cava
26 Right brachiocephalic vein
27 Brachiocephalic artery ; notice that there are two brachiocephalic veins, but only a single brachiocephalic artery
28 Left brachiocephalic vein
29 Left common carotid artery
30 Left subclavian artery
31 Interventricular septum (largely removed)

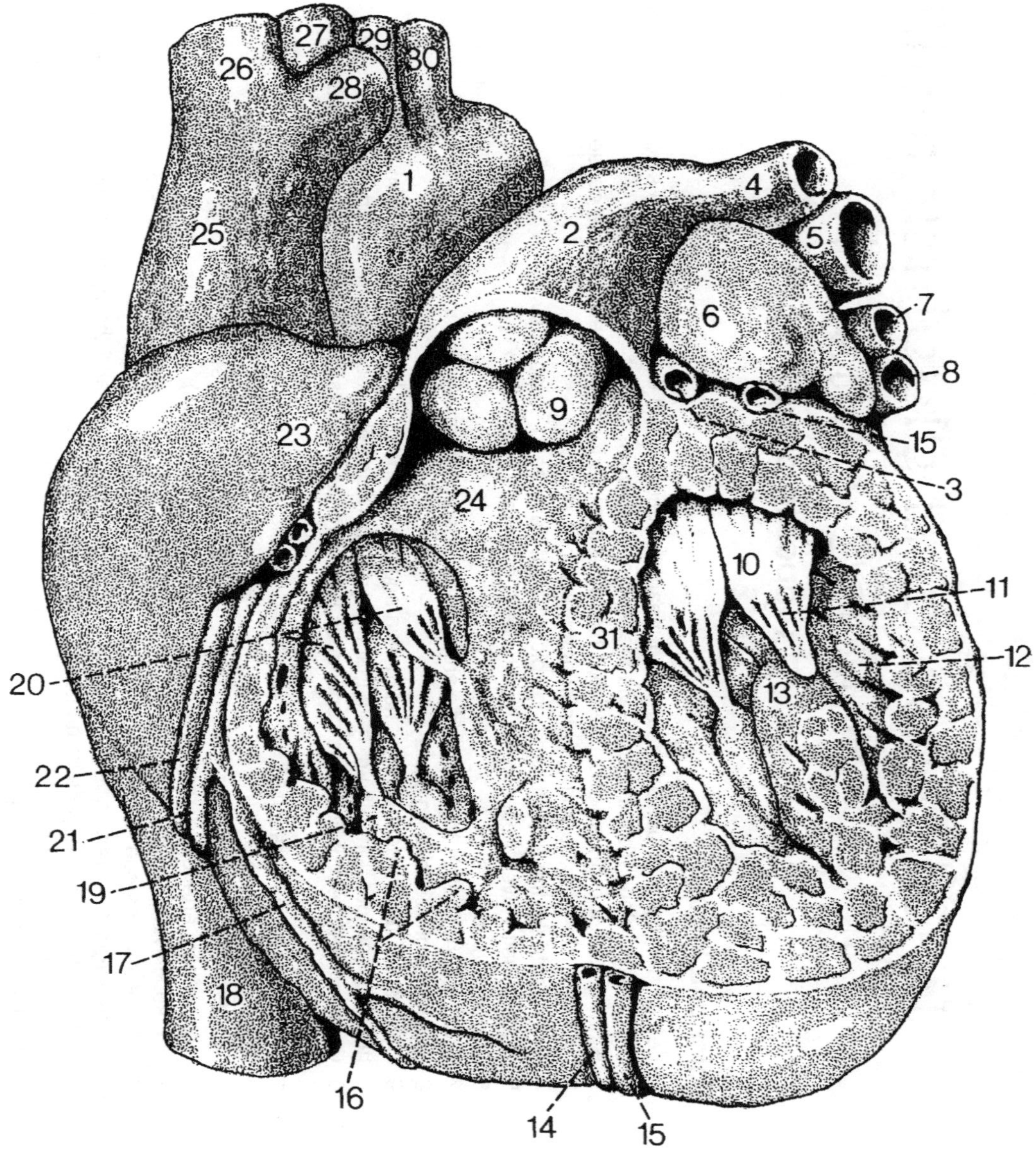

Th-31 Base and diaphragmatic surface of heart

(opposite page)

Color and label

1 Left atrium (**base** or posterior surface of heart); it occupies the oblique pericardial sinus; it receives the oxygenated blood from the lungs via the 4 pulmonary veins.
2 Right atrium; it receives deoxygenated blood via the inferior and superior venae cavae.
3 Left ventricle (diaphragmatic or inferior surface of heart)
4 Right ventricle; the epicardium and epicardial fat have been stripped away.
5 Cusp of half valve at opening of inferior vena cava into right atrium
6 Superior vena cava
7 Arch of aorta; notice that the aortic arch curves posteriorly as well as to the left.
8 Beginning of descending aorta
9 Coronary sinus; largest intrinsic heart vein and main conduit of blood returning from the substance of the heart; opens into right atrium; note that the great cardiac vein becomes the coronary sinus.
10 Great cardiac vein; it becomes continuous with coronary sinus approximately 2.5 cm from the right atrium.
11 Circumflex artery (branch of left coronary artery)
12 Right coronary artery
13 Small (or lesser) cardiac vein; note that it empties into coronary sinus.
14 Ligamentum arteriosum (remains of the fetal ductus arteriosum)
15 Left subclavian artery
16 Left common carotid artery
17 Brachiocephalic artery; gives rise to the right subclavian artery and the right common carotid artery.
18 Opening (orifice) of azygos vein into the superior vena cava
19 Right pulmonary artery
20 Right superior pulmonary vein
21 Right inferior pulmonary vein
22 Posterior interventricular artery
23 Middle cardiac vein
24 **Apex** of heart
25 Left posterior ventricular branch of circumflex artery
26 Posterior vein of left ventricle
27 Superior left pulmonary vein
28 Left pulmonary artery
29 Inferior left pulmonary vein

Th-31 Base and diaphragmatic surface of heart

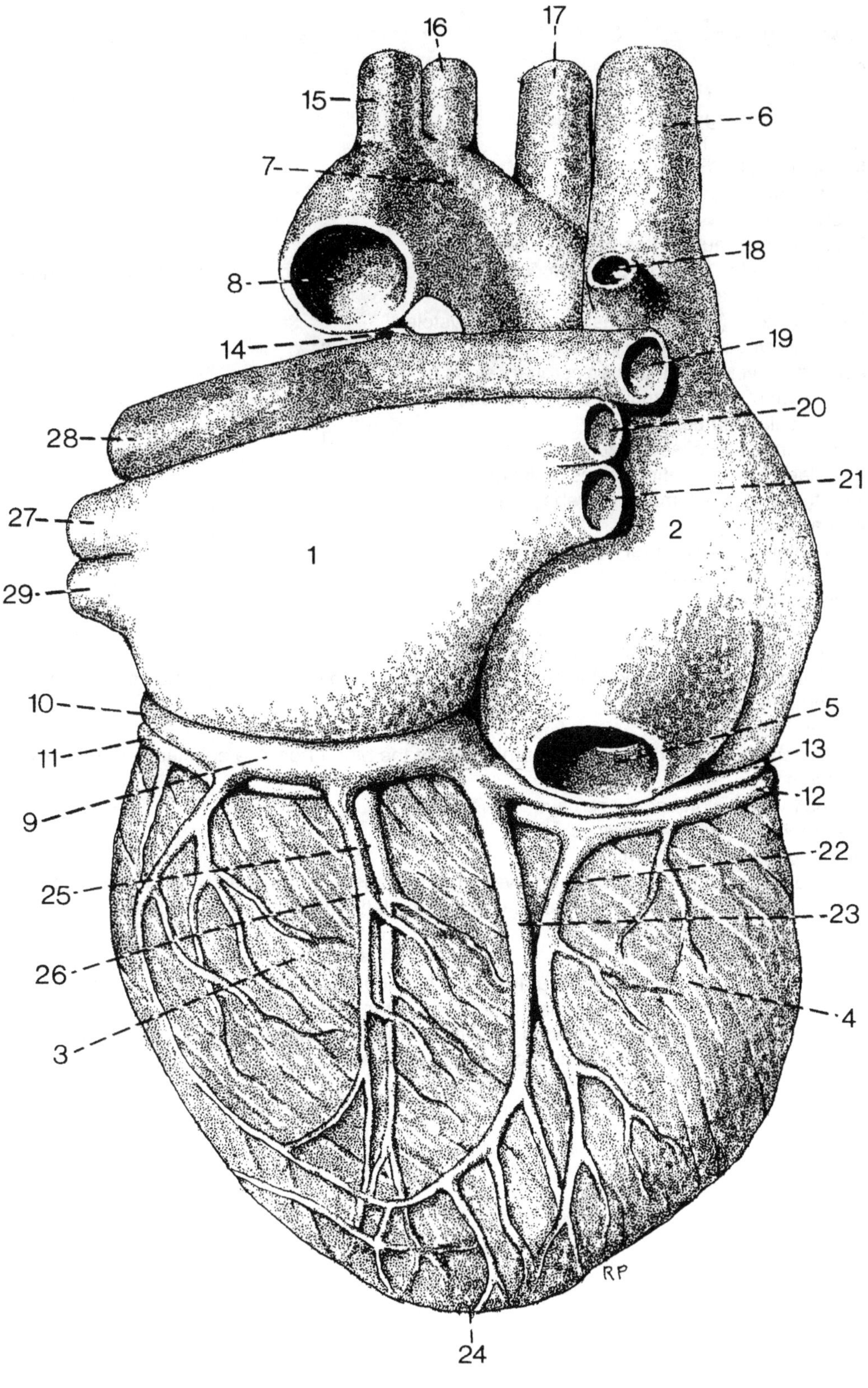

Th-32 Right atrium and right ventricle

(opposite page)

Color and label

1 Inferior vena cava
2 Superior vena cava
3 Azygos vein ending in superior vena cava
4 Right brachiocephalic vein
5 Left brachiocephalic vein
6 Ascending aorta
7 Pulmonary trunk
8 Left auricle (right auricle has been cut away)
9 Pectinate muscles (*musculi pectinati*, "comblike" muscles; *pecten*, Latin, comb) in right atrium
10 Right coronary artery
11 Pulmonary valve (closed in diastole; open in systole)
12 Anterior interventricular artery (branch of left coronary artery)
13 Great cardiac vein; continues as coronary sinus
14 Infundibulum of right ventricle (conus arteriosus)
15 Interventricular septum
16 Chordae tendineae of septal cusp (leaflet)
17 Trabeculae carneae (Latin, beams of flesh)
18 Moderator band (septomarginal trabecula)
19 Great cardiac vein
20 Anterior interventricular artery
21 Anterior papillary muscle
22 Chordae tendineae
23 Posterior papillary muscle
24 Anterior cusp of tricuspid valve (right atrioventricular valve)
25 Fibrous ring around right atrioventricular orifice (anchors the bases of tricuspid valve cusps or leaflets)
26 Right coronary artery
27 Small cardiac vein
28 Orifice (opening) of coronary sinus; returns most of the blood from the substance of the heart to the right atrium
29 Valve (half valve) of inferior vena cava
30 Crista terminalis (cut in two places)
31 Limbus (border) of fossa ovalis
32 Fossa ovalis (site of the fetal **foramen ovale** that fuctions as a one-way valve, directing oxygenated blood from the right atrium through the interatrial wall to the left atrium; closed after birth)
33 Sinuatrial node (pacemaker)
34 Septal cusp of tricuspid valve
35 Triangle of Koch (site of **atrioventricular node**); bounded by (1) base of septal leaflet of tricuspid valve, (2) anterior margin of orifice of coronary sinus, and (3) tendon of Todaro
36 Tendon of Todaro; rounded collagenous bundle that may be palpated extending from the valve of the inferior vena cava to the right fibrous trigone

Th-32 Right atrium and right ventricle

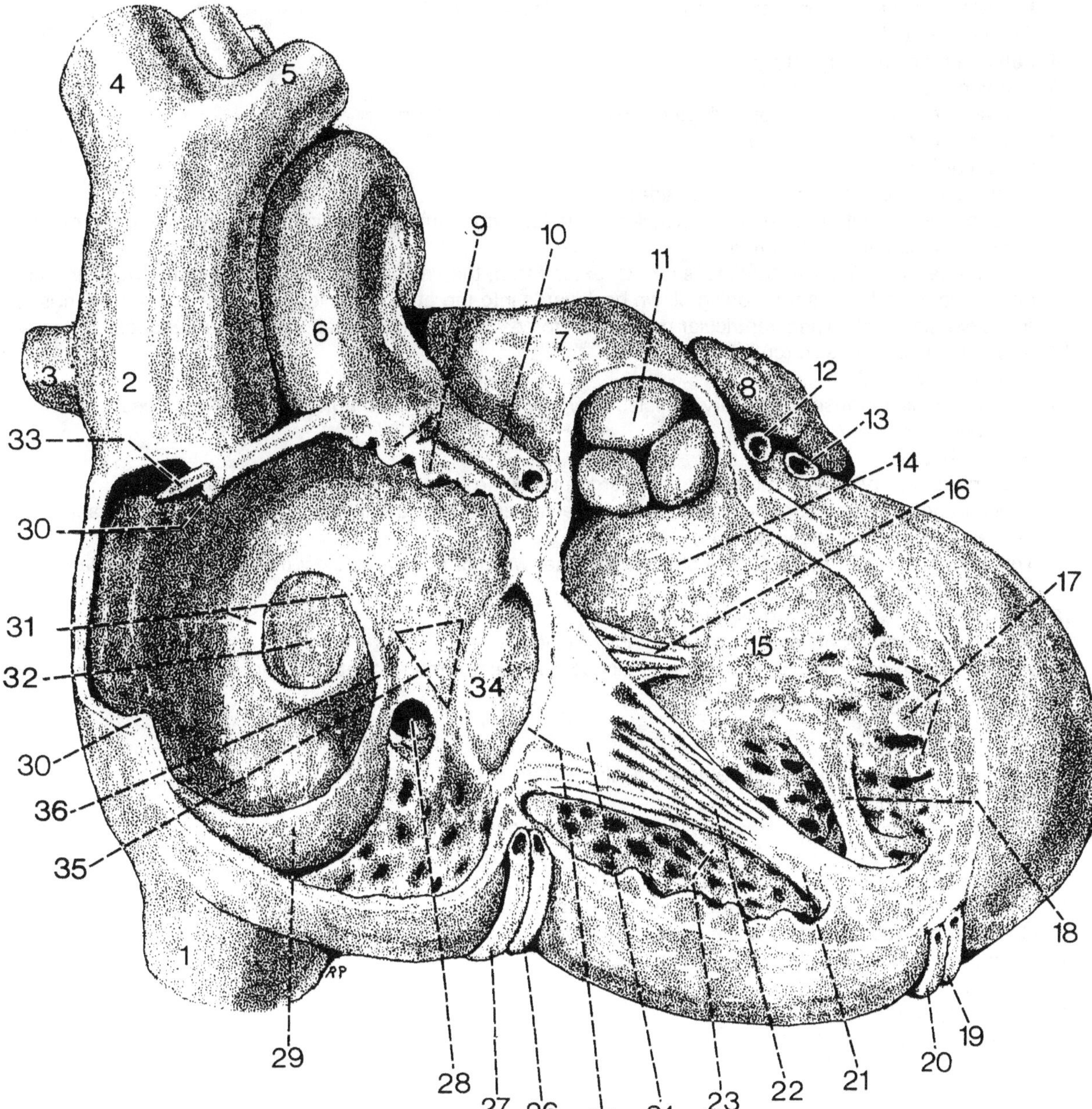

Right atrium Right ventricle

Th-33 Left ventricle

(opposite page)

Color and label

1 Arch of aorta
2 Ligamentum arteriosum; remnant of embryonic ductus arteriosus which shunted blood from pulmonary artery to aorta; normally it closes and becomes ligamentous after birth.
3 Pulmonary trunk
4 Left inferior pulmonary artery
5 Left superior pulmonary artery
6 Left auricle; ear-like atrial appendage or outpouching of left atrium
7 Anterior interventricular artery
8 Great cardiac vein
9 Aortic valve (viewed from ventricular side)
10 Anterior cusp of mitral valve; this valve closes the left artrioventricular orifice during systole and prevents the reflux of blood into the left atrium.
11 Chordae tendineae; these tendinous chords extend from the valve cusps (or leaflets) to the papillary muscles and prevent the leaflets from being blown backwards into the atrium; the leaflets have no intrinsic muscles and close passively when ventricular contraction forces blood against their ventricular surfaces.
12 Apex of papillary muscle (cut)
13 Wall of left ventricle
14 Anterior papillary muscle; papillary muscles may have more than one apical nipple-like process, as shown here.
15 Apex of heart
16 Posterior papillary muscle; note that the chordae tendinae from both papillary muscles attach to both the anterior and posterior mitral valve cusps; thus the initial papillary muscle contraction causes apposition of the valve cusps.
17 Trabeculae carneae; muscular bundles on the inner walls of both ventricles; the two auricles contain the musculi pectinati.
18 Interventricular septum (largely removed)
19 Trabeculae carneae on interior wall of right ventricle
20 Posterior cusp and chordae tendineae of tricuspid valve; guards right atrioventricular orifice
21 Papillary muscle
22 Right marginal artery
23 Interior of right ventricle
24 Right atrium seen through right atrioventricular orifice
25 Wall of right ventricle
26 Anterior valve cusp and chordae tendineae of tricuspid valve
27 Lesser cardiac vein
28 Right coronary artery
29 Septal cusp and chordae tendinae of tricuspid valve
30 Conus arteriosus of right ventricle (infundibulum)
31 Pulmonary valve (viewed from ventricular aspect)
32 Superior vena cava
33 Ascending aorta
34 Right brachiocephalic vein
35 Brachiocephalic artery
36 Left brachiocephalic vein
37 Left common carotid artery
38 Left subclavian artery

Th-33 Left ventricle

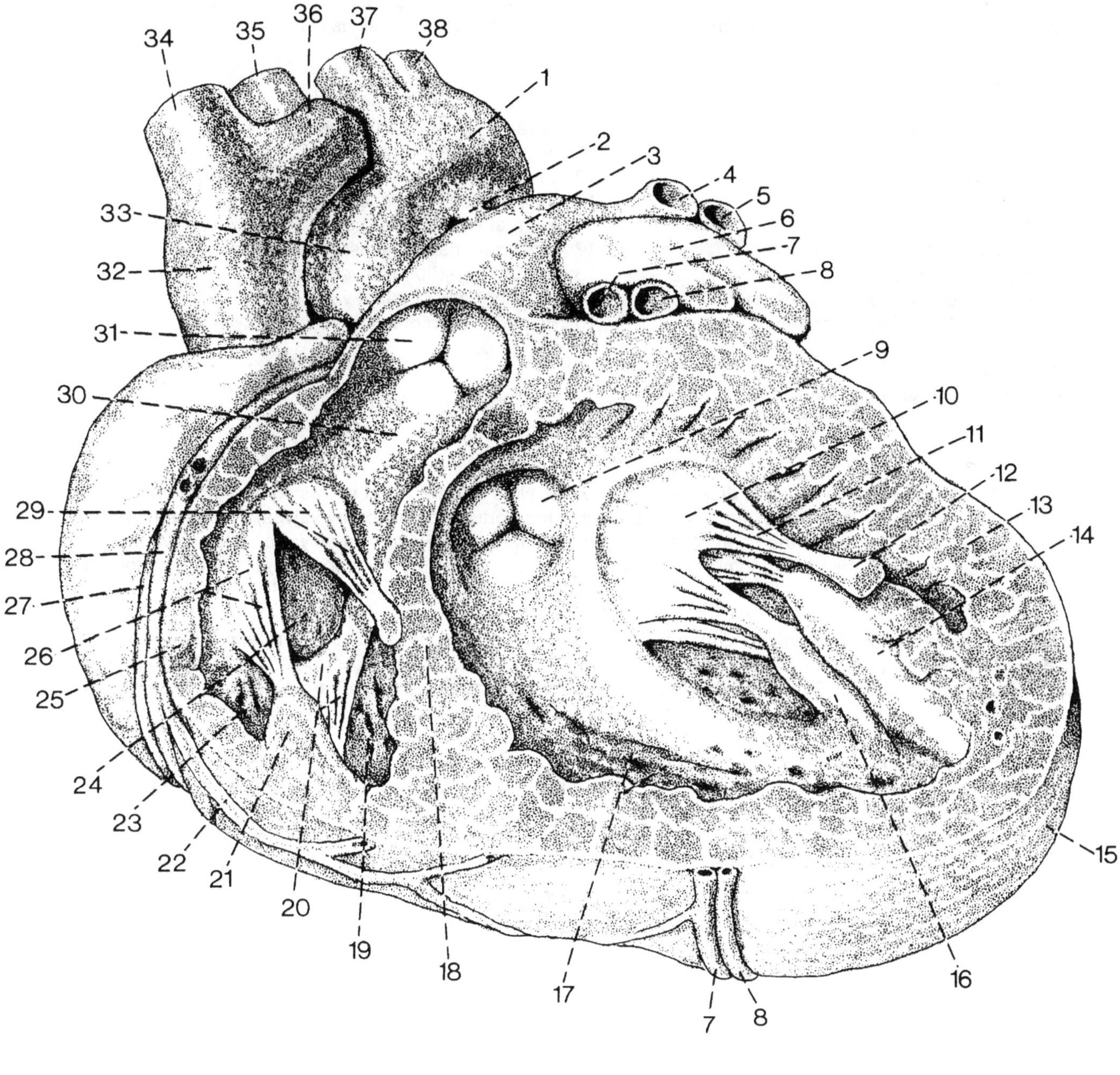

Th-34 Heart valves and valve action

(opposite page)

Top figure shows the four heart valves viewed from the posterior aspect. Both the right and left atria have been removed (the atria lie **posterior** to the ventricles). The aorta and the pulmonary trunk have been cut just above their valves. Note that the two coronary arteries arise from the aorta; the right coronary artery (5) arises from the right aortic sinus (6) and the left coronary artery (7) arises from the left aortic sinus (8).

Color and label

1 Pulmonary valve
2 Aortic valve
3 Tricuspid valve (right atrioventricular valve)
4 Mitral valve (bicuspid or left atrioventricular valve)
5 Right coronary artery
6 Right aortic valvule and sinus and origin (orifice) of right coronary artery
7 Left coronary artery
8 Left aortic valvule and sinus and origin of left coronary artery
9 Anterior interventricular branch of left coronary artery
10 Circumflex branch of left coronary artery
11 Anterior cusp of tricuspid valve (right atrioventricular valve)
12 Posterior cusp of tricuspid valve
13 Septal cusp (not always present)
14 Anterior cusp of mitral valve
15 Posterior cusp of mitral valve

Bottom figure shows valve action in **diastole** and **systole**. Note that the heart valves consist of strong thin membranous leaflets or cusps (they are called valvules in the aortic and pulmonary valves) that have no muscle. They are shaped so that when the heart contracts, blood will flow in one direction only; from atria to ventricles, and from ventricles into the aorta and pulmonary trunk. They are closed by the blood being pushed **backwards** against the cusps.

Diastole. The heart muscle (myocardium) in the walls of both the atria and ventricles is **relaxed.** The **atrioventricular (AV) valves** (tricuspid and mitral) are both **open** (1 and 2) allowing blood to pass from the atria to the ventricles (arrows 1 and 2). The two **semilunar valves** (aortic 3 and pulmonary 4) are **closed** because the pressure in the aorta and pulmonary trunk is higher than that in the ventricles.

Systole. The atria and especially the **ventricles contract** forcing blood out of the heart and into the aorta and pulmonary trunk (arrows 3 and 4). The **mitral and tricuspid valves** are **closed** (5 and 6) and, once the pressure in the ventricles exceeds the pressure in the two great arteries, the **aortic and pulmonary valves** are forced **open** (7 and 8). The elastic walls of the aorta and pulmonary arteries bulge outward and absorb part of the systolic pressure wave and smooth out the pulse. Two-thirds of the time the heart is in distole and one-third it is in systole.

RA Right atrium
RV Right ventricule
LA Left atrium
PT Pulmonary trunk
A Aorta

Th-34 Heart valve action

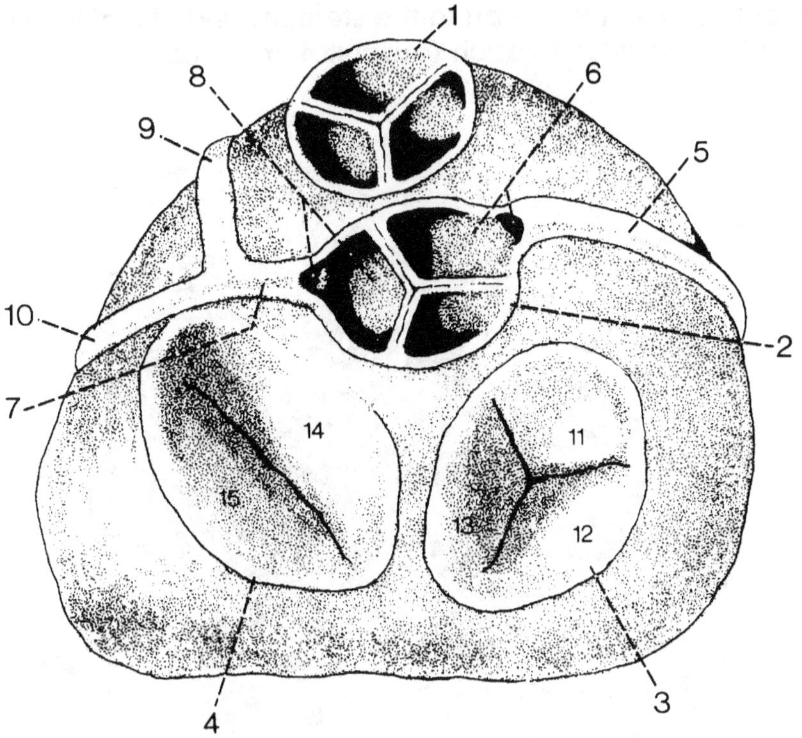

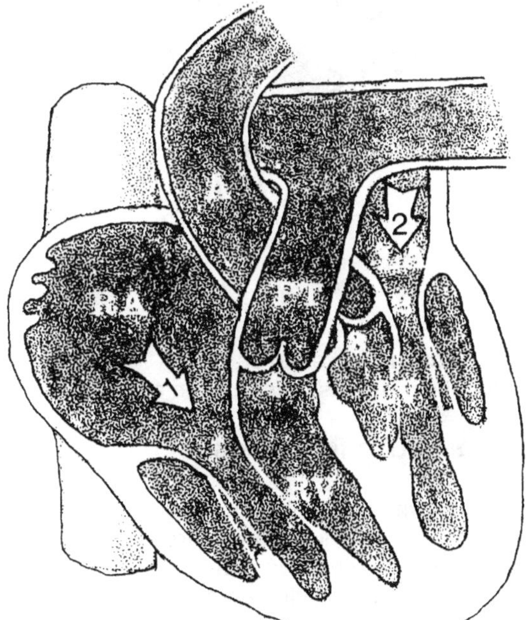

Diastole

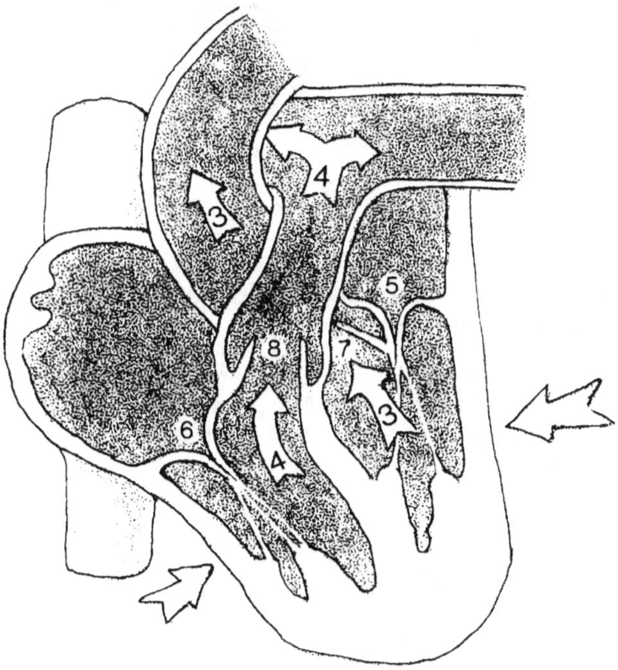

Systole

Th-35 The four heart valves

Relation of the four valves of the heart to the sternum and ribs of the anterior thoracic wall and the best locations to listen to each (auscultation areas)

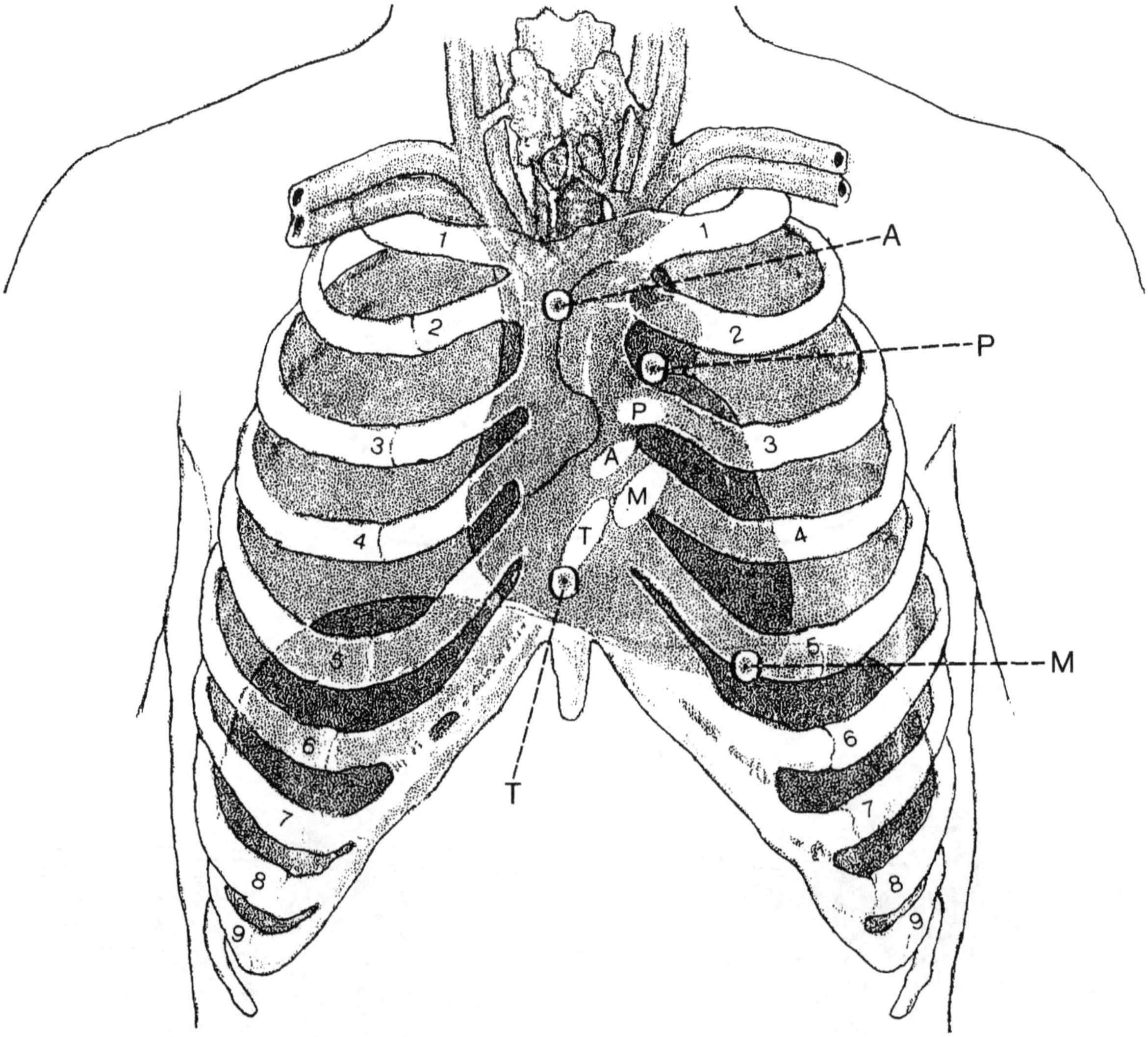

Color and label the position of the four heart valves (ellipses with letters T, P, M, A)

T Tricuspid valve; color blue; guards the right atrioventricular orifice; prevents backflow of blood from right ventricle to right atrium.

P Pulmonary valve; color blue; prevents backflow of blood from pulmonary trunk to right ventricle.

M Mitral valve; color red; guards left atrioventridcular orifice; prevents backflow of blood from left ventricle to left atrium.

A Aortic valve; color red; prevents backflow of blood from aorta to left ventricle.

White circles connected to letters indicate the best position to listen to each of the four heart valves (auscultation areas).

Label auscultation areas

T Tricuspid valve auscultation area
P Pulmonary valve auscultation area
M Mitral valve auscultation area
A Aortic valve auscultation area

Muscle: An etymological cartoon

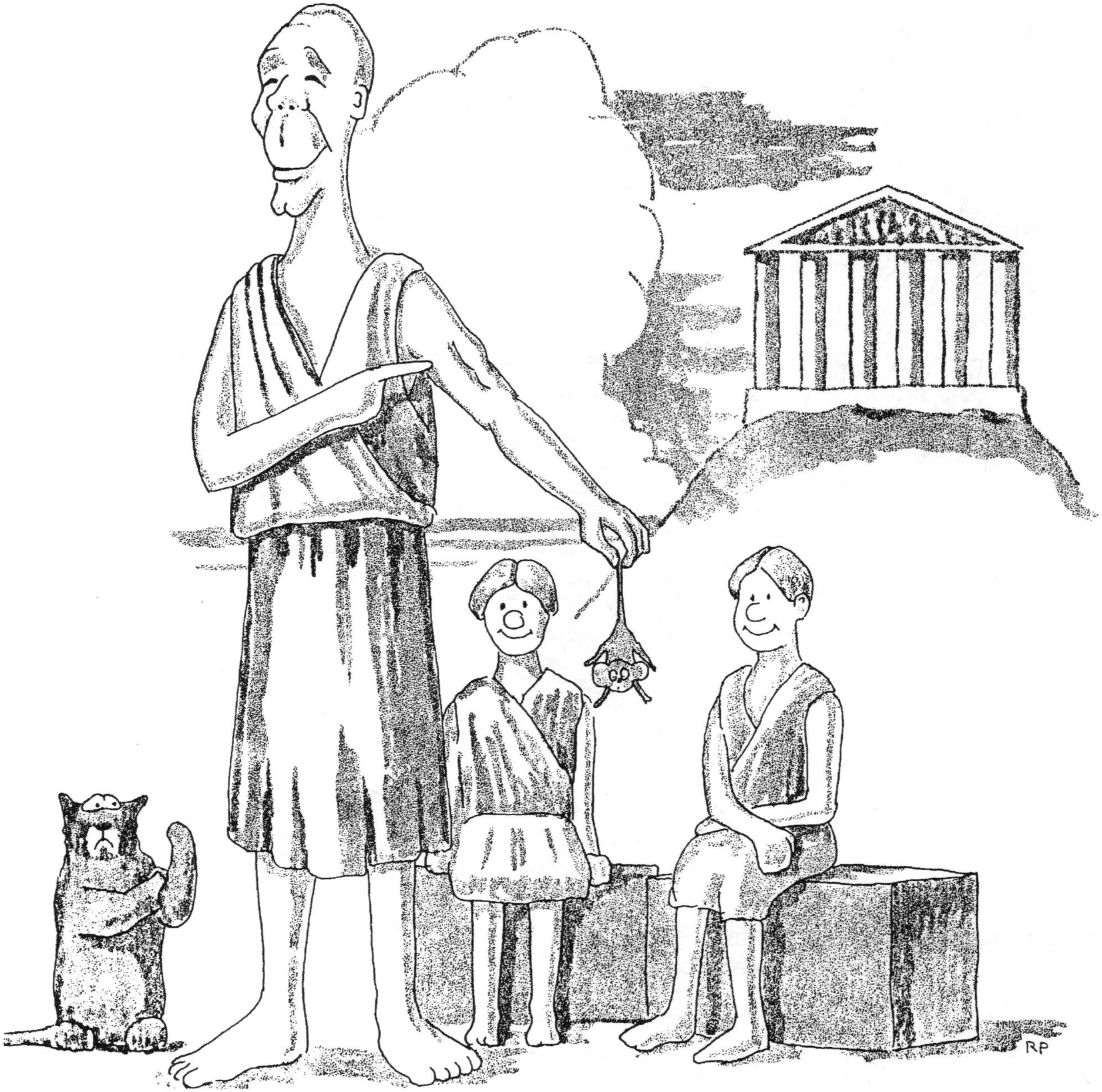

To the ancient Greeks and Romans, contracted muscle looked like small mice running under the skin, so they named the fleshy red bundles of the body musculi, which means "little mice," *musculus* being the diminutive of *mus*, mouse.

A pedagogue, or teacher, orginally meant a leader of children and is derived from *pais*, a child, and *agogos*, to lead; hence, a leader of children.

Acropolis means a "high city," from *akron*, peak, and *polis*, city. The acromion is the lateral peak or extremity of the shoulder blade or scapula (*akron*, peak, and *omos*, shoulder). Acrophobia is the fear of heights. Akron, Ohio is built upon a hill.

Th-36 Coronary arteries (most common pattern)

Anterior view of heart
Shaded vessels are on posterior surface

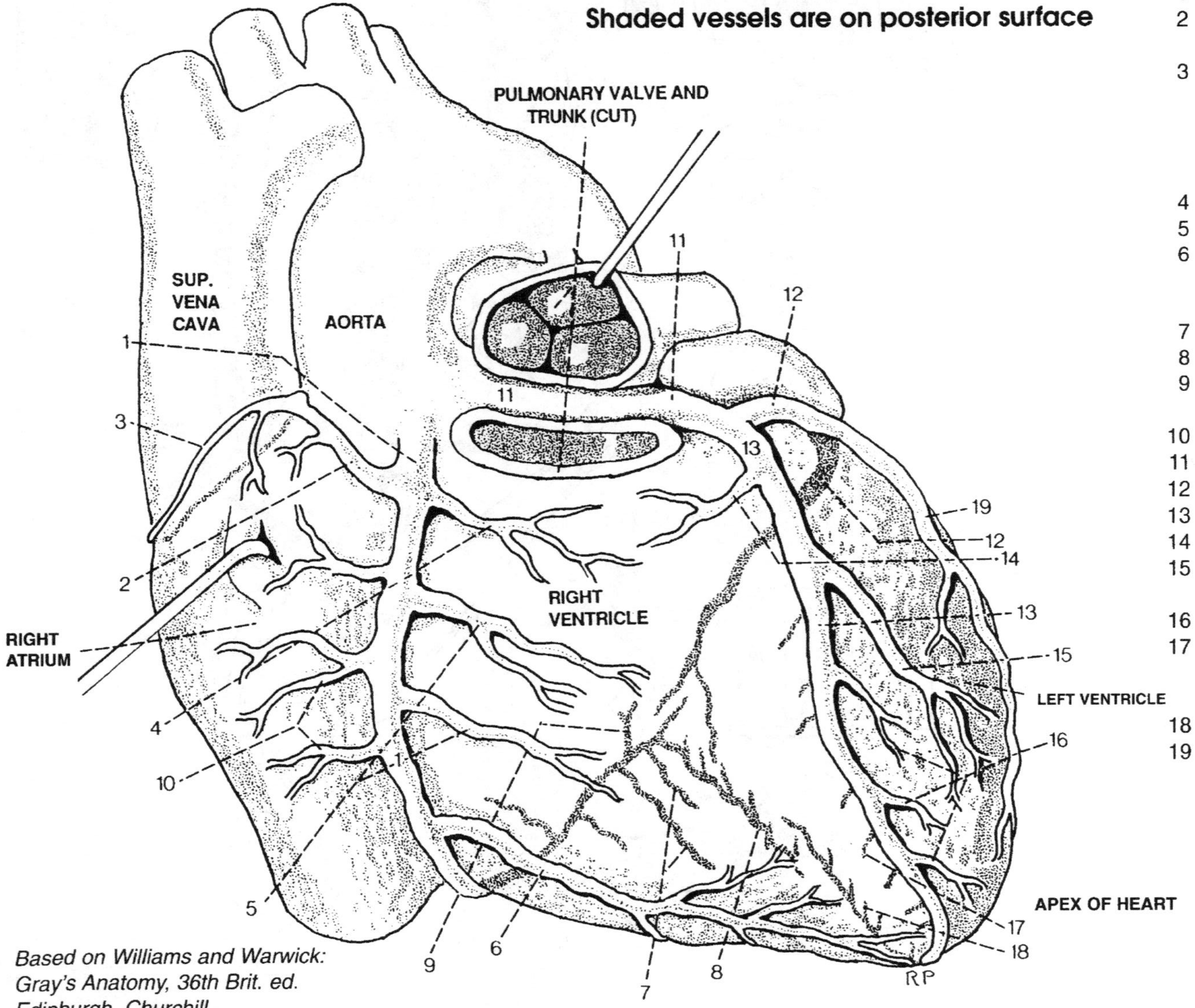

Based on Williams and Warwick: Gray's Anatomy, 36th Brit. ed. Edinburgh, Churchill Livingstone, 1980, pp 669-673

Color and label

1 Right coronary artery
2 Main atrial branch (usually called artery of sinuatrial node)
3 Sinuatrial nodal artery (arises from right coronary artery in 55% of hearts examined; from circumflex branch of left coronary artery in 45% of hearts)
4 Right conus artery
5 Right anterior ventricular rami
6 Right marginal artery (reaches apex of heart in 93% of hearts examined)
7 Right posterior ventricular rami
8 Posterior interventricular artery
9 Atrioventricular nodal artery (supplies AV node)
10 Anterior atrial rami
11 Left coronary artery
12 Circumflex artery
13 Anterior interventricular artery
14 Left conus artery
15 Left diagonal artery (present in 33-50% of hearts)
16 Left anterior ventricular arteries
17 Anterior septal rami (supplies anterior part of interventricular septum)
18 Posterior septal arteries
19 Left marginal artery (present in 90% of hearts)

Th-37 Coronary veins

Venous drainage of the walls of the heart

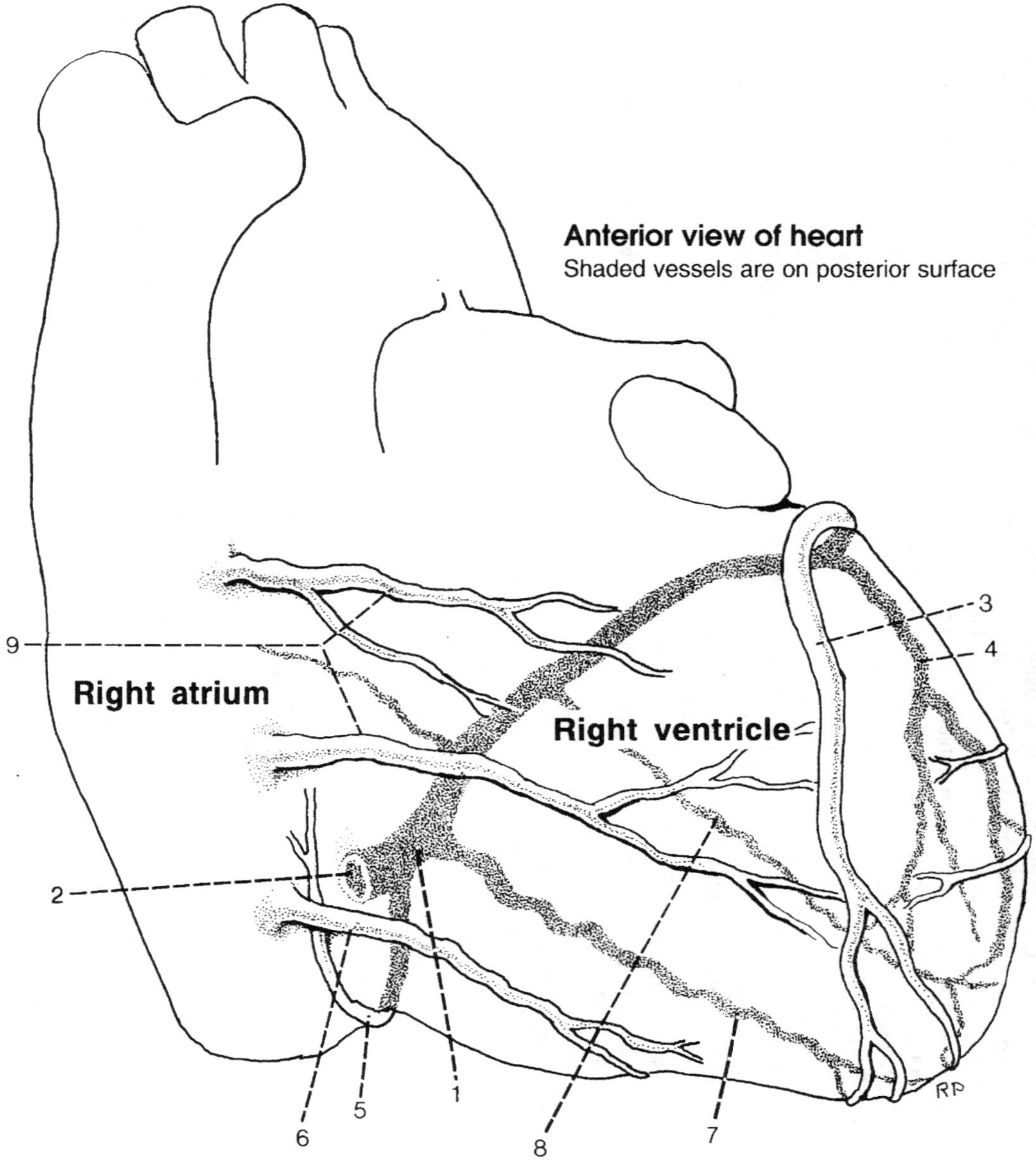

Anterior view of heart

Shaded vessels are on posterior surface

Color and label

1 Coronary sinus (on posterior surface of the heart); the coronary sinus is the main vein that drains blood from the substance (walls) of the heart.
2 Orifice (opening) of the coronary sinus into the right atrium
3 Great cardiac vein
4 Left marginal vein
5 Small cardiac vein
6 Right marginal vein; usually ends in right atrium as shown here; less frequently it drains into small cardiac vein, which then drains into coronary sinus.
7 Middle cardiac vein
8 Posterior vein of left ventricle
9 Anterior cardiac veins; notice these usually drain directly into the right atrium and not into the coronary sinus as do most of the cardiac veins.

The patterns of both veins and arteries vary considerably from one individual to another. Veins vary in their layout considerably more than arteries; the dissector should not expect to encounter arteries and veins especially the latter, exactly like those presented here.

Venae cordis minimae are small veins in the walls of the heart; they return blood from the walls of the heart directly into the chambers. Their openings, termed foramina venarum minimarum, are found in all four chambers, but chiefly in the atria.

Th-38 Cardiac conducting system
(opposite page)

Color and label

1 Sinuatrial node (pacemaker); it initiates the cyclic wave of myocardial depolarization and contraction; its center is traversed by the sinoatrial nodal artery (nodal central artery); it receives a rich supply of sympathetic and parasympathetic nerves which can either speed up or slow down its rate of dischage.
2 Atrioventricular node; its discharge sets off a rapid-moving depolarization down the atrioventricular bundle.
3 Atrioventricular (common) bundle (of His); in membranous part of interventricular septum; notice that the atrioventricular bundle has penetrated the right fibrous trigone.
4 Right atrioventricular bundle branch
5 Left atrioventricular bundle branch
6 Subendocardial plexus of Purkinje cells in left ventricle; these form the terminal branches of left atrioventricular bundle.
7 Right bundle within moderator band (septomarginal trabecula); the papillary muscles contract immediately before ventricular wall contraction, thus pulling the atrioventricular valve leaflets closer together and allowing their concave surfaces to catch the initial force of systolic ventricular blood, which causes the leaflets to "balloon" backward into the closed position. In addition, during ventricular systole, tension on the chordae tendineae by the contracted papillary muscles prevents the valve leaflets from being blown backward into the atria and blood from being regurgitated into the atria.
8 Subendocardial plexus of Purkinje cells in right ventricle; as is the case in the left ventricle, these comprise the terminal branches of right atrioventricular bundle.
9 Pulmonary valve
10 Ascending aorta
11 Superior vena cava
12 Termination of the superior vena cava
13 Tendon of Todaro; a rounded subendocardial collagenous bundle extending from the right fibrous trigone (see figure 38) to the valve of the inferior vena cava; it forms part of the triangle of Koch, which marks the site of the atrioventricular node (see figure 31).
14 Orifice and valve of the coronary sinus
15 Termination and valve of the inferior vena cava
16 Base and posterior leaflet of tricuspid valve; both the septal leaflet and the anterior leaflet have been removed
17 Moderator band (septomarginal trabecula)
18 Posterior papillary muscle of left ventricle
19 Interventricular septum (muscular part)
20 Base and posterior leaflet of mitral valve
21 Right fibrous trigone (part of cardiac skeleton); the small opening in the right fibrous trigone through which the atrioventricular bundle passes affords the only connection between the atria and the ventricles; otherwise, the fibrous cardiac skeleton completely blocks atrial excitation from reaching the ventricles.

The existence and the exact role of "internodal tracts" connecting the sinuatrial node to the atrioventricular node have been intensely debated since the beginning of the 20th century. Early investigators identified what they believed to be three internodal tracts in the wall of the right atrium, an anterior, a middle, and a posterior. One investigator reported finding specialized cardiac cells in one tract that he felt supported the existence of a rapid-conducting pathway between the two nodes. However, current thinking dismisses the existence of any specialized tracts in the right atrium, and that the spread of atrial excitation, unlike that in the ventricles, travels from one myocardial cell to another across the atrial wall. Compact bundles of parallel myocardial cells in the atrial wall probably convey the excitatory impulse slightly faster than the excitatory wave that travels through the greater part of the wall.

Th-38 Cardiac conducting system

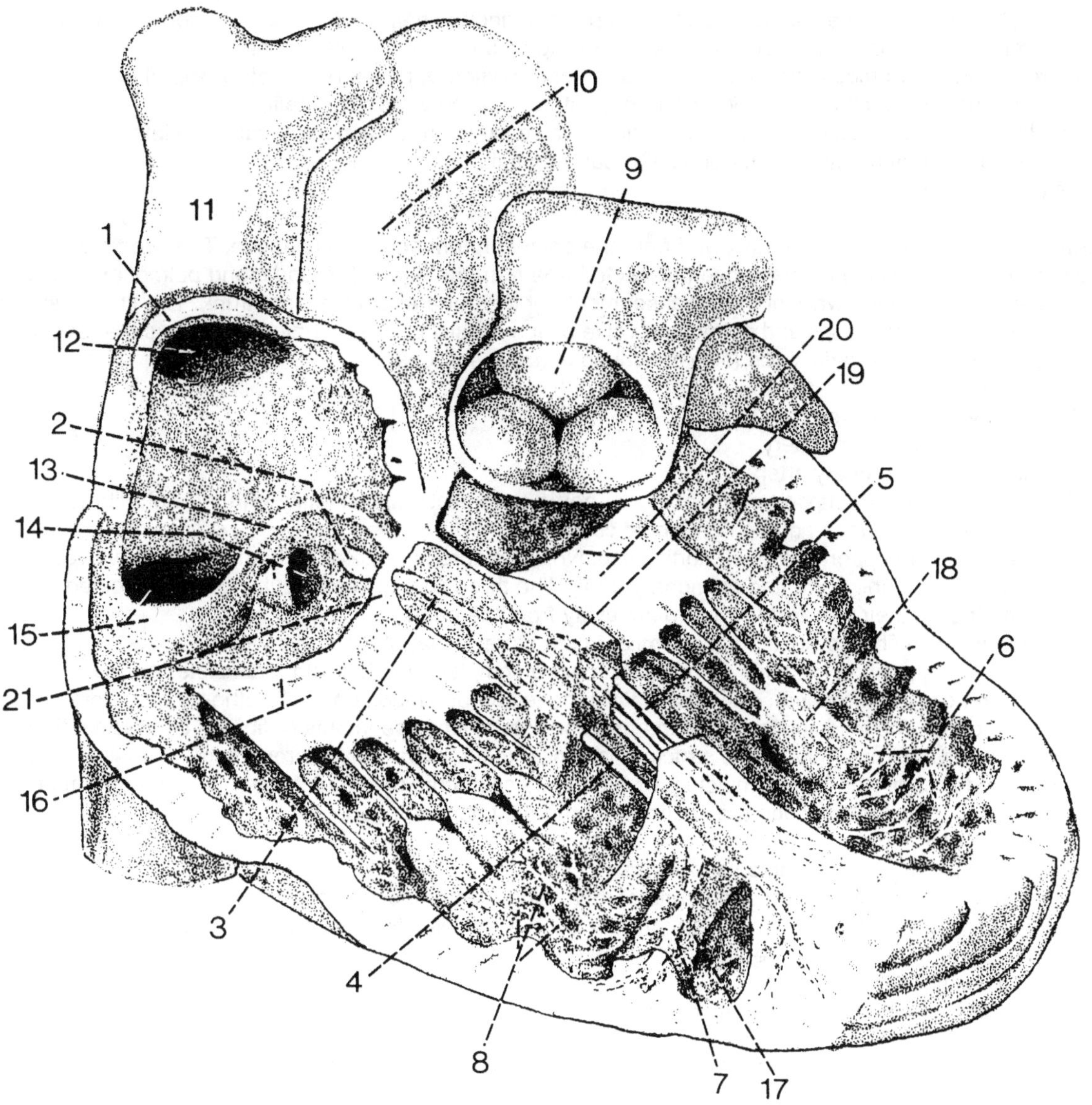

Th-39 Cardiac fibrous skeleton

(opposite page)

Label the indicated structures

Figure A. Posterior view (from atrial aspect) of four heart valves with their fibrous supporting skeleton. The atria have been removed.

1 Fibrous attachment of pulmonary valve cusps: **a,** anterior cusp; **r,** right cusp; **l,** left cusp (actually, left posterior)
2 Fibrous attachment for aortic valve cusps: **r,** right (actually, right-anterior) cusp; **p,** posterior cusp; **l,** left cusp;
3 Right fibrous trigone (central fibrous body; it appears trigone-shaped only when cut coplanar with the atrioventricular orifices; see figure B, below). Strongest part of fibrous skeleton.
4 Fibrous annulus of tricuspid valve leaflets: **a,** anterior leaflet; **p,** posterior leaflet; **s,** septal leaflet.
5 Fibrous annulus of mitral (bicuspid) valve: **p,** posterior leaflet; **a,** anterior leaflet.
6 Tendon of the infundibulum; extends from aortic valve skeleton to pulmonary valve skeleton
7 Site of passage of atrioventricular bundle through right fibrous trigone
8 Left fibrous trigone

Figure B. Fibrous cardiac skeleton viewed from the posterior right and slightly above. The two fibrous rings (tricuspid and mitral valve annuli) have been dissected free from the heart. The aortic and pulmonary valve fibrous supports are shown in the walls of the initial segments of the aorta and pulmonary trunk. The fibrous supports for both the aortic valve cusps and pulmonary valve cusps consist of three semicircular loops that anchor the semilunar cusps to the arterial walls (also described as triple scallops).

1 Aorta initial segment
2 Pulmonary trunk initial segment
3 Opening of left coronary artery
4 Opening of right coronary artery
5 Posterior semicircular support of the posterior aortic cusp. Note its continuity with the right fibrous trigone.
6 Right semicircular support of the right aortic cusp
7 Left semicircular support of the left aortic cusp. Note the fibrous skeleton of both semilunar valves are within the walls of the aorta and pulmonary trunk. The three fibrous semicircular loops are joined to each other at their free ends, which point away from the heart.
8 Pulmonary valve fibrous skeleton; it is similar in structure to that of the aortic valve.
9 Mitral valve fibrous ring (annulus fibrosus). It is not a complete ring but rather consists of two curved prongs (fila coronaria), one arising from the left fibrous trigone and the other arising from the right fibrous trigone. The incomplete part of the ring consists of small segments of fibrous connective tissue.
10 Tricuspid valve fibrous annulus; its structure is similar to the mitral valve fibrous ring. It consists mainly of two curved prongs with an incomplete part filled in by segments of fibrous tissue. It differs from that of the mitral valve in that both prongs are anchored to the right fibrous trigone.
11 Atrioventricular node
12 Membranous part of interventricular septum
13 Atrioventricular bundle (AV common bundle) traversing membranous part of interventricular septum
14 Right and left AV bundle branches (cut); the AV bundle divides into these two branches at the edge of the muscular interventricular septum (not shown).
15 Left fibrous trigone
16 Right fibrous trigone (central fibrous body)

After Williams et al., Gray's Anatomy, 38th British edition, 1995, with slight modification

Figure C. Front view of the heart with the anterior wall largely removed to show the position of the fibrous supporting elements: **T,** tricuspid valve; **M,** mitral valve; **A,** aortic valve; **P,** pulmonary valve. Note the three-loop configuration of both the aortic and pulmonary valve fibrous sleletons. As the ascending aorta leaves the heart, its valve is directed up, right, and slightly forward, whereas the pulmonary valve is directed slightly up, to the left and backward, so that the two valves are situated at right angles to one another.

Figure D. The initial segments of the ascending aorta (A) and the pulmonary trunk (P) viewed from the front. Note their 90-degree relation to each other.

Th-39 Cardiac fibrous skeleton

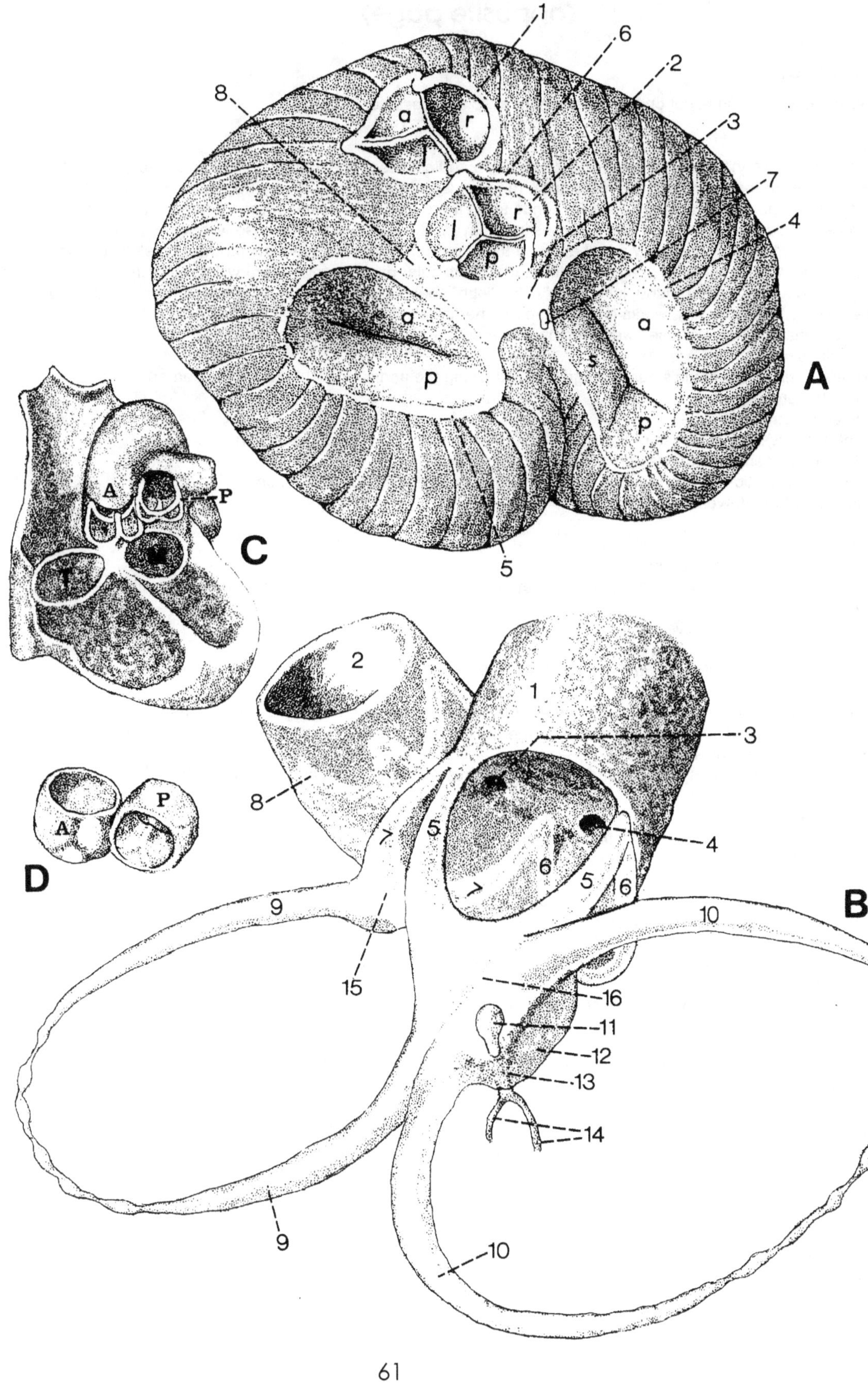

Th-40 Aortic valve and its fibrous support
(opposite page)

Color and label

Figure A. Initial segment of aorta cut open between right cusp and posterior cusp
1 Right aortic cusp
2 Left aortic cusp
3 Posterior (non-coronary) cusp. The three cusps and three aortic sinuses are named according to the origins of the coronary arteries. In the adult heart the **right cusp** (and sinus) are actually more anterior than right, the **left** is actually posterior, and the **posterior** tends to be more right than posterior (see figures C and D below). ` The cusps are folds of endocardium with a fibrous inner layer. The cusps, as is the case with mitral and tricuspid valve leaflets, have no muscle. Rather they are shaped so that higher pressure from the left ventricle (systolic ejection) will force them open. Whereas higher pressure in the aorta (ventricular diastolic relaxation) will force them to close (causing the "dupp" heart sound in "lubb-dupp, lubb-dupp". The "lubb" sound is the ventricular contraction and the closing of the AV valves. The pulmonary valve works in the same manner in relation to the right ventricle.
4 Right aortic sinus (the aortic sinuses were originally named the *sinuses of Valsalva*)
5 Left aortic sinus
6 Posterior aortic sinus; the aortic sinuses bulge outward giving the aortic root a tri-bulbous appearance.
7 Orifice of right coronary artery
8 Orifice of left coronary artery
9 Nodule (*of Arantius*); a small mass of fibrous tissue on the midpoint of the cusp free border
10 Lunule; thin translucent area of cusp on either side of the nodule
11 Triangular area of aortic wall between the cusp attachments. There are three of these.
12 Membranous part of interventricular septum
13 Left ventricle
14 Right ventricle
15 Muscular part of interventricular septum
16 Subaortic curtain (intervalvular septum); between left cusp and non-coronary cusp. It is continous with the anterior leaflet of the mitral valve.
17 Anterior leaflet of the mitral valve
18 Aortic wall (beginning of ascending aorta)
After Williams et al., Gray's Anatomy, 38th British edition, 1995.

Figure B. Fibrous support for aortic valve cusps; dissected from aorta; viewed from right posterior aspect
1 Posterior cusp semicircular support; it arises from the right fibrous trigone
2 Right cusp semicircular support
3 Left cusp semicircular support; note all three semicircular supports are joined at their apices (10)
4 Right fibrous trigone
5 Left fibrous trigone
6 Anterior curved prong of tricuspid valve fibrous annulus (cut)
7 Posterior curved prong of tricuspid valve fibrous annulus (cut)
8 Posterior curved prong of mitral valve fibrous annulus (cut)
9 Anterior curved prong of mitral valve fibrous annulus (cut)
10 Joined apices of left and right semicircular fibrous loops (also described as three "triple scallops")

Figure C. Aorta valve **closed** viewed from above (aortic aspect); note apposed boundaries of the 3 cusps form a triradiate pattern.
1 Right cusp and sinus (each sinus is enclosed by the outer aortic wall and the inner ladle-shaped cusp).
2 Left cusp and sinus
3 Posterior cusp and sinus
4 Left coronary artery dividing into the anterior interventricular artery (5) and circumflex artery (6)
7 Right coronary artery

Figure D. Aortic valve in **open** position (ventricular systole). Aortic diameter increases during ventricular ejection. The free edges of the three cusps become taut and straight as the aortic wall expands, causing localized vortices of ejected blood in each sinus and insuring that the orifices of the coronary arteries remain open. All four heart valve fibrous supports are deformable and change shape considerably as the valves alternately open and close.
1 Right cusp
2 Left cusp
3 Posterior cusp
4 Left ventricle viewed through open aortic valve

Th-40 Aortic valve and its fibrous support

A

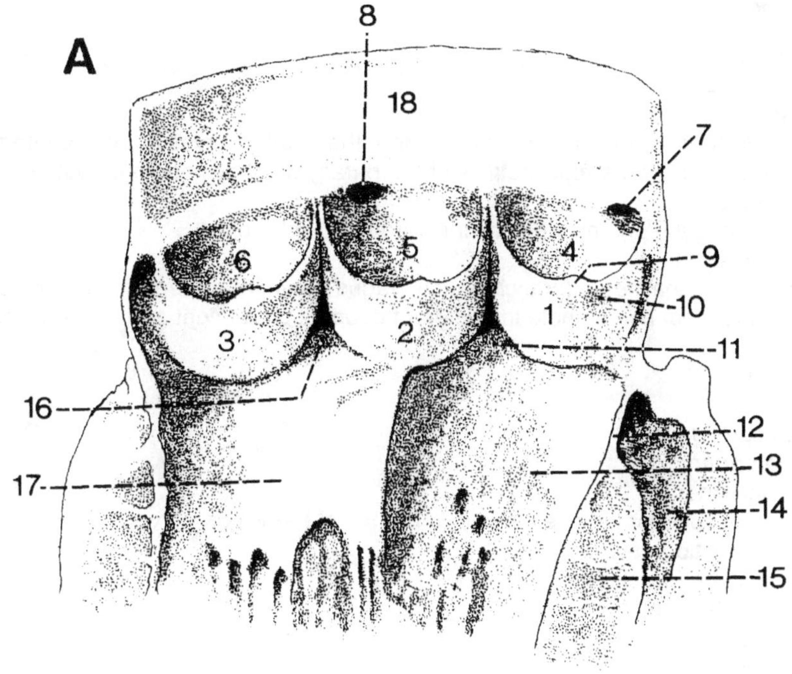

B

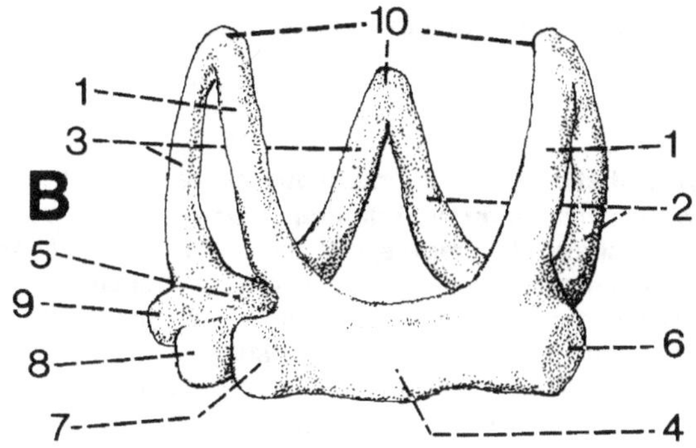

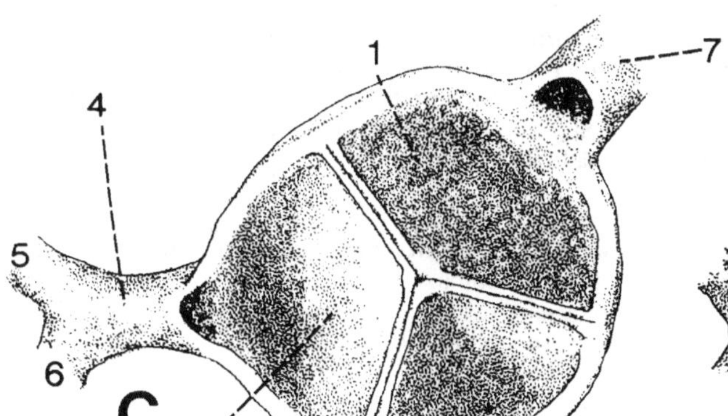

C

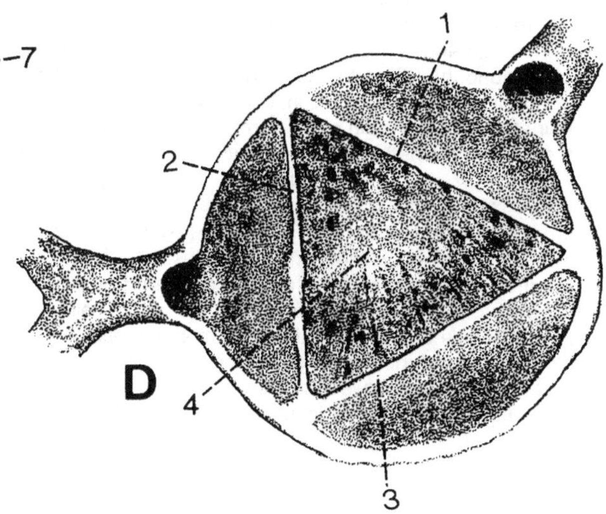

D

Th-41 Nerves to the heart

(opposite page)

Color and label

1 Heart (right ventricle)
2 Superior vena cava
3 Arch of aorta
4 Left vagus nerve (CN X, cranial nerve number ten; the cranial nerves are designated by Roman numerals; the two vagus nerves are the main outflow of the parasympathetic nervous system).
5 Right vagus nerve
6 Right phrenic nerve; the phrenic nerves innervate the diaphragm.
7 Left phrenic nerve
8 Right recurrent laryngeal nerve (branch of right vagus nerve; "recurrent" means "runs backward")
9 Left recurrent laryngeal nerve; note the different courses of the right and left recurrent larygeal nerves.
10 Cardiac plexus*
11 Pulmonary trunk
12 Trachea
13 Left common carotid artery
14 Left subclavian artery
15 Right subclavian artery
16 Internal branch of superior laryngeal nerve (a branch of the vagus nerve)
17 Right common carotid artery
18 Left anterior scalene muscle
19 Thyroid gland (right lobe)
20 Cricoid cartilage
21 Thyroid cartilage
22 Superior larngeal branch of vagus nerve
23 Superior thyroid artery
24 External laryngeal branch of superior laryngeal branch of vagus nerve
25 Internal jugular vein
26 Hyoid cartilage

*Cardiac plexus consists of both **sympathetic** and **parasympathetic nerve fibers**. The **preganglionic sympathetic** fibers originate bilaterally from nerve cell bodies in the **intermediolateral column** of the upper thoracic spinal cord gray matter. They leave the spinal cord with the ventral root of thoracic spinal nerves. Most of the fibers quickly exit the spinal nerve and enter the sympathetic trunk where most preganglionic fibers synapse upon postganglionic nerve cell bodies in the **sympathetic chain ganglia**. However, some preganglionic sympathetic fibers pass through the chain ganglia without synapsing and synapse instead upon sympathetic nerve cell bodies in the **cardiac plexus** (prevertebral ganglia). Postganglionic fibers from the ganglia then penetrate the heart and end mainly in the region of the SA node and AV node. They accelerate the heart beat and increase the force of systolic contraction. The preganglionic parasympathetic nerve fibers arise from **nuclei** in the brain stem **medulla** and travel within the vagus nerve and its cardiac branches, which supply the cardiac plexus with **parasympathetic fibers** that intermingle with sympathetc fibers. The parasympathetic fibers leave the cardiac plexus, penetrate the heart and synapse upon **postganglionic parasympathetic neurons** in the **walls of the right atrium** clustered mainly around the SA node and AV node. They have a slowing effect on the rate of the heart beat and an inhibitory effect on the force of the heart contraction. It is impossibe to distinguish sympathetic fibers from parasympathetic fibers by gross examination. The initiation of the cardiac cycle is myogenic; the physiologic demands of the body are conveyed to the heart by the parasympathetic and sympathetic nervous system, which modulate its rate and strength.

A **plexus** is a network of interlacing nerves or blood vessels.
A **nerve** is a collection of nerve cell fibers (axons) **outside** the central nervous system (brain and spinal cord; CNS). Larger nerves contain blood vessels and are enclosed by strong connective tissue sheaths.
A **ganglion** is a group of nerve cell bodies **outside** the central nervous system.
A neuroanatomical **nucleus** is a collection of nerve cell bodies within the central nervous system.
A **tract** is bundle of axons **within** the central nervous system.
A **synapse** is the **functional contact** between one nerve cell and another nerve cell or muscle fiber or gland. Most synapses occur at the junction between the tiny bulbous endings of axons of one neuron and the dendrites and cell body of another. It is the point where the nerve impulse is transmitted from one nerve cell to another.

Th-41 Nerves to the heart

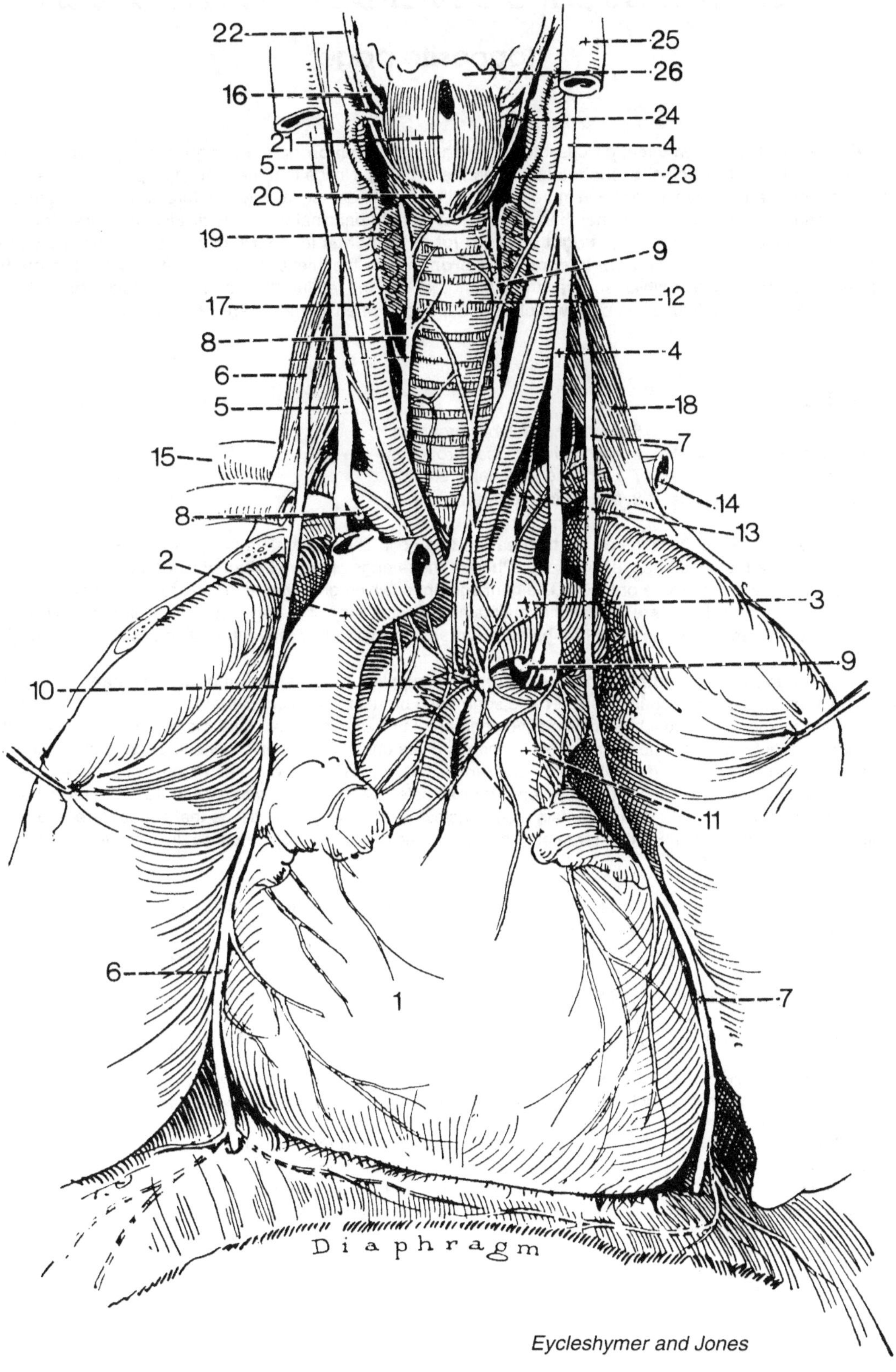

Eycleshymer and Jones

Th-42 Trachea, bronchi, and mediastinal surface of the lungs

(opposite page)

Figure A. The windpipe, or **trachea,** divides into two main or **principal bronchi**: the **right principal bronchus** supplying the right lung and the **left principal bronchus** supplying the left lung. Notice that the right principal bronchus is larger in diameter and more vertical than the left and more in line with the trachea, explaining why foreign objects usually become lodged in the right principal bronchus rather than in the left. The right principal bronchus divides into **three lobar bronchi** that each supply a lobe of the right lung: a **right superior lobar bronchus** to the superior lobe, a **right middle lobar bronchus** to the middle lobe, and a **right inferior lobar bronchus** to the inferior lobe. The **left principal bronchus** divides into a **superior lobar bronchus** which supplies the superior lobe of the left lung and an **inferior lobar bronchus** that supplies the inferior lobe. The left lung has only two lobes, a superior and an inferior, there being no middle lobe or horizontal fissure.

Color and label

1 Trachea
2 Right principal bronchus
3 Left principal bronchus
4 Right superior lobar bronchus
5 Right middle lobar bronchus
6 Right inferior lobar bronchus
7 Left superior lobar bronchus
8 Left inferior lobar bronchus

Notice the transverse rings of cartilage on the trachea* and bronchi. These rings are incomplete posteriorly, the void being filled by the nonstriated (smooth) tracheal muscle. Although these rings appear C-shaped when cut horizontally, they may bifurcate or fuse with the ring above or below. The cartilage rings, which give way to irregular plates of cartilage in the smaller branches of the bronchial tree, are essential in maintaining the patency of the air-conducting tubes and keeping them from collapsing as the air pressure inside them falls below the pressure exerted by the surrounding tissue during inspiration.

The lobar bronchi give off **segmental bronchi**, each of which supplies a **bronchopulmonary segment** of lung tissue. In the right lung the superior lobar bronchus gives off three segmental bronchi, the middle lobar bronchus gives off two segmental bronchi, and the inferior lobar bronchus gives off five segmental bronchi. In the left lung the superior lobar bronchus usually gives off four segmental bronchi and inferior lobar bronchus gives off five segmental bronchi. Each segmental bronchus has a designated number 1-10 plus B (for bronchus); for example, B1, B2, B3. Likewise each bronchopulmonary segment has the corresponding number 1-10 plus S (for segment); for example, S1,S2, S3 (figures 42 and 43). The bronchopulmonary segments are important in that they each contain a self-enclosed segment of lung tissue that is separated from its adjoining segments by connective tissue partitions (or septa) that allow single segments to be surgically removed—if diseased—leaving the rest of the lung intact.

*The word *trachea* comes from the Greek *tracheia,* which means "rough". Aristotle, who believed that the arteries contained air, named the trachea the "rough artery" as opposed to the arteries which he called the "smooth arteries". "Artery" was soon dropped from its name but *tracheia* persisted and became the accepted name for the windpipe.

Figures B and C. Medial surface of lungs

Color and label

1 Pleura surrounding hilum of both lungs
The hilum is the point where structures enter and leave the lung
2 Principal bronchus
3 Pulmonary artery
4 Pulmonary veins
5 Pulmonary ligament
6 Oblique fissure
7 Horizontal fissure (right lung only)
8 Diaphragmatic (inferior) surface
9 Groove for azygos vein (right lung)
10 Groove for aorta (left lung)
11 Anterior sharp margin and anterior surface
12 Posterior surface and round margin

Th-42 Trachea, bronchi, and mediastinal surface of the lungs

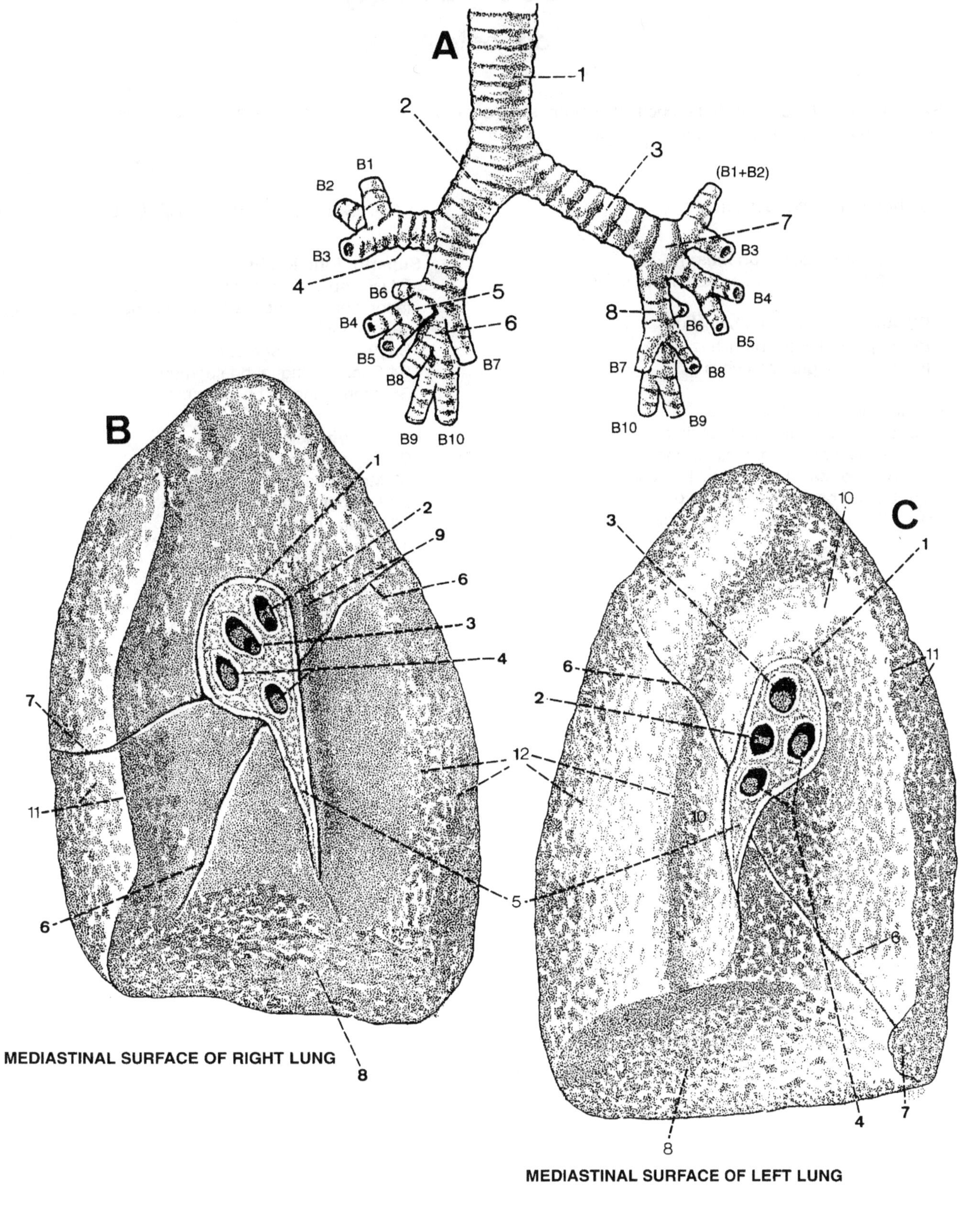

Th-43 Bronchopulmonary segments Left Lung

(opposite page)

Each segmental bronchus and bronchopulmonary segment (bp) is designated by a letter and a number in addition to a name that indicates its position.

Segmental bronchi

Left superior lobar bronchus
B1+B2 Apicoposterior segmental bronchus

B3 Anterior segmental bronchus
B4 Superior lingual bronchus
B5 Inferior lingual bronchus

Left inferior lobar bronchus
B6 Superior segmental bronchus
B7 Medial basal segmental bronchus
B8 Anterior basal segmental bronchus
B9 Lateral basal segmental bronchus
B10 Posterior basal segmental bronchus

Bronchopulmonary (bp) segments

Superior lobe left lung
S1+S2 Apicoposterior bp segment
(segments S1 and S2 are often supplied by a single segmental bronchus)
S3 Anterior bp segment
S4 Superior lingual bp segment
S5 Inferior lingual bp segment

Inferior lobe left lung
S6 Superior bp segment
S7 Medial basal bp segment
S8 Anterior basal bp segment
S9 Lateral basal bp segment
S10 Posterior basal bp segment

Th-43 Bronchopulmonary segments Left Lung

Lateral surface

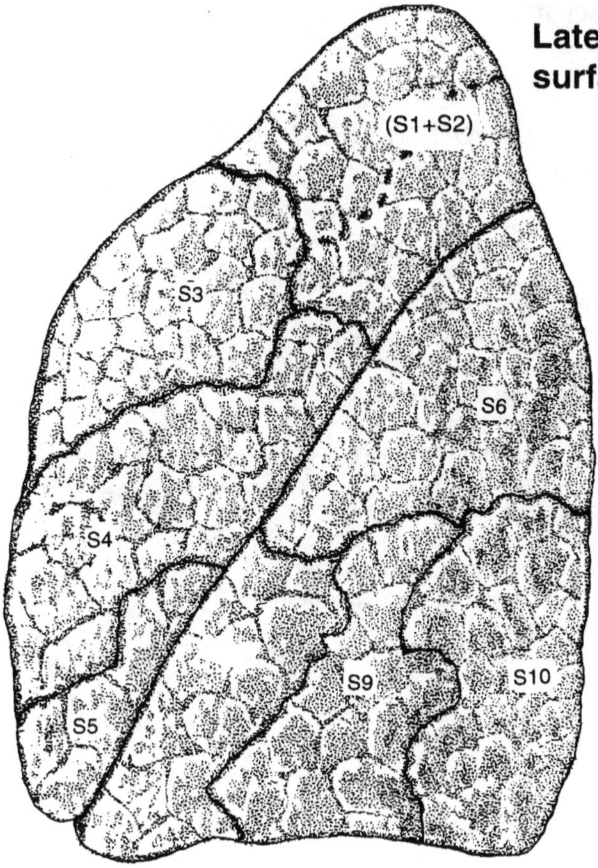

The left lung consists of only two lobes separated by the oblique fissure. Usually the upper lobe contains only four bronchopulmonary segments, as opposed to the right superior lobe which contains five. Segments S1 and S2 are supplied by a single segmental bronchus and, hence, function as a single segment. The lower lobe usually contains five segments, although bronchopulmonary segment S7 is missing in the lung pictured here.

After E. Pernkopf

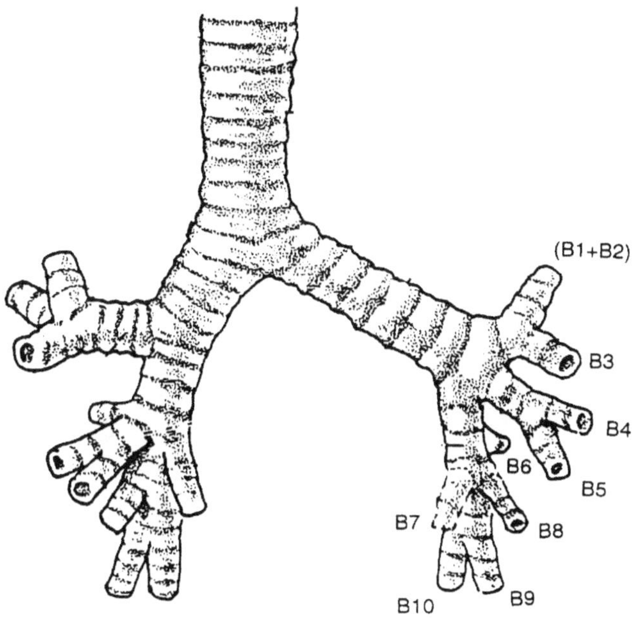

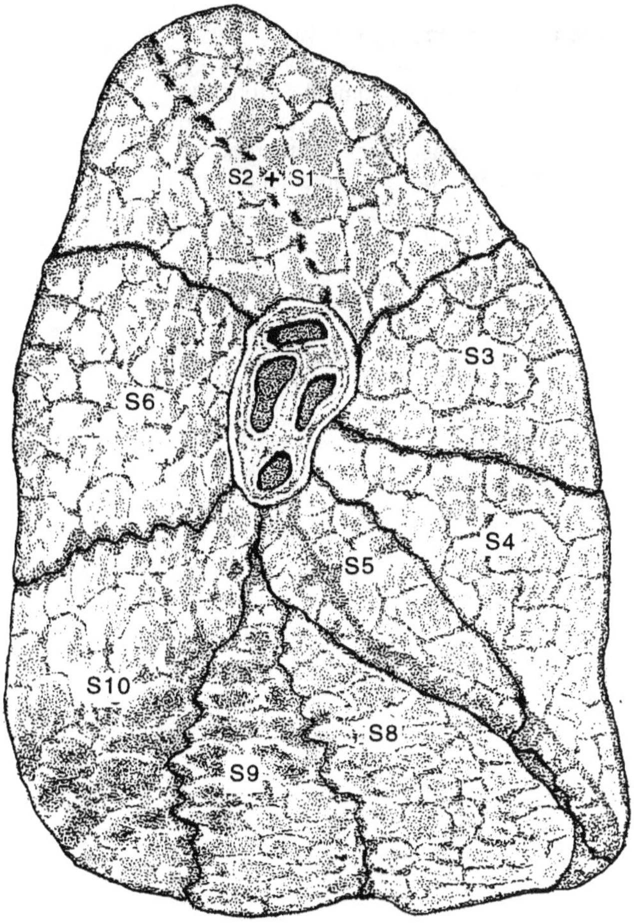

Medial and diaphragmatic surfaces

Color each segmental bronchus (B1-B10) the same color as the bronchopulmonary segment (S1-S10) that it supplies

Th-44 Bronchopulmonary segments Right Lung

(opposite page)

Segmental bronchi

Right superior lobar bronchus
- B1 Apicoposterior segmental bronchus
- B2 Posterior segmental bronchus
- B3 Anterior segmental bronchus

Right middle lobar bronchus
- B4 Lateral segmental brnchus
- B5 Medial segmental bronchus

Right inferior lobar bronchus
- B6 Superior segmental bronchus
- B7 Medial basal segmental bronchus
- B8 Anterior basal segmental bronchus
- B9 Lateral basal segmental bronchus
- B10 Posterior basal segmental bronchus

Bronchopulmonary (bp) segments

Superior lobe right lung
- S1 Apicoposterior bp segment
- S2 Posterior bp segment
- S3 Anterior bp segment

Middle lobe right lung
- S4 Lateral bp segment
- S5 Medial bp segment

Inferior lobe right lung
- S6 Superior bp segment
- S7 Medial basal bp segment
- S8 Anterior basal bp segment
- S9 Lateral basal bp segment
- S10 Posterior basal bp segment

Th-44 Bronchopulmonary segments Right Lung

Color each segmental bronchus (B1-B10) the same color as the bronchopulmonary segment (S1-S10) that it supplies

The right lung differs from the left lobe by having three lobes instead of two and a horizontal fissure (which may not always be present) in addition to an oblique fissure. The boundaries of the bronchopulmonary segments are not visible on the surface of the lung as pictured here. Each broncho-pulmonary segment is a self-contained unit of respiratory tissue which, if diseased, may be surgically excised rather than having a whole lobe or the entire lung removed. The right upper lobe has three segments, the middle lobe has two segments, and the inferior lobe has five segments.

After E. Pernkopf

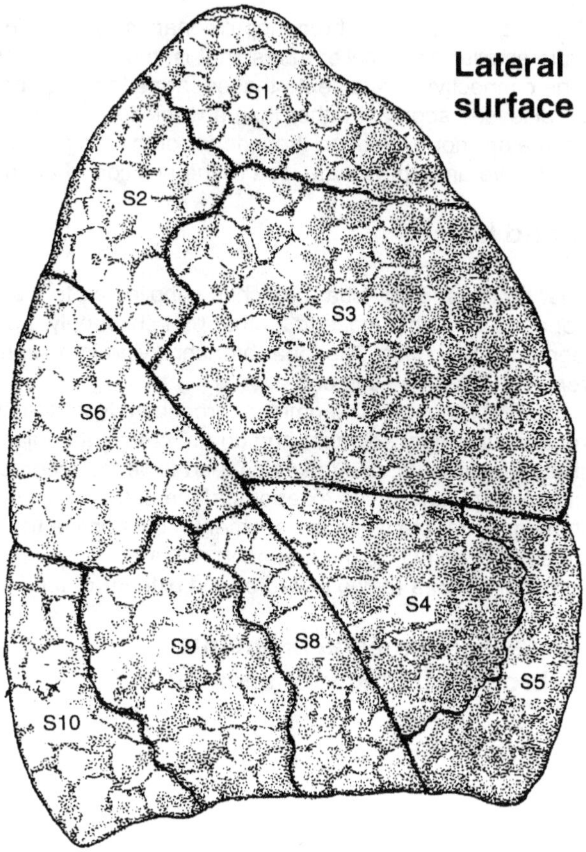

Lateral surface

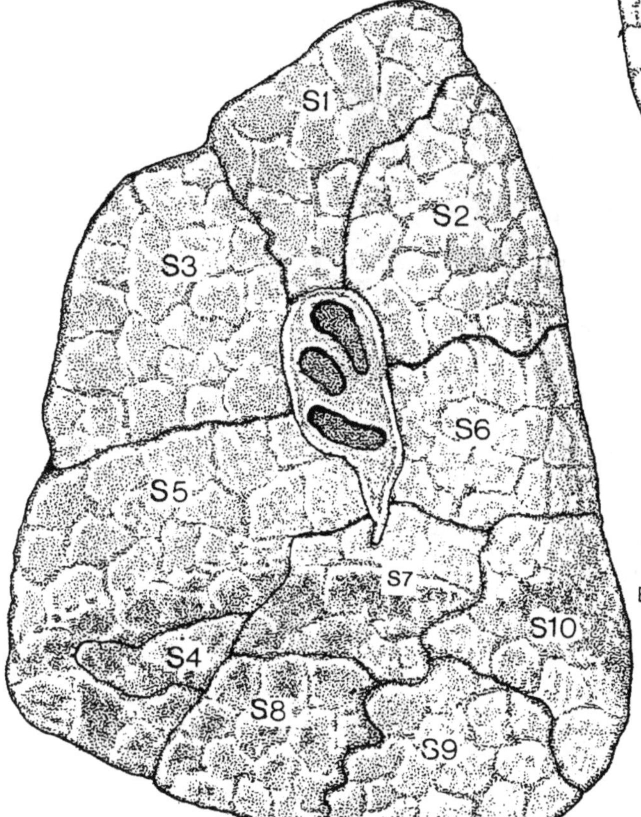

Medial and diaphragmatic surfaces

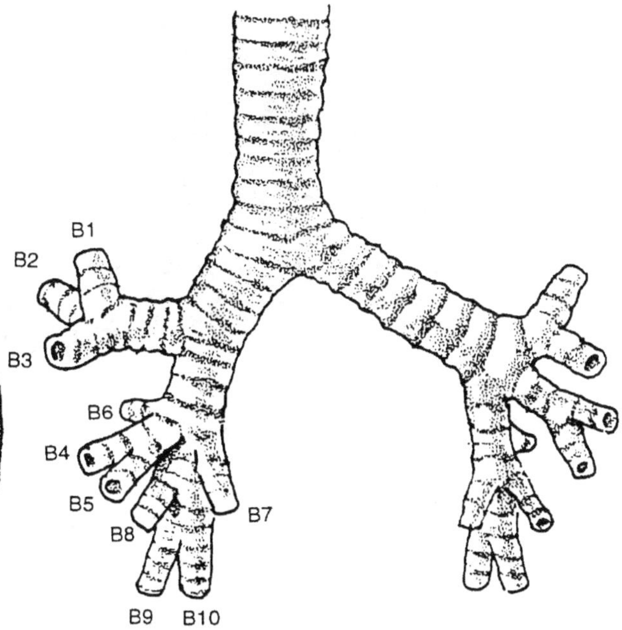

Th-45A Bronchopulmonary segment

Air passages

The air passages in 9 to 10 bronchopulmonary segments in each lung are self-contained branching tubes that divide into smaller and smaller tubes; that is, they do not pass into adjacent segments, but rather remain entirely within the connective tissue septa that separate the segments from one another. In cases of disease or damage, a single diseased segment rather than a whole lobe may be surgically excised. Unfortunately, the exact positions of the septa are not evident on the exterior of the lungs. The dissector should, however, appreciate their importance and have an approximate idea of the position of each segment.

Color and label

1 Lobar broncus. Each lobar bronchus supplies air to a single lobe of the lungs; the 3 lobar bronchi supply the 3 lobes in the right lung, and 2 lobar bronchi supply the 2 lobes in the left lung.
2 Segmental bronchus. The lobar bronchi divide into segmental bronchi, each of which supplies a single bronchopulmonary segment.
3 Divisions (branches) of segmental bronchus. Note that the air passageways remain entirely within the bronchopulmonary segment and do not cross into adjacent segments. The arteries sometimes extend into adjacent segments, and the veins tend to lie intersegmentally between the segments as well as under the pulmonary pleura on the exterior surface of the lungs (see opposite page).
4 Intersegmental (between the segments) connective tissue septa (partitions)
5 Intrasegmental (within the segment) septa
6 Pulmonary pleura (being pulled off the exterior of the lung)

Air passage (segmental bronchus) in one bronchopulmonary segment

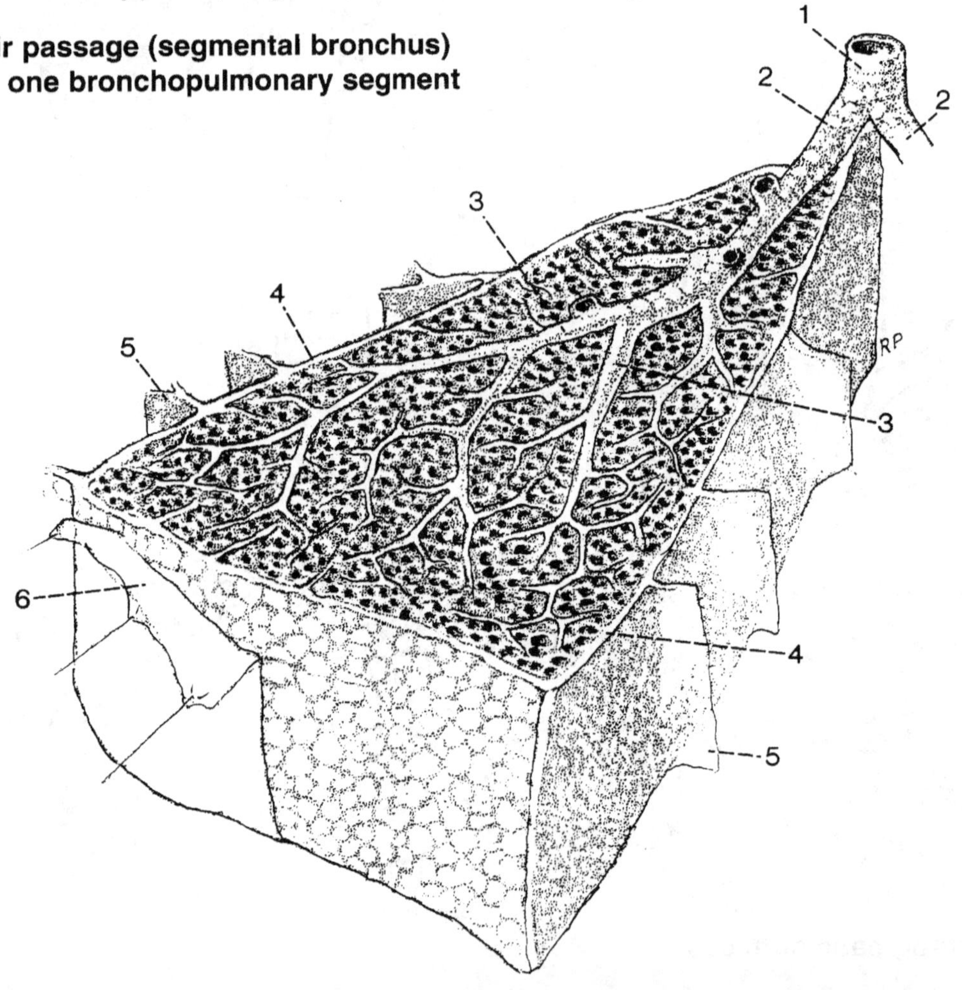

Th-45B Bronchopulmonary segment

Color and label

1 Lobar bronchus (branch of principal bronchus)
2 Segmental bronchus (branch of lobar bronchus)
3 Lobar artery (branch of pulmonary artery)
4 Segmental artery (branch of lobar artery)
5 Branch (tributary) of pulmonary vein
6 Intersegmental (between segments) vein
7 Venous plexus in connective tissue intersegmental septum (partition between bronchopulmonary segments)
8 Subpleural venous plexus
9 Arteries penetrating septum and entering adjacent segment
10 Connective tissue septum between segments
11 Pleura (reflected)
12 Septa extending into segment and into adjacent segments (not shown)

Air passage (segmental bronchus) and accompanying blood vessels in one bronchopulmonary segment

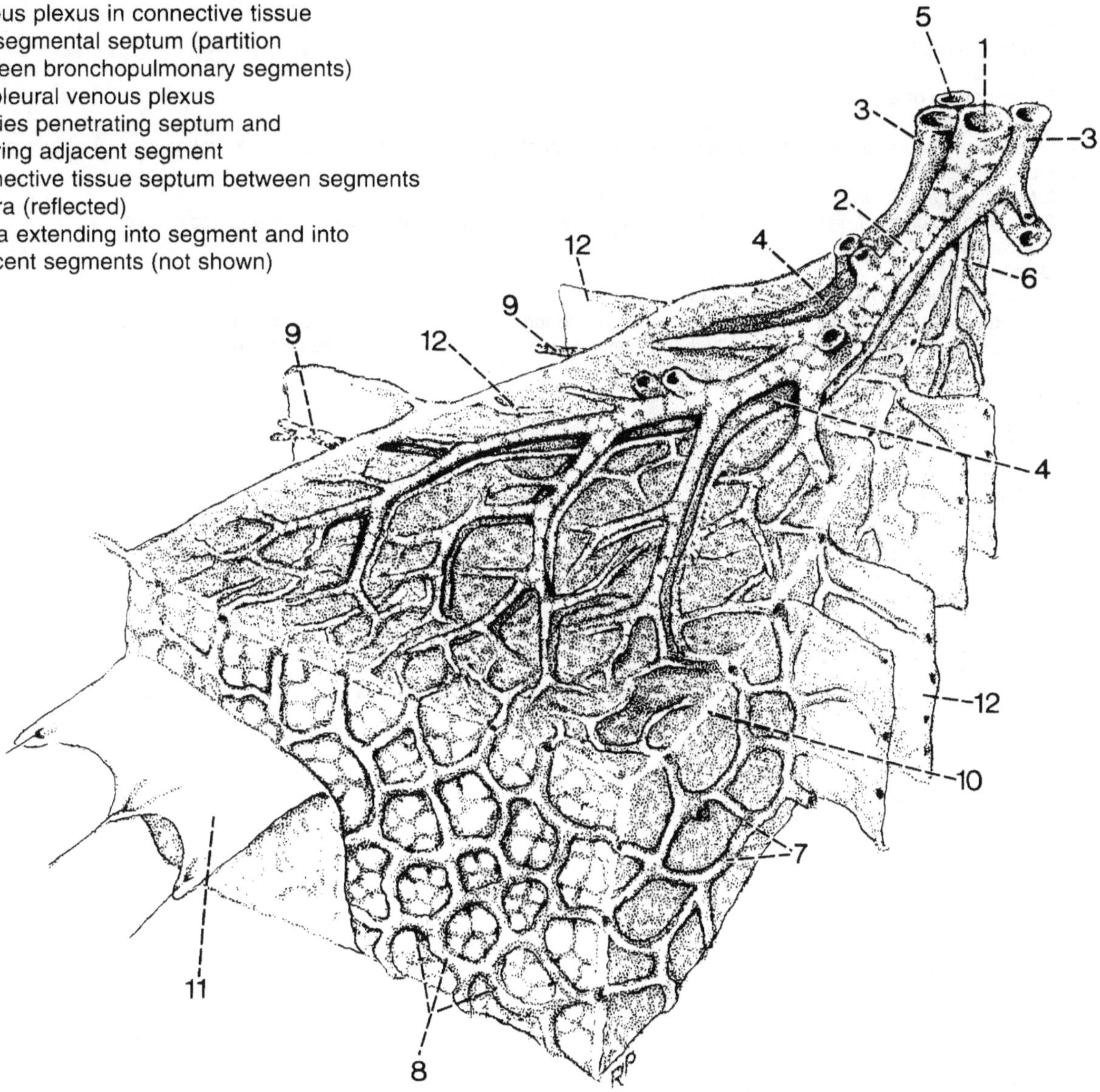

The right lung usually contains ten bronchopulmonary (BP) segments and the left lung usually has nine segments. Each BP segment has its own self-contained air supply consisting of a single segmental bronchus (2) and its progressively smaller branches. The segmental artery, which may be more than one (3), tends to accompany the segmental bronchus and its descendant divisions. Arteries occasionally become intersegmental and enter adjacent segments (9). The smaller veins are intrasegmental and drain peripherally into the larger intersegmental veins that course in the connective tissue septums (6,7). The veins also form venous plexuses beneath the pleura (11).

Th-46 Lungs and pleura

(opposite page)

The pleura is a serous membrane that invests the lungs and lines the inside of the rib cage. The **pulmonary** pleura covers the lungs and the **parietal** pleura lines the inside of the chest cavity. The parietal pleura is made up of: 1) the costal pleura, which lines the inside of the ribs; 2) the diaphragmatic pleura, which covers the upper surface of the diaphragm, and 3) the mediastinal pleura, which covers most of the pericardium. The pleura is actually two closed sacs that the lungs grow into just as the heart pushes into the pericardium. The actual space in the pleural sacs (pleural cavity) is a potential space that contains only a little serous fluid that allows the pulmonary pleura covering the lungs to slide against the parietal pleura.

Color and label

Figure A. Front view of lungs
1 Thymus gland (remnant)
2 Pulmonary (visceral) pleura (invests the lungs; reflected)
3 Superior lobe of left lung
4 Cardiac notch
5 Mediastinal pleura (fused to pericardium; part of the parietal pleura); note that the two pleural sacs are totally separate.
6 Oblique fissure
7 Inferior lobe of left lung
8 Reflection (folding) of diaphragmatic pleura with costal pleura forming the costodiaphragmatic recess
9 Pericardium
10 Diaphragm
11 Diaphragmatic pleura (fused to top of diaphragm)
12 Costodiaphragmatic recess of right lung. Note that the lung does not completely occupy the recess and that the pleura extends more caudally than does the lung. During normal breathing the lung will push partly into this recess and withdraw with every breath.
13 Inferior lobe of right lung
14 Oblique fissure
15 Middle lobe of right lung
16 Horizontal fissure
17 Parietal pleura (cut edge)
18 Superior lobe of right lung
19 Pulmonary pleura (reflected)

Figure B. Inferior view of lungs and heart
1 Heart
2 Inferior lobe of left lung
3 Oblique fissure
4 Pericardiacophrenic artery and vein ("sandwiched" between the pericardium and the mediastinal pleura)
5 Phrenic nerve (also "sandwiched")
6 Left lung (inferior surface of inferior lobe)
7 Aorta (giving rise to two posterior intercostal arteries)
8 Sympathetic trunk
9 Azygos vein receiving two posterior intercostal veins
10 Thoracic duct
11 Esophagus and esophageal plexus (on its exterior)
12 Inferior vena cava
13 Inferior lobe of right lung
14 Oblique fissure
15 Superior lobe of right lung
16 Phrenic nerve and accompanying pericardiacophrenic artery and vein

Figure C. Bifurcation of the trachea into right and left principal bronchi. Cut coronally. Viewed from behind
1 Trachea (wind pipe)
2 Right main bronchus; note it is larger and more vertical than the left main bronchus.
3 Left main bronchus; note it is more horizontal than the right main bronchus
4 Carina (keel-like projection at bifurcation); foreign objects often become lodged on the carina.

Th-46 Lungs and pleura

A

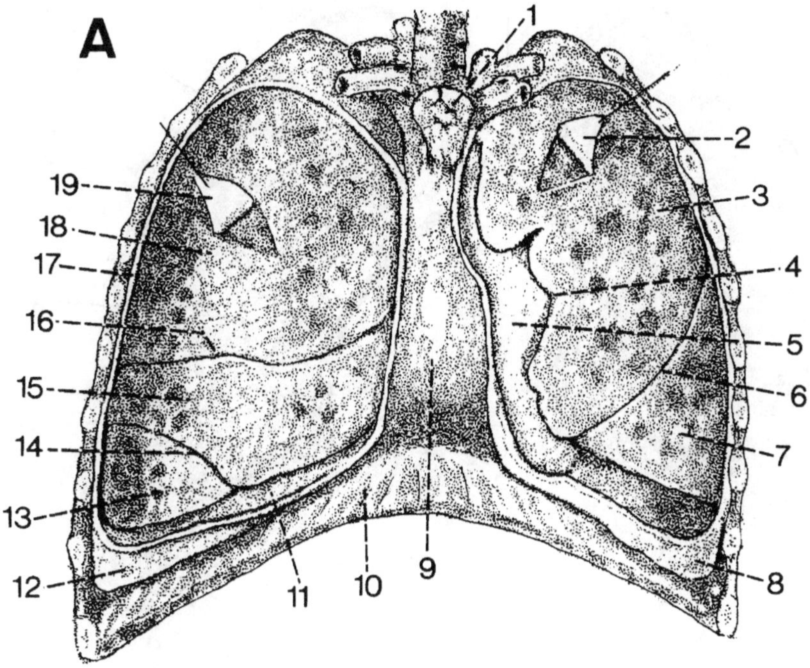

C

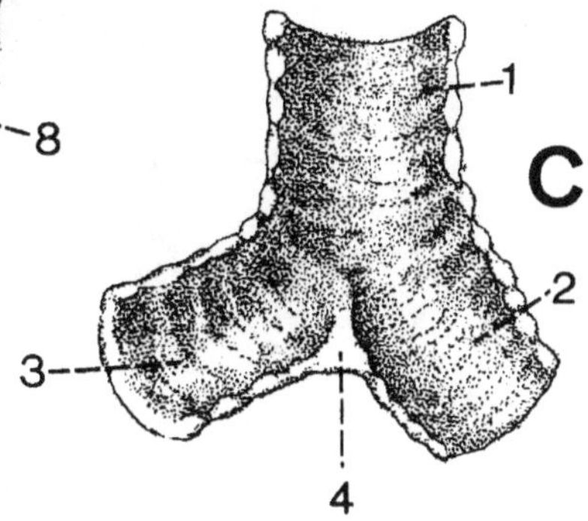

B

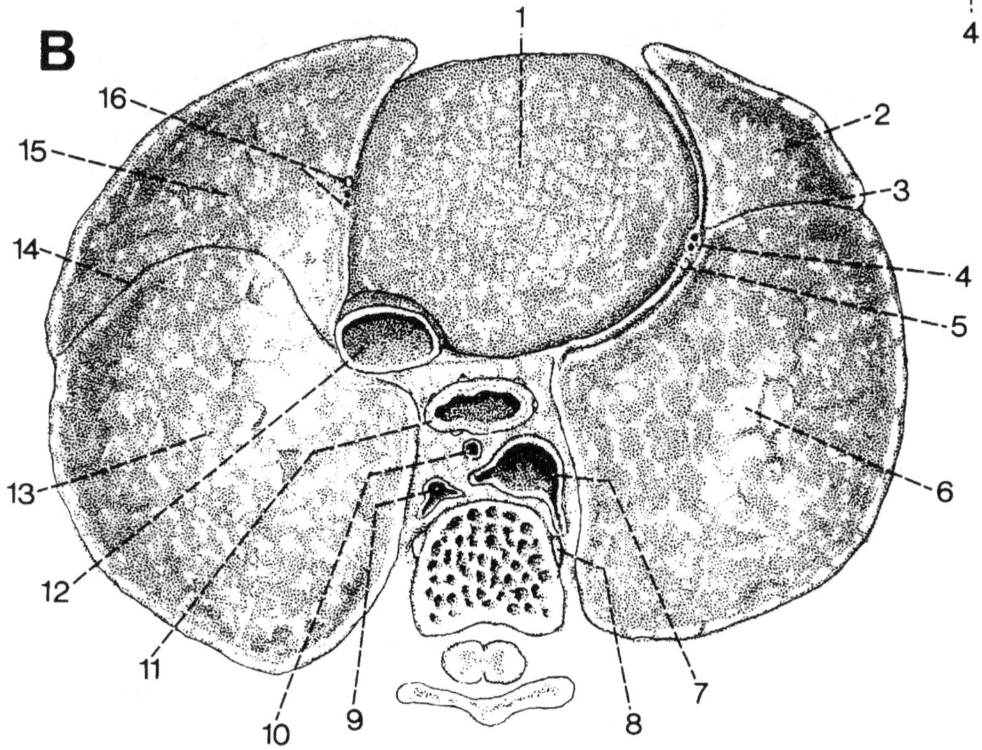

Th-47 The pleura and pleural recesses

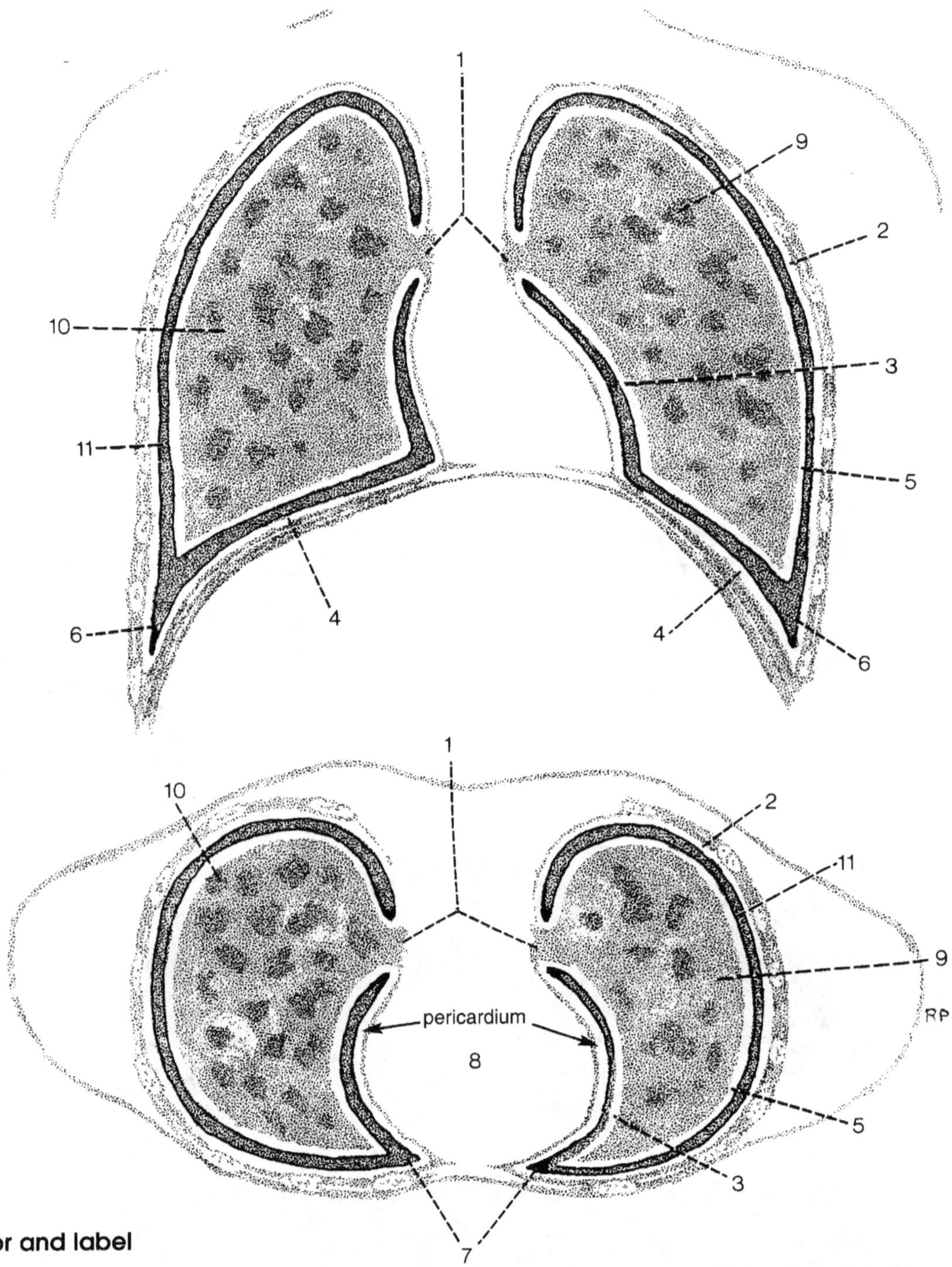

Color and label

1 Roots of lung; these contain the principal bronchi, arteries, veins, nerves, and lymphatics entering and leaving the lungs
2 Costal pleura
3 Mediastinal pleura (fused to pericardium)
4 Diaphragmatic pleura
5 Pulmonary (visceral) pleura
6 Costodiaphragmatic recess; normally only a slit. Note that it extends considerably further caudally than does the lung.
7 Costomediastinal recess; also only a slit. The recesses are important in that their accidental puncture may introduce infection into the pleural cavity
8 Heart
9 Left lung
10 Right lung
11 Pleural cavity (a potential space)

Th-48 Trachea, esophagus and vagus nerve

Posterior aspect

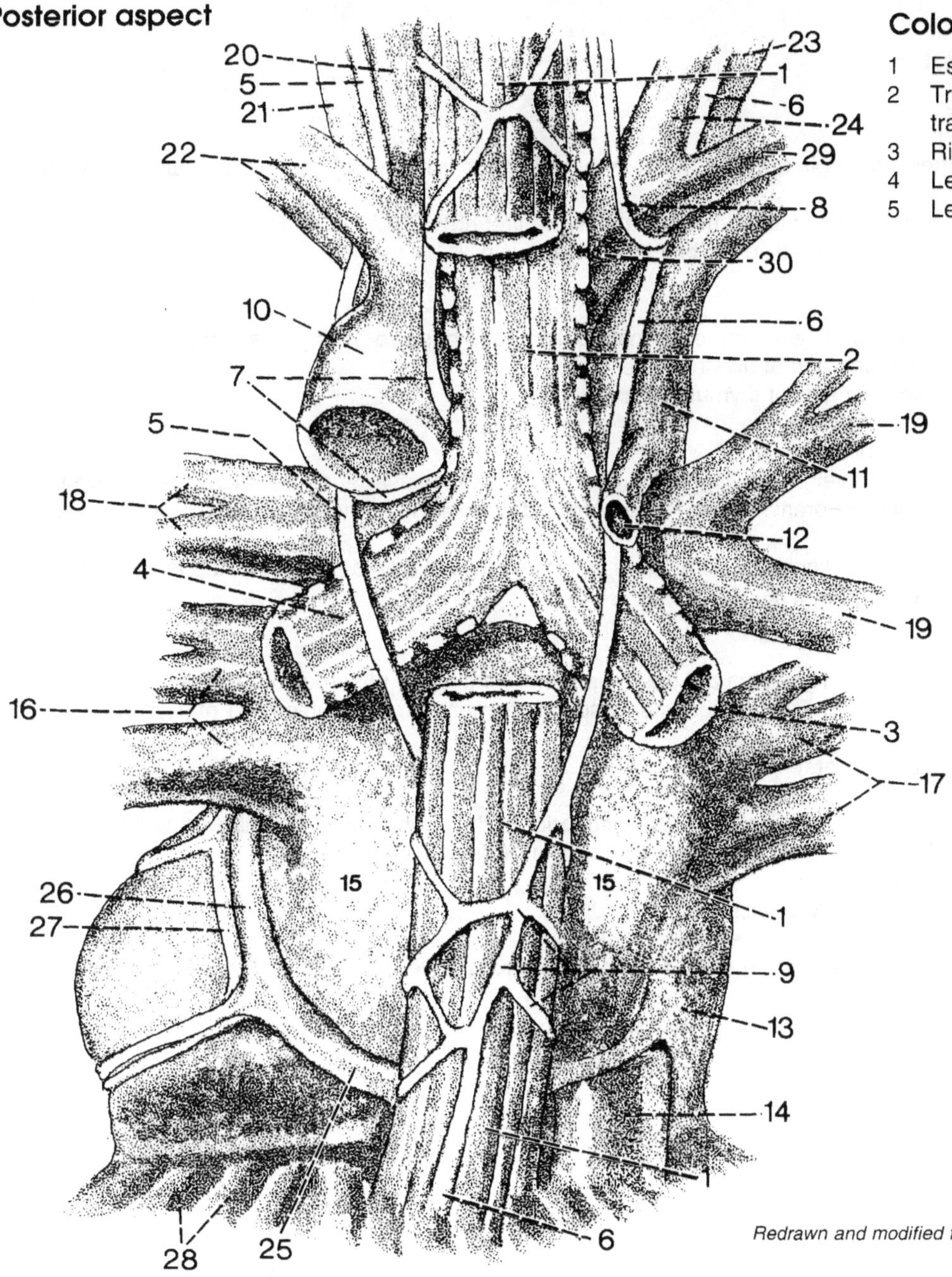

Redrawn and modified from Thorek figure 221

Color and label

1 Esophagus (section removed)
2 Trachea (posterior surface; tracheal muscle)
3 Right principal bronchus
4 Left principal bronchus
5 Left vagus nerve
6 Right vagus nerve
7 Left recurrent laryngeal nerve
8 Right recurrent laryngeal nerve
9 Esophageal plexus
10 Arch of aorta
11 Superior vena cava
12 Azygos vein
13 Right atrium
14 Inferior vena cava
15 Left atrium
16 Left pulmonary veins (red)
17 Right pulmonary veins (red)
18 Left pulmonary arteries (blue)
19 Right pulmonary arteries (blue)
20 Left common carotid artery
21 Internal jugular vein
22 Left subclavian artery and vein
23 Right jugular vein
24 Right common carotid artery
25 Coronary sinus
26 Great cardiac vein
27 Circumflex artery
28 Diaphragm
29 Right subclavian artery
30 Brachiocephalic artery

Th-49 Right mediastinum

Right lung has been removed (opposite page)

Color and label

1 Right vagus nerve
2 Internal jugular vein
3 Internal thoracic artery; its origin is variable, but it usually arises from the first part of the subclavian artery
4 Subclavian vein
5 Cupula of pleura; covers apex of lung (the part above the first rib)
6 Internal thoracic vein; usually ends in the brachiocephalic vein
7 Manubrium
8 Vagus nerve
9 Anterior intercostal artery and vein (cut); each intercostal space has two pairs of these vessels: one pair below the rib above and one pair above the lower rib
10 Superior vena cava and remains of thymus gland
11 Ascending aorta
12 Lobar branches of right pulmonary artery
13 Internal thoracic artery and vein; note cut origins of anterior intercostal arteries and veins. The internal thoracic vessels also give off branches to the sternum and perforating branches to the pectoralis major muscle and to the breast
14 Phrenic nerve with pericardiacophrenic artery and vein (mediastinal pleura has been stripped away)
15 Pericardium and cut edge of parietal pleura
16 Sternum (body)
17 Pulmonary veins
18 Pulmonary ligament; visceral ligaments are made up of a double layer of serous membrane — here it is pleura — and connective tissue. In the abdomen visceral ligaments are a double layer of peritoneum.
19 Diaphragm
20 Greater splanchnic nerve (roots)
21 Intercostal nerve
22 Intercostal vein, artery, and nerve (**vein** is usually superior to the **artery,** which lies above the **nerve**; a useful mnemonic — from top to bottom — is VAN for vein, artery, and nerve).
23 Sympathetic ganglionated trunk
24 Right superior and inferior lobar bronchi
25 Azygos vein and azygos arch
26 Superior intercostal vein; note it is larger than the other intercostal veins
27 Trachea
28 Posterior intercostal vein, artery, and intercostal nerve
29 First rib
30 Right subclavian artery
31 Right common carotid artery

Th-49 Right mediastinum

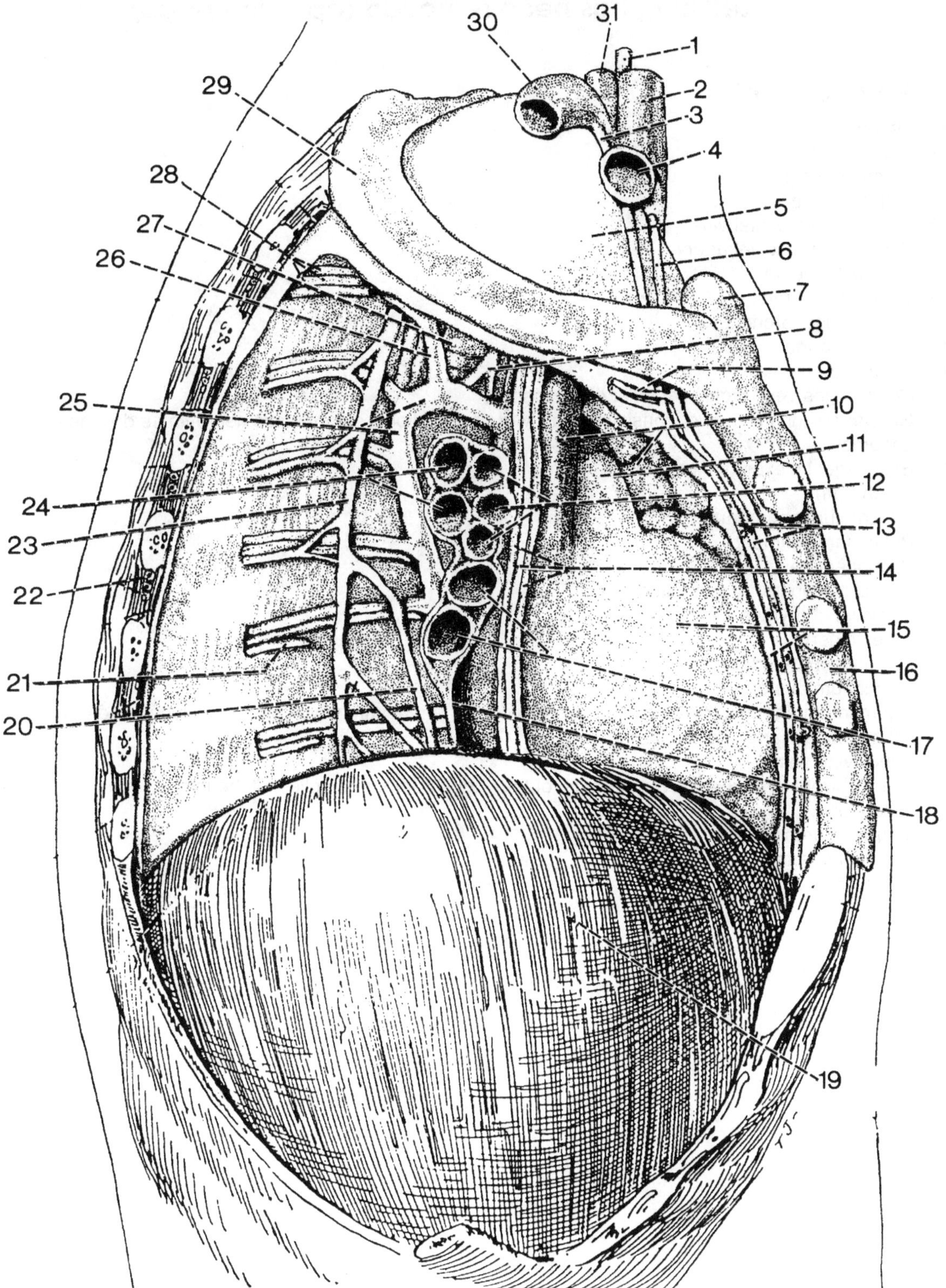

Eycleshymer and Jones with modification

Th-50 Left mediastinum

Left lung has been removed (opposite page)

Color and label

1 First rib
2 Arch of aorta
3 Sympathetic ganglion
4 Left vagus nerve
5 Posterior intercostal vein
6 Posterior intercostal artery
7 Intercostal nerve
8 Sympathetic trunk
9 Left principal bronchus
10 Thoracic aorta
11 Esophagus
12 Hemiazygos vein; highly variable; often absent.
13 Greater splanchnic nerve; consisting mainly of preganglionic sympathetic nerve fibers destined for the abdomen.
14 Esophageal plexus (vagus nerve)
15 Diaphragm
16 Pericardium and heart
17 Pulmonary ligament
18 Pulmonary veins
19 Pericardiacophrenic artery and vein
20 Remains of thymus gland
21 Phrenic nerve
22 Left pulmonary artery
23 Manubrium of sternum
24 Ligamentum arteriosum; remains of the fetal ductus arteriosum which shunted oxygenated blood from the left pulmonary artery to the aorta.
25 Subclavian vein
26 Left recurrent laryngeal nerve; a branch of the vagus nerve; it supplies all the intrinsic muscles of the larynx except one.
27 Internal thoracic artery
28 Subclavian artery
29 Cupula of the pleura

Th-50 Left mediastinum

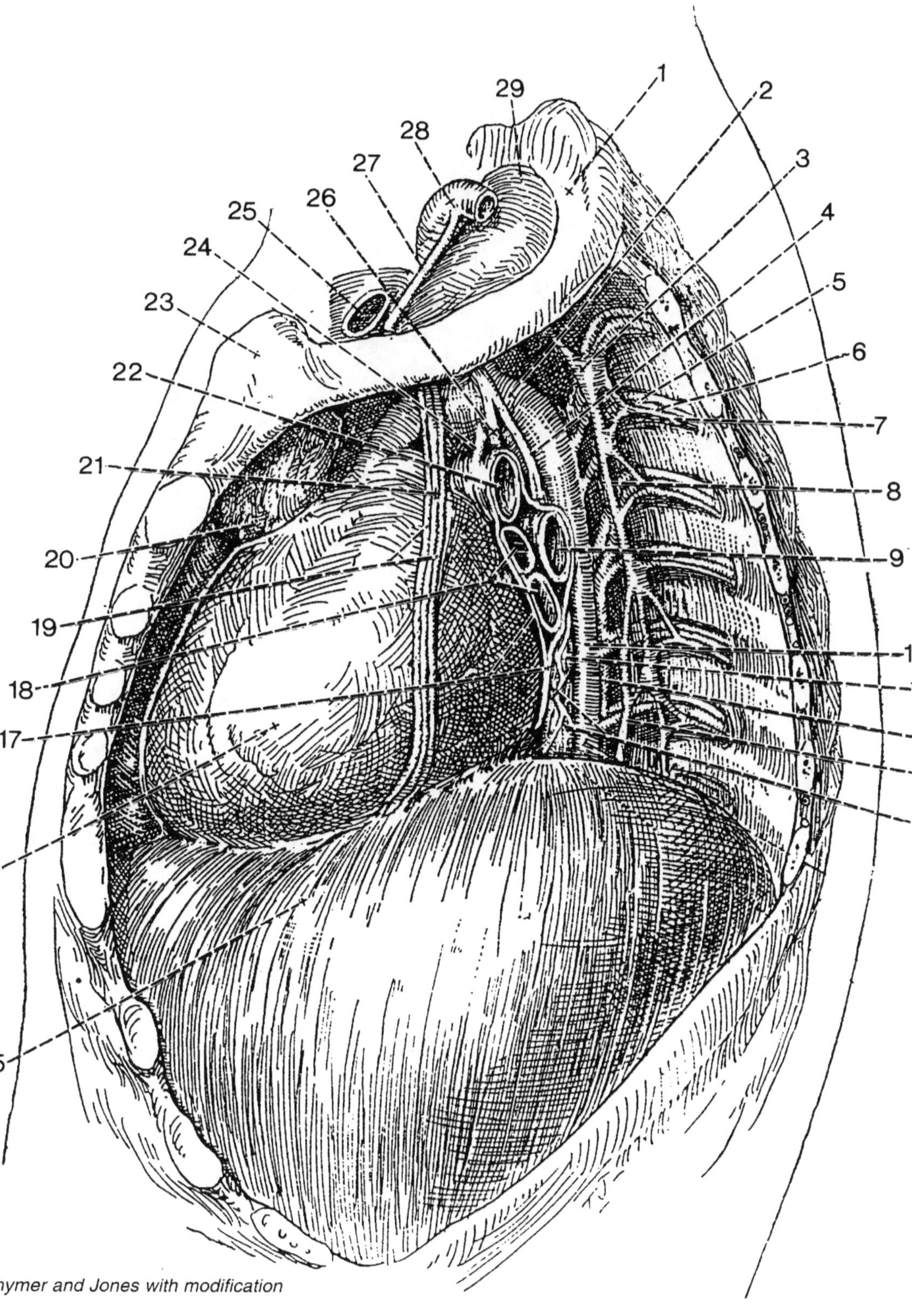

Eycleshymer and Jones with modification

Th-51 Diaphragm

Viewed from below

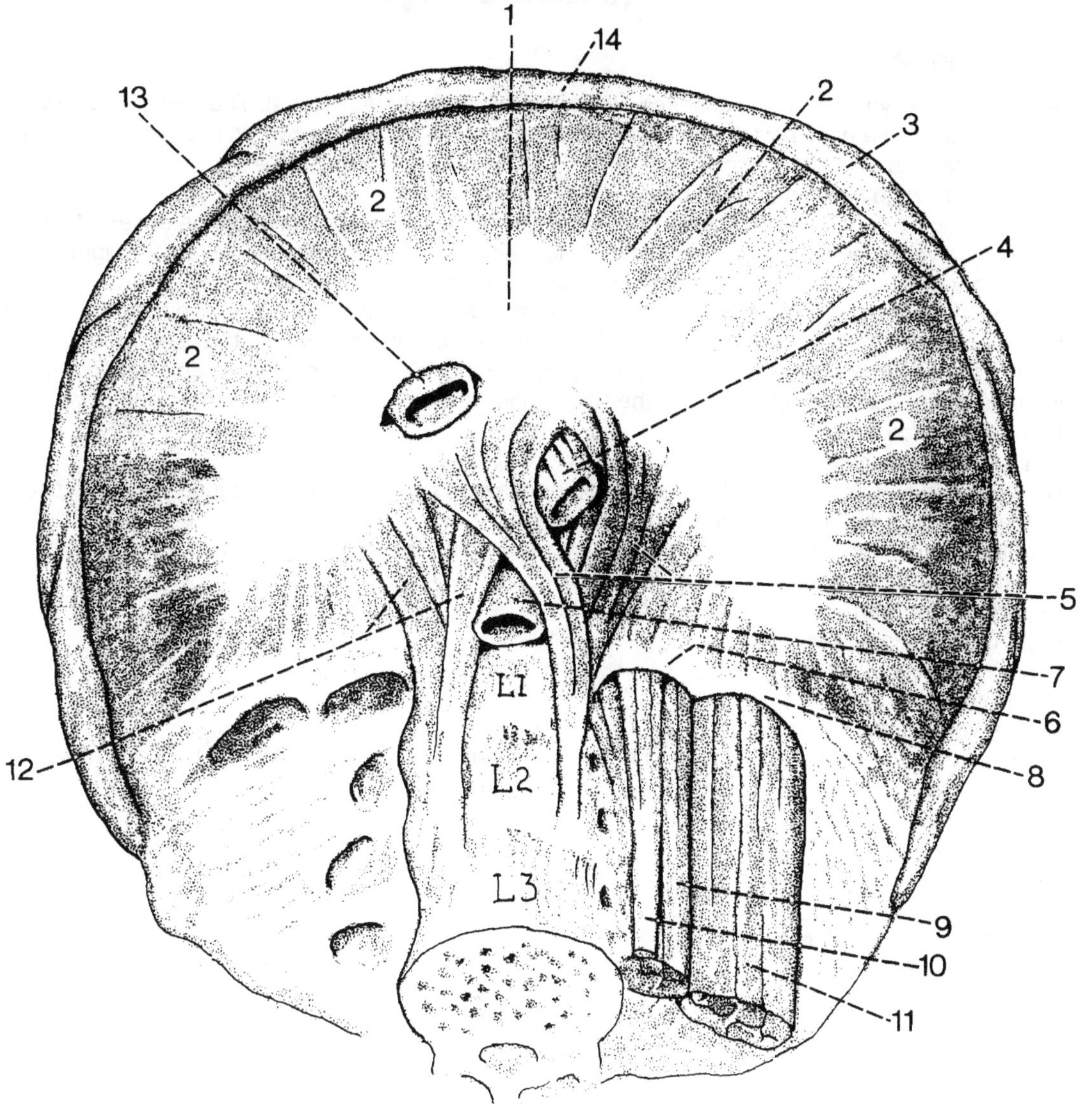

Color and label

1 Central tendon; a strong fibrous sheet into which the peripheral muscular diaphragm inserts. It forms the superior part of the dome-shaped diaphragm. It is pulled down with each inspiration (diaphragmatic contraction) and rises up with each expiration (diaphragmatic relaxation).
2 Muscular part of diaphragm. The diaphragm arises from the sternum (14), the lower border of the rib cage (3), the right (12) and left crura (5), and the medial (7) and lateral (8) arcuate ligaments.
3 Rib cage lower border
4 Esophagus. The right and left vagus nerves pass with the esophagus into the abdomen. A hiatal hernia is the protrusion of part of the stomach through the esophageal hiatus into the thorax.
5 Left crura of diaphragm
6 Medial arcuate ligament
7 Aorta; the thoracic duct and occasionally the azygos vein pass through the aortic opening. The aorta actually enters the abdomen **behind** the diaphragm and **not through** it.
8 Lateral arcuate ligament
9 Psoas major muscle
10 Psoas minor muscle (tendon)
11 Quadratus lumborum muscle
12 Right crura of the diaphragm
13 Inferior vena cava
14 Sternum (xiphoid process)

Th-52 Azygos vein and its tributaries

(opposite page)

Color and label

1 Azygos vein. Azygos means "not paired, without a twin or a mate" (Greek). The name probably arose because the hemiazygos and accessory hemiazygos veins, even when present, do not present a symmetrical mirror-image "twin".
2 Opening of azygos vein into the superior vena cava
3 Hemiazygos vein. The hemiazygos and accessory hemiazygos veins may both be absent. In this situation the azygos vein receives the posterior intercostal veins from the left side as well as the right side.
4 Accessory hemiazygos vein. The azygos system of veins is highly variable.
5 Horizontal connecting vein draining hemiazygos vein on the left into the azygos vein on the right
6 Left superior intercostal vein. The second, third, and sometimes the fourth intercostal veins unite to form the superior intercostal vein, which drains into the left brachiocephalic vein. The right superior intercostal vein joins the azygos vein where it begins its arch towards the superior vena cava.
7 Posterior intercostal vein
8 Left ascending lumbar vein
9 Right ascending lumbar vein. The azygos and hemiazygos veins begin at the junction of the ascending lumbar vein and the subcostal vein (not shown).
10 Left ascending lumbar vein connecting with left renal vein. The lumbar veins drain mainly into the superior vena cava by way of the azygos system.
11 Superior vena cava
12 Right brachiocephalic vein
13 Left brachiocephalic vein
14 Right renal vein
15 Inferior vena cava
16 Portion of inferior vena cava receiving hepatic veins. This portion is surrounded by the liver, which has been removed.
17 Lumbar vein
18 Aorta (cut)
19 Diaphragm
20 Esophagus (cut)
21 Pectoralis major muscle
22 Pectoralis minor muscle
23 Right kidney
24 Left kidney

Th-52 Azygos vein and its tributaries

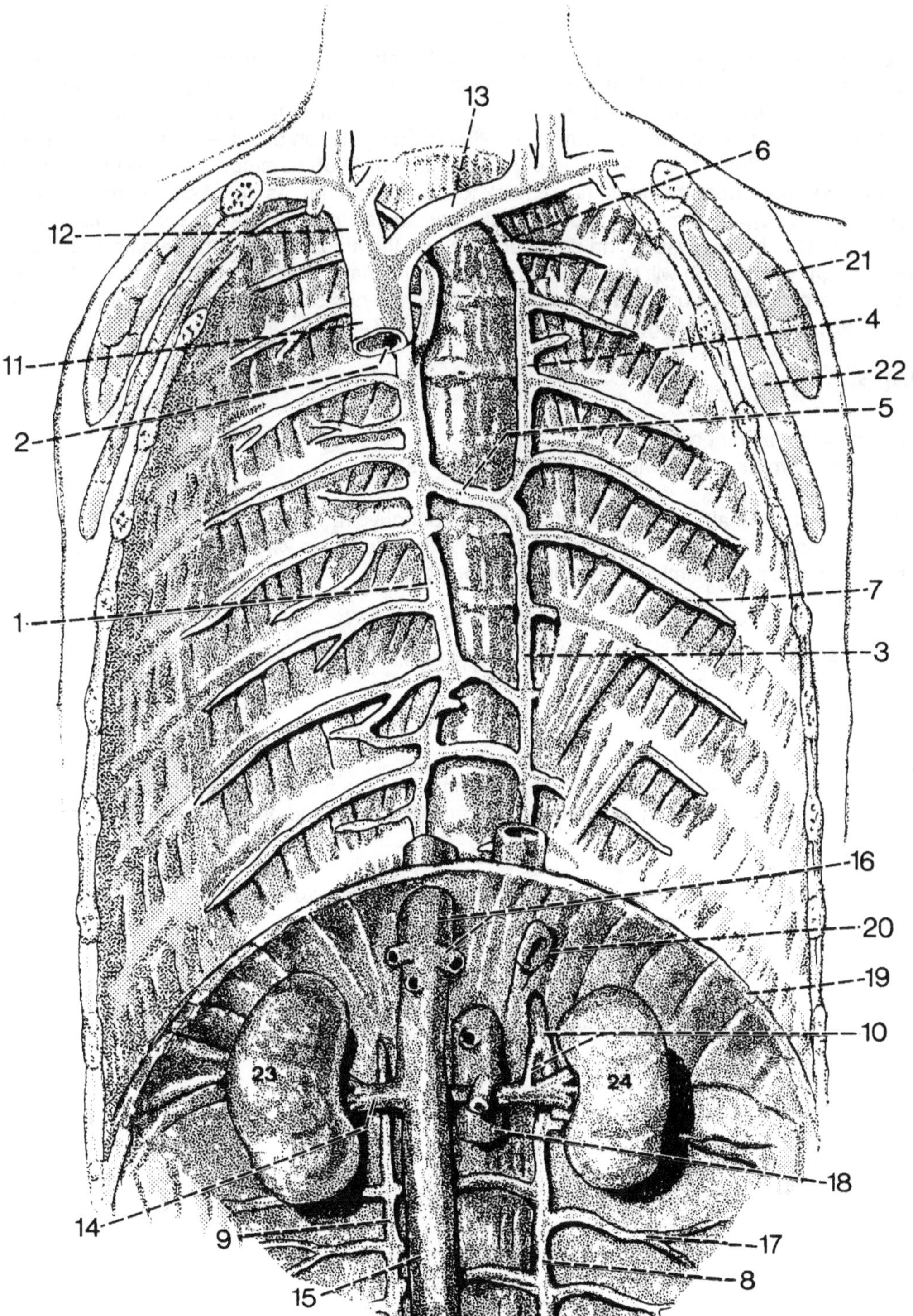

Th-53 Blood flow in the fetus

(opposite page)

Fetal blood gains its oxygen and gives off its carbon dioxide in the placenta (1). Oxygen-rich blood is carried from the placenta to the fetus by the umbilical vein (2). The umbilical vein enters the abdomen and ends in the liver where it attaches to the left branch of the portal vein. A short shunt within the liver, the ductus venosus (5), conveys the blood to the inferior vena cava (6) which empties the oxygen-rich blood — along with some oxygen-poor blood from the fetus's abdomen and legs — into the right atrium (7) of the heart. The superior vena cava also returns oxygen-poor blood from the arms, head, neck to the right atrium. As blood enters the right atrium, a considerable portion of the oxygen-rich blood passes through two holes in the interatrial septum (8) (see figure 54), into the left atrium (10), thus bypassing the right ventricle and the lungs. Most of the remaining oxygen-rich blood ejected by the right ventricle (9) will be shunted from the pulmonary trunk (12) to the aorta (13) by a connection between the pulmonary trunk and the aortic arch (14), the ductus arteriosus (13) (figure B); thus only a small portion of oxygenated blood will go to the lungs.

Color and label

Figure A

1 Placenta (blood oxygenated here)
2 Umbilical vein (within umbilical cord with two umbilical arteries)
3 Umbilicus
4 Umbilical vein (intra-abdominal); attaches to left branch of portal vein.
5 Ductus venosus; venous shunt in liver that connects end of umbilcal vein with inferior vena cava; closes after birth; its origin is encircled by a muscular sphincter.
6 Inferior vena cava
7 Right atrium
8 Foramen ovale (opening in fetal interatrial septum; closes after birth) (see figure 54)
9 Right ventricle)
10 Left atrium
11 Left ventricle
12 Pulmonary trunk
13 Ductus arteriosus; shunts oxygen-rich blood from pulmonary trunk to arch of aorta; the great vessels arising from the aortic arch will convey oxygenated blood to the head and neck; closes after birth.
14 Aorta
15 Internal iliac artery
16 Umbilical arteries. These close off and become ligamentous after birth except for the proximal portions that become parts of the superior vesical arteries.
17 Liver
18 Portal vein

Figure B Fetal heart showing the ductus arteriosus diverting oxygen-rich blood from the pulmonary trunk to the aortic arch

Th-53 Blood flow in the fetus

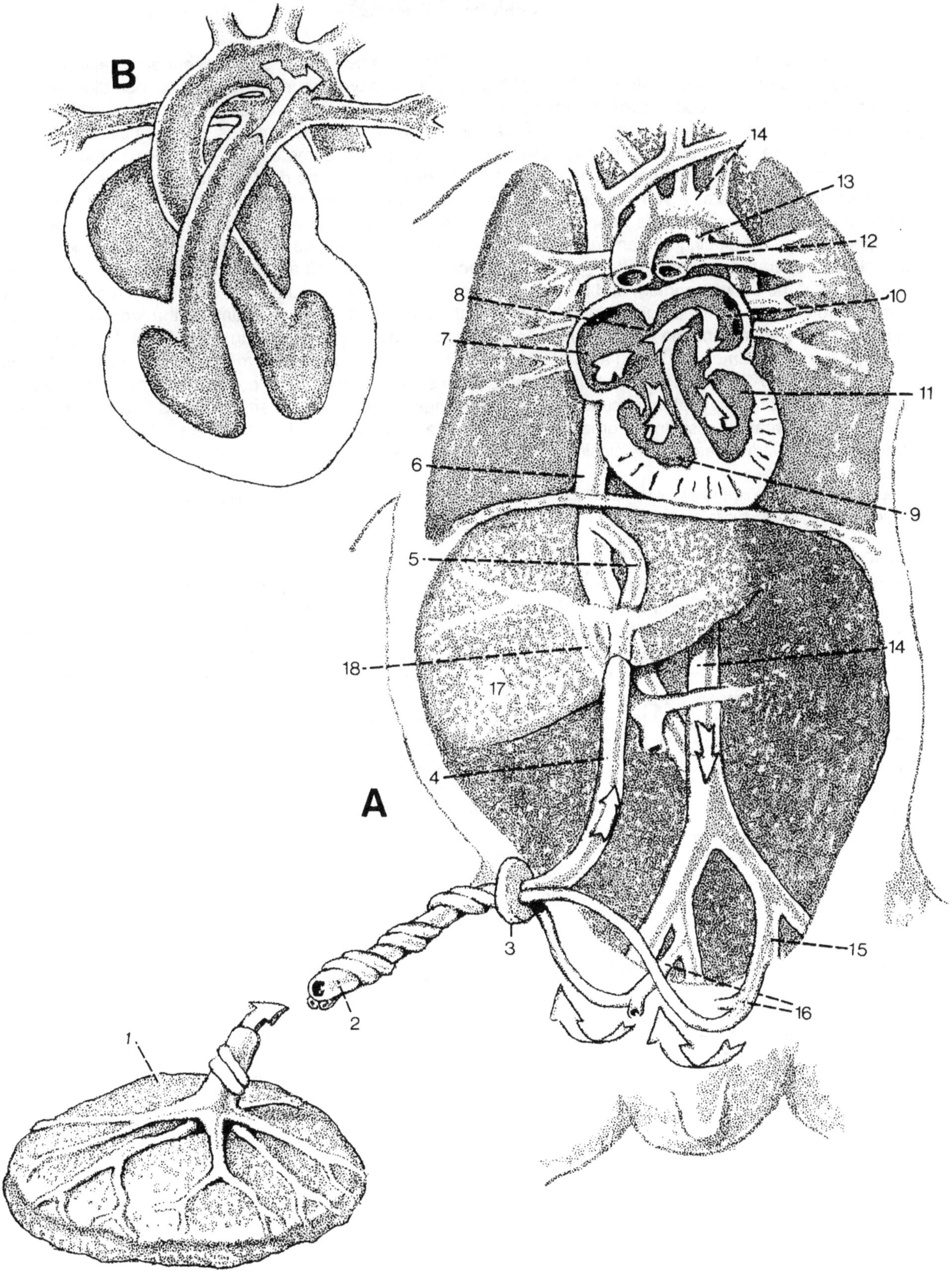

Th-54 Fetal heart in late development

(opposite page)

During intrauterine development the lungs are nonfunctional, contain no air, and consequently relatively little blood is pumped to the lungs before birth. Fetal blood gains its oxygen and gives off its carbon dioxide in the placenta. Oxygen-rich blood is carried from the placenta to the fetus by the umbilical vein. The umbilical vein enters the abdomen and ends in the liver where a short shunt, the ductus venosus, conveys the blood to the inferior vena cava, which empties the oxygen-rich blood—along with some oxygen-poor blood from the fetus's abdomen and legs—into the right atrium of the heart. As blood enters the right atrium, the limbus (L. edge) of the foramen ovale acts as a vane which deflects a considerable portion of the oxygen-rich blood through two holes, the foramen ovale and the foramen secundum, to the left atrium, thus bypassing the right ventricle and the lungs. In the developing human heart the right and left atria remain confluent with each other and are not completely separated until after birth. The wall between the right and left atria, the interatrial septum, is formed by two septa, the septum primum and the septum secundum. The two septa each develop with an opening that allows blood to flow from the right atrium directly into the left atrium. The two foramina, the foramen secundum* in the septum primum and the foramen ovale in the septum secundum, are not in line so that the septum primum covers the foramen ovale and acts as a one-way valve that allows blood to flow only from the right atrium to the left atrium. After birth the definitive adult interatrial septum is formed by coalescence of the two septa, the septum primum and the septum secundum. Once the lungs are inflated with air, the blood flow to the lungs is dramatically increased, resulting in greater pressure in the left atrium which forces the septum primum against the septum secundum, essentially closing off the foramen ovale.

*The septum primum initially forms with a ventral transitory foramen, the foramen primum, which disappears when a second dorsal foramen, the foramen secundum, subsequently develops in the septum primum.

Color and label

Figure A. The internal configuration of fetal heart in late pregnancy (opposite page)

1 Oxygenated blood entering the right atrium from the inferior vena cava
2 Oxygenated blood passing through two openings (foramina) and entering the left artium. This blood will enter the left ventricle where it will be ejected out of the heart through the aorta.
3 Oxygenated blood remaining in the right atrium. This blood will enter the right ventricle and be ejected through the pulmonary trunk
4 Limbus (L. edge, border) of the foramen ovale acting as a deflecting vane
5 Septum secundum
6 Foramen secundum
7 Septum primum
8 Superior vena cava
9 Orifices of right pulmonary veins
10 Left pulmonary veins
11 Mitral valve
12 Chordae tendineae
13 Papillary muscle
14 Trabeculae carneae in left ventricle
15 Interventricular septum (muscular part)
16 Right ventricle
17 Tricuspid valve
18 Valve of inferior vena cava
19 Crista terminalis
20 Orifice of coronary sinus

Redrawn from Patten, Foundations of Embryology, New York, McGraw-Hill, 1958, p. 524.

Figure B. After birth interatrial septum separates the two atria

1 Septum primum joining with septum secundum and sealing off the foramen ovale
2 Septum secundum
3 Fossa ovalis (L. *fossa*, a depression). The closed foramen ovale becomes the fossa ovalis. Its floor is formed by the septum primum.
4 Oxygen-depleted blood entering inferior vena cava. Oxygen-rich blood is then returned from the lungs to the left atrium.
5 Superior vena cava

Th-54 Fetal heart in late development

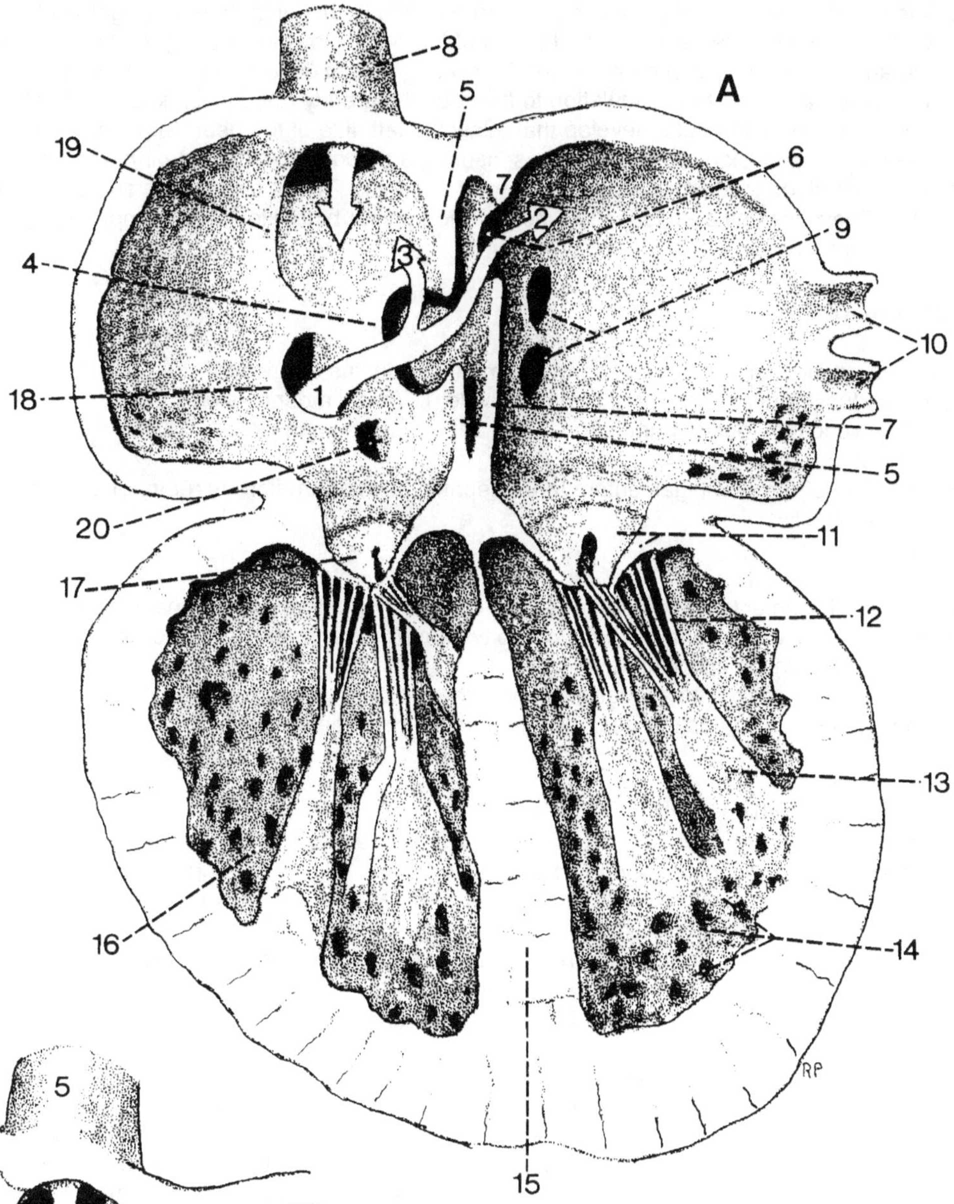

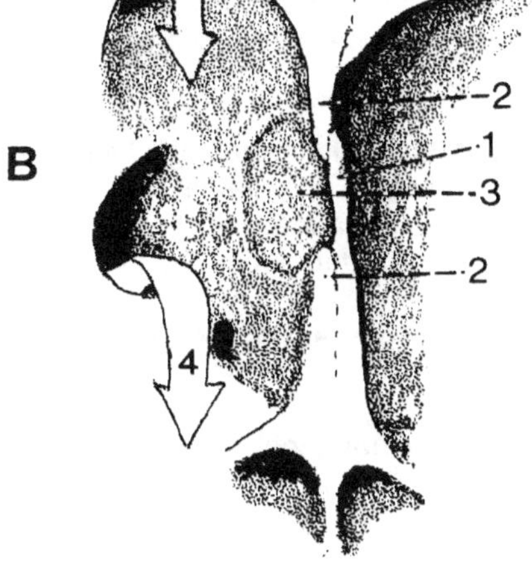

Th-55 Circulatory changes after birth

(opposite page)

From the time of birth until death the volume of blood pumped to the lungs from the right ventricle equals the volume of blood pumped by the left ventricle to the rest of the body. However, during fetal development the lungs contain no air and require only enough blood for their own physical development; consequently the pulmonary circulation is considerably less than circulation to the rest of the body (the systemic circulation). To rectify this imbalance two shunts or "short cuts" develop that allow the left side of the heart to pump a volume of blood equal to that pumped by the right side of the heart, thus insuring a smooth transition at birth from maternal/placental oxygenation of fetal blood to that of oxygenation by air-breathing. These circulatory "short cuts" persist throughout intrauterine life. They close off and cease to function shortly after birth. However, complete anatomical closure may take weeks or months.

Color and label

Figure A

1 Ligamentum arteriosum (postpartum fibrous remnant of ductus arteriosus)
2 Fossa ovalis (postpartum remnant of foramen ovale; L. *fossa*, a depression)
3 Ligamentum venosum (postpartum fibrous remnant of ductus venosus)
4 Left branch of portal vein
5 Round ligament of the liver (ligamentum teres hepatis; postpartum fibrous remnant of intra-abdominal portion of the umbilical vein)
6 Umbilicus
7 Aorta
8 Medial umbilical ligaments in extraperitoneal fat on inside of anterior abdominal wall (postpartum remnants of the intra-abdominal portions of the two umbilical arteries). These close shut just past the origin of their last branch up to the umbilicus.
9 Superior vesical (L. *vesica*, the bladder) arteries; the proximal portions of the umbilical arteries remain patent (open) and function as the beginning lengths of the superior vesical arteries.
10 Bladder
11 Portal vein
12 Inferior vena cava (behind liver)
13 Aortic arch
14 Left pulmonary artery (ductus arteriosus connects the aortic arch to the origin of the left pulmonary artery)

Figure B

Blood flow in the aorta and pulmonary arteries after closure of the ductus arteriosus

1 Ligamentum arteriosum
2 Pulmonary trunk
3 Aortic arch
4 Left pulmonary artery

The foramen ovale becomes the fossa ovalis.
This foramen, along with the foramen secundum (figure 53), conveys blood from the right atrium to the left atrium. A series of three trans-septal foramina develop in the fetus. The first foramen (foramen primum) disappears when the second (foramen secundum) appears. The second and third foramina (foramen secundum and foramen ovale) work together and persist until birth when the increased blood flow from the fully functional lungs and pulmonary veins increases the pressure in the left atrium, forcing shut the valve-like flap and functionally closing off the two foramina in the interatrial septum. Failure to anatomically fuse is not uncommon and is not critical as long the flap covers the foramen ovale.

The ductus arteriosus becomes the ligamentum arteriosum.
This shunt conveys blood from the pulmonary trunk to the aortic arch. With the first breath the lungs expand. Resistance to arterial blood in the pulmonary arteries falls significantly, resulting in a dramatic increase in circulation to the lungs, and blood is no longer forced from the pulmonary trunk to the aorta. Functional closure of the ductus arteriosus occurs a few hours or days after birth, although complete obliteration of the lumen takes 6 to 8 weeks.

The intra-abdominal portion of the umbilical vein becomes the round ligament of the liver. Although no longer functional, the lumen of the round ligament usually persists into adulthood.

The ductus venosus becomes the ligamentum venosum.

The intra-abdominal portion of the umbilical arteries becomes the medial umbilical ligaments or plicae (folds).

Th-55 Circulatory changes after birth

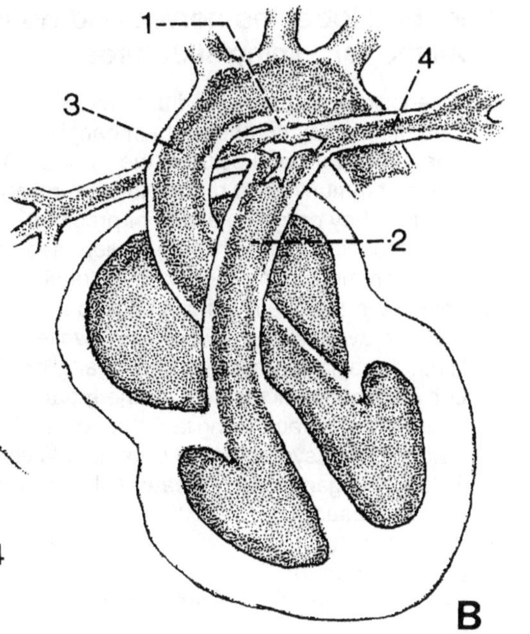

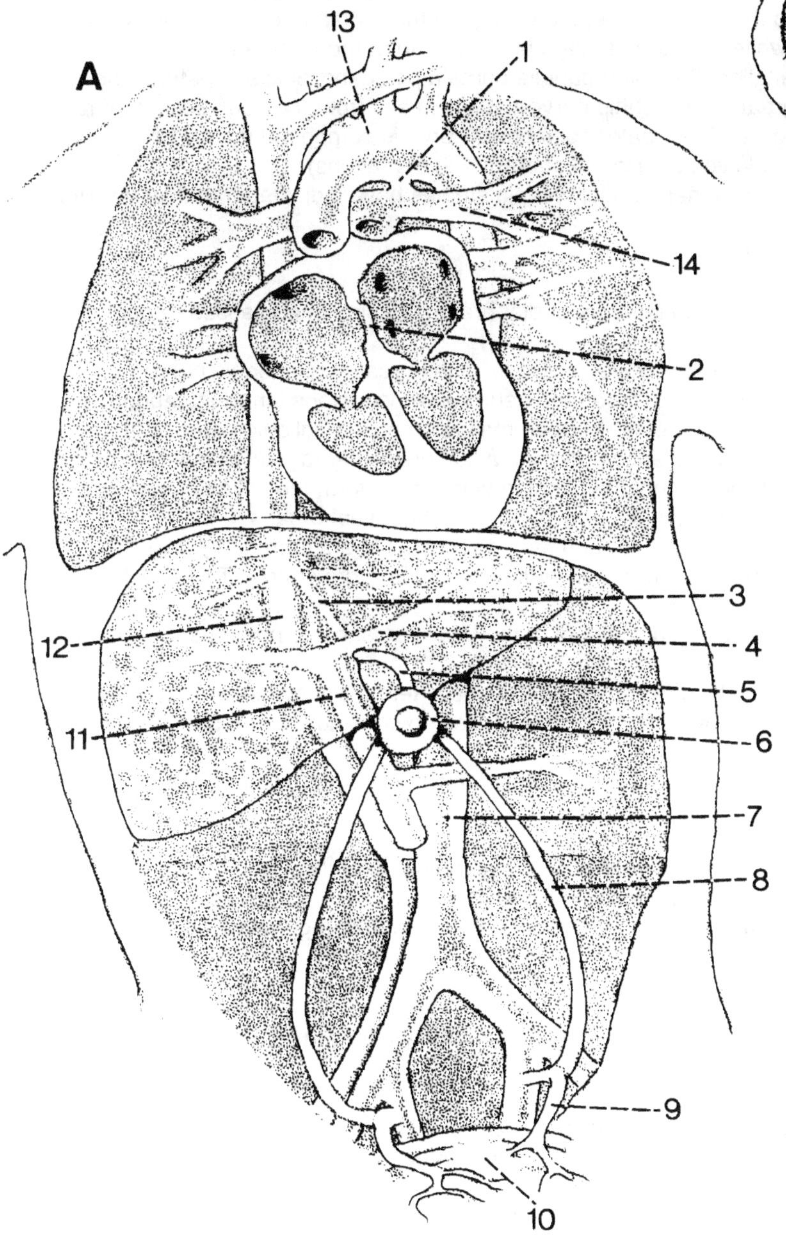

Th-56 Thoracic splanchnic nerves

(opposite page)

Color and label the nerves and ganglia
Label the remaining structures

1 Anterior ramus (also called anterior primary division) of thoracic nerve 5 (= 5th intercostal nerve)
2 Fifth thoracic sympathetic chain ganglion; there are usually 11 thoracic sympathetic chain ganglia on each side of the vertebral column; the sympathetic chain lies beneath the parietal pleura.
3 White communicating ramus; these rami connect the spinal nerves to the adjacent sympathetic chain ganglia; they carry the axons of preganglionic sympathetic neurons from the spinal nerve to the corresponding sympathetic ganglion (see figure 56).
4 Gray communicating ramus; these rami convey the unmyelinated axons of the postganglionic sympathetic neurons in the chain ganglia back to the spinal nerve; there may be more than one gray ramus or a gray ramus may fuse with a white rami; white rami tend to lie more lateral than the gray rami.
5 Ninth thoracic sympathetic chain ganglion; the chain ganglia contain postganglionic sympathetic neurons.
6 Left greater splanchnic nerve; the greater splanchnic nerve usually arises from the coalescence of rami (or roots) from thoracic ganglia 5 through 9. The greater splanchnic nerve is comprised mainly of preganglionic sympathetic fibers* in addition to visceral afferent** fibers (axons).
7 Splanchnic ganglion on greater splanchnic nerve; microscopic studies have indicated that this ganglion is always present.
8 Aorta (cut)
9 Diaphragm (cut)
10 Left greater splanchnic nerve passing through left crus of diaphragm; it sometimes passes through the diaphragm with the aorta.
11 Adrenal (suprarenal) gland (left and right). It receives fibers from the greater splanchnic nerve.
12 Left celiac ganglion; it contains postganglionic sympathetc neurons whose axons innervate abdominal viscera. The axons in the greater splanchnic nerve synapse mainly on postganglionic neurons in the celiac ganglion; however, some greater splanchnic axons also supply the adrenal gland, and other axons continue through the celiac ganglion without synapsing where they form the celiac plexus and synapse in other ganglia. Axons from these ganglia end in various abdominal organs.
13 Lowest splanchnic nerve (not always present) (right and left); it receives fibers from ganglion T12.
14 Lesser splanchnic nerve (right and left); it usually receives fibers (axons) from ganglia T10 and T11, which mainly end in the aorticorenal ganglion.
15 Aorticorenal ganglion (right and left); preganglionic fibers in the lesser splanchnic nerve usually end here upon postganglionic neurons.
16 Renal plexus; axons in the lowest splanchnic (when present) usually terminally synapse on this plexus. Activation of sympathetic fibers to the kidneys causes renal vessels to constrict, thus restricting blood to the kidney and subsequent water loss.
17 Right celiac ganglion; most preganglionic fibers in greater splanchic nerve synapse upon postganglionic sympathetic neurons in this ganglion.
18 Greater splanchnic nerve (right)
19 Ramus (or root) of greater splanchnic nerve from 8th thoracic ganglion; in addition to efferent fibers, these rami contain visceral afferent** fibers traveling back to the spinal cord.
20 Sympathetic trunk; the trunk on each side contains ascending and descending preganglionic axons.

***Fiber** and **axon** are used synonymously here.

****Afferent** and **efferent** applied to nerves mean, respectively, "running toward" and "running away from" the CNS, that is, the brain and spinal cord.

Sympathetic activation causes: conversion of glycogen to glucose in the liver
inhibition of gastric secretion in the stomach
inhibition of intestinal peristalsis
contraction of the spleen, thus expelling more blood into the general circulation
contraction of urinary sphincters, thus retaining body water

Th-56 Thoracic splanchnic nerves

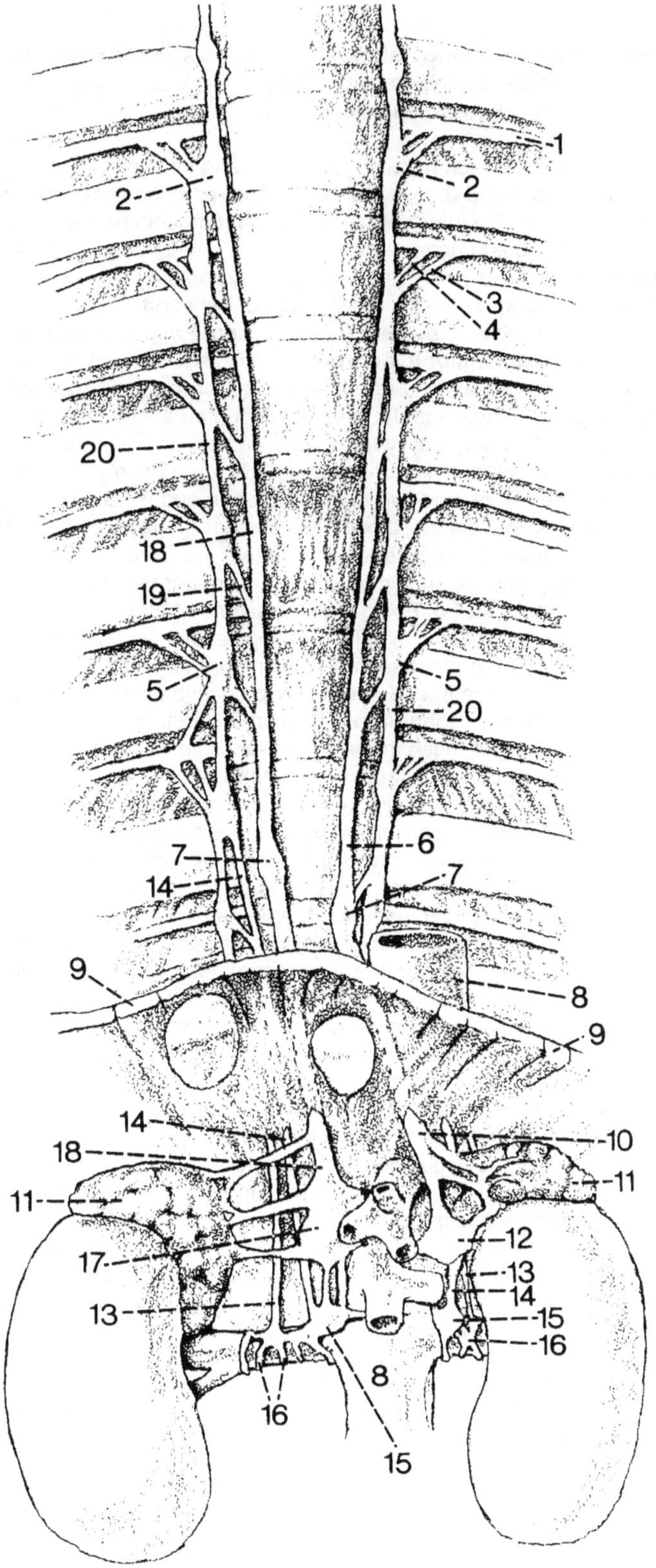

Th-57 Autonomic nervous system

(opposite page)

Use a different color for each of the following autonomic neurons and their axons:

Preganglionic sympathetic	Preganglionic parasympathetic	Visceral afferent
Postganglionic sympathetic	Postganglionic parasympathetic	

For simplification each category is represented by a single neuron and its axon.
Preganglionic sympathetic neurons 1 and 3 have cell bodies (somata) in the lateral gray column of the thoracic spinal cord where they form two groups, the intermediolateral and intermediomedial. These preganglionic sympathetic neurons are present only in the thoracic and upper lumbar region of the spinal cord (T1-L2). Starting with **preganglionic sympathetic neuron 1**, color its cell body (soma) and its axon as it exits the spinal cord via the anterior root. Trace its axon as it then leaves the thoracic spinal nerve by way of the short white communicating ramus—these axons are lightly myelinated, hence its white appearance—and synapses upon **postganglionic sympathetic neuron 2** in a sympathetic chain ganglion. **Postganglionic neuron 2** sends its axon back to the thoracic spinal nerve via a gray communicating ramus. Postganglionic axons are unmyelinated, hence their gray appearance. The distinction between white (myelinated) and gray (unmyelinated) nerve fibers can be ascertained only by microscopic inspection. However, white communicating branches are usually further lateral than are the gray rami, which may number more than one. Axons of postganglionic sympathetic neurons such as neuron 2 axon will travel within thoracic spinal nerve to the body wall or within nerves to the limbs and eventually end upon and modulate—depending upon the physiologic state and the ambient temperature—sweat glands, blood vessels near the skin, and hair follicles. Return to **preganglionic sympathetic neuron 3**. Color and trace its axon as it enters the sympathetic ganglion, but instead of synapsing in this ganglion, it ascends within the sympathetic trunk to the superior cervical gangion where it synapses upon **postganglionic sympathetic neurons 4 and 5**. Postganglionic axons of neurons 4 descend to innervate the heart (increase the rate and strength of contraction and dilate coronary vessels) via the cardiac plexus. Postganglionic fibers of **neurons 5** form the **carotid plexus (6)** around the internal carotid artery and ascend into the head where they will affect the size of the pupil in the eye (enlarge it) and inhibit tear production in the lacrimal glands and saliva in the salivary glands. Color and trace the course of **preganglionic neuron 7** into its ganglion where it synapses upon **postganglionic neurons 8, 9, and 10**. The axons of these three neurons re-enter the corresponding spinal nerve and travel in it to its area of distribution. **Sudomotor neuron 8** causes myoepithelial cells on sweat glands to contract, thus expeling sweat. **Pilomotor neuron 9** activates arrector pili muscle of hair on skin. **Neuron 10** modulates cutaneous blood flow. Note that **Neuron 11** passes through its ganglion without synapsing and becomes a **thoracic splanchnic nerve**. These preganglionic fibers pass behind the diaphragm and enter the abdomen where they synapse upon irregular aggregates of sympathetic ganglia (prevertebral ganglia) such as the celiac ganglion (also called solar ganglion). **Postganglionic neurons 12 and 13** in these sympathetic ganglia have a wide distribution to the abdominal viscera where they have a mainly inhibitory effect (constrict abdominal blood vessels, inhibit peristalsis, etc.). The cell body of **visceral afferent neuron 14** is a typical unipolar first-order sensory neuron (with a single process that divides like a T) found in the dorsal root ganglion. It relays diffuse visceral pain (tummy ache) and functions in gastrointestinal reflexes. **Neuron 15** in the opposite lateral gray column gives rise to another preganglionic splanchnic fiber; however, this one ends, not in a ganglion, but in the medulla of the adrenal (suprarenal) gland where it synapses upon **chromaffin cell 16,** which synthesizes epinephrine (adrenalin) and norepinephrine (noradrenalin), which are distributed by blood vessels throughout the body. Thus, should circumstances demand it, these two blood-borne catecholamines can greatly augment the effect of the sympathetic system. **Neuron 17** represents a **preganglionic parasympathetic neuron cell body** in one of the brain stem nuclei* of the vagus nerve. Axons from somata such as 17 travel within the vagus nerve and supply a very wide range of viscera in both the thorax and abdomen. The preganglionic parasympathetic fibers in the vagus nerve are much longer that the postganglionic fibers whose postganglionic cell bodies lie either in plexuses very close to the target organ or within the walls of the organ itself as does **postganglionic parasympathetic neuron 18**. Aggregates of these postganglionic neurons in the walls of target organs are termed intramural (L. within the walls) ganglia . The parasympathetic system tends to conserve and build up free energy. It promotes digestion, assimilation, secretion of glands, peristalsis, and the conversion of glucose to glycogen. Some researchers feel that in addition to the sympathetic and parasympathetic nervous systems, the extensive intrinsic neuronal network in the gastrointestinal tract constitutes a third division of the visceral nervous system, the enteric nervous system. Supportive evidence for a third autonomous division includes experiments demonstrating that transplanted intestine can function after being totally separated from all sympathetic and parasympathetic nervous control.

*A neuroanatomical nucleus is an aggregate of neurons in the CNS.

Th-57 Autonomic nervous system

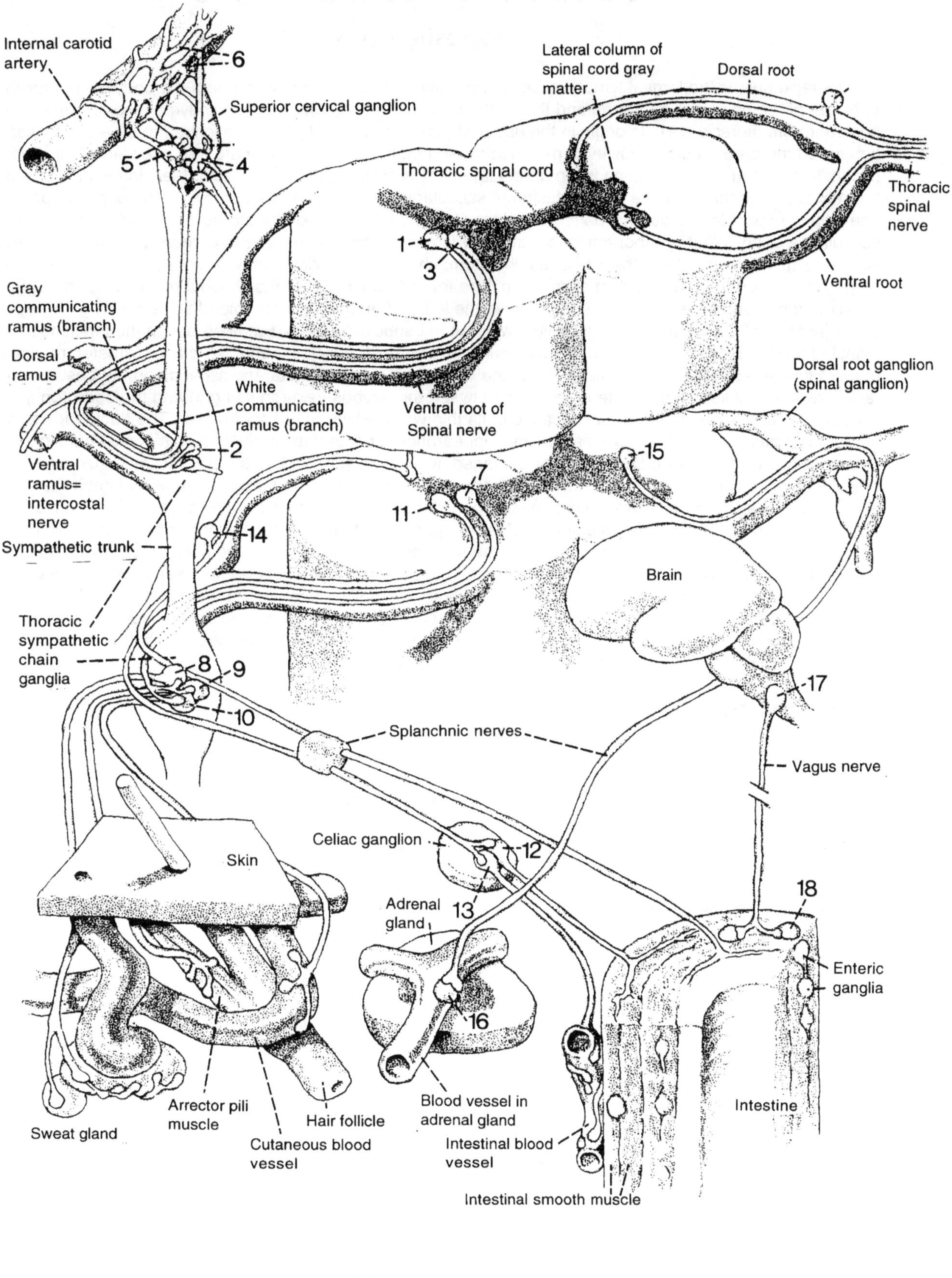

Th-58 Thoracic duct and related structures

(opposite page)

The thoracic duct is the largest lymph vessel in the body. It drains all the lymph from the body except for the right half of the head, the right arm, and the right half of the thorax, which drain into lymphatic duct(s) on the posterior right thoracic wall. Its origin in the upper abdomen has usually been described to be a thin-walled dilation called the cisterna chyli. However, more recent and thorough studies indicate that a "cisternal" dilation occurs in only 1 in 5 bodies. Even when an enlargement is present it tends to assume a wide variety of shapes. It rarely assumes the form of a simple, fusiform, saccular dilation such as that drawn on the opposite page. Thus one should expect to find various patterns and forms at the beginning of the thoracic duct rather than a single saccular swelling. What is important is that at its abdominal origin the thoracic duct receives lymphatic trunks carrying lymph from the legs, the intestines, the stomach, and the abdominal wall. These lymphatic trunks converge and end on the thoracic duct at its origin. The thoracic duct carries the lymph it receives up through the thorax to the base of the neck where it arches to the left and empties into the blood stream through an opening at the junction of the left internal jugular vein with the left subclavian vein. Fat absorbed in the intestines from digested food reaches the venous blood by this route. The duct, which is about 0.5 cm in diameter, reaches the thorax by passing through the aortic hiatus of the diaphragm with the aorta and ascends on the posterior thoracic wall where it lies on the vertebral column between the azygos vein (on its right) and the aorta (on its left). It is easy to overlook the thoracic duct because of its thin walls, which may appear clear. The duct tends to have numerous small dilations that give it a varicose appearance, and as it ascends it takes a somewhat zig-zag course. Should the thoracic duct be cut or damaged, lymph will spill out into the pleural cavity (usually the left). This condition is called chylothorax. Chyle (Gk. *chylos*, juice) is the name for the white milky lymph that appears after a fatty meal. This white lymph contains tiny particles of digested fat called chylomicrons, which were absorbed in the intestines. The greater part of the lymphatic system, with the exception of the thoracic duct and some of the larger lymph nodes, is too small to be seen by gross dissection. One should appreciate that lymphatic vessels accompany blood vessels throughout the body. The lymphatic system serves a vital function in producing lymphocytes and antibodies that fight disease. In addition it returns to the general circulation the protein-laden extracellular fluid that has extravasated from capillaries. As mentioned above, it also transports digested fat from the intestines to the venous blood flow. The term *lymphatics* usually refers to both the lymphatic vessels as well as the lymph nodes situated along their course.

Color and label

1. Cisterna chyli (present only in 20% of cases)
2. Abdominal lymph nodes in afferent lymphatic trunks
3. Outline of aortic hiatus (aorta removed)
4. Thoracic duct
5. Posterior intercostal arteries (cut at origins from aorta, which has been removed)
6. Left subclavian vein
7. Left internal jugular vein
8. Left brachiocephalic vein
9. Superior vena cava
10. Sympathetic trunk
11. Azygos vein

Th-58 Thoracic duct and related structures

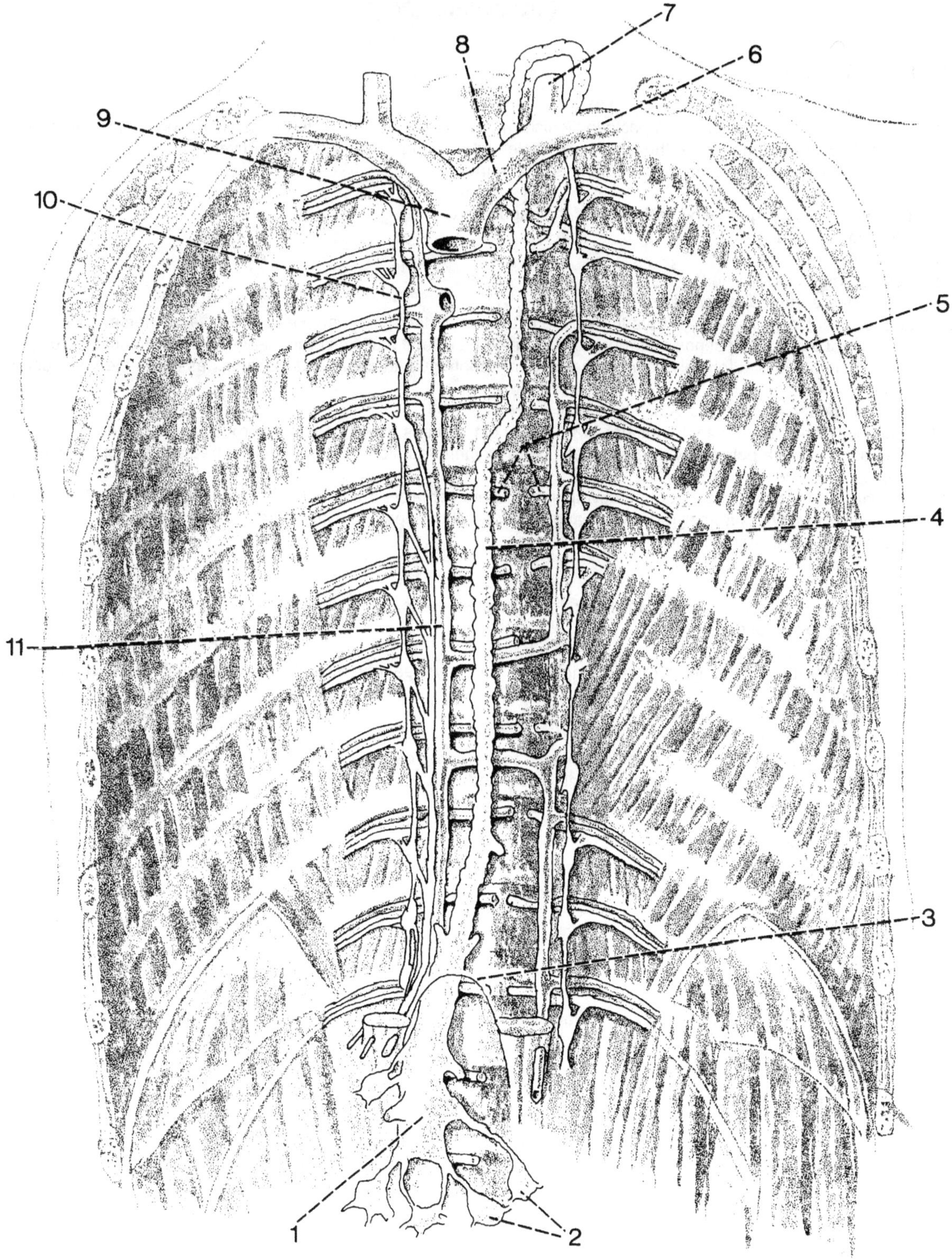

Th-59 Mediastinum after removal of heart and pericardium

The great vessels have been severed.
(opposite page)

Color and label

1 Left internal jugular vein
2 Left middle cervical ganglion (its postganglionic sympathetic axons innervate the cervical region, upper arm, and heart)
3 Thoracic duct (it terminates in the junction of the left internal jugular and subclavian vein)
4 Internal thoracic artery (formerly: internal mammary artery)
5 Thoracic duct
6 Left recurrent laryngeal nerve (a branch of the vagus nerve)
7 Left subclavian artery
8 Vagus nerve
9 Left common carotid artery
10 Arch of the aorta (cut at top of arch)
11 Left recurrent laryngeal nerve (note that as the left recurrent laryngeal nerve leaves the vagus nerve, it winds around the arch of the aorta; it sends motor branches to all the skeletal muscles of the larynx except the cricothyroid; it also sends sensory and autonomic fibers to the cervical esophagus, trachea, and the larynx as far as the vocal cords)
12 Left bronchus
13 Left pulmonary artery
14 Bronchial artery (these vary in number, size, and origin; there is usually one right bronchial artery and two left bronchial arteries; unlike the pulmonary arteries, these carry oxygenated blood to the bronchial tree and the bronchial lymph nodes)
15 Esophageal plexus (a network of parasympathetic fibers partially embedded in the exterior of the esophagus joined by sympathetic fibers from sympathetic ganglia by way of the posterior pulmonary plexus)
16 Descending aorta (thoracic part)
17 Esophagus
18 Thoracic duct
19 Azygos vein (note it receives venous blood from the posterior intercostal veins)
20 Right common carotid artery
21 Right internal jugular vein
22 Right recurrent laryngeal nerve (note the right recurrent laryngeal nerve winds around the right subclavian artery)
23 Right vagus nerve
24 Right subclavian artery
25 Right subclavian vein
26 Right brachial plexus (motor and sensory nerves to the upper extremity)
27 Right phrenic nerve with pericardiacophrenic artery and vein
28 Azygos vein (cut at its junction with the superior vena cava)
29 Right bronchus (note its division into superior, middle, and inferior lobar bronchi)
30 Branches of right pulmonary artery
31 Superior lobar bronchus
32 Right vagus nerve
33 Right middle lobar bronchus
34 Right superior pulmonary vein
35 Right inferior lobar bronchus
36 Right inferior pulmonary vein
37 Greater splanchnic nerve
38 Phrenic nerve with pericardiacophrenic artery and vein (note their "sandwiched" position between the pericardium and mediastinal pleura)
39 Base of pericardium (adherent to central tendon of diaphragm)
40 Inferior vena cava
41 Apex of right lung
42 Left lung

Th-59 Mediastinum after removal of heart and pericardium

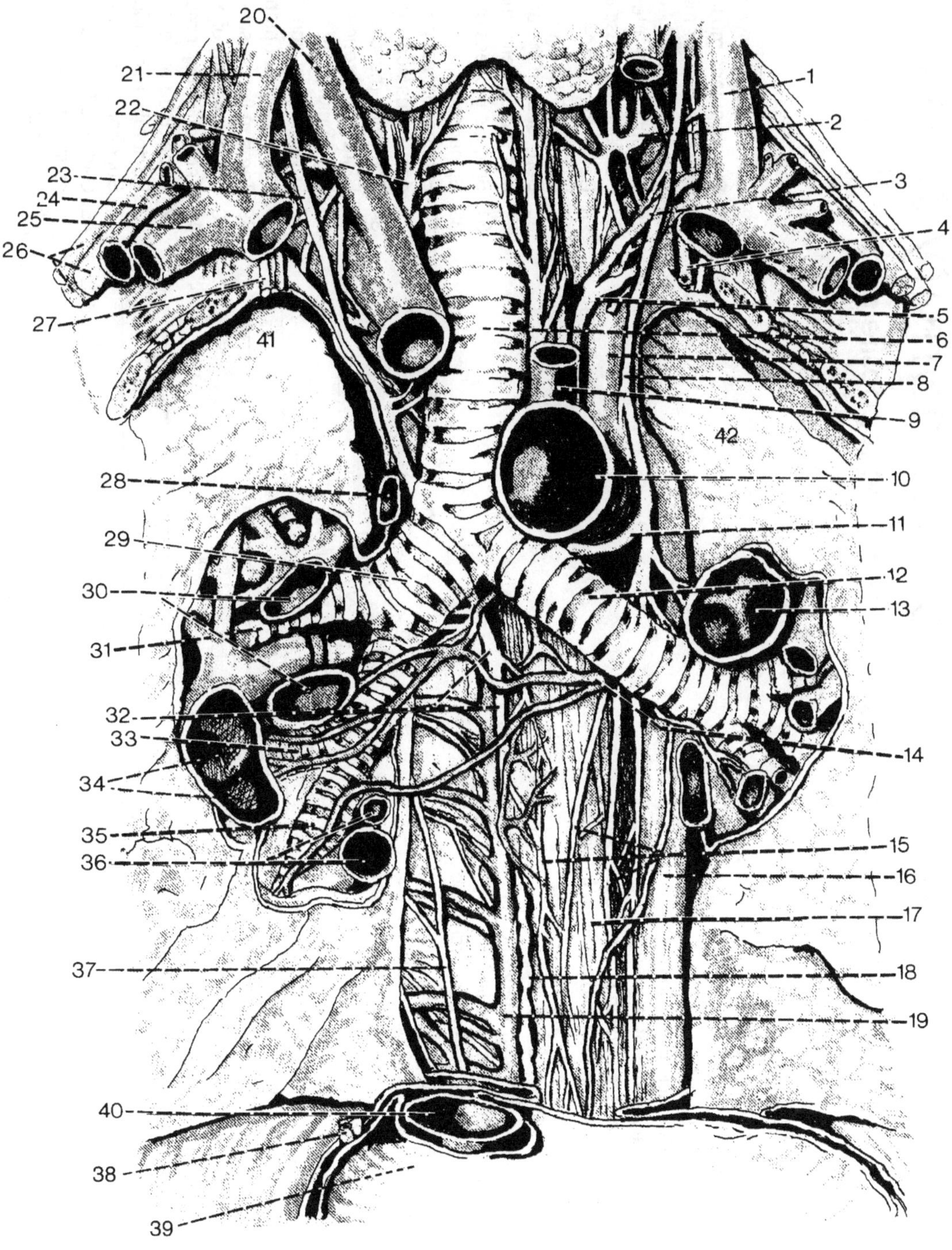

Redrawn from Tondury

Th-60 Cross section of thorax level of bifurcation of pulmonary trunk

(Looking up from below) (opposite page)

Color and label

1 Remnant of thymus gland and prepericardial fat
2 Sternum (body)
3 Ascending aorta
4 Internal thoracic vein and artery
5 Pulmonary trunk; bifurcation into right and left pulmonary arteries
6 Left main bronchus (note cartilage in walls)
7 Upper lobe of left lung
8 Left phrenic nerve with pericardiacophrenic artery and vein (these three structures lie sandwiched between pericardial sac and mediastinal pleura)
9 Short head of biceps brachii muscle
10 Long head of biceps brachii and tendon
11 Coracobrachialis muscle
12 Humerus of left arm
13 Deltoid muscle
14 Tendon of latissimus dorsi muscle
15 Lateral head of triceps brachii muscle
16 Long head of triceps brachii
17 Radial nerve
18 Brachial artery
19 Basilic vein
20 Ulnar nerve
21 Median nerve

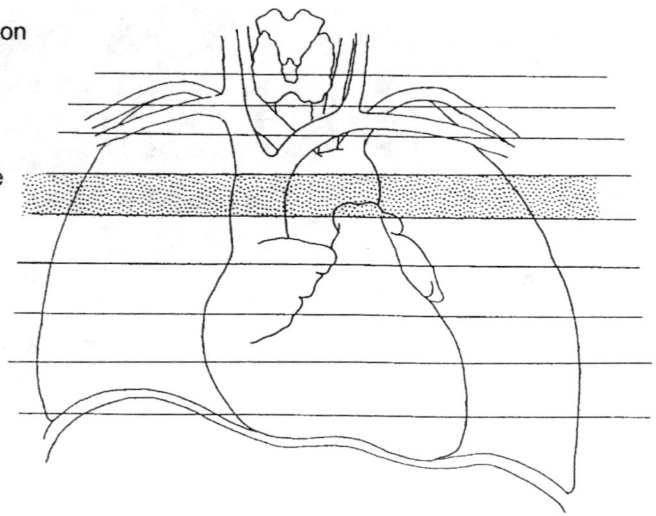

22 Left scapula
23 Subscapularis muscle
24 Serratus anterior muscle
25 Lower lobe of left lung
26 Left pulmonary artery
27 Semispinalis muscle
28 Descending aorta
29 Head of rib sixth rib
30 Body of sixth thoracic vertebra and sympathetic trunk
31 Spinous process of vertebra T5
32 Spinal cord
33 Esophagus, azygos vein, and right vagus nerve (in between)
34 Trapezius muscle
35 Right main bronchus
36 Right pulmonary artery
37 Lower lobe of right lung
38 Right scapula (inferior angle)
39 Teres major muscle
40 Oblique fissure of right lung
41 Pectoralis major muscle
42 Upper lobe of right lung
43 Pectoralis minor muscle
44 Superior vena cava
45 Cartilage forming keel-like carina at bifurcation of trachea
46 Left vagus nerve

Th-60 Cross section of thorax level of bifurcation of pulmonary trunk

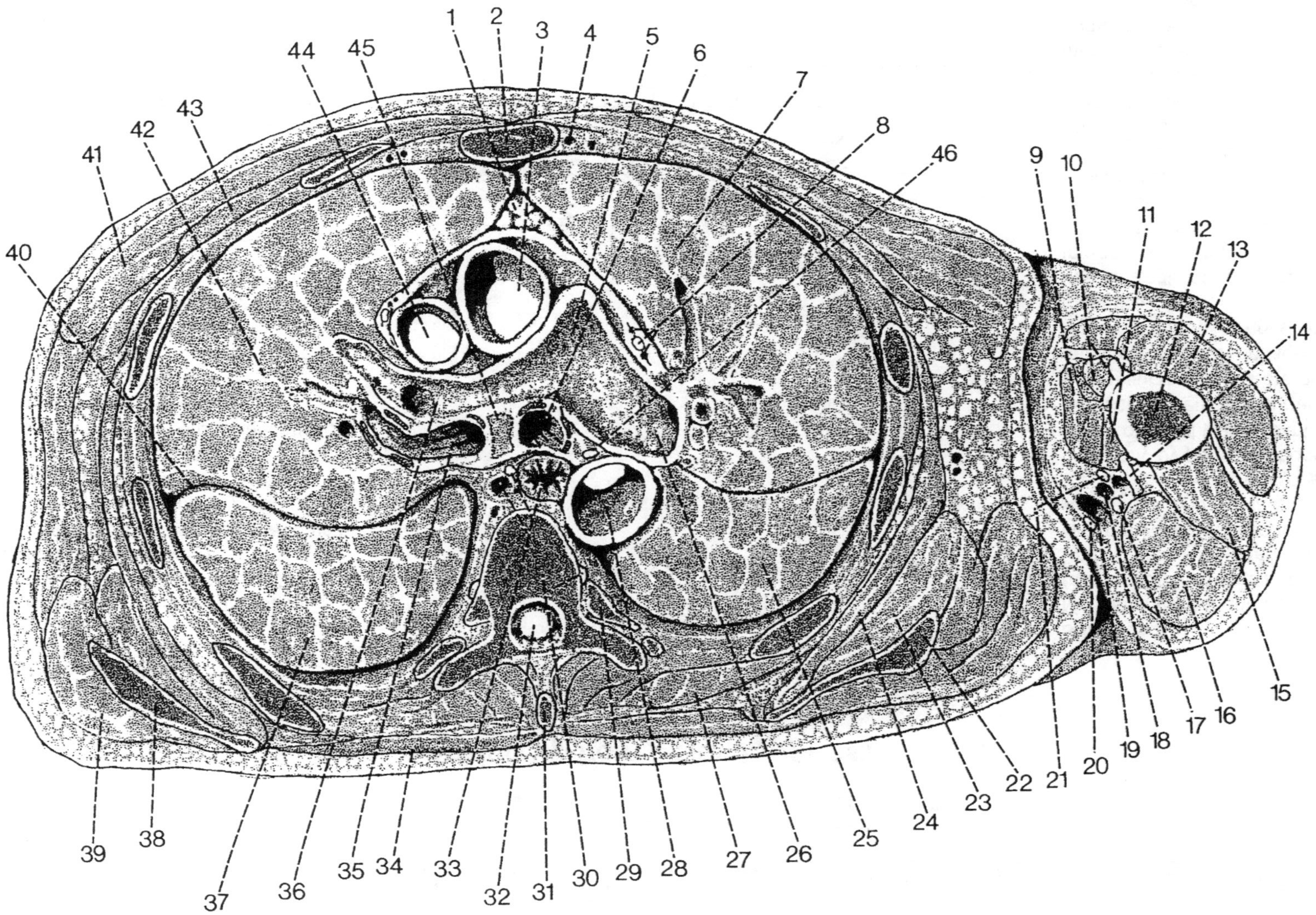

Th-61 Cross section of thorax just below pulmonary valve

(Looking up from below) (opposite page)

Color and label

1 Sternum (body)
2 Pulmonary valve seen through infundibulum of right ventricle
3 Left phrenic nerve with pericardiacophrenic artery and vein
4 Superior left pulmonary vein leading into left atrium
5 Left inferior lobar bronchus surrounded with bronchial cartilage
6 Superior lobe of left lung
7 Intercostal muscles
8 Lymph nodes
9 Inferior lobe of left lung
10 Serratus anterior muscle
11 Latissimus dorsi muscle
12 Teres major muscle
13 Subscapularis muscle
14 Scapula (inferior angle)
15 Infraspinatus muscle
16 Esophagus (surrounded by anterior and posterior esophageal plexuses formed by left and right vagus nerves)
17 Rhomboideus major muscle
18 Trapezius muscle
19 Aorta (descending thoracic)
20 Sympathetic trunk
21 Azygos vein
22 Spinous process of thoracic vertebra T6

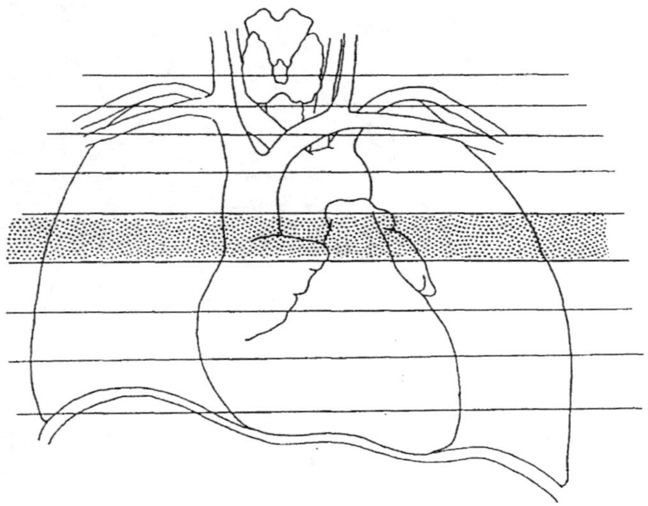

23 Spinal cord
24 Multifidus (deep) and semispinalis (more superficial) back muscles
25 Body of thoracic vertebra T7
26 Right inferior lobar bronchus with cartilage in its wall
27 Pleural space or cavity (bounded externally by parietal pleura on inside of chest wall and internally by visceral pleura on surface of lung; both pleural spaces here are greatly enlarged due to shrinkage of the lungs)
28 Right pulmonary artery dividing into lobar branches
29 Inferior angle of right scapula
30 Inferior lobe of right lung
31 Intercostal vein, artery, and nerve
32 Middle lobe of right lung
33 Oblique fissure
34 Superior lobe of right lung
35 Superior vena cava
36 Pectoralis major muscle
37 Left atrium (superior part)
38 Internal thoracic artery and paired veins
39 Ascending aorta
40 Prepericardial fat with remnants of thymus gland
41 Thoracic duct

Th-61 Cross section of thorax just below pulmonary valve (Looking up from below)

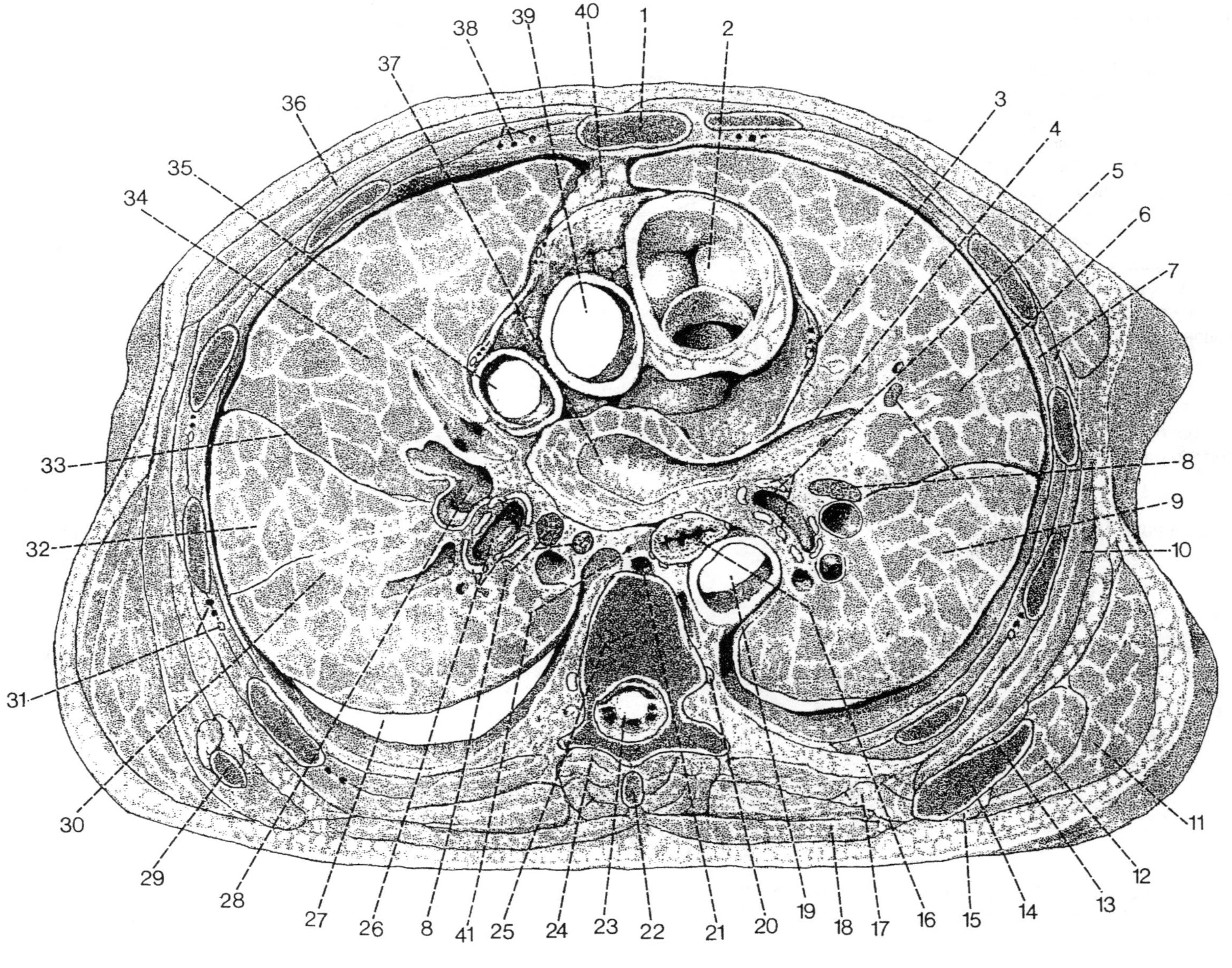

Th-62 Cross section of thorax just below aortic valve

(Looking up from below) (opposite page)

Color and label

1 Body of sternum
2 Right ventricle of heart
3 Fourth costal cartilage
4 Aortic valve (viewed from ventricular side)
5 Great cardiac vein
6 Anterior interventricular branch of left coronary artery; also called left anterior descending or LAD
7 Left ventricle (narrow outflow tract leading to aorta)
8 Wall of left ventricle
9 Superior lobe of left lung
10 Pericardium (fused with pleura)
11 Sixth intercostal vein, artery, and nerve below 6th rib (appear posterior to rib in horizontal section)
12 Portion of anterior cusp of mitral valve (bicuspid or left atrioventricular valve)
13 Lower lobe of left lung
14 Coronary sinus
15 Esophagus
16 Longissimus muscle (part of erector spinae muscle)
17 Aorta (descending thoracic part)
18 Spinal cord
19 Spinous process of vertebra T7
20 Body of thoracic vertebra T8
21 Sympathetic trunk
22 Azygos vein receiving left intercostal vein

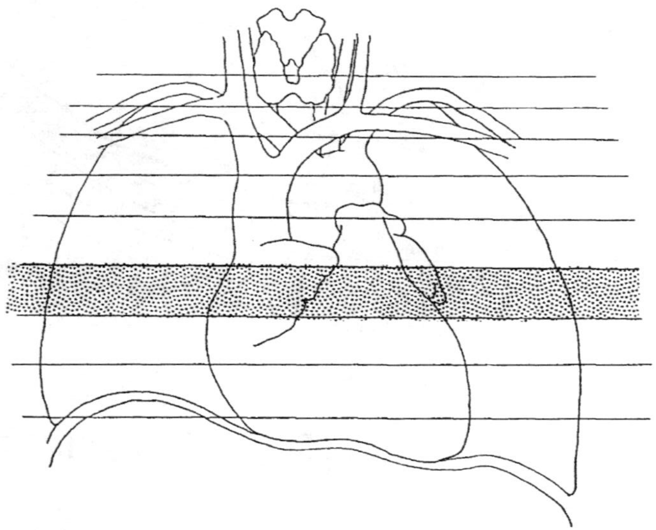

23 Right pulmonary veins emptying into left atrium
24 Left atrium
25 Latissimus dorsi
26 Serratus anterior muscle
27 Pleural cavity (greatly expanded due to shrinkage of lung)
28 Middle lobe of right lung
29 Phrenic nerve with pericardiacophrenic artery and vein (between fused pericardium and pleura)
30 Opening of superior vena cava into right atrium
31 Pectinate muscles (musculi pectinati) in right auricle (an out-pouching or appendage of the right atrium)
32 Internal thoracic artery and vein (vein is doubled)
33 Costomediastinal recess of pleural space (parietal pleura is reflected from inside of chest wall onto outside of pericardial sac)
34 Small cardiac vein
35 Right coronary artery
36 Circumflex branch of left coronary artery
37 Crista terminalis (leader points to approximate site of SA node) (pacemaker)
38 Oblique fissure of right lung
39 Thoracic duct

Th-62 Cross section of thorax just below aortic valve (Looking up from below)

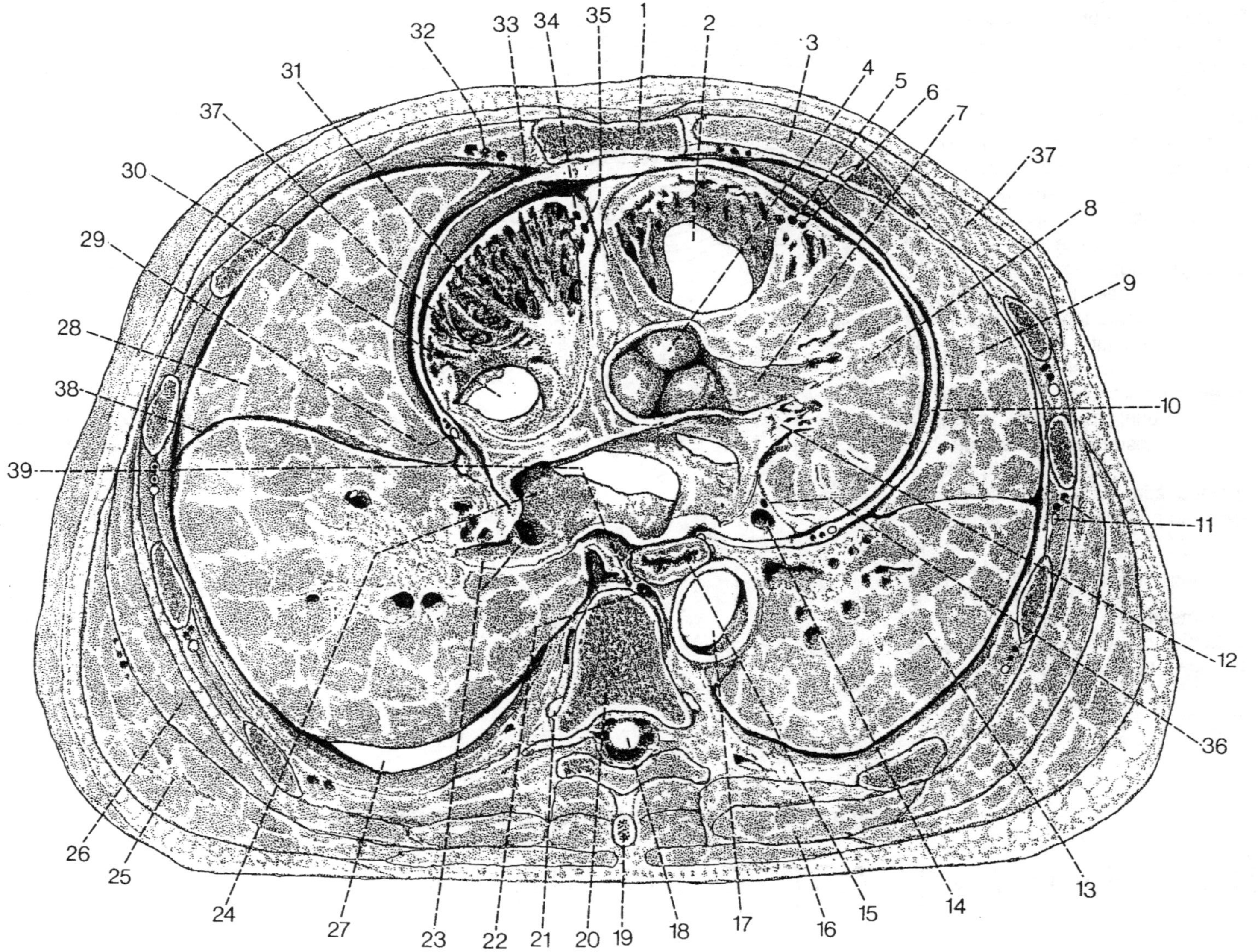

Th-63 Cross section of thorax at level of male nipple

(Looking up from below) (opposite page)

Color and label

1 Right ventricle of heart
2 Body of sternum
3 Interventricular septum
4 Left ventricle and trabeculae carneae (muscular bundles on the inside walls of both ventricles)
5 Male nipple (papilla)
6 Anterior papillary muscle in left ventricle
7 Left phrenic nerve with pericardiacophrenic artery and vein (between pericardium and pleura)
8 Upper lobe of left lung
9 Oblique fissure in left lung
10 Chordae tendineae
11 Serratus anterior muscle
12 Anterior cusp of mitral (bicuspid) valve (left AV valve)
13 Left atrium (small portion)
14 Lower lobe of left lung
15 Coronary sinus (largest intrinsic heart vein)
16 Descending aorta and hemiazygos vein receiving left posterior intercostal vein
17 Semispinalis (superficial) and erector spinae muscles
18 Spinal nerve T8
19 Body and lamina of thoracic vertebra T8

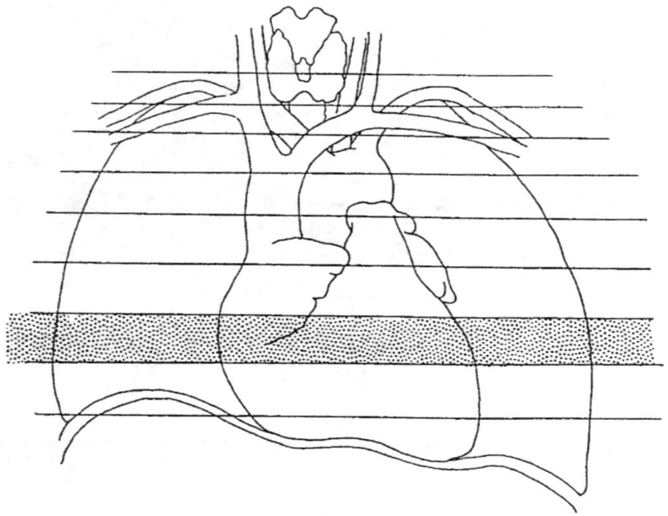

20 Spinal cord and internal venous plexus
21 Spinous process of thoracic vertebra T7
22 Azygos vein and right posterior intercostal vein
23 Sympathetic trunk
24 Trapezius muscle
25 Esophagus (surrounded by esophageal plexus mainly from vagal nerve fibers) and thoracic duct
26 Latissimus dorsi muscle
27 Lower lobe of right lung
28 Intercostal vein, artery, and nerve
29 Intercostal muscles
30 Upper lobe of right lung
31 Pectoralis major muscle
32 Right atrium of heart
33 Internal thoracic artery and veins (doubled)
34 Costal cartilage
35 Anterior cusp of tricusid valve (right AV valve)
36 Pericardium (pericardial sac); made up of internal thin parietal serous pericardium and outer strong fibrous pericardium; on either side the pericardium is fused with the thin parietal (or mediastinal) pleura. Phrenic nerve and accompanying vessels are “sandwiched” between pericardium and pleura
37 Posterior cusp of mitral valve
38 Enlarged pleural cavity due to shrinkage of lungs

Th-63 Cross section of thorax at level of male nipple

(Looking up from below)

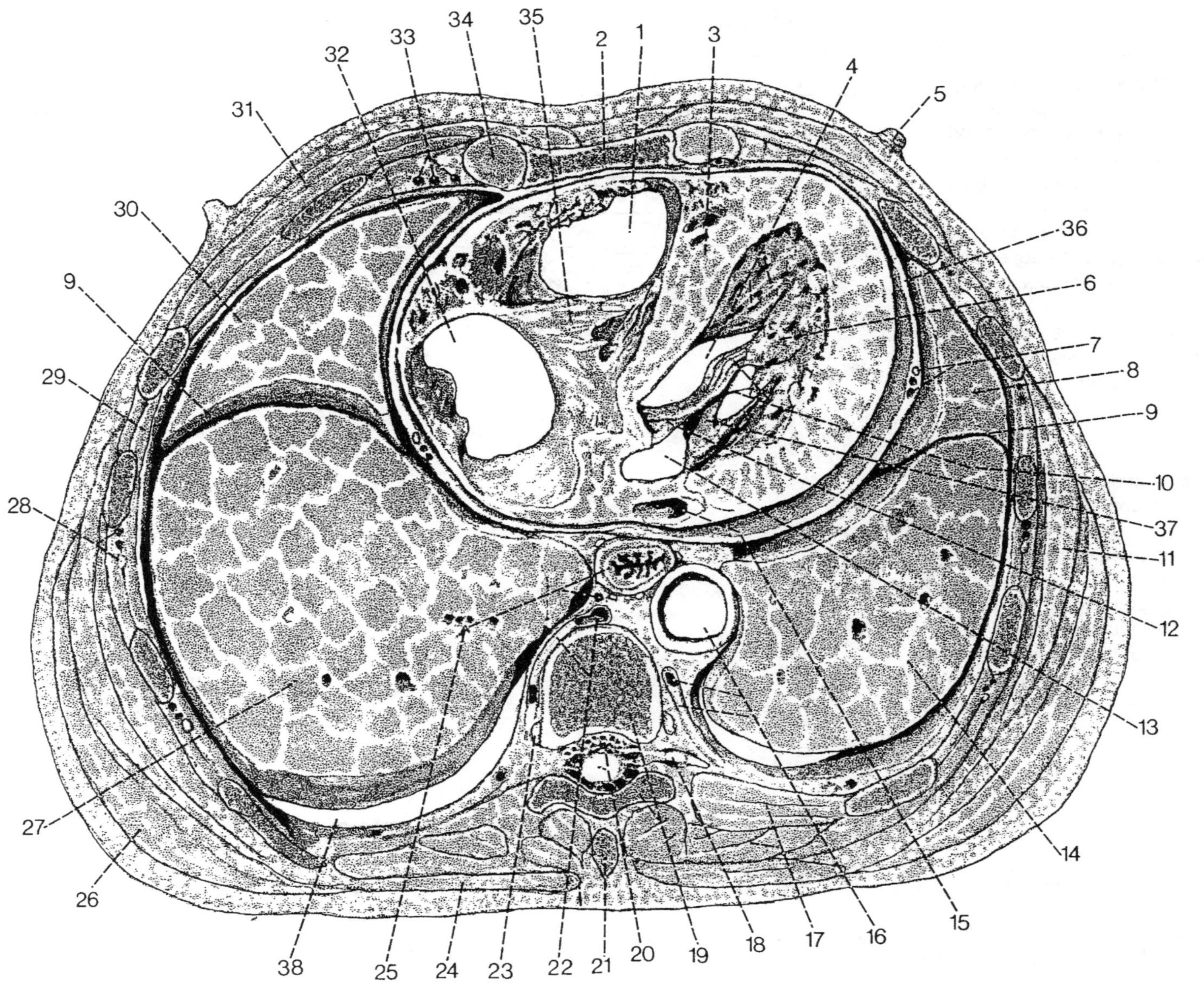

Th-64 Cross section of thorax with right dome of diaphragm and right lobe of liver

(Looking up from below) (opposite page)

Color and label

1 Inferior vena cava (arrow in right atriium points to superior lip of vena caval "half valve")
2 Thoracic aorta and thoracic duct
3 Right atrium
4 Right ventricle
5 Left ventricle
6 Esophagus (surrounded by esophageal plexus)
7 Pectoralis major muscle
8 Interventricular septum (muscular part)
9 Pleural space (in life it is a potential space containing only a little serous fluid
10 Cusp of mitral valve
11 Lower part (lingula) of upper lobe of left lung
12 Left phrenic nerve, pericardiacophrenic artery and vein
13 Coronary sinus (main vein draining blood from the walls of the heart to the right atrium)
14 External and internal intercostal muscles
15 Lower lobe of left lung
16 Latissimus dorsi muscle
17 Sympathetic trunk
18 Azygos vein receiving posterior intercostal vein
19 Spinous process of thoracic vertebra T8
20 Spinal cord
21 Body of thoracic vertebra T9

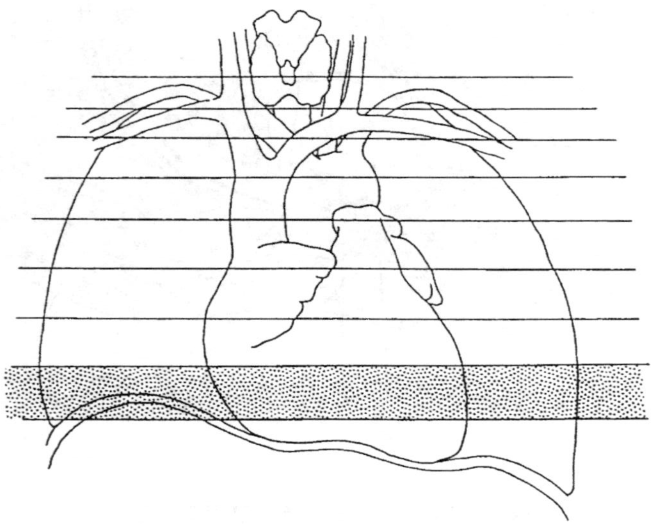

22 Intercostal nerve (ventral or anterior ramus) of spinal nerve T9
23 Bare area of liver (not covered with peritoneum and firmly adhering to underside of diaphragm)
24 Right lobe of liver (its most superior part, causing right dome of diaphragm to be higher than left)
25 Diaphragm (right dome)
26 Intercostal vein (nearest to rib), artery, and nerve
27 Ninth rib
28 Serratus anterior muscle
29 Lower lobe of right lung
30 Pericardial sac (fibrous pericardium lined internally with thin serous layer; fused laterally with the pleural membrane)
31 Internal thoracic artery and vein
32 Middle lobe of right lung
33 Costal cartilage
34 Right phrenic nerve with pericardiacophrenic artery and vein (between fused pericardial sac and pleura)
35 Anterior intercostal artery and vein (from internal thoracic artery)
36 Pectinate muscles in right auricle
37 Costal cartilage
38 Sternum
39 Anterior cusp and chordae tendineae of tricuspid valve

Th-64 Cross section of thorax with right dome of diaphragm and right lobe of liver

(Looking up from below)

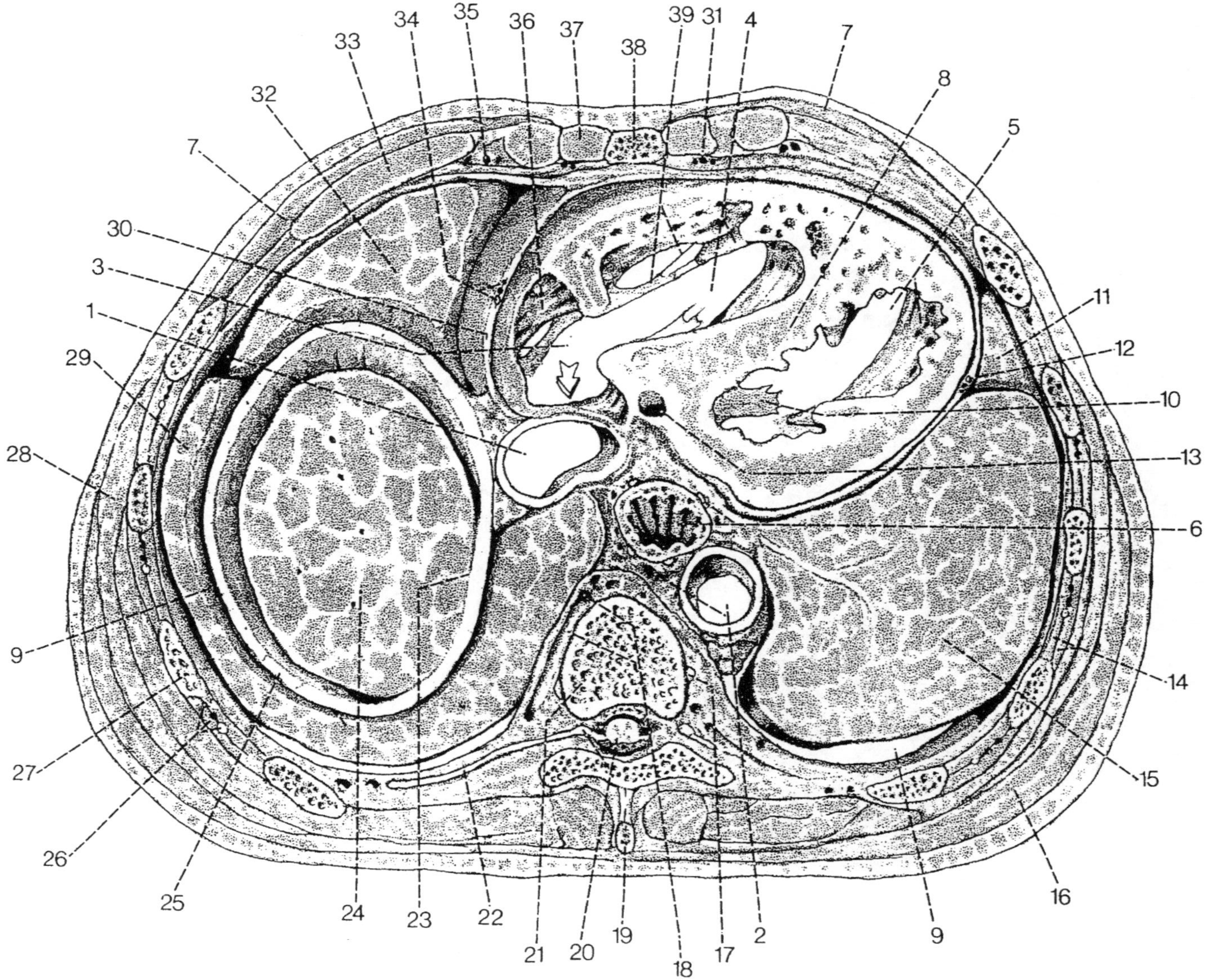

Part II: The Abdomen

Duodenum (etymological cartoon)

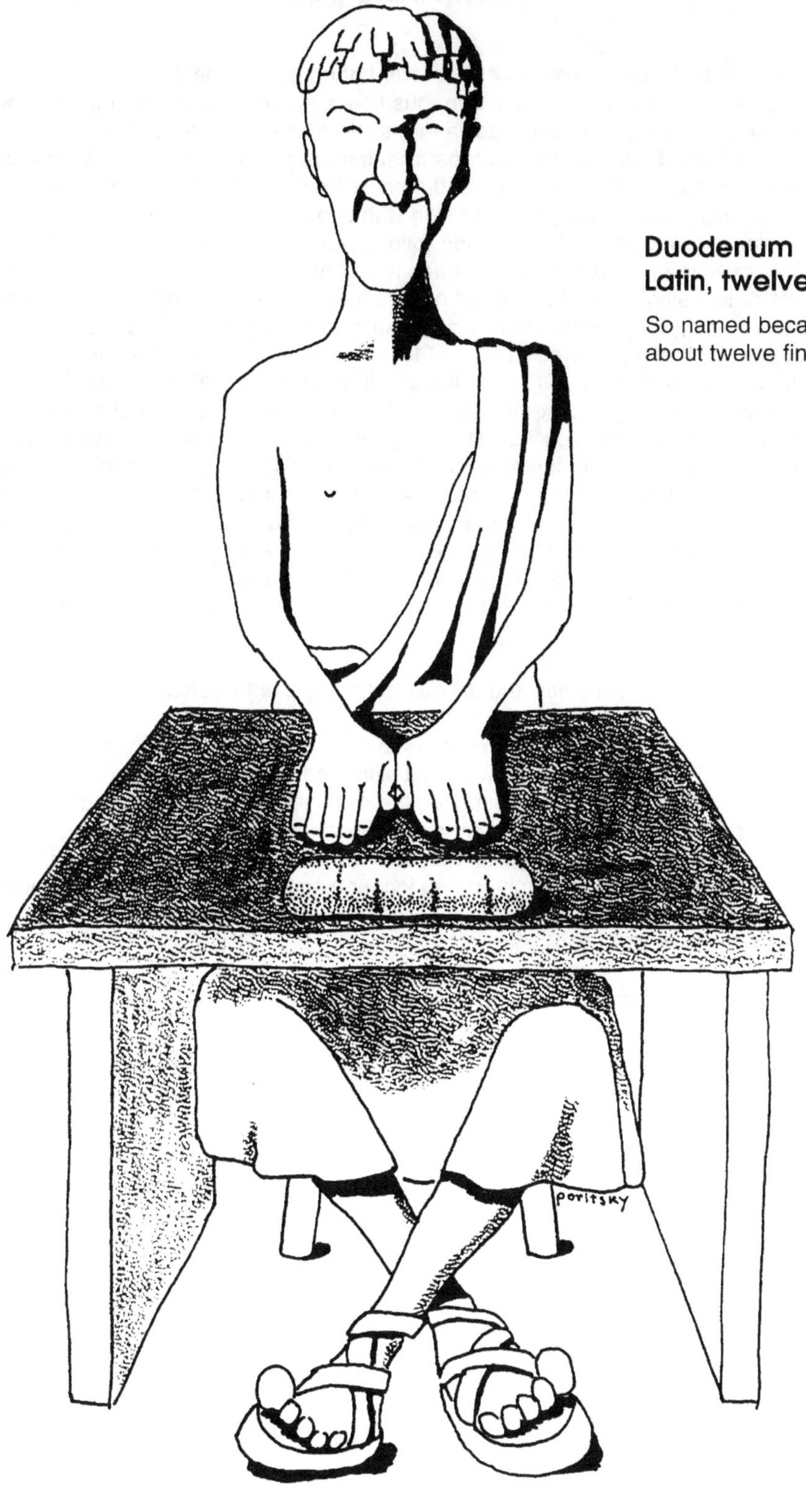

Duodenum
Latin, twelve

So named because its length is about twelve fingerbreadths

Ab-1 Segmental innervation of the skin of the anterior trunk

(opposite page)

The right side (viewer's left) shows the bands of skin called dermatomes, each of which is supplied by the cutaneous* branches of a single spinal nerve. The cutaneous fibers in each nerve pass through the underlying muscles and deep fascia and enter the superficial fascia in 2 sites: as medial anterior branches and as lateral branches (shown on left side). Each branch emerges from the deep fascia as a white cord about 2 mm thick. It then ramifies in the superficial fascia into smaller and smaller branches which eventually become microscopic. These spread out and supply the deep layer of the skin with sensory fibers (pain, touch, and temperature) along with fibers to sweat glands (sudomotor), hair follicles (pilomotor), and cutaneous blood vessels (vasomotor). There is considerable overlap in the distribution of each spinal nerve, which sends branches into adjacent dermatomes, so that injury to a single spinal nerve will not result in a loss of sensation to skin area in question. Note that the nipple is usually supplied by the anterior branch of the 4th thoracic verve (T4), and the umbilicus (belly button) is supplied by the 10th thoracic nerve (T10). The lower 5 thoracic nerves (intercostal nerves T7–T11) along with the subcostal nerve (T12) and the first lumbar nerve (L1) innervate the anterolateral abdominal wall muscles. These nerves begin as ventral (primary) rami of spinal nerves and travel between the muscles of the body wall which they supply. Nerves T5-T11 supply the lower intercostal muscles including the muscles of the innermost layer. They then continue downward and medially and supply the transversus abdominis, the internal and external oblique muscles, and finally the rectus abdominis. Should the nerve to a muscle be accidentally severed, the muscle will be paralyzed, and if the damaged nerve is unable to regenerate into the affected muscle, the muscle will eventually atrophy and be replaced by connective tissue. Herpes zoster† (shingles)‡ is an acute viral disease which attacks the sensory cells in a dorsal root ganglia. One of its most striking symptoms is the eruption of smallpox-like vesicles in a dermatomic distribution that corresponds to the distribution of the affected sensory nerve cells.

SC, supraclavicular nerves; these are small and difficult to find by blunt dissection.

VAL, ventral axial line; the original midline in the embryonic developing arm; note there is a "jump" from cervical nerve C4 to thoracic nerve T2 along this line, leaving out skin areas supplied by cervical nerves C6,C7, C8, and thoracic nerve T1. In the embryo these nerves supplied the distal tip of the arm bud which was to become the future hand and forelimb. As the developing arm grew out, the strips of cutaneous innervation no longer kept the original band-like pattern. These nerves elongated with their cutaneous endings supplying discrete dermatomes that encompassed just the hand or the forelimb and no longer extended as a continuous band back to the thorax.

*Cutaneous, pertaining to the skin, L. *cutis*, skin

†Herpes is Greek for to creep, to crawl; zoster is Greek for a belt, a girdle.

‡The word shingles is derived from the Middle English schingles, an alteration of the medieval Latin *cingulus* from the Latin *cingulum*, a belt, a girdle; from *cingere*, to tie about, to gird.

Ab-1 Segmental innervation of the skin of the anterior trunk

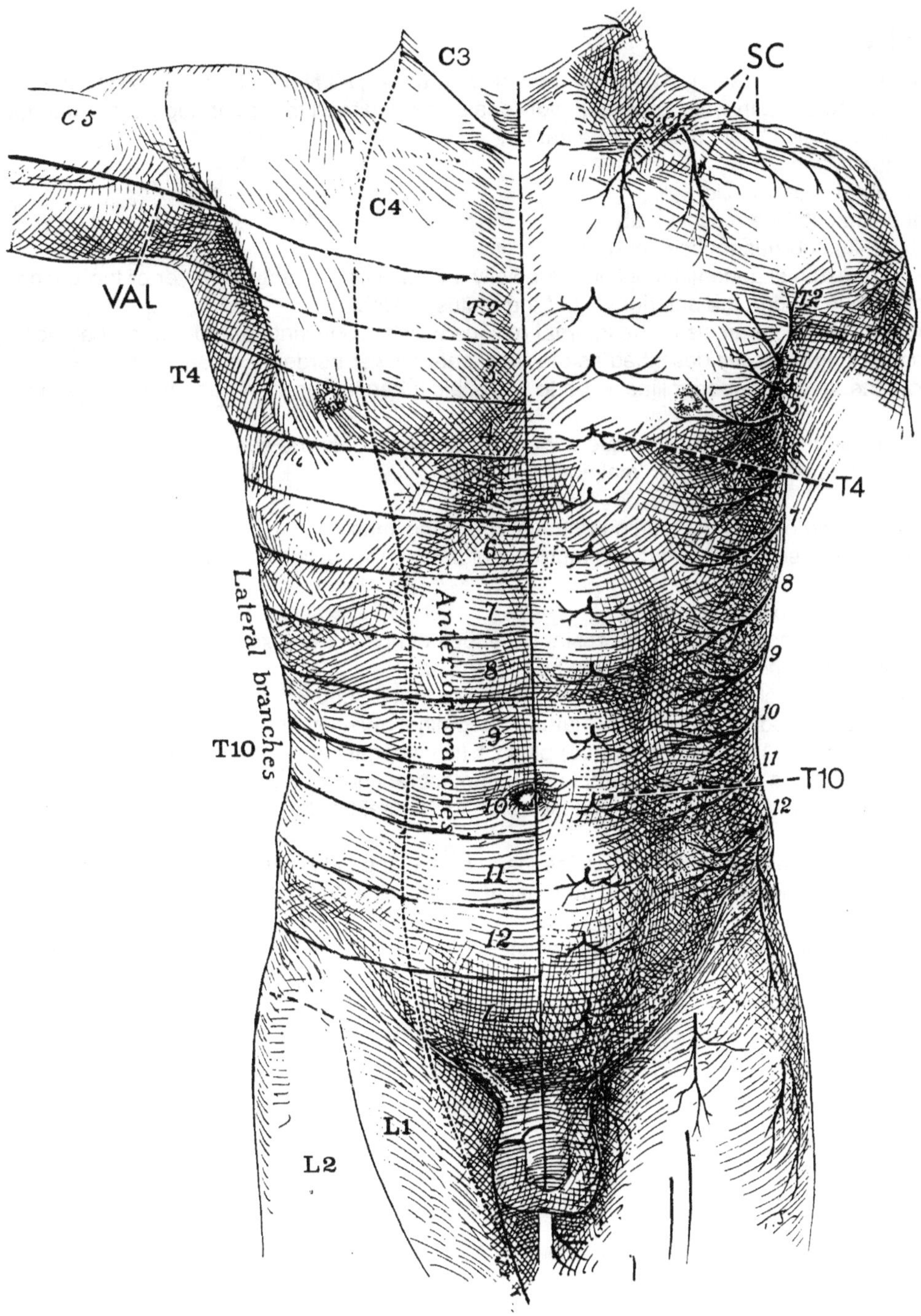

Eycleshymer and Jones

Ab-2 Muscles of the anterior and lateral abdominal walls I
(opposite page)

Color and label

1 Rectus abdominis; note its segmental arrangement with (usually) 3 fibrous bands between the segments (tendinous intersections). In well-developed individuals, the enlarged muscular segments often give the anterior abdomen wall a "washboard" appearance.
2 Tendinous intersection
3 Transversus abdominis muscle
4 Internal abdominal oblique muscle (cut)
5 External abdominal oblique muscle (cut)
6 Aponeurosis* of external abdominal oblique; medially it fuses with the anterior layer of the aponeurosis of the internal oblique to form the anterior wall of the rectus sheath.
7 Anterior layer of the aponeurosis of the internal oblique which divides into anterior and posterior layers
8 Inguinal ligament; traditionally described as the "thickened" lower border of external oblique aponeurosis; it extends from the anterior superior iliac spine to the pubic tubercle; recent reports have questioned any thickening.
9 Superficial inguinal ring in external oblique aponeurosis; opening for the spermatic cord in males and the round ligament in females; bigger on males
10 Pubic tubercle
11 Pubic symphysis and pubic crest; origin of rectus abdominis muscle
12 Conjoint tendon; formed by the fused aponeuroses of the internal oblique and the transversus abdominis muscles
13 Anterior superior iliac spine
14 Insertion of the rectus abdominis on the costal cartilages of ribs 5-7 and xiphoid process
15 Origin of external abdominal oblique muscle from ribs 5-12
16 Anterior cutaneous branch of intercostal nerve T12; note that it supplies a band of skin that includes the umbilicus. The rectus abdominis and the 3 lateral abdominal muscles are innervated by thoracic (intercostal) nerves T5-T12 (subcostal nerve) plus L1 (iliohypogastric nerve). Cutaneous branches of these nerves also supply strips of skin; for example, cutaneous branches of nerve T4 supply the nipple.
17 Linea semilunaris; a curved depression that indicates the lateral border of the rectus abdominis muscle and the rectus sheath.
18 Linea alba; all three lateral abdominal muscles insert on the linea alba by way of their aponeuroses. All 6 muscles working together will draw in the abdominal wall (suck in the gut).

*An aponeurosis is a strong flat tendinous sheet which acts as an extension of its attached muscle.

Ab-2 Muscles of the anterior and lateral abdominal walls I

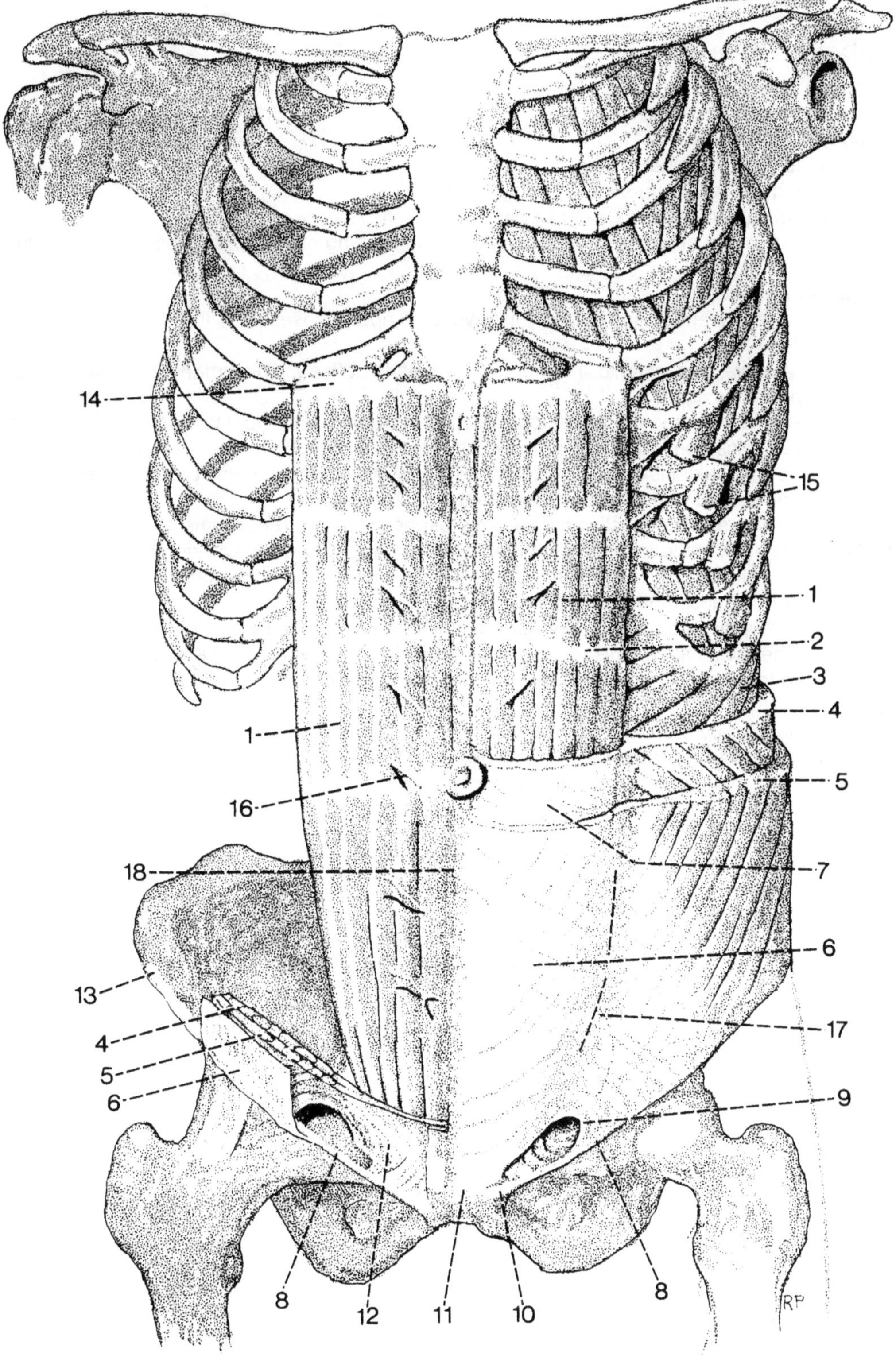

Ab-3 Muscles of the anterior and lateral abdominal walls II

(opposite page)

Color and label

1 Rectus abdominis muscle
2 Tendinous intersection
3 External abdominal oblique muscle
4 Aponeurosis of external abdominal oblique (a small piece; fusing with aponeurosis of internal oblique)
5 Internal abdominal oblique muscle
6 Anterior and posterior layers of rectus sheath formed by the splitting of the aponeurosis of the internal oblique
7 Transversus abdominis muscle
8 Aponeurosis of transversus abdominis (cut; at this level all 3 aponeuroses pass in front of the rectus abdominis)
9 Arcuate line (*linea arcuata*; a crescentic line, not always clearly defined, which marks the lower border of the posterior layer of the rectus sheath)
10 Linea alba; midline fibrous insertion of the 3 aponeuroses from the 3 flat abdominal muscles on each side; this avascular strip extends from the xiphoid process to the pubic symphysis; it is free of all but the tiniest blood vessels, and a surgical incision in the midline will sever no nerves to muscles since the nerves travel from the posterior spinal cord within the body wall to the anterior midline.
11 Transversalis fascia; a layer of connective tissue lying just beneath the transversus abdominis muscle and external to the peritoneum; in the lower third of the rectus abdominis sheath, where there is no posterior fibrous layer, the transversalis fascia forms the posterior layer of the rectus sheath.
12 Superior epigastric artery; accompanied by 2 or more veins (not shown)
13 Inferior epigastric artery; the inferior and superior epigastric arteries, along with their accompanying veins, anastomose within the rectus abdominis muscle, thus providing potential side channels (collateral circulation) for blood to reach the legs and lower trunk in the case of an obstructed aorta.
14 Inguinal ligament
15 Conjoined tendon; formed by the fused aponeuroses of the internal oblique and the transversus muscles
16 Opening in the internal oblique for the spermatic cord
17 Superficial inguinal ring in the external oblique aponeurosis
18 Spermatic cord with fibers of cremaster muscle
19 Testis
20 Pyramidalis muscle; absent in approximately 20% of cases
21 Posterior layer of rectus sheath

Ab-3 Muscles of the anterior and lateral abdominal walls II

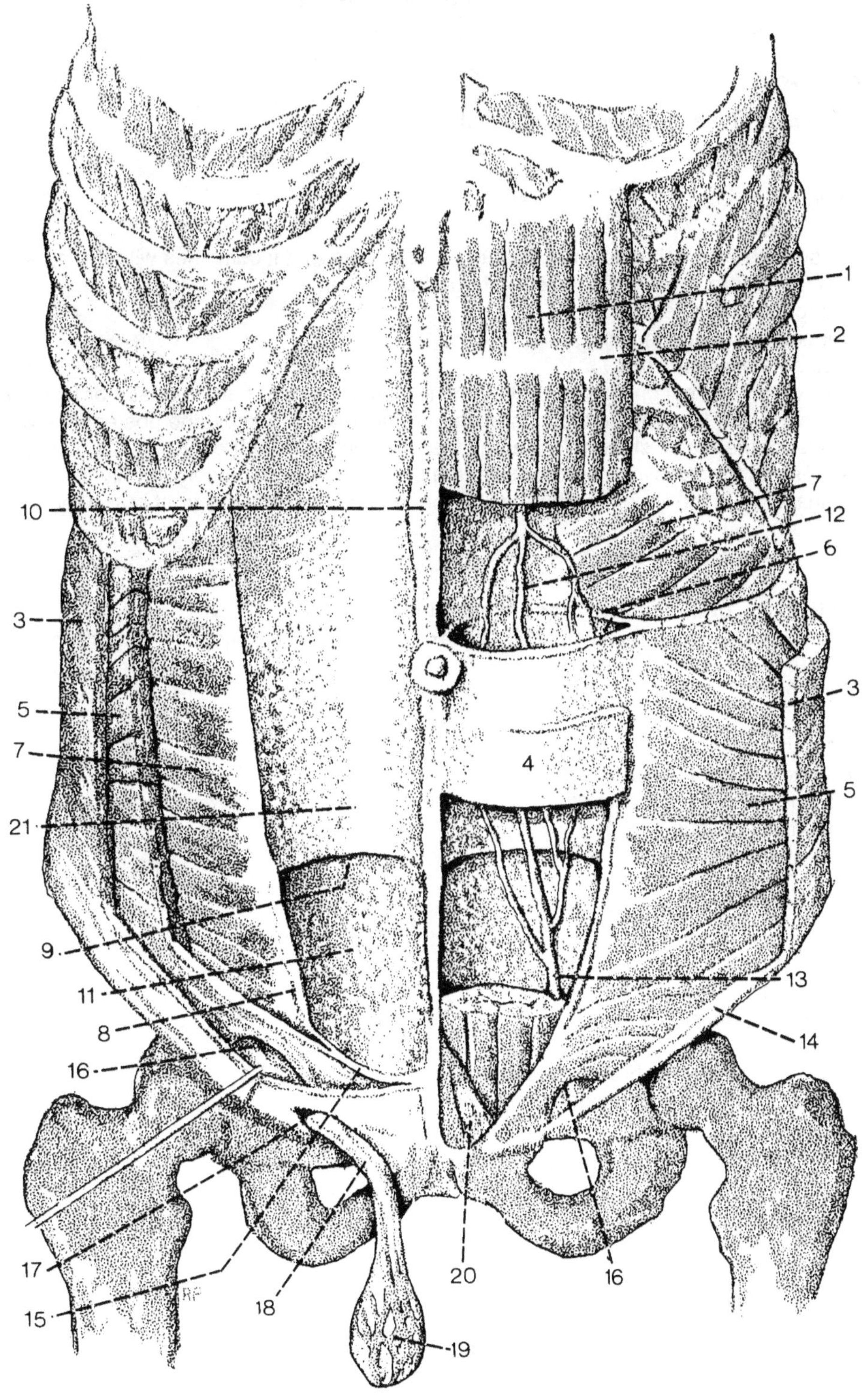

Ab-4 Muscles and layers of the anterior abdominal wall
(opposite page)

Color and label

Figure A. Muscles of the anterior abdominal wall

1 Umbilicus
2 Rectus abdominis muscle
3 Tendinous intersection
4 Aponeurosis of the external abdominal oblique muscle; note that it combines with the aponeurosis of the internal oblique to form the anterior layer of the rectus sheath.
5 External abdominal oblique muscle
6 Internal abdominal oblique muscle
7 Transversus abdominis muscle
8 Aponeurosis of the internal oblique; note that it splits into an anterior and a posterior layer with the former becoming the anterior layer of the rectus sheath and the latter becoming the posterior layer.
9 Posterior layer of the rectus sheath; formed by the posterior layer of the internal oblique aponeurosis and the aponeurosis of the transversus abdominis; the posterior layer is present in only the upper two-thirds of the abdominal wall; in the lower one-third, all 3 aponeuroses pass to the front of the rectus abdominis muscles.
10 Anterior layer of the rectus sheath

Figure B. The 9 layers of the anterior abdominal wall
The deep fascia surrounding the muscles has been exaggerated in thickness and partially removed on the right side (viewer's left).

1 Skin
2 Superficial fascia fatty layer (Camper's)
3 Superficial fascia fibrous layer (Scarpa's)
4 External abdominal oblique muscle
5 Internal abdominal oblique muscle
6 Transversus abdominis muscle
7 Transversalis fascia
8 Extraperitoneal (preperitoneal) fat
9 Peritoneum (parietal layer which lines the inside of the walls)
10 Rectus abdominis muscles
11 Anterior layer of the rectus sheath
12 Posterior layer of the rectus sheath
13 Linea alba
14 Aponeurosis of the external oblique muscle
15 Intestine; covered with visceral peritoneum or serosa

Ab-4 Muscles and layers of the anterior abdominal wall

A

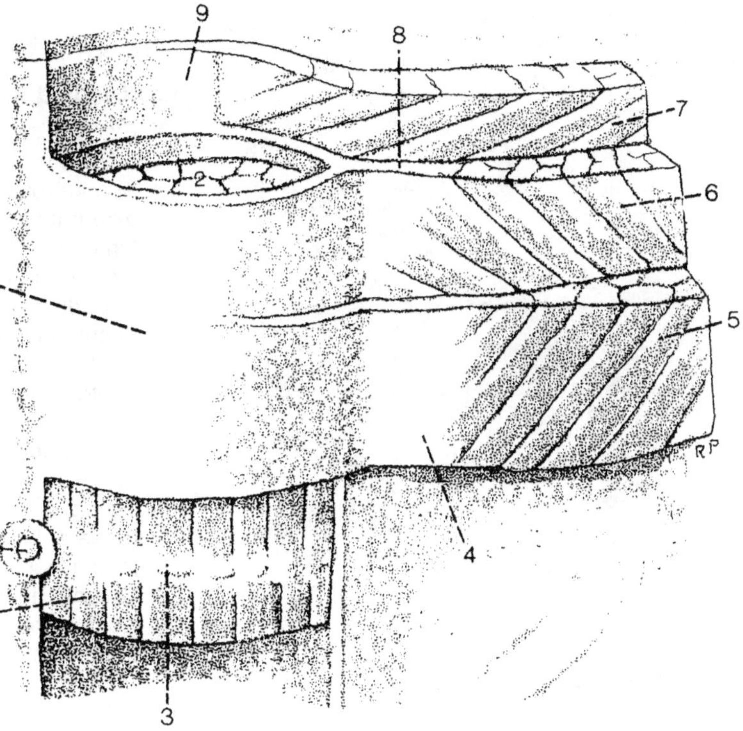

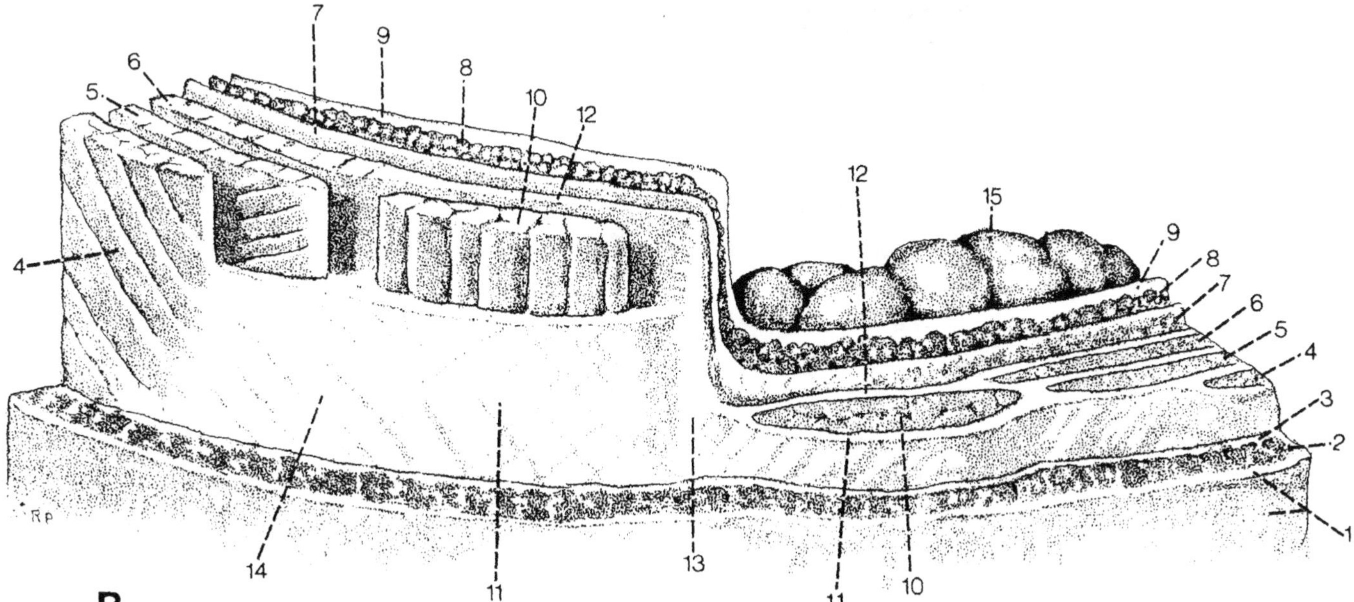

B

Ab-5 External abdominal oblique aponeurosis and superficial inguinal ring

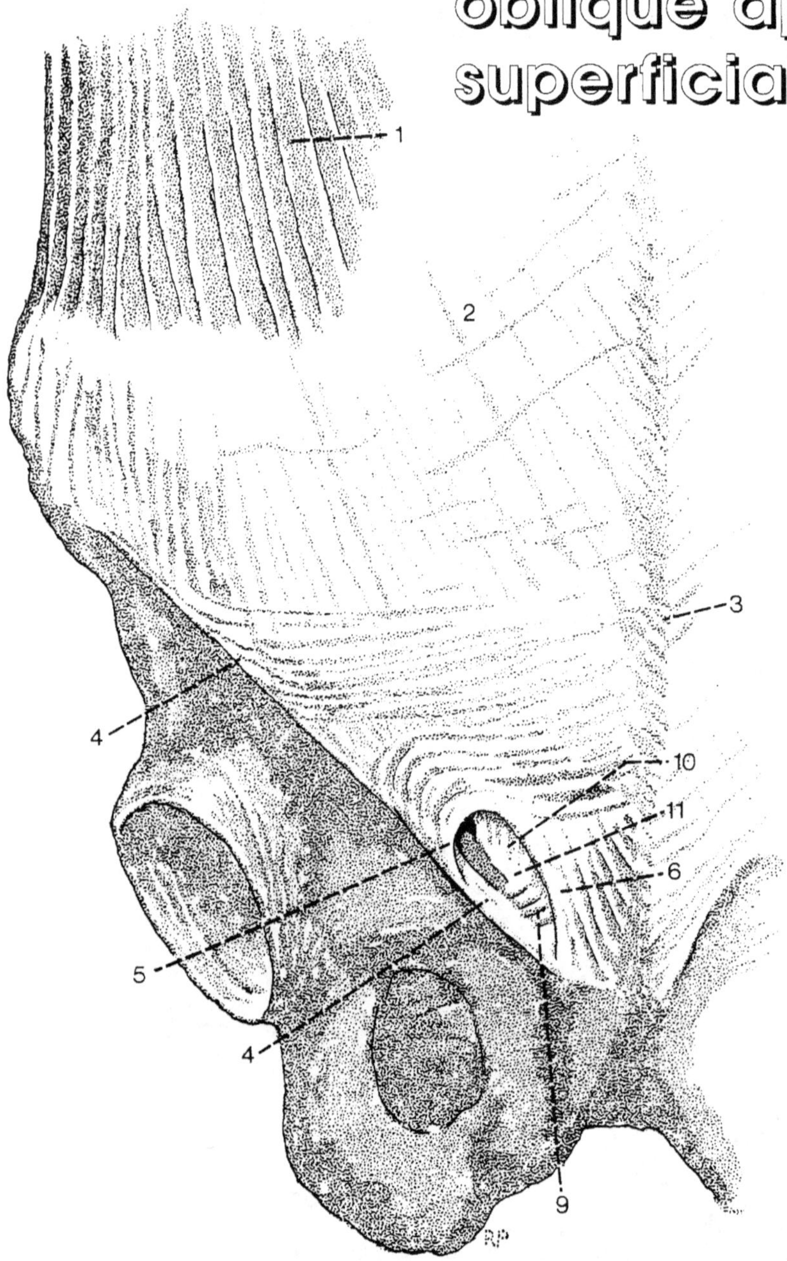

Redrawn from Moore

Color and label

1 External abdominal oblique muscle
2 Aponeurosis of external oblique
3 Linea alba
4 Inguinal ligament
5 Superficial inguinal ring; opening for spermatic cord in males; for round ligament of uterus in females
6 Medial crus; attached to the pubic crest and in front of the pubic symphysis
7 Lateral crus; attached to the pubic tubercle
8 Intercrural fibers
9 Lacunar ligament
10 Conjoint tendon attached to pectineal ligament
11 Pectineal ligament

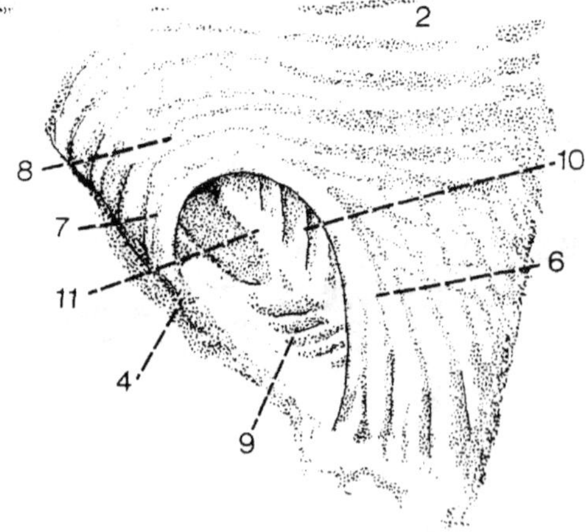

Ab-6 Inguinal canal dissection

Color and label

1 Aponeurosis of external abdominal oblique (cut)
2 Inguinal ligament; lower border of external oblique aponeurosis
3 Aponeurosis of internal abdominal oblique (cut)
4 Aponeurosis of transversus abdominis; note that all 3 aponeuroses pass in front of the rectus abdominis muscle at this level.
5 Anterior layer of rectus sheath
6 Conjoint tendon; formed by the arched lower borders of the aponeuroses of the internal oblique and the transversus abdominis
7 Spermatic cord; round ligament of the uterus in the female
8 Deep inguinal ring in the transversalis fascia
9 Transversalis fascia
10 Interfoveolar ligament
11 Internal abdominal oblique muscle
12 Transversus abdominis muscle
13 Extraperitoneal fat
14 Rectus abdominis muscle
15 Peritoneum
16 External spermatic fascia; continuous with deep fascia of external oblique
17 Cremasteric fascia and cremasteric muscle; continuous with internal oblique
18 Internal spermatic fascia; continuous with transversalis fascia
19 Vas (ductus) deferens
20 Testicular artery surrounded by pampiniform plexus of testicular vein; countercurrent heat exchange cools blood to the testis
21 Inferior epigastric artery and vein(s)
22 Femoral vein
23 Femoral artery
24 Great saphenous vein
25 Saphenous hiatus (opening)
26 Fascia lata (deep fascia of the thigh)
27 Subcutaneous fat (superficial fascia)
28 Superficial inguinal ring

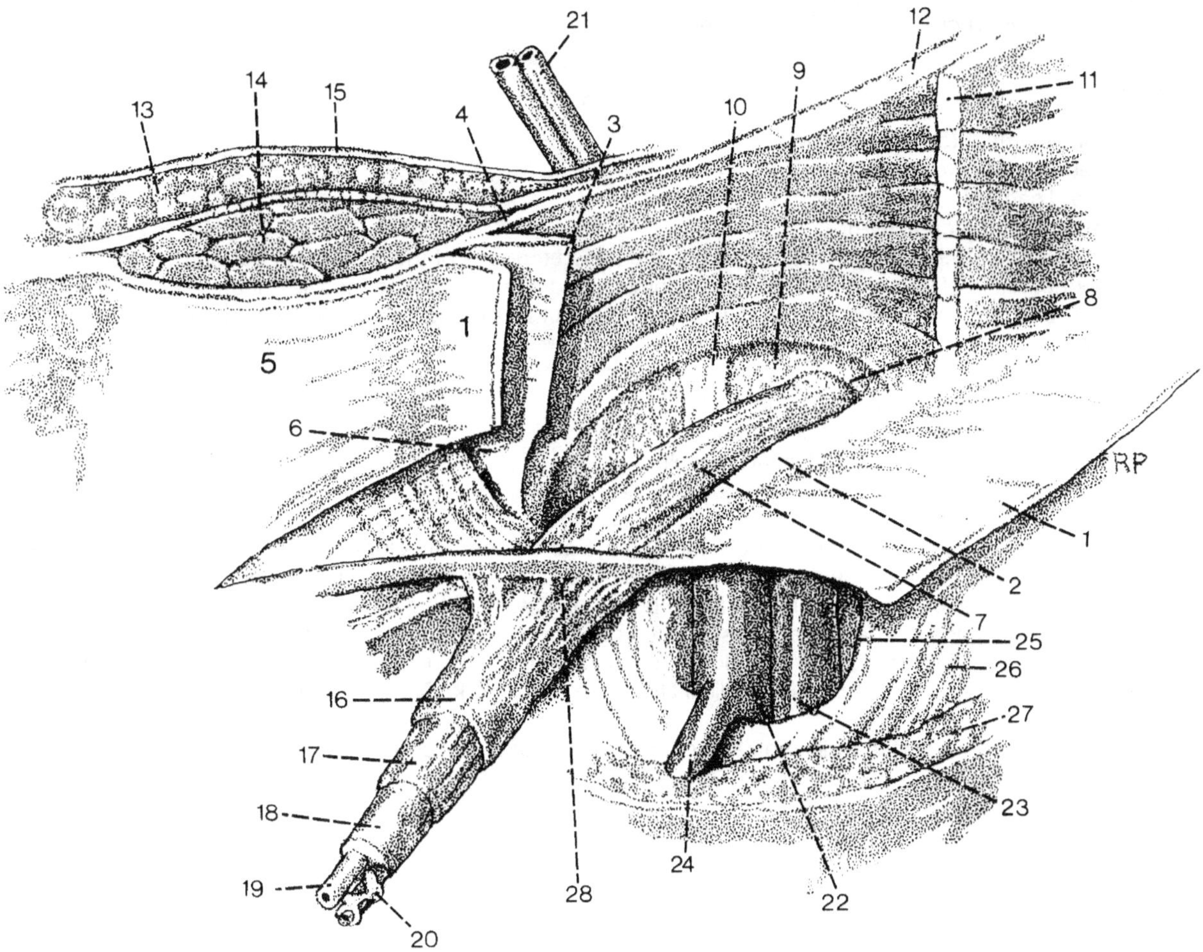

Ab-7 Inguinal ligament and related structures

(opposite page)

Color and label

Figure A

1 Inguinal ligament; hammock-like free lower edge of the aponeurosis of the external abdominal oblique muscle; it extends from the anterior superior iliac spine to the pubic tubercle; attached to the deep fascia of thigh (fascia lata).
2 Aponeurosis of the external abdominal oblique; it has been cut above the inguinal ligament, pulled forward, and partially dissected free of the inguinal ligament on the left.
3 Lacunar ligament; triangular extension of the medial end of the inguinal ligament extending to the pectineal ligament; its apex is attached medially to the pubic tubercle and its lateral concave base forms the medial border of the femoral ring; the spermatic cord passes over it; its superior surface forms the floor of the inguinal canal medially.
4 Reflex ligament; a poorly developed triangular band usually fused with either the conjoint tendon directly behind it or with the aponeurosis of the external oblique directly in front of it;* it has been reflected backwards on the left side.
5 Pectineal ligament; a strong fibrous band extending laterally from the base of the lacunar ligament along the pecten pubis (*pecten*, Latin, a comb); the conjoint tendon inserts upon it.
6 Superficial inguinal ring; the spermatic cord in the male and the round ligament of the uterus in the female and the ilioinguinal nerve in both sexes pass through it.
7 Lateral (inferior) crus of superficial inguinal ring
8 Medial (superior) crus of superficial inguinal ring

Figure B

1 Inguinal ligament (cut on left side)
2 Aponeurosis of external oblique
3 Lacunar ligament
4 Reflex ligament (see above)
5 Conjoint tendon (falx** inguinalis); formed by the joined tendons of the medial inferior borders of the aponeuroses of both the transversus abdominis and internal oblique muscles; it arches over the spermatic cord in males and the round ligament of the uterus in the female and inserts on the pectineal ligament.
6 Superficial inguinal ring
7 Lateral crus of the superficial inguinal ring
8 Medial crus of the superficial inguinal ring
9 Aponeurosis of transversus abdominis muscle
10 Aponeurosis of internal abdominal oblique muscle

*The reflex ligament has been decribed by some authors as a poorly developed expansion of the lateral crus of the inguinal ligament which passes medially and upward behind the medial end of the superficial inguinal ring in front of the conjoint tendon, feebly reinforcing the posterior wall of the inguinal canal and interweaving with similar fibers from the opposite side. Others describe it as a poorly developed triangular band of the external oblique aponeurosis of one side that crosses the midline, passes behind the superficial inguinal ring of the opposite, and inserts on the pectineal line. Churchill's Medical Dictionary, New York, Churchill Livingstone, 1989.

***Falx*, Latin, a sickle, a scythe (falciform, arched, in the form of a sickle or scythe)

Ab-7 Inguinal ligament and related structures

A

B

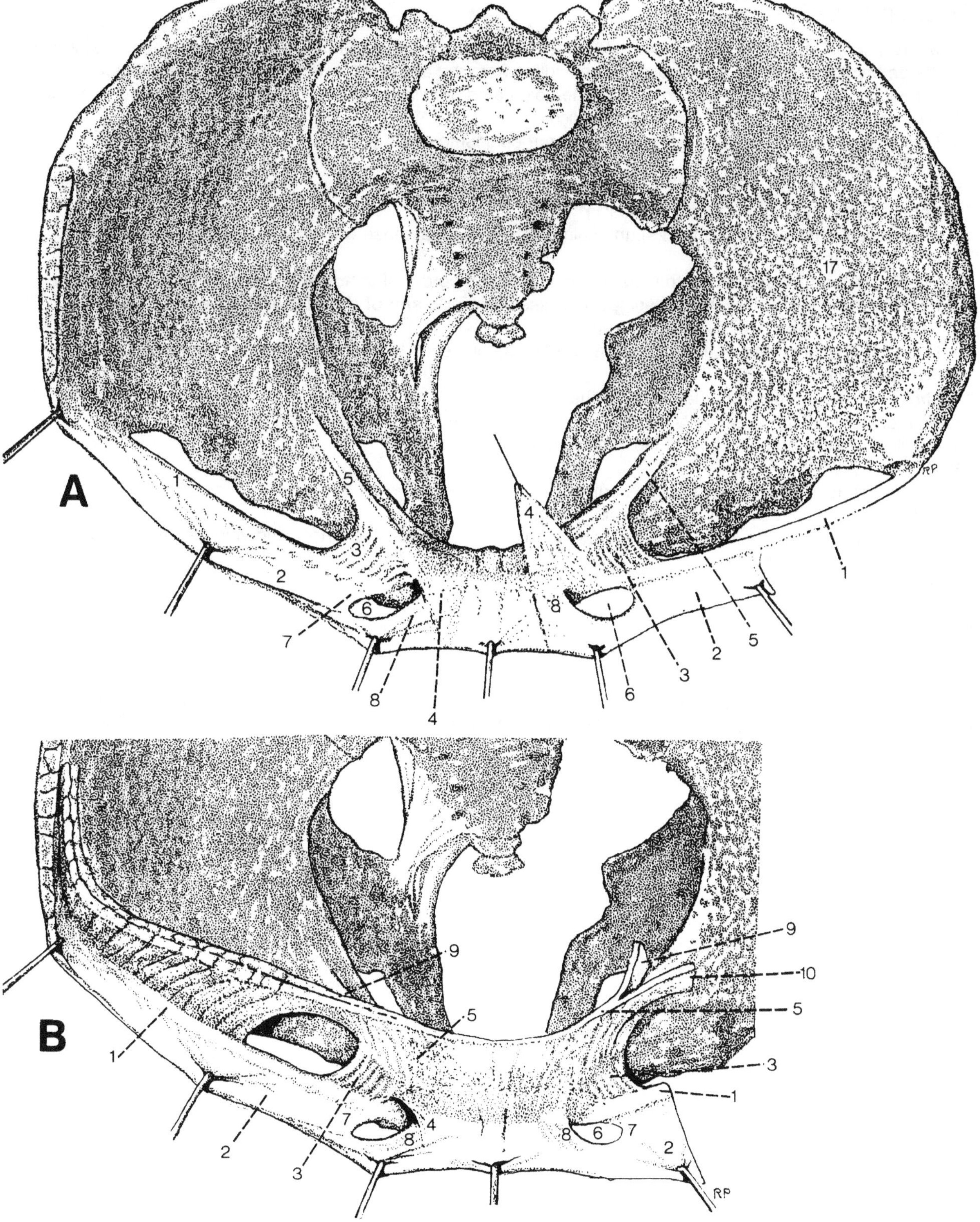

Ab-8 Lower anterior abdomen wall viewed from the inside

(opposite page)

Color and label

1 Median umbilical fold (or *plica*, Latin, fold); a raised fold of peritoneum formed by the ligamentous remains of the embryologic urachus,* extending in the midline from the apex of the urinary bladder to the umbilicus.
2 Medial umbilical fold (or plica); formed by the obliterated umbilical artery extending from the superior vesical (*vesica*, Latin, a bladder) artery to the umbilicus
3 Lateral umbilical fold (or plica); formed by inferior epigastric artery and vein
4 Rectus abdominis muscle
5 Umbilicus
6 Lateral border of rectus abdominis muscle
7 Inferior epigastric artery and vein(s); the vein is often doubled; these will anastomose with the superior epigastric vessels
8 Inguinal trigone, Hesselbach's triangle; formed by lateral border of rectus abdominis medially, by inguinal ligament inferiorly, and by inferior epigastric vessels laterally; **site of direct inguinal hernia.**
9 Parietal peritoneum partially stripped away
10 Deep inguinal ring; **site of indirect inguinal hernia**; this tends to be much larger in males than in females.
11 Testicular artery and vein
12 Ureter; conveys urine from the kidney to the bladder
13 Vas (ductus) deferens; conveys semen from the testis to the protate gland
14 Seminal vesicle; secretes part of the seminal fluid
15 Prostate gland
16 Urinary bladder; under parietal peritoneum
17 External iliac vein; becomes femoral vein in thigh
18 External iliac artery; becomes femoral artery in thigh; the external iliac artery and vein give rise to the inferior epigastric artery and vein.
19 Iliopsoas muscle
20 Femoral nerve
21 Deep inguinal ring
22 Parietal peritoneum

*Urachus: the vestigial distal part of the embryonic allantois. The lumen of the urachus is obliterated early in human embryos and becomes the cord-like median umbilical fold. The proximal part of the sausage-like allantois forms the bladder.

Ab-8 Lower anterior abdomen wall viewed from the inside

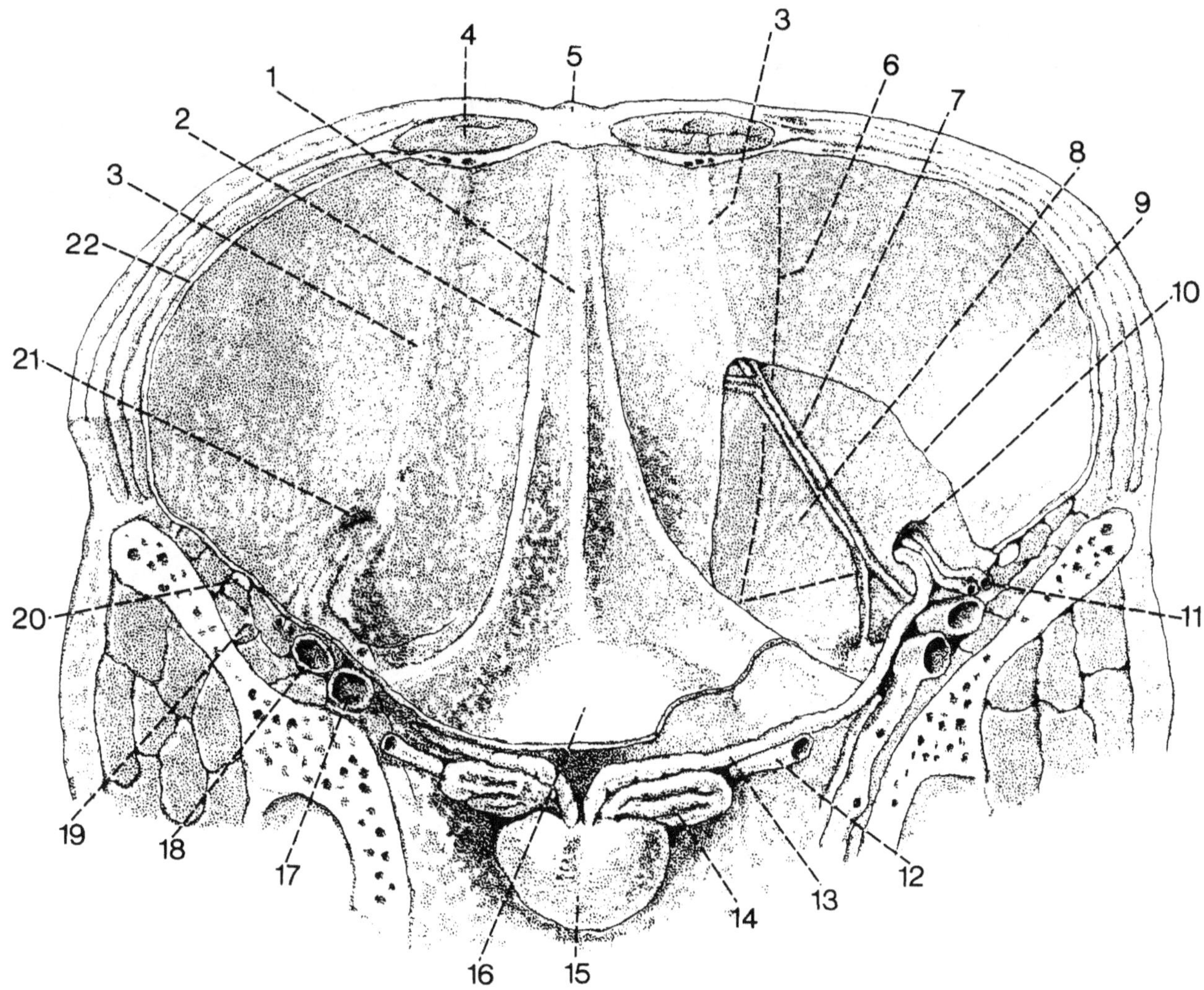

Redrawn and modified from Eycleshymer and Jones

Ab-9 Thoracic and abdominal viscera after removal of anterior thoracic and abdominal walls

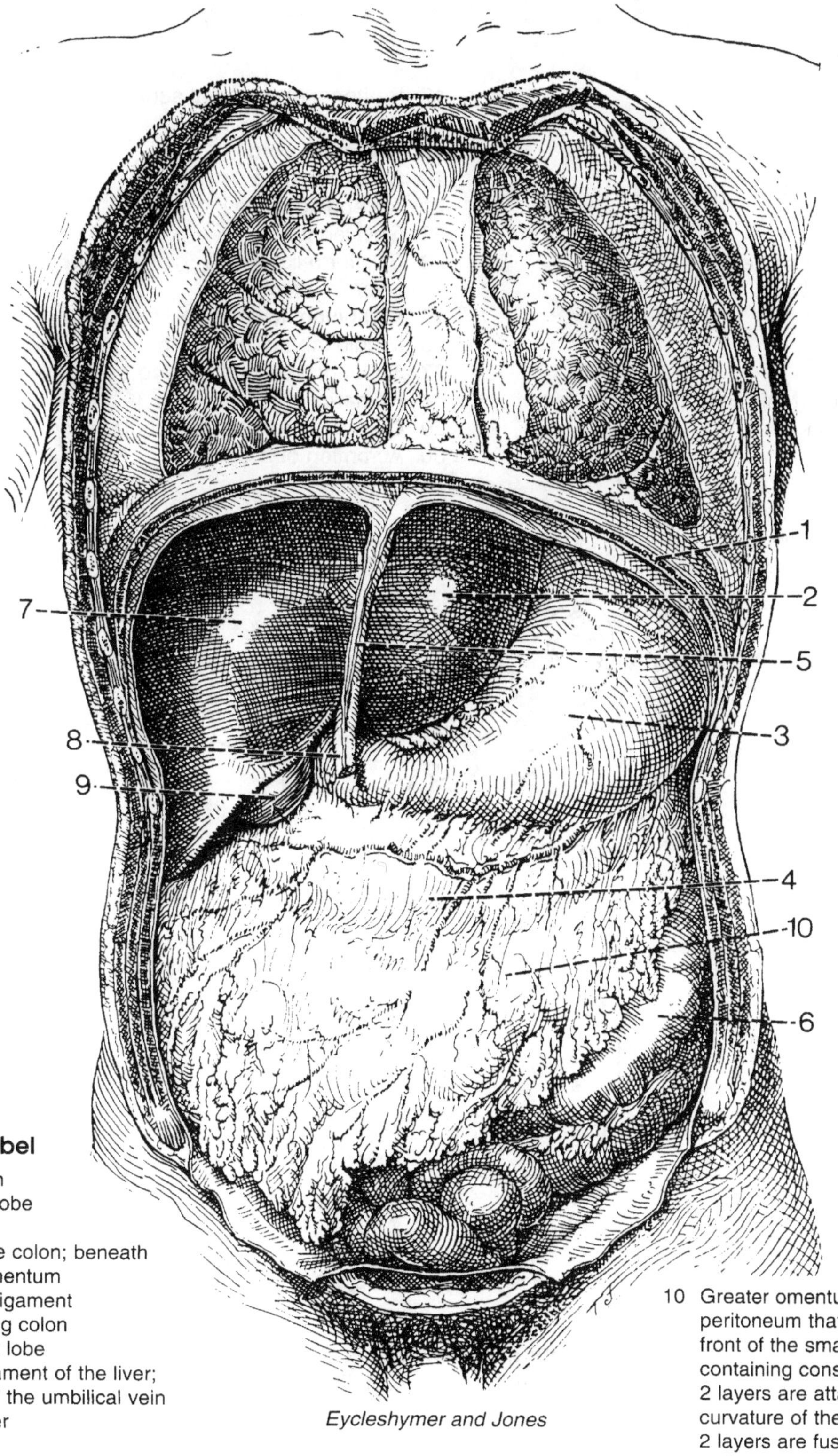

Eycleshymer and Jones

Color and label

1 Diaphragm
2 Liver; left lobe
3 Stomach
4 Transverse colon; beneath greater omentum
5 Falciform ligament
6 Descending colon
7 Liver; right lobe
8 Round ligament of the liver; remains of the umbilical vein
9 Gallbladder
10 Greater omentum; a double layer of peritoneum that is folded on itself in front of the small intestine; usually containing considerable fat; the anterior 2 layers are attached to the greater curvature of the stomach; the posterior 2 layers are fused to the transverse colon and mesocolon.

Ab-10 Thorax and abdominal viscera

In relation to the skeleton - Anterior view

(opposite page)

Color and label

1 Trachea
2 Esophagus
3 Left common carotid artery
4 Left subclavian artery
5 Clavicle
6 Manubrium
7 Pericardium covering heart
8 Left lung; lower lobe
9 Diaphragm
10 Spleen
11 Stomach
12 Transverse colon (tenia coli)
13 Descending colon
14 Inguinal ligament
15 Femoral nerve
16 Femoral artery (lateral) and femoral vein (medial)
17 Peritoneum (external surface)
18 Bladder
19 Spermatic cord
20 Small intestine
21 Ascending colon
22 Gallbladder
23 Falciform ligament
24 Liver (right lobe)
25 Right lung; lower lobe
26 Middle lobe of right lung
27 Superior lobe of right lung
28 Humerus
29 Coracoid process of scapula
30 Acromion of scapula
31 Clavicle

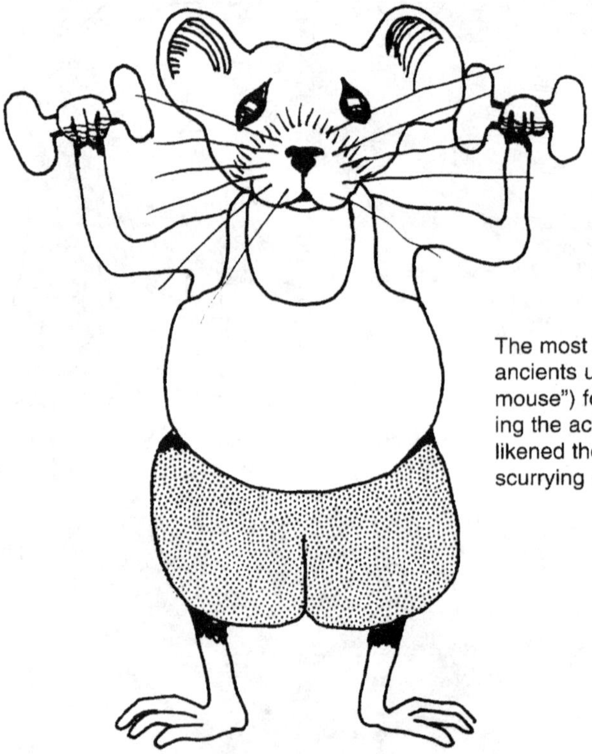

The most likely explanation of why the ancients used the term *musculus* ("little mouse") for muscles is that, not knowing the actual function of muscles, they likened their contraction to little mice scurrying under the skin.

The word **muscle** originally meant "little mouse" (Latin, *mus*, mouse; *musculus*, little mouse)

Ab-10 Thorax and abdominal viscera

In relation to the skeleton

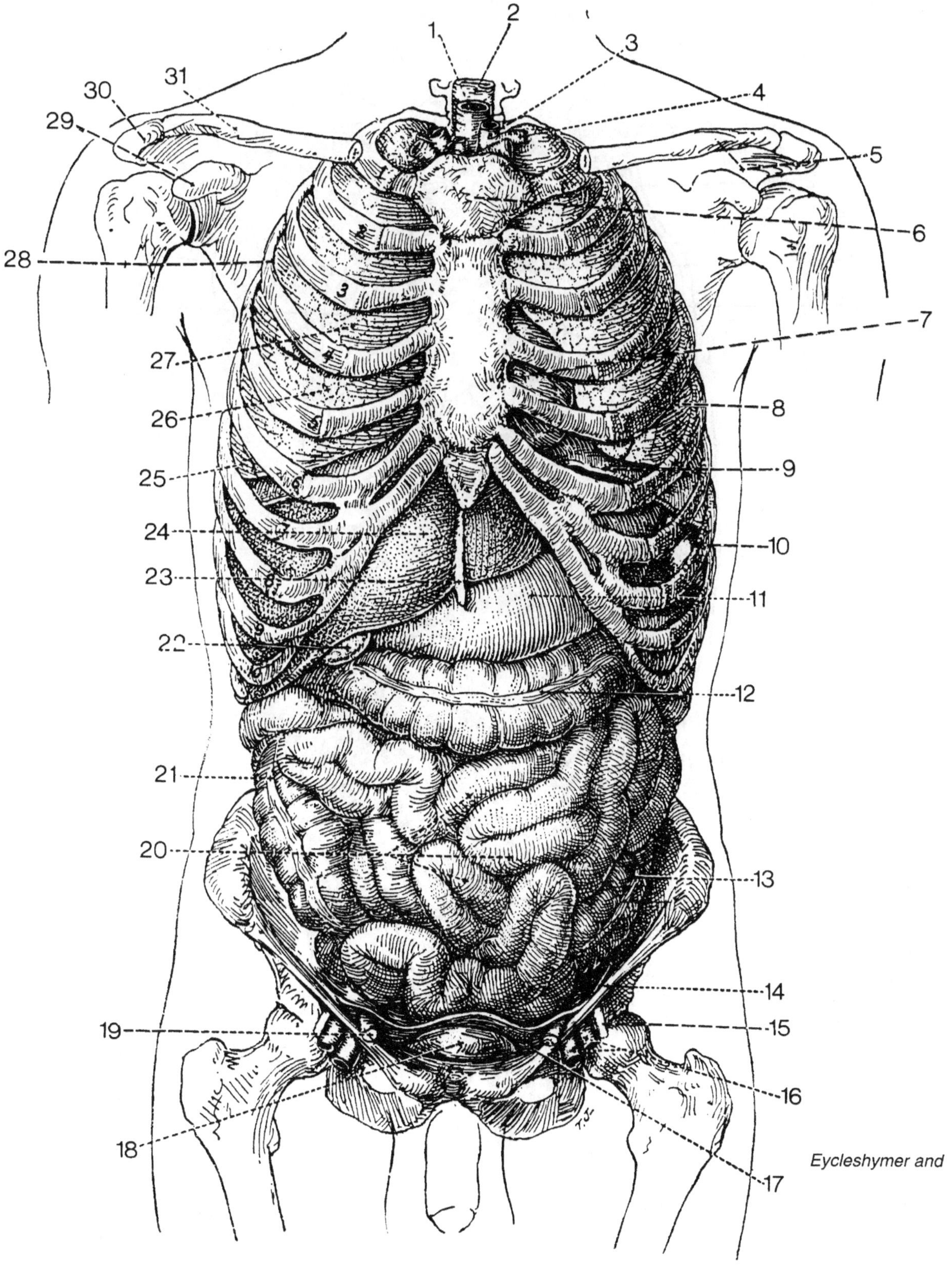

Eycleshymer and Jones

Ab-11 Frontal (coronal) section of the trunk

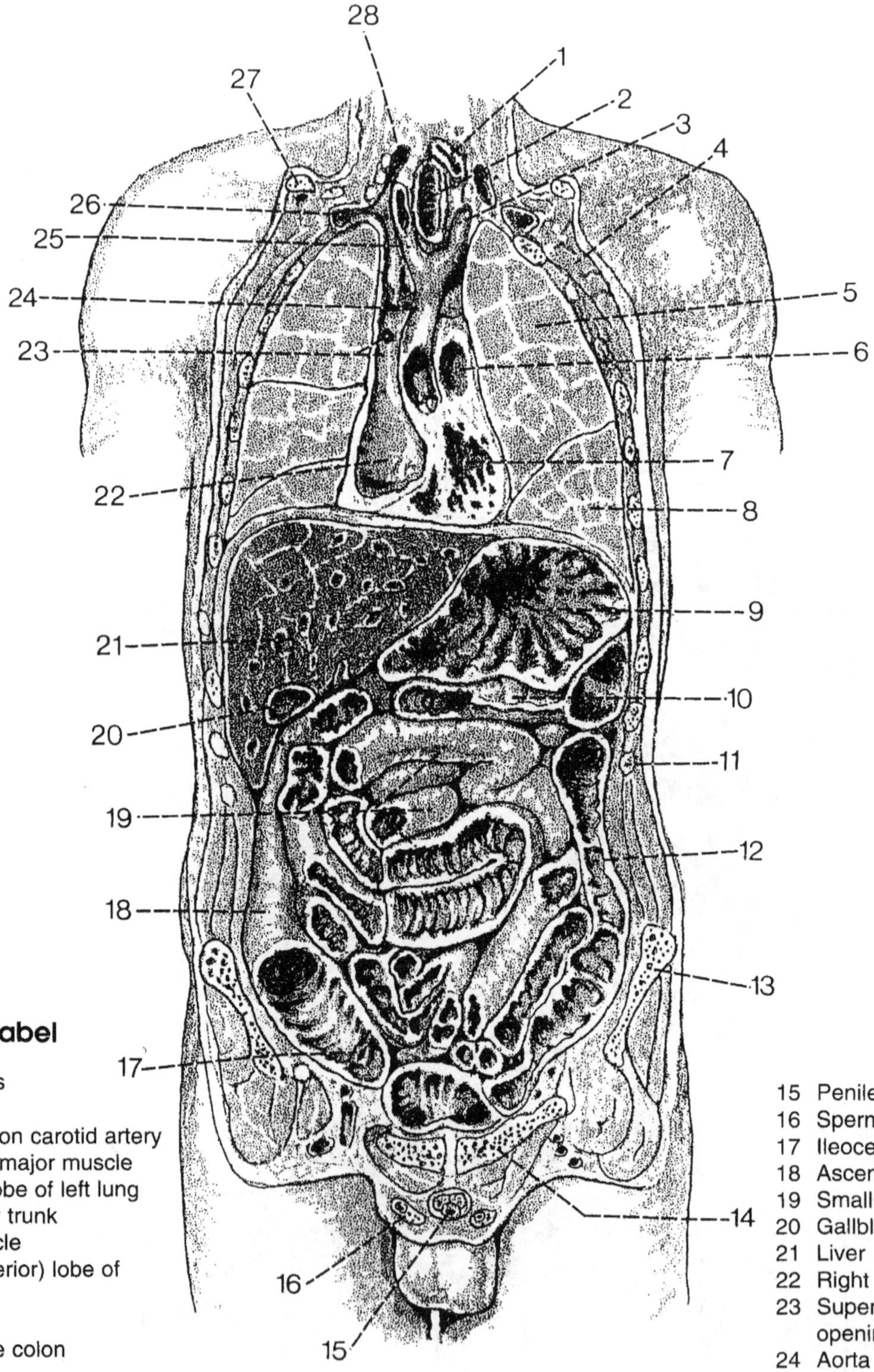

Redrawn and modified from Eycleshymer and Jones

Color and label

1 Esophagus
2 Trachea
3 Left common carotid artery
4 Pectoralis major muscle
5 Superior lobe of left lung
6 Pulmonary trunk
7 Left ventricle
8 Lower (inferior) lobe of left lung
9 Stomach
10 Transverse colon
11 Rib 10
12 Descending colon
13 Ilium
14 Pubis
15 Penile (spongy) urethra
16 Spermatic cord
17 Ileocecal valve
18 Ascending colon
19 Small intestine
20 Gallbladder
21 Liver
22 Right atrium
23 Superior vena cava with opening of azygos vein
24 Aorta (ascending)
25 Brachiocephalic artery
26 Subclavian vein
27 Clavicle (cut)
28 Internal jugular vein

Ab-12 Thoracic and abdominal viscera

Left aspect

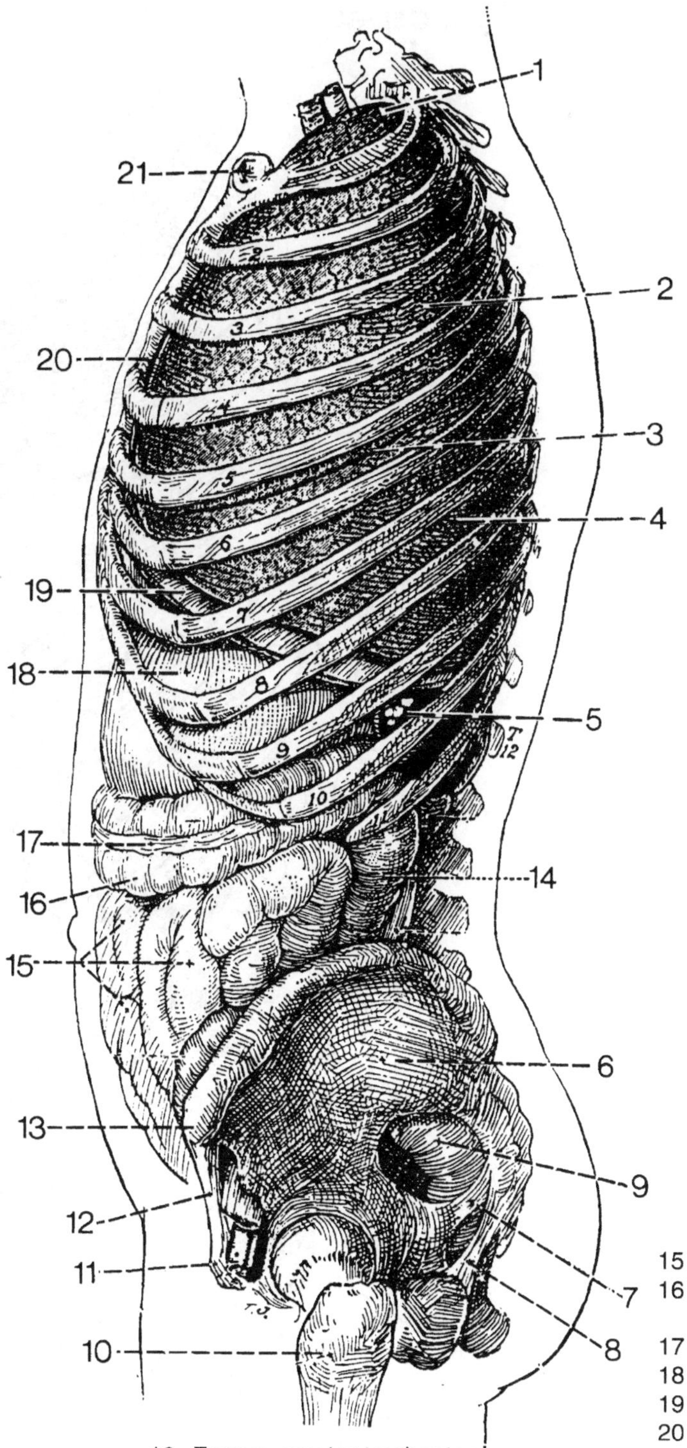

Eycleshymer and Jones

Color and label

1 Apex
2 Upper lobe of lung
3 Oblique fissure
4 Lower lobe of lung
5 Spleen
6 Ilium
7 Sacrospinous ligament
8 Sacrotuberous ligament
9 Rectum (viewed through greater sciatic foramen)
10 Femur; greater trochanter
11 Pubic tubercle
12 Inguinal ligament
13 Anterior superior iliac spine
14 Descending colon
15 Small intestine
16 Saccules (haustra) of transverse colon
17 Tenia coli
18 Stomach
19 Diaphragm
20 Sternum
21 Manubrium; clavicular notch

Ab-13 Thoracic and abdominal viscera

Right aspect

Color and label

1 Cervical vertebra 7
2 Apex of right lung
3 Upper lobe of right lung
4 Middle lobe
5 Oblique fissure
6 Lower lobe
7 Gallbladder
8 Stomach
9 Transverse colon
10 Small intestine
11 Anterior superior iliac spine
12 Femur; greater trochanter
13 Ischial tuberosity
14 External anal sphincter
15 Sacrotuberous ligament
16 Sacrospinous ligament
17 Ilium
18 Ascending colon; tenia coli
19 Right kidney
20 Head of femur
21 Liver
22 Diaphragm
23 Horizontal fissure

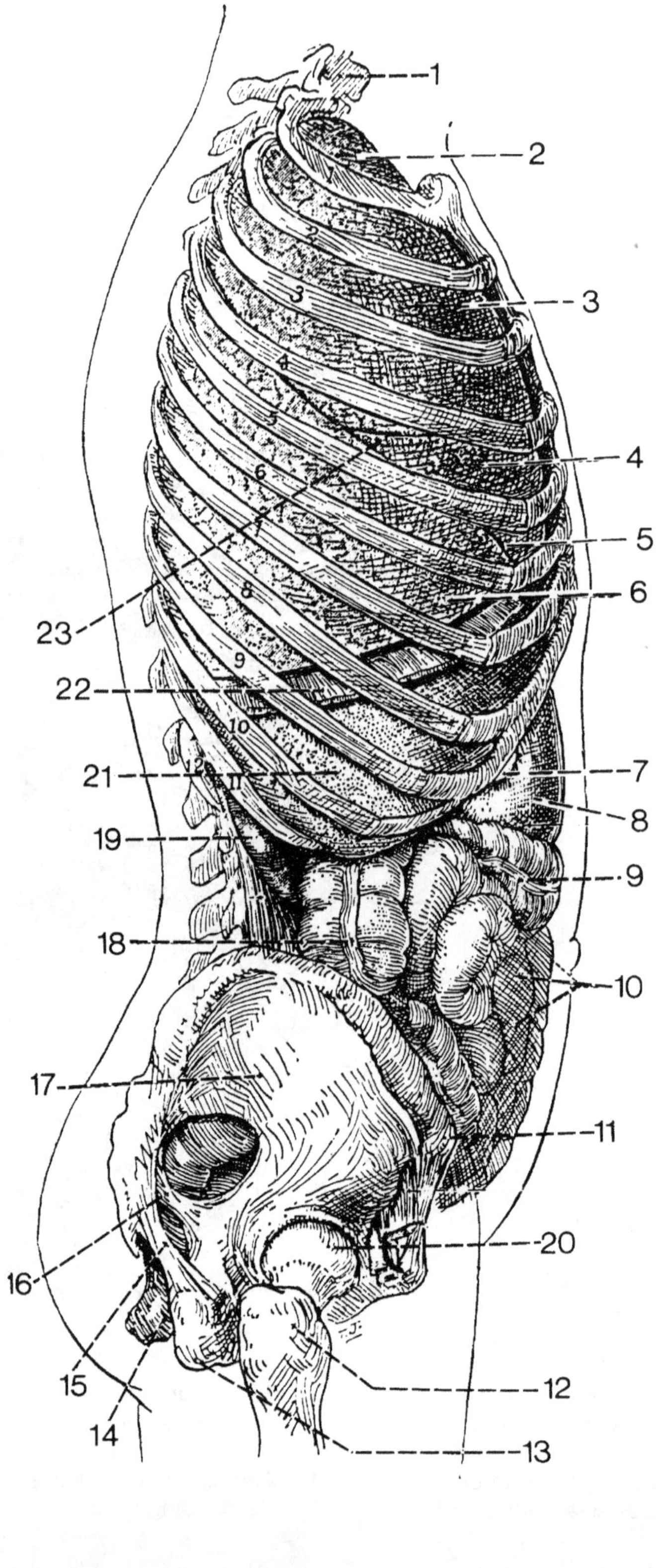

Ab-14 Thoracic and abdominal viscera

In relation to the skeleton — Posterior view

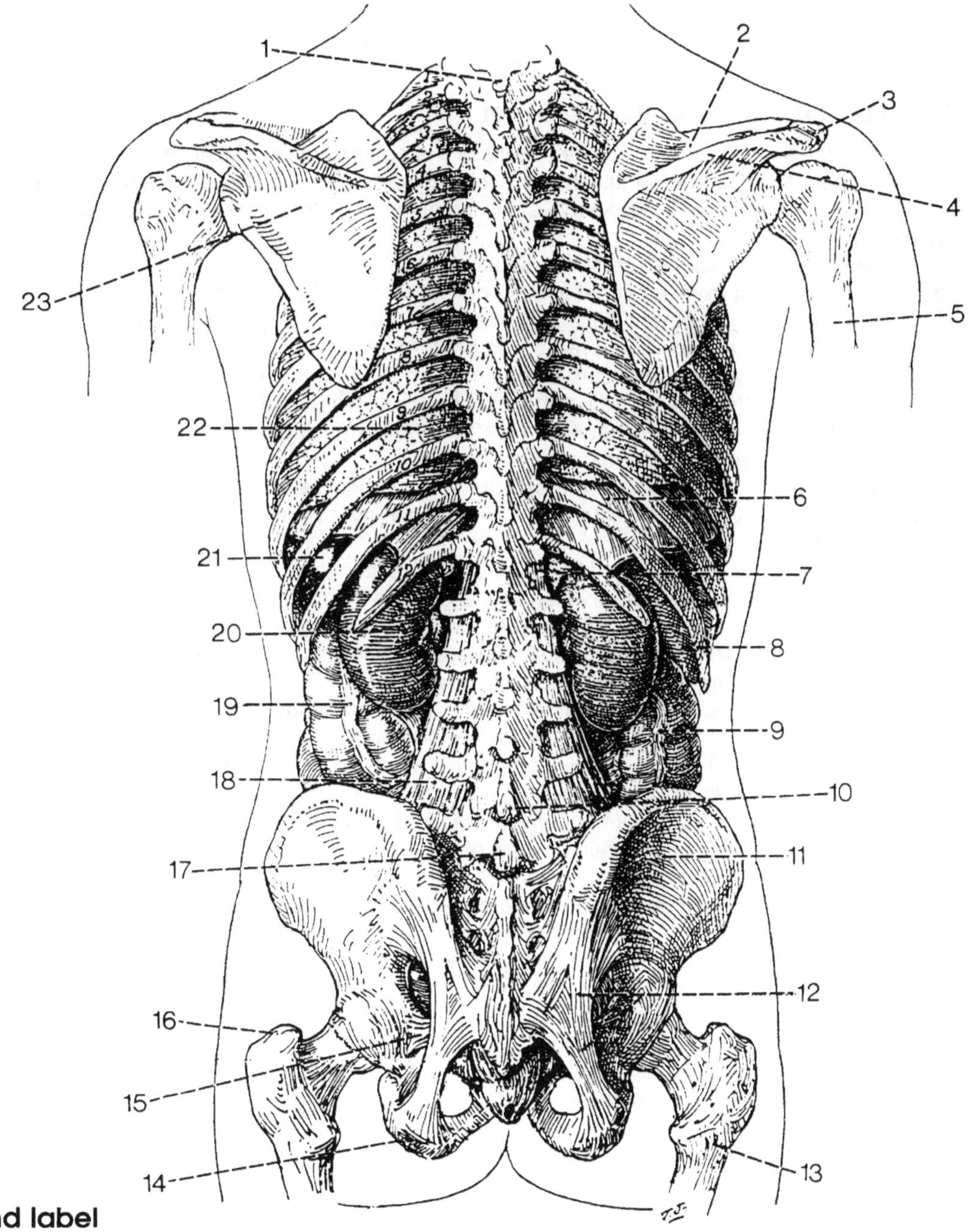

Color and label

1 Thoracic vertebra 1
2 Scapula (supraspinous fossa)
3 Acromion
4 Spine of scapula
5 Humerus
6 Diaphragm
7 Adrenal gland
8 Liver
9 Ascending colon
10 Fifth lumbar vertebra spinous process
11 Ilium of coxal (hip) bone
12 Sacrospinous ligament
13 Femur
14 Ischial tuberosity
15 Sacrospinous ligament
16 Greater trochanter
17 Median sacral crest (fused spinous processes)
18 Psoas major muscle
19 Tenia coli of descending colon
20 Left kidney
21 Spleen
22 Left lung; lower lung
23 Infraspinous fossa of scapula

Ab-15 Midsagittal section of the female peritoneal cavity

(opposite page)

Trace the lining and covering of the peritoneum

1 Parietal peritoneum; lines the inner surface of the walls of the abdominopelvic cavity; the free surface of the peritoneum is lined with a single layer of flattened mesothelial cells that secrete serous fluid that allows the peritoneal-covered organs, such as the stomach, small intestines, and transverse colon, to freely slide against each other.
2 Peritoneum (parietal) lining inferior surface of the diaphragm
3 Peritoneum (visceral) covering the liver; its reflection (folding) from the liver on to the inferior surface of the diaphragm forms the **coronary ligament,** which attaches the liver to the diaphragm. The **bare area** of the liver is that portion of the liver surface not covered with peritoneum.
4 Lesser omentum; a double layer of peritoneum extending from the liver to the lesser curvature of the stomach; it forms part of the anterior wall of the lesser bursa (lesser sac).
5 Peritoneum (visceral); forming the outermost layer (serosa) of the stomach; the stomach, like the liver, is almost completely covered with peritoneum.
6 Greater omentum; anterior layer; note that the greater omentum consists of a double layer of peritoneum that is folded on itself in front of the small intestines; the anterior layer is suspended from the greater curvature of the stomach.
7 Greater omentum; posterior layer; note that the posterior layer ascends and adheres to the transverse colon and the anterior layer of the transverse mesocolon. In early embryonic development, a cavity is present between the anterior and posterior layers of the greater omentum as indicated in the accompanying illustration. However, in late pregnancy this cavity is obliterated below the level of the transverse colon as the layers fuse, the internal layers of mesothelium disappear, and fat is deposited in the greater omentum.
8 Transverse mesocolon; the mesentery of the large intestine is called the **mesocolon**. Like the mesentery of the small intestine, it is a double layer of peritoneum. Here it attaches the transverse colon to the posterior abdominal wall. It contains blood vessels, nerves, lymph nodes, and lymphatic vessels that supply the transverse colon, and varying amounts of fat. Unlike the ascending and descending colon, which are both fused to the posterior abdominal wall and have no mesocolon, the transverse meso colon gives the transverse colon has a certain amount of mobility.
9 Peritoneum (parietal) lining the posterior abdominal wall; here covering the pancreas; organs such as the kidneys, which lie behind the peritoneum, or are covered with peritoneum only on their anterior surface such as the pancreas, are considered to be **retroperitoneal**.
10 Mesentery; this is a double layer of peritoneum with connective tissue support that attaches the major part of the small intestines (the jejunum and ileum) to the posterior abdominal wall. It contains a rich network of blood vessels, nerves, lymph nodes, and lymph vessels (here called lacteals).
11 Serosal layer of peritoneum on the small intestine
12 Peritoneum covering anterior surface of the duodenum; this part of the duodenum is retroperitoneal.
13 Peritoneum (parietal) on posterior abdominal wall
14 Peritoneum covering the uterus (tunica serosa, perimetrium)
15 Omental bursa (lesser sac); this is the peritoneal-enclosed space behind the liver and stomach (indicated by the vertical arrow).
16 Omental foramen (epiploic foramen, foramen of Winslow); connects the omental bursa with the remainder of the peritoneal cavity.
17 Rectouterine pouch (excavatio rectouterine, pouch of Douglas)
18 Vesicouterine pouch (excavatio vesicouterina)

Ab-15 Midsagittal section of the female peritoneal cavity

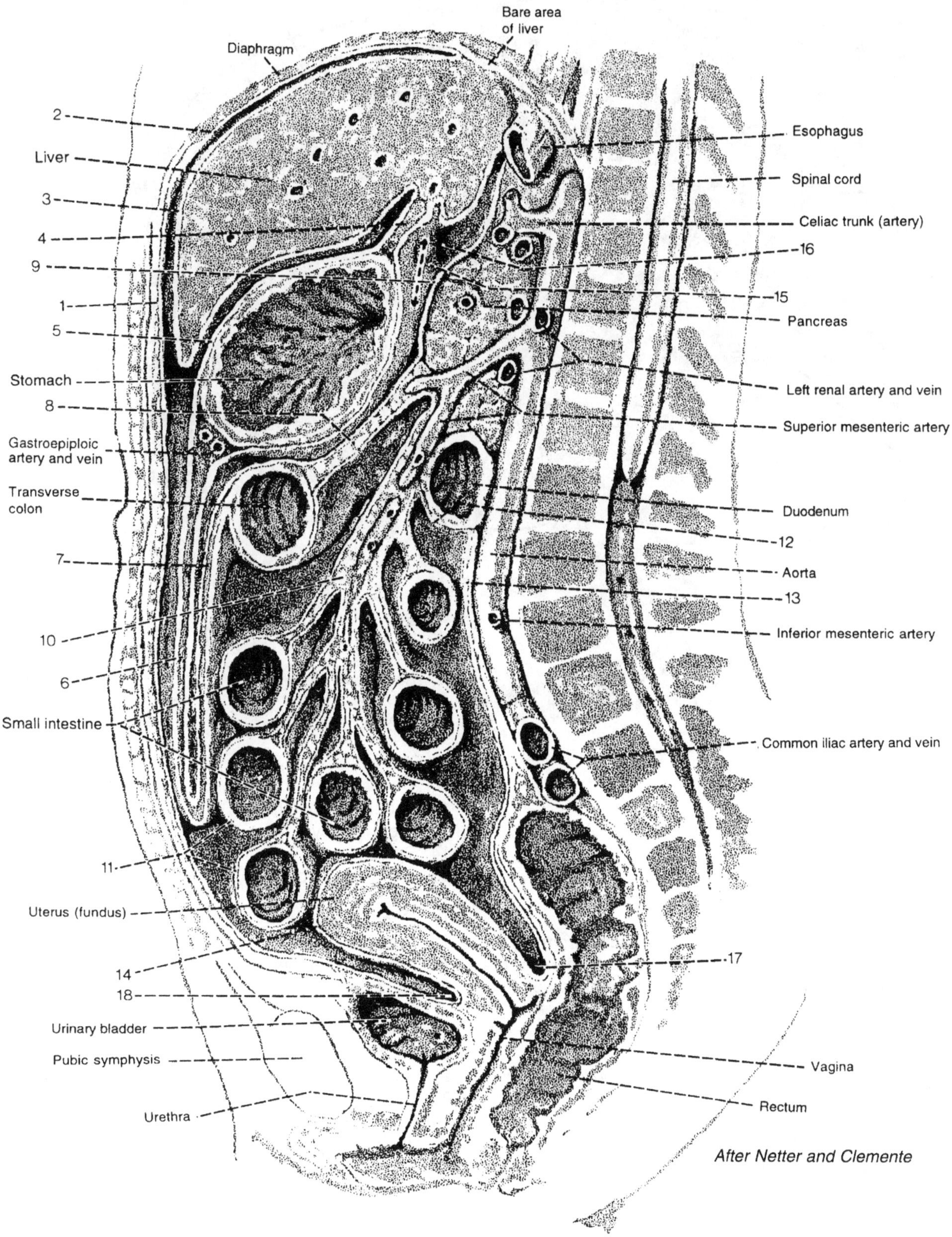

After Netter and Clemente

Ab-16 The stomach

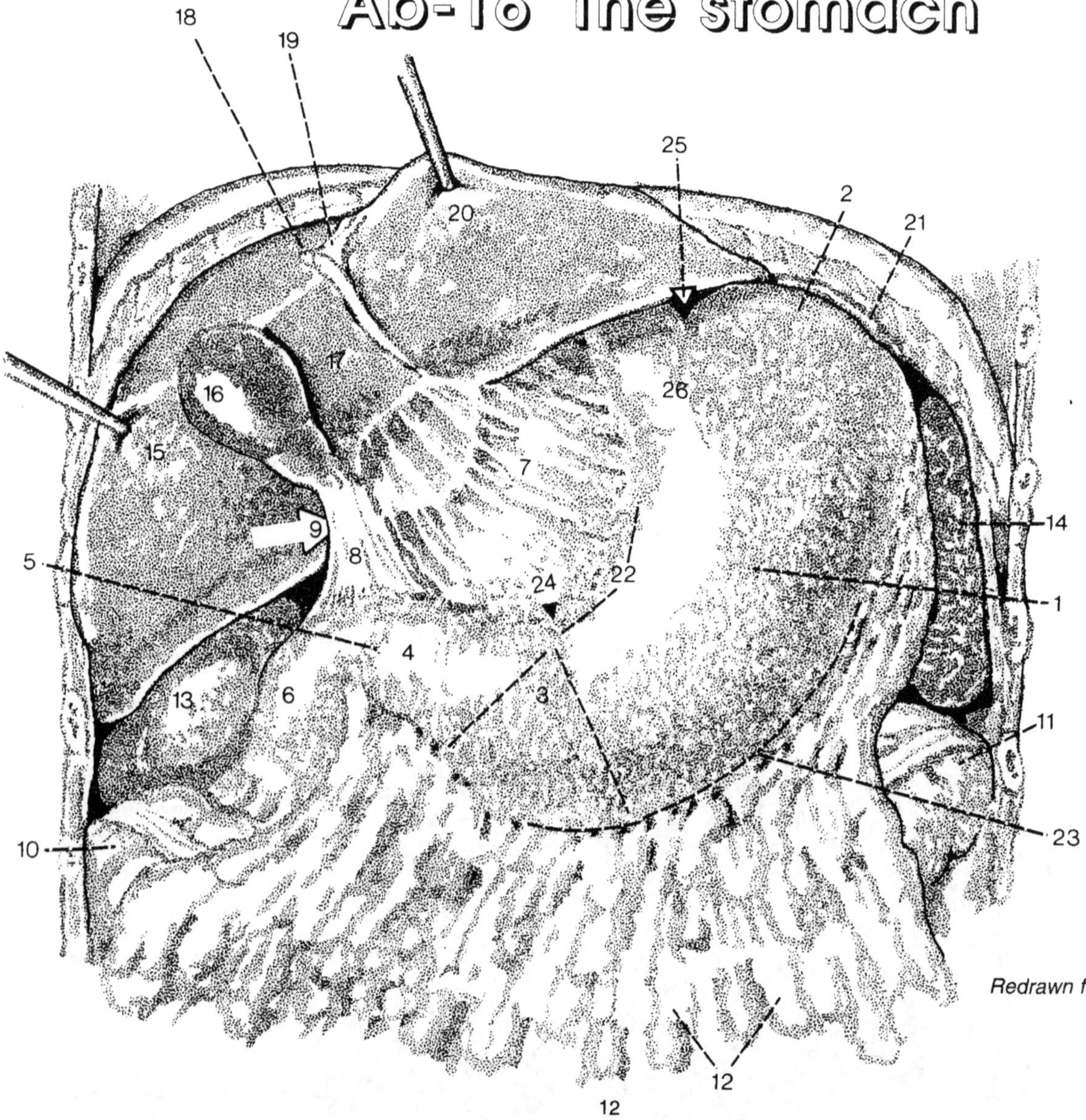

Redrawn from Netter

Color and label

1 Stomach (body, corpus)
2 Stomach (fundus)
3 Stomach (pyloric antrum)
4 Stomach (pyloric canal)
5 Stomach (pyloric sphincter)
6 Duodenum
7 Lesser omentum; peritoneum extending from the liver to the lesser curvature of stomach; this part of the lesser omentum is also called the hepatogastric ligament.
8 Hepatoduodenal ligament; part of the lesser omentum; consists of peritoneum surrounding the common bile duct, the proper hepatic artery, and the portal vein.
9 Arrow in omental foramen (former names: epiploic foramen, foramen of Winslow)
10 Right (hepatic) flexture of colon
11 Left (splenic) flexture of colon
12 Greater omentum
13 Right kidney
14 Spleen
15 Liver; right lobe
16 Gallbladder
17 Liver; quadrate lobe
18 Round ligament of the liver; remnant of umbilical vein
19 Falciform ligament
20 Liver; left lobe
21 Diaphragm
22 Lesser curvature of stomach
23 Greater curvature of stomach
24 Angular incisure (notch, indentation) of stomach
25 Cardiac incisure of stomach
26 Cardiac part of stomach; pars cardiaca gastris; an area 3-4 cm wide that surrounds and includes the esophageal opening (cardiac orifice) into the stomach.

Ab-17 Blood supply of the stomach

Color and label

1 Abdominal aorta
2 Celiac trunk; a very short artery that immediately divides into 3 branches; it is the sole source of arterial blood to the stomach.
3 Common hepatic artery
4 Proper hepatic artery
5 Right gastric artery; note its origin from the proper hepatic artery
6 Gastroduodenal artery
7 Superior pancreaticoduodenal arteries (anterior and posterior); these supply both the head of the pancreas (not shown) and the upper duodenum.
8 Left gastric artery
9 Esophageal branch of left gastric artery
10 Splenic artery (posterior to stomach)
11 Short gastric arteries
12 Left gastro-epiploic artery (its new name is gastro-omental artery)
13 Spleen
14 Esophagus
15 Right gastro-omental (gastro-epiploic) artery

Note the anastomoses between the right and left gastric arteries as well as between the right and left gastroepiploic arteries.

After Hollinshead and Rosse

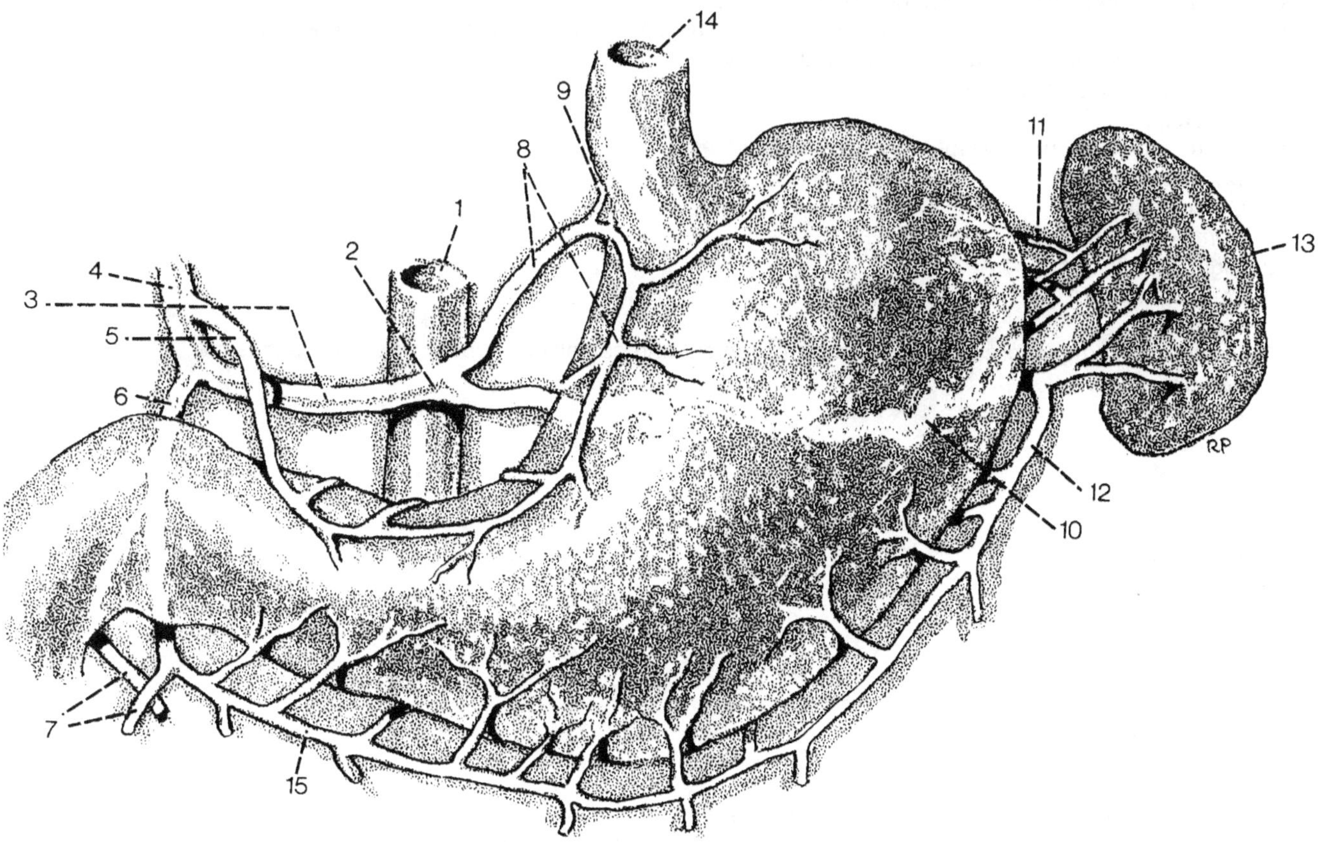

Ab-18 Stomach, duodenum, and pancreas

(opposite page)

Color and label

1 Esophagus
2 Cardiac orifice and cardiac region of stomach
3 Fundus of stomach; left dome-shaped part of stomach superior to horizontal plane X—X; usually filled with air.
4 Body of stomach
5 Pyloric antrum
6 Pyloric canal
7 Pyloric opening
8 Pyloric sphincter (*pylorus*, Greek for gatekeeper)
9 Duodenum; first or superior part, "duodenal bulb"
10 Duodenum; second or descending part
11 Duodenum; third or horizontal part
12 Duodenum; fourth or ascending part
13 Probe in greater duodenal papilla; opening for common bile duct and pancreatic duct; these 2 ducts may unite and end as a single duct or they may end as 2 very close but separate ducts within the papilla.
14 Lesser duodenal papilla; opening of accesssory pancreatic duct
15 Pancreatic duct; the head of the pancreas, which "nestles" into the C-shape of the duodenum, has been partially removed to reveal the 2 pancreatic ducts.
16 Accessory pancreatic duct
17 Pancreas
18 Circular folds of duodenal mucosa (plicae circulares)*
19 Common bile duct
20 Cystic duct
21 Common hepatic duct
22 Right hepatic duct
23 Left hepatic duct
24 Gallbladder
25 Gastric folds (rugae, plicae, ridges); these flatten out and partially disappear when stomach is full and distended.
26 Aorta
27 Celiac trunk
28 Left gastric artery
29 Splenic artery
30 Common bile duct
31 Proper hepatic artery
32 Left hepatic artery
33 Right hepatic artery
34 Middle hepatic artery
35 Right gastric artery
36 Gastroduodenal artery
37 Superior mesenteric vein
38 Superior mesenteric artery

* Plicae circulares: circular folds of mucous membrane which project into the lumen of the small intestine whether it is empty or distended. They may extend partly or totally around the circumference of the lumen. They first appear in the second part of the duodenum. They are most numerous in the proximal half of the jejunum, after which they decrease in both size and in number so that they are absent in the end of the ileum. They were formerly called valves of Kerckring. Churchill's Illustrated Medical Dictionary, New York, Churchill Livingstone, 1989.

Ab-18 Stomach, duodenum, and pancreas

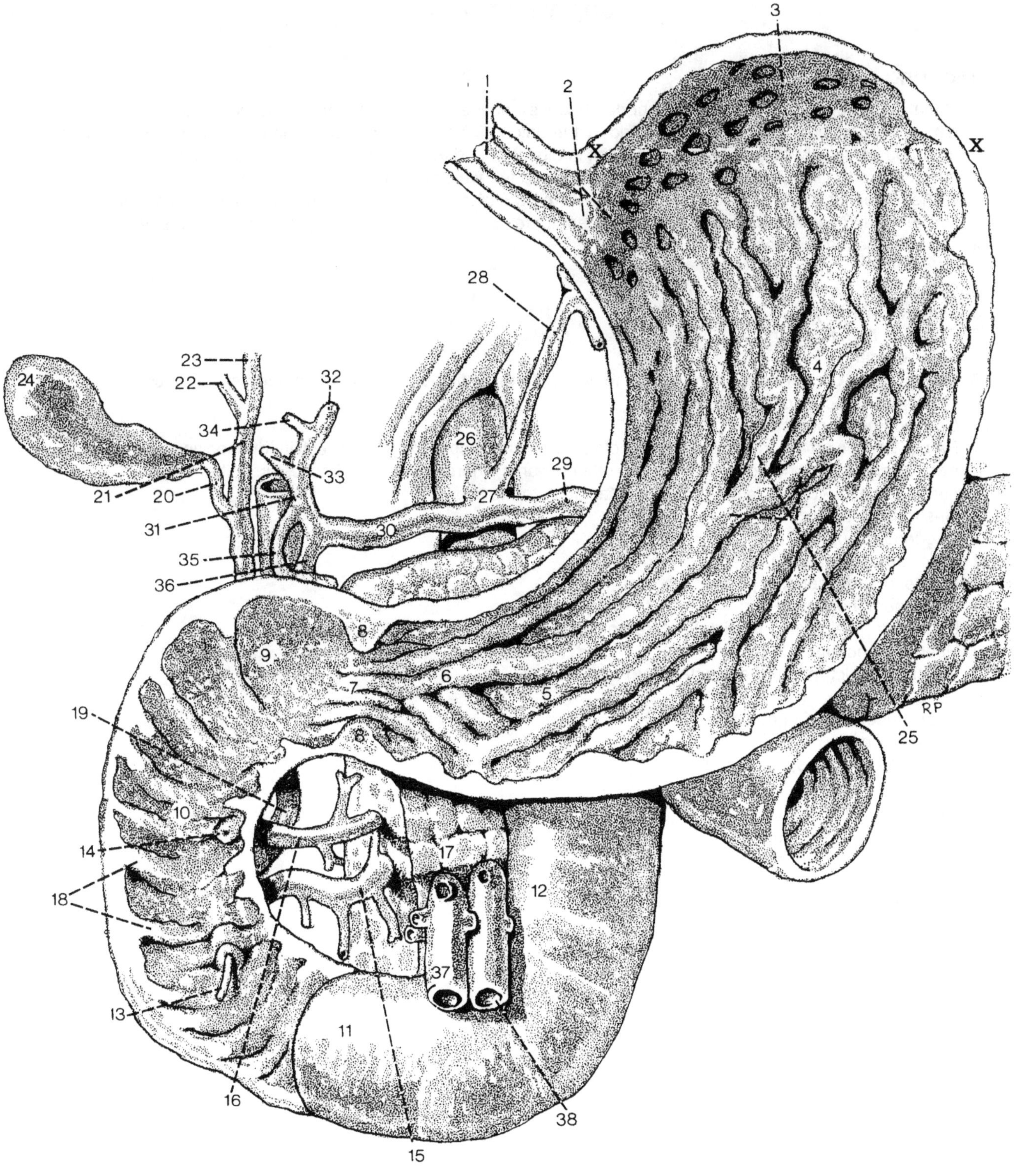

Ab-19 Pancreas, duodenum, and spleen

Stomach has been removed and the liver raised (opposite page)

Color and label

1 Portal vein (hepatic portal vein, vena portae hepatis); notice that the portal vein is rather large in diameter but short in length, being formed by the union of the superior mesenteric vein and the splenic vein. It carries practically all the venous blood rich in digested and absorbed food from the stomach and intestines to the liver, with the exception of absorbed fat, which is conveyed by the lymphatic vessels to one of the large veins in the neck. The spleen sends products from the breakdown of red blood cells to the liver. Unlike regular veins, the hepatic portal vein terminates in the liver by dividing into smaller and smaller veins.
2 Superior mesenteric vein
3 Splenic vein
4 Celiac trunk (celiac artery)
5 Left gastric artery
6 Common hepatic artery
7 Splenic artery
8 Common bile duct; note it is formed by the union of the cystic duct and the common hepatic duct.
9 Cystic duct (duct of gallbladder)
10 Common hepatic duct
11 Proper hepatic artery; in anatomic terminology, the word proper implies exclusivity or specifically "its own" artery, that is, not to be shared with other organs; whereas *common* implies, in spite of its name, *hepatic*—it goes to other organs in addition to the liver
12 Gastroduodenal artery
13 Duodenum; superior part
14 Major duodenal papilla
15 Duodenum; descending part
16 Duodenum; horizontal part
17 Beginning of jejunum; just distal (nearer to the anus) to the duodenojejunal flexture
18 Head of pancreas
19 Pancreatic duct (partially dissected free)
20 Tail of pancreas
21 Liver (underside of right lobe)
22 Cystic artery
23 Gallbladder (fundus)
24 Inferior vena cava
25 Abdominal aorta
26 Adrenal (suprarenal) gland
27 Splenic artery and vein
28 Spleen
29 Left kidney
30 Superior mesenteric artery
31 Right kidney

Ab-19 Pancreas, duodenum, and spleen

Stomach has been removed and the liver raised

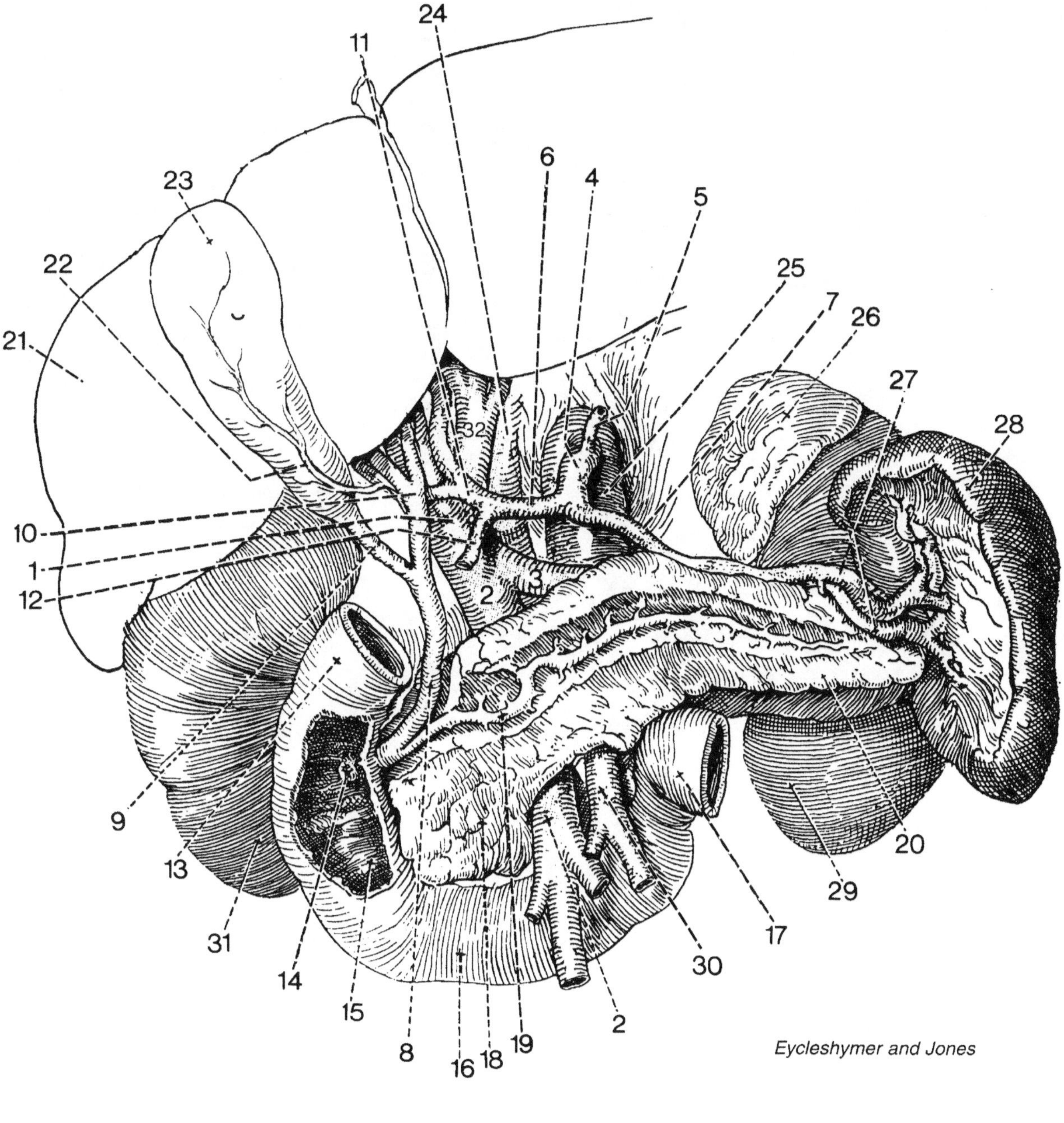

Eycleshymer and Jones

Some Latin anatomic terms

1 Tibia means a flute or pipe as well as the shinbone. The ancients probably made flutelike instruments from the shinbones of animals.

2 Fenestra is Latin for window. Fenstrated means to contain little windows, as in fenestrated capillaries.

3 Crista galli is Latin for cock's comb and is the name of the bony ridge at the top of the ethmoid bone.

4 Rostrum means a beak or snout, or a ship's prow. The speaker's platform in the forum was decorated with the prows of ships captured in battle. Rostral means toward the nose.

5 Alveolus is Latin for a little hollow or bucket and is the diminutive of alveus, which could mean a trough, boat, hold of a ship, bathtub, bed of a stream, beehive, or gaming table.

6 Pecten is Latin for comb. Pectinate means comb-like. The pectinate muscles in the heart suggested a comb to earlier anatomists.

7 Putamen is Latin for "that which falls off with paring," such as a husk or a shell. The putamen is a mass of nerve cells in the brain in the shape of a shell.

8 Speculum is Latin for mirror. A speculum in medicine is an instrument with which a physician can examine passages and the interior of the body.

9 Acetabulum is the bony socket of the hip joint. It is derived from *acetum*, vinegar, and probably *poculum*, cup; hence, it means vinegar cup.

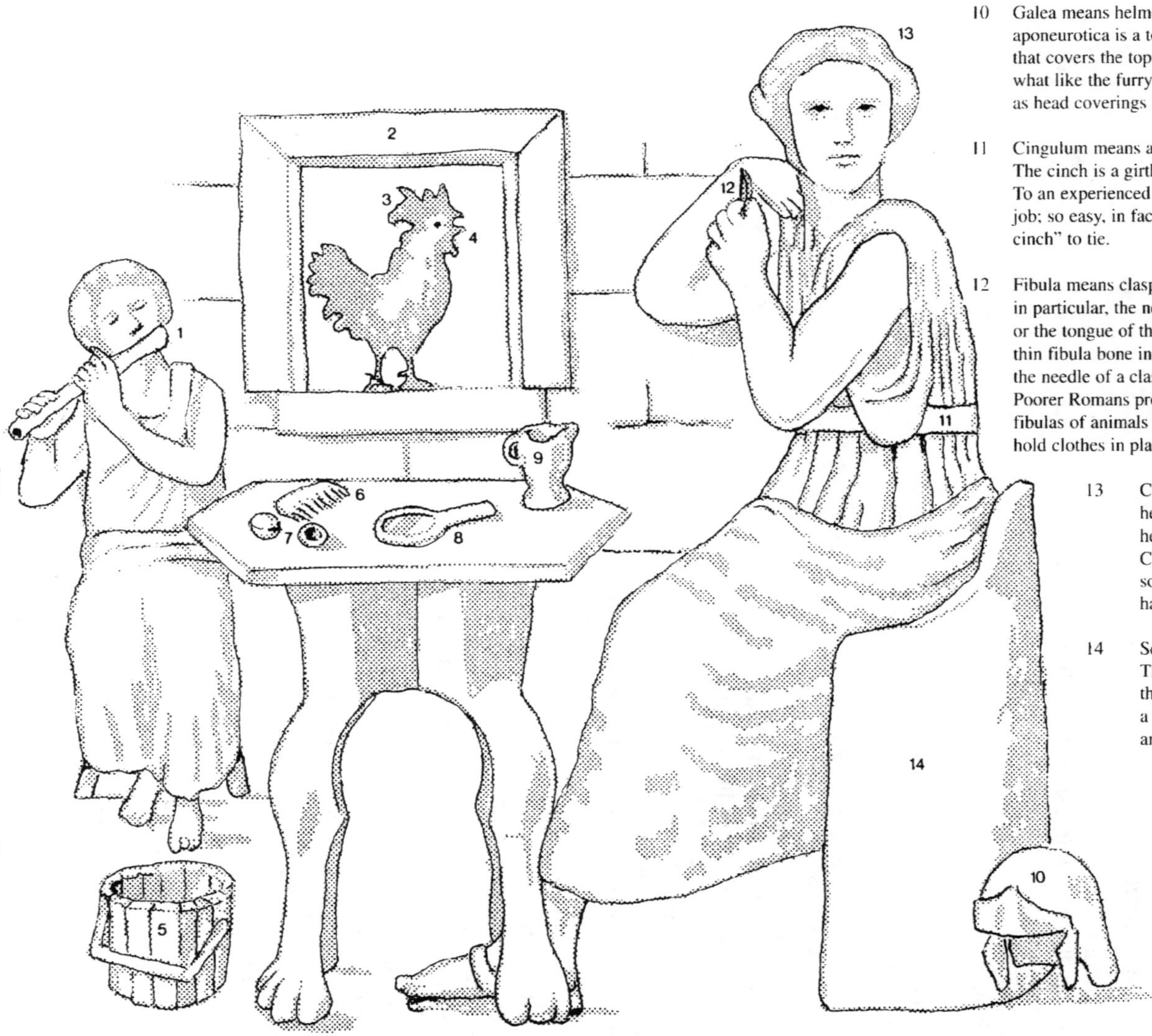

10 Galea means helmet. The galea aponeurotica is a tough membrane that covers the top of the skull somewhat like the furry animal skins used as head coverings by ancient soldiers.

11 Cingulum means a girdle or sword belt. The cinch is a girth or a saddle or pack. To an experienced hand it was an easy job; so easy, in fact, that "it was a cinch" to tie.

12 Fibula means clasp, brooch, or buckle; in particular, the needle of the clasp or the tongue of the buckle. The long, thin fibula bone in the leg resembled the needle of a clasp to the Romans. Poorer Romans probably used the fibulas of animals as straight pins to hold clothes in place.

13 Capillus is Latin for hair of the head, being derived from *caput*, head, and *pilus*, hair. Capillaries are blood vessels so thin they were likened to the hair of the head.

14 Sella means a chair or stool. The sella turcica, which houses the pituitary gland, suggested a Turkish saddle to the ancient anatomists.

Ab-20 Celiac trunk and its branches

(opposite page)

Color and label

1 Gallbladder
2 Fundus of stomach (most of stomach removed)
3 Spleen
4 Duodenum
5 Jejunum
6 Pancreas
7 Celiac trunk
8 Left gastric artery
9 Splenic artery
10 Common hepatic artery
11 Proper hepatic artery
12 Right gastric artery (cut)
13 Right branch of proper hepatic artery
14 Middle branch of proper hepatic artery
15 Left branch of proper hepatic artery
16 Supraduodenal artery
17 Gastroduodenal artery
18 Anterior superior pancreaticoduodenal artery
19 Posterior superior pancreaticoduodenal artery
20 Dorsal pancreatic artery
21 Great pancreatic artery
22 Artery of tail of pancreas
23 Short gastric artery
24 Left gastro-epiploic (gastro-omental) artery
25 Inferior pancreatic artery
26 Inferior phrenic artery
27 Inferior pancreaticoduodenal artery
28 Posterior inferior pancreaticoduodenal artery
29 Anterior inferior pancreaticoduodenal artery
30 Right gastro-epiploic (gastro-omental) artery
31 Cystic artery
32 Common bile duct
33 Cystic duct
34 Common hepatic duct
35 Portal vein
36 Superior mesenteric vein
37 Superior mesenteric artery
38 Middle colic artery
39 Cut edge of transverse mesocolon and dorsal layer of greater omentum
40 Cut edge of root of mesentery

Ab-20 Celiac trunk and its branches

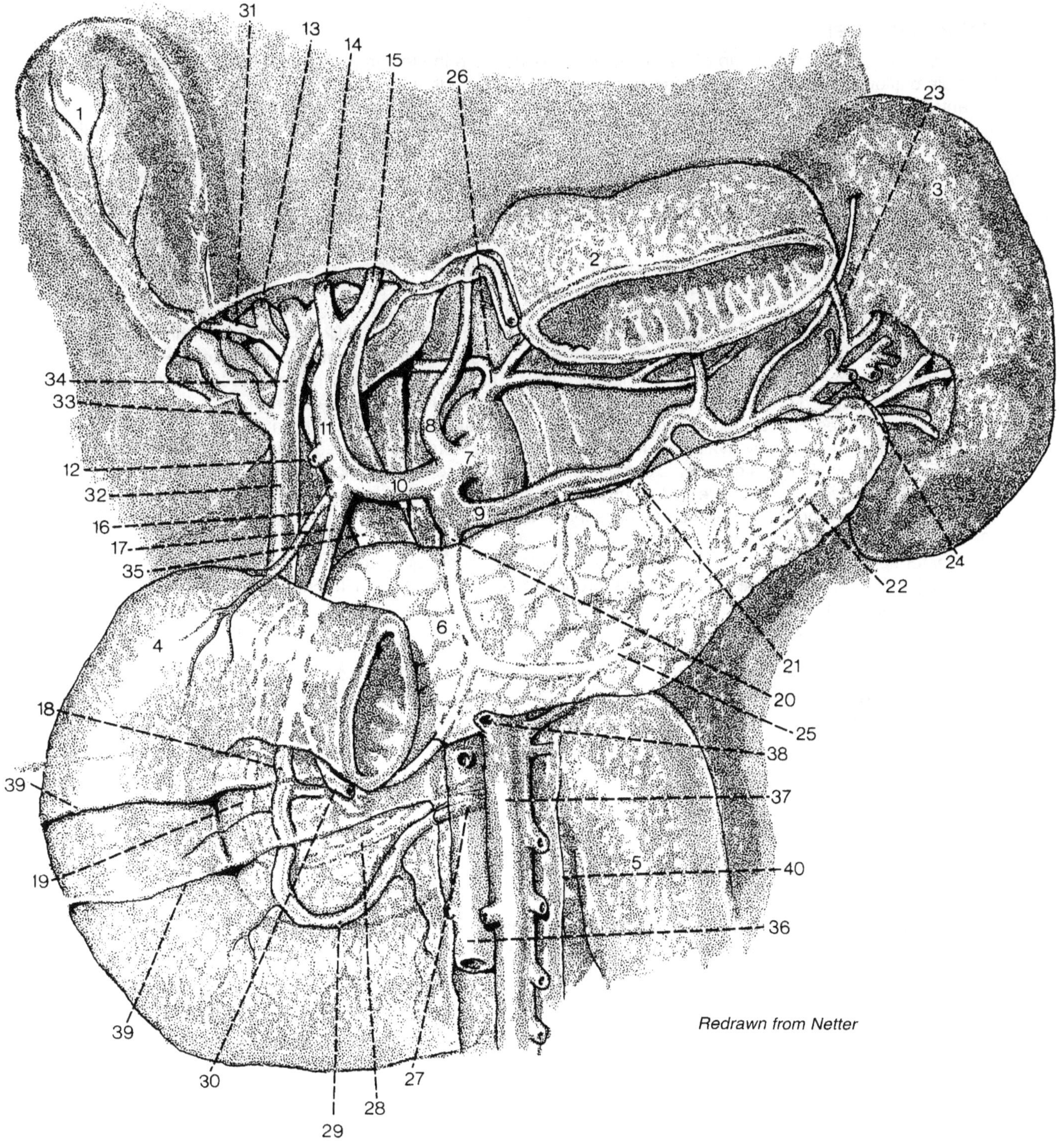

Redrawn from Netter

Ab-21 Nerve supply of the stomach

(opposite page)

Color and label

1 Anterior vagal trunk; made up of mainly nerve fibers from the the left vagus nerve. The vagus nerve is the main outflow of the **parasympathetic nervous system**. Note that it enters the abdomen as 2 trunks, an anterior and a posterior, the latter formed mainly by the right vagus nerve, both closely applied to the esophagus. It consists of preganglionic parasympathetic fibers headed to postganglionic neurons within the walls of the stomach and intestines, which in turn will send their axons to digestive glands and smooth muscle of the alimentary tract. Vagal stimulation causes secretion of the gastric glands and motility (peristalsis) of the musculature in the walls of the stomach.
2 Hepatic branch of anterior vagal trunk; note that it lies between the two layers of peritoneum that comprise the lesser omentum.
3 Celiac branch of posterior vagal trunk. Here parasympathetic fibers from the vagus nerve intermingle with, and subsequently travel with, sympathetic neurons as part of the celiac plexus.
4 Celiac ganglia. Note that these 2 ganglia lie on the aorta on either side of the (arterial) celiac trunk. These ganglia contain postganglionic **sympathetic** neuron cell bodies. Unlike vagal fibers, which stimulate the digestive glands to secrete and promote peristalsis, the sympathetic fibers arising from these ganglia have an inhibitory effect on the digestive tract. These postganglionic neurons receive preganglionic sympathetic fibers by way of the thoracic greater splanchnic nerves (7) and also from some lumbar splanchnic nerves. Stimulation of sympathetic fibers to the liver causes breakdown of glycogen to glucose, thus affording more readily available energy to the body as would be required during physical exertion.
5 Aorticorenal ganglion; postganglionic sympathetic neurons receive preganglionic fibers from the lesser thoracic splanchnic nerve and in turn send their fibers to the kidney where they have the effect of inhibiting the production of urine and conserving water.
6 Superior mesenteric ganglion
7 Greater splanchnic nerve. These fibers arise from preganglionic sympathetic cell bodies at levels T5-T9 in the thoracic spinal cord and pass through the diaphragm to end in the celiac ganglia.
8 Lesser splanchnic nerve
9 Greater anterior gastric nerve
10 Vagal branch to pylorus via hepatic plexus
11 Plexus on left gastric artery
12 Plexus on splenic artery
13 Plexus on common hepatic artery
14 Hepatic plexus
15 Plexus on gastro-epiploic artery
16 Superior mesenteric plexus
17 Lesser omentum, anterior leaf
18 Right crus of diaphragm
19 Inferior vena cava
20 Aorta and subphrenic arteries on underside of diaphragm

The autonomic nerve fibers, such as those derived from the vagus nerve and the celiac ganglia, are extremely thin and difficult to find by gross dissection.

Ab-21 Nerve supply of the stomach

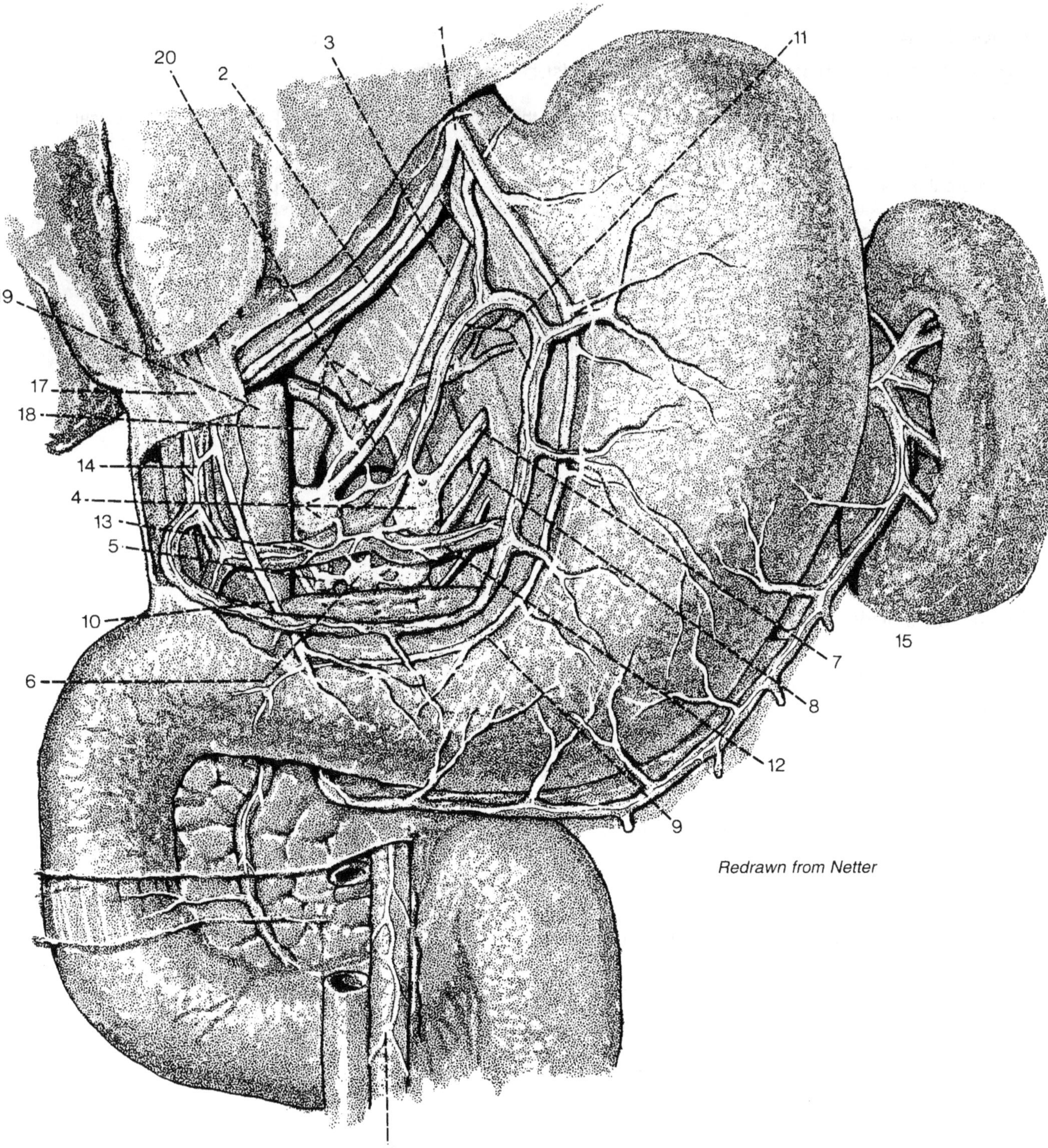

Redrawn from Netter

Ab-22 The liver (hepar)

(opposite page)

Color and label

Figure A. Diaphragmatic surface (anterior/superior surface)

1 Round ligament of the liver; intra-abdominal portion of the obliterated umbilical vein. This part of the umbilical vein extends from the umbilicus to the liver where it forms a fissure on the underside of the liver. During fetal life the umbilical vein conveyed oxygenated blood and nutrients from the mother's placenta to the fetal liver where the major portion of its blood flowed into the ductus venosus, which in turn emptied directly into the inferior vena. Although nonfunctional after birth, the lumen of the round ligament persists and may be used to inject substances directly into the liver.
2 Falciform ligament (sickle-shaped, *falx*, Latin, a sickle or scythe). The round ligament forms its inferior border.
3 Anterior leaf (peritoneal reflection) of coronary ligament extending from right lobe of liver to the diaphragm; also called upper layer of coronary ligament.
4 Left coronary ligament extending from left lobe of liver to the diaphram; on the left lobe, the anterior and posterior layers tend to fuse into a single layer (see figure B below)
5 Right triangular ligament
6 Left triangular ligament
7 Fibrous hepatic annex; this may contain liver tissue.
8 Right lobe* of liver
9 Left lobe* of liver
10 Fundus of gallbladder
11 Bare area of the liver; not covered by peritoneum and adhering to diaphragm by areolar tissue

Figure B. Posterior surface of liver

1 Falciform ligament
2 Anterior (or superior layer) of right coronary ligament
3 Right triangular ligament
4 Left triangular ligament
5 Fibrous hepatic annex
6 Bare area of liver
7 Inferior vena cava; notice that it is held firmly against the liver in a deep groove by the ligament of the inferior vena cava (13), which surrounds it posteriorly, and also by the 3 hepatic veins that empty into it.
8 Left lobe*
9 Right lobe*
10 Caudate lobe; the caudate lobe is so named not because it is more caudal than the quadrate lobe, which it is actually superior to, but rather because it has a tail-like extension or *cauda* (Latin, tail).
11 Right hepatic vein emptying into the inferior vena cava
12 Esophageal impression
13 Ligament of inferior vena; may contain liver tissue.

*The long-held anatomical description of the liver as consisting of 4 lobes was based upon its gross appearance. However, this designation of 4 lobes does not coincide with or accurately relate to the internal distribution of the hepatic veins and the branches of the portal vein.

Ab-22 The liver (hepar)

A

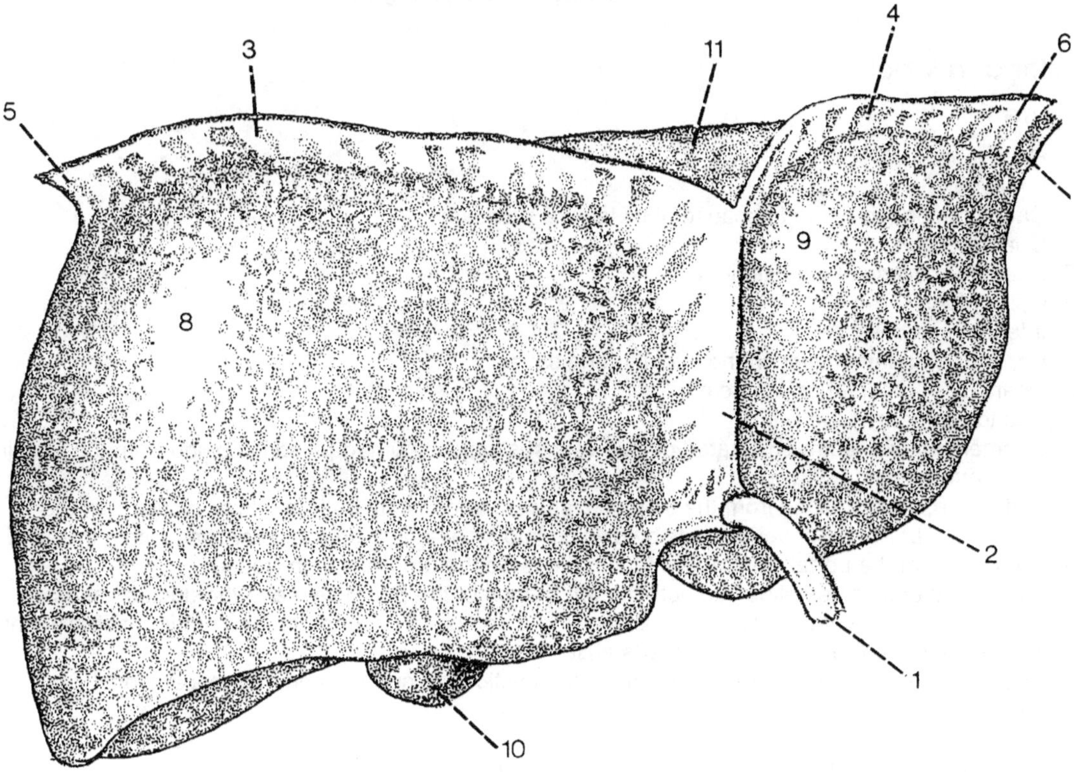

B

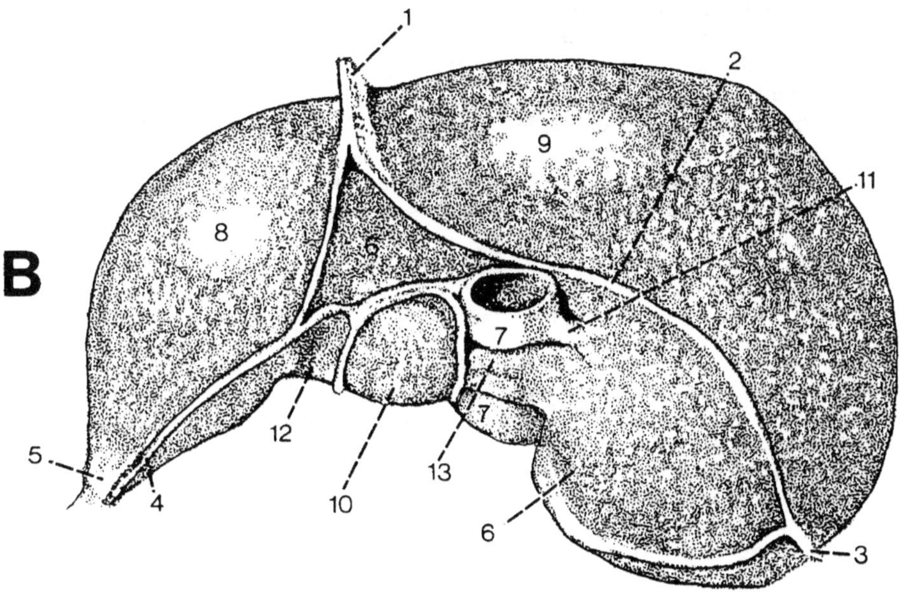

Ab-23 Liver

Visceral (posterior/inferior) surface
(opposite page)

Color and label

Figure A

1 Right lobe
2 Left lobe
3 Caudate lobe (so named because of its tail-like process)
4 Quadrate lobe
5 Caudate process of caudate lobe
6 Gallbladder
7 Inferior vena cava
8 Hepatic veins terminating in the inferior vena cava
9 Ligament of the inferior vena cava
10 Round ligament of the liver
11 Ligamentum venosum; obliterated ductus venosus which shunted placental blood from the umbilical vein to the inferior vena cava.
12 Portal vein; carries blood from the stomach, spleen, and intestines to the liver. Notice that the portal vein, unlike other veins, ends by divding into smaller and smaller branches within the liver.
13 Left branch of the portal vein; notice that in the fetus the umbilical vein (round ligament after birth) empties into both the left branch of the portal vein and the ductus venosus (ligamentum venosum after birth), thus allowing a portion of oxygen-rich and nutrient-rich placental blood to be diverted to the fetal liver as needs arise.
14 Common bile duct; formed by the joining of the cystic duct and the common hepatic duct.
15 Cystic duct
16 Aorta
17 Celiac trunk (actually arising from the **front** of the aorta)
18 Common hepatic artery
19 Proper hepatic artery (*proper* here means "its own"; that is, it supplies just the liver)
20 Right posterior layer of the coronary ligament
21 Left posterior layer of the coronary ligament
22 Right triangular ligament
23 Left triangular ligament
24 Lesser omentum (cut, vertical part, hepatogastric ligament). This extends from the liver to the lesser curvature of the stomach.
25 Lesser omentum (cut, horizontal part, hepatoduodenal ligament); this part contains the portal vein, proper hepatic artery, and the bile ducts between its two layers. It extends from the transverse porta hepatis to the duodenum.

Figure B

1 Right lobe
2 Left lobe
3 Caudate lobe
4 Quadrate lobe
5 Round ligament of the liver
6 Ligamentum venosum
7 Portal vein
8 Left branch of portal vein
9 Inferior vena cava
10 Bare area of liver
11 Porta hepatis (gate of the liver, Latin); this transverse fissure forms the horizontal bar of the H-shape on the visceral surface of the liver. The hepatic ducts, portal vein, and proper hepatic artery pass through it.
12 Proper hepatic artery
13 Hepatic duct
14 Fossa for gallbladder (gallbladder removed)

Ab-23 Liver

(visceral surface)

A

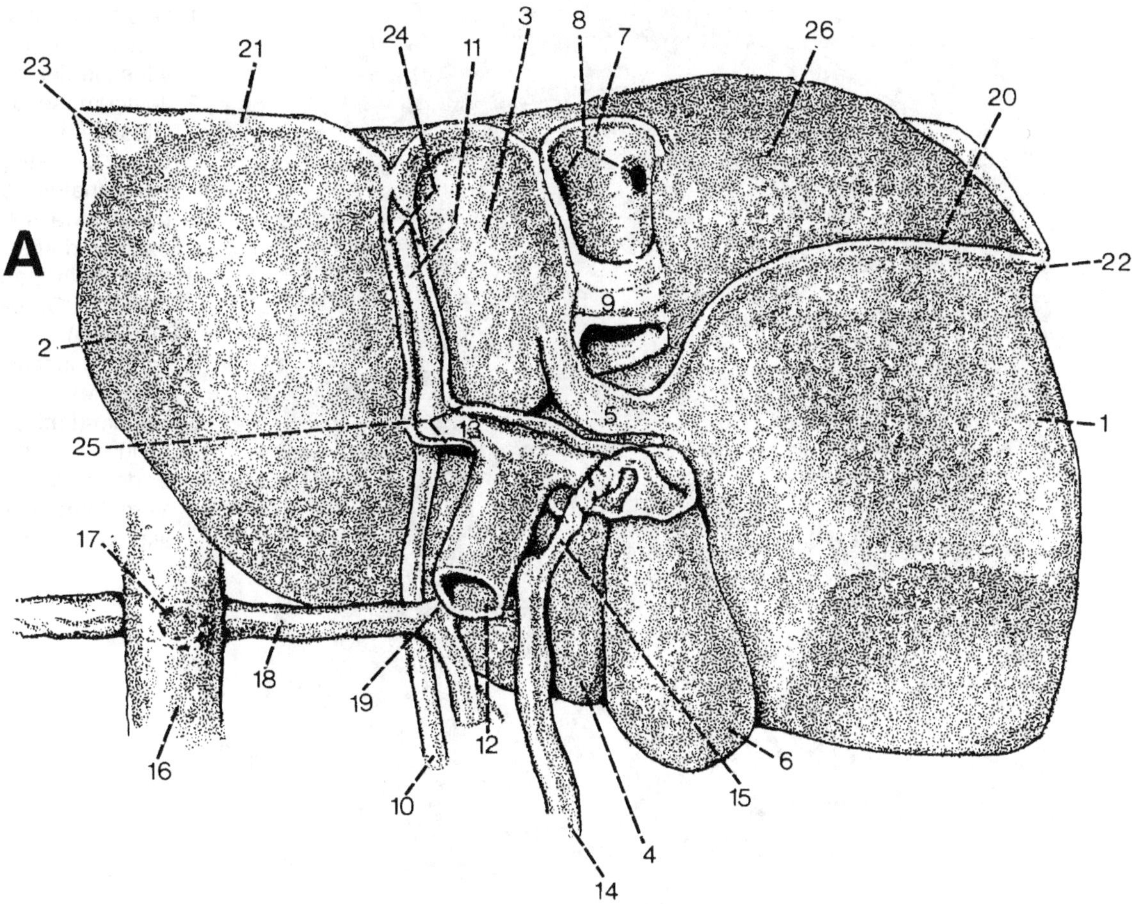

B

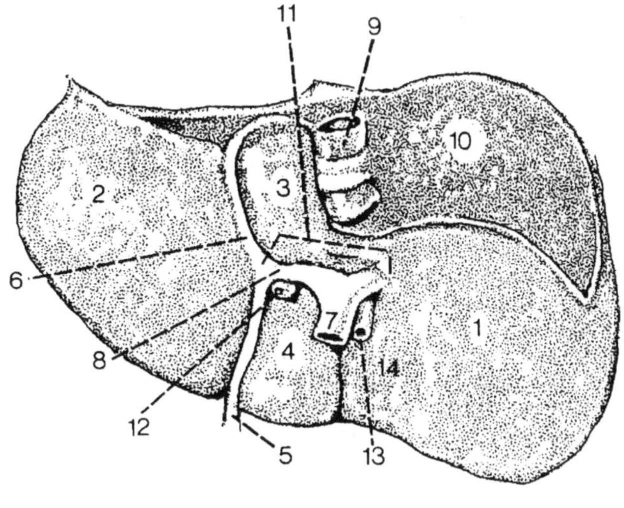

Ab-24A The intestines I

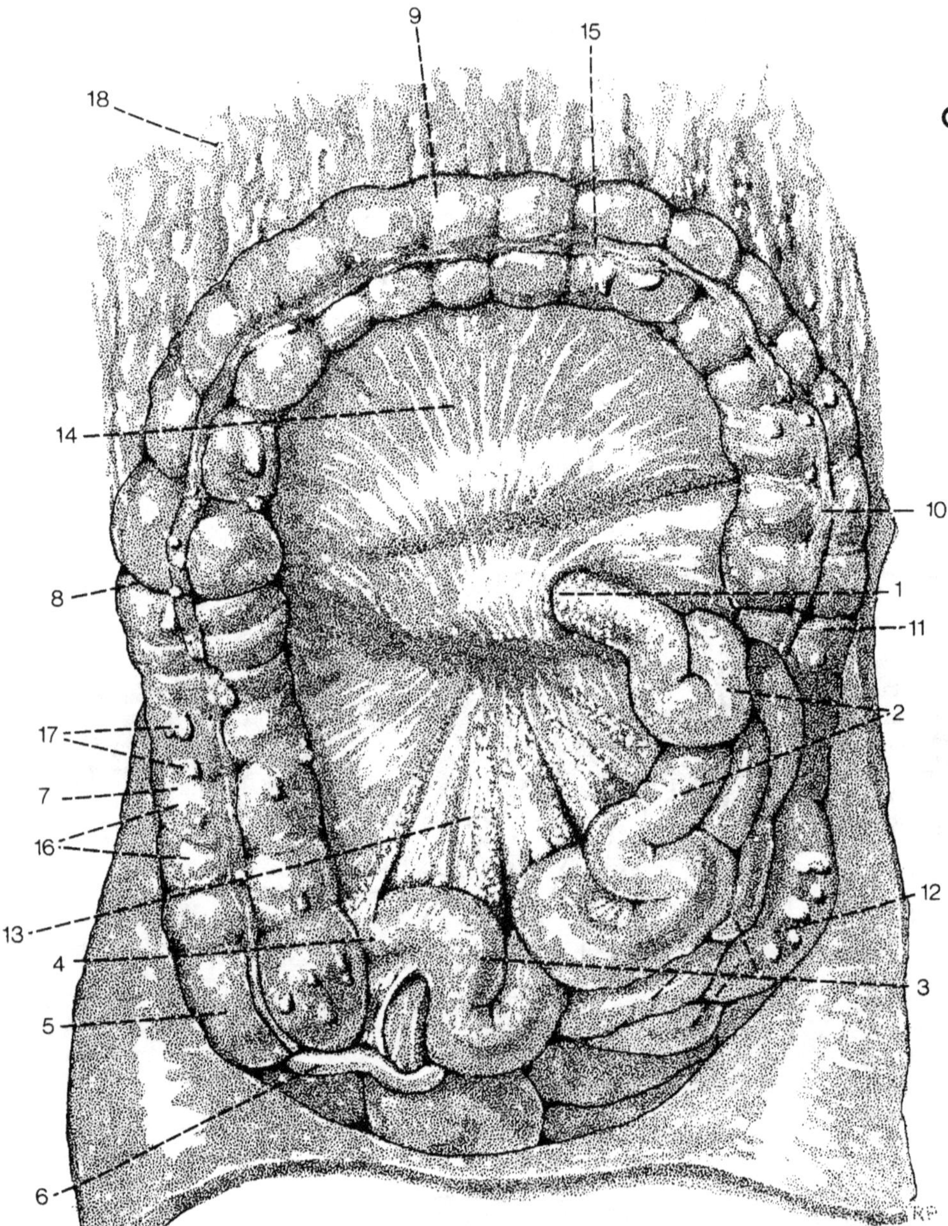

Color and label

1 Duodenojejunal flexure; beginning of mesenteric small intestine (jejunum and ileum)
2 Jejunum (second part of small intestine; Latin, *jejunus*, empty or fasting, from the early anatomists' finding that it was always empty when examined after death)
3 Ileum (third part of small intestine; Greek, *eileo*, to twist or roll up)
4 Ileocolic junction (end of small intestine)
5 Cecum (Latin, *caecus*, blind, as in a blind passageway or dead end)
6 Vermiform appendix (worm-like, Latin, *vermis*, worm)
7 Ascending colon (the large intestine or bowel is also called the colon)
8 Right colic flexture
9 Transverse colon
10 Left colic flexture
11 Descending colon
12 Sigmoid colon (named by its supposed resemblance to the Greek letter sigma)
13 Mesentery; attaches the jejunum and ileum to the posterior abdominal wall.
14 Transverse mesocolon; attaches transverse colon posteriorly.
15 Tenia coli (longitudinal strip of smooth muscle)
16 Haustra coli (outpouchings on colon)
17 Epiploic appendices (new name: omental appendices). These are small fatty appendices unique to the large intestine.
18 Greater omentum (raised up)

Ab-24B The intestines II

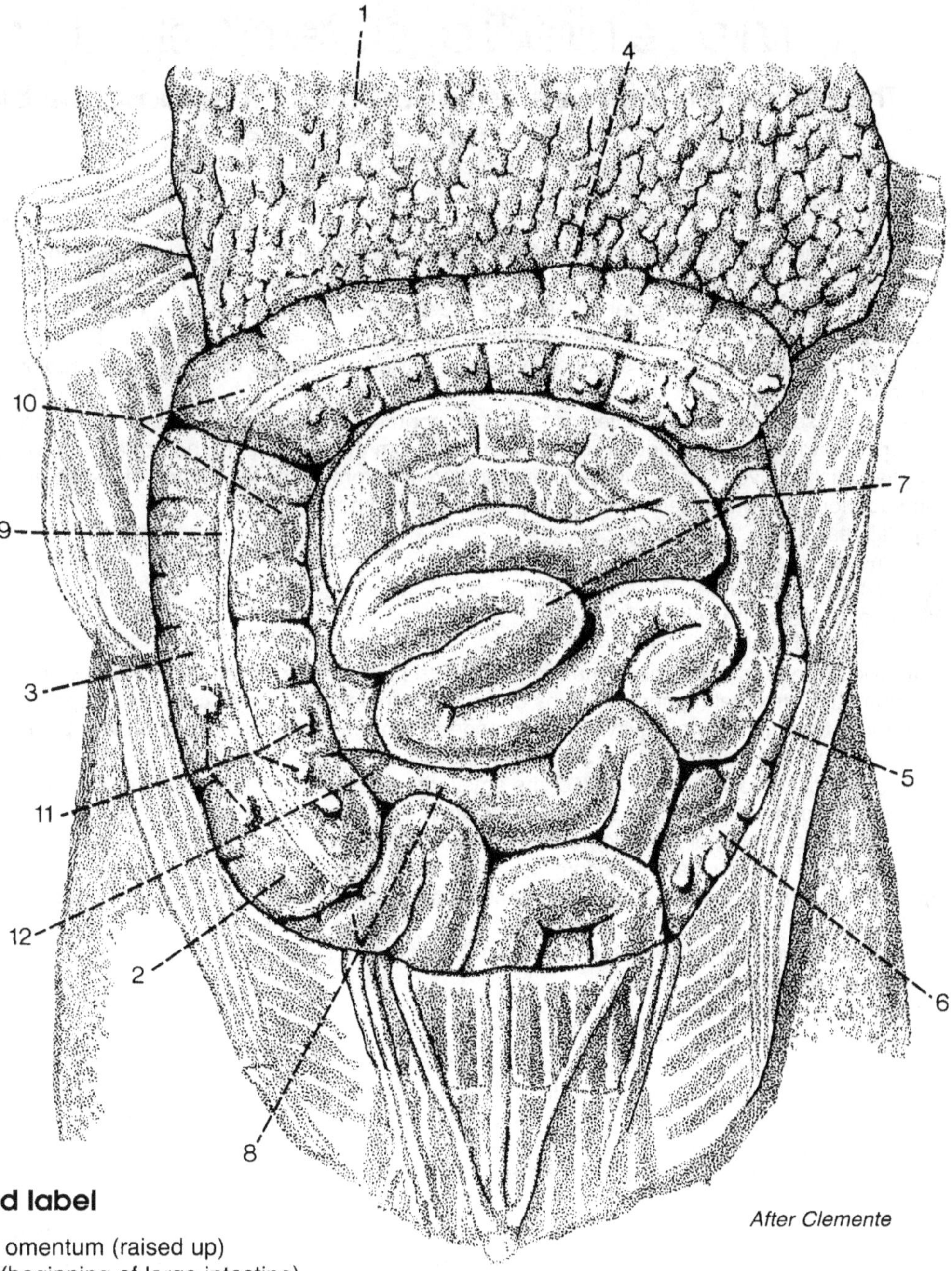

After Clemente

Color and label

1 Greater omentum (raised up)
2 Cecum (beginning of large intestine)
3 Ascending colon (large intestine)
4 Transverse colon
5 Descending colon
6 Sigmoid colon
7 Jejunum (second part of small intestine)
8 Ileum (third part of small intestine)
9 Teniae coli (three longitudinal strips of smooth muscle on the large intestine)*
10 Haustra coli (outpouchings or sacculations)*
11 Appendices epiploicae (small fatty globs)*
12 Termination of the ileum (emptying into the large intestine)

* These are found only on the large intestine or colon.

Ab-25 Distribution of the superior mesenteric artery and vein

The mesentery has been stripped away to expose the blood vessels (opposite page)

Color and label

1 Superior mesenteric artery. Branches of this large artery supply the major portion of the intestines: the lower half of the duodenum*, all of the jejunum and ileum, the ascending colon, and the right half of the transverse colon. The remainder of the large intestine (left half of transverse colon, descending colon, and sigmoid colon) is supplied by branches of the smaller inferior mesenteric artery. Branches of the latter anastomose with those of the superior mesenteric artery within the transverse mesocolon (the mesentery of the large intestine).

2 Superior mesenteric vein. This vein is the major contributor of venous blood to the hepatic portal system. It carries the digested and absorbed food from the intestine to the portal vein, which then empties into the liver. The relatively short portal vein is formed by the joining of the splenic vein with the superior mesenteric vein behind the pancreas (not shown).

3 Jejunal vessels

4 Ileal vessels

5 Ileocolic artery and vein

6 Right colic artery and vein

7 Midcolic artery and vein (branches)

8 Left colic artery and vein. These are branches of the inferior mesenteric artery and vein.

9 Jejunum; the proximal (upper) two-fifths of the small intestine. It forms coils and loops mainly in the upper left quadrant of the abdominal cavity. It is suspended from the posterior abdominal wall by its mesentery, which allows its coils enough mobility to slide past each other.

10 Ileum. The distal (lower) three-fifths of the small intestine. Like the jejunum, it has a mesentery, which permits its coils and loops to change their shape and position.

11 Cecum; the beginning of the colon or large intestine

12 Termination of the ileum at the cecum

13 Appendix epiploica: these small fatty appendages are present only on the large intestine and are helpful in identifying it.

14 Lymph node; the interconnecting lymph channels (lymphatics) are too small to be seen with the naked eye unless specially stained.

15 Transverse colon (raised up)

16 Greater omentum (raised up)

17 Transverse mesocolon. The transverse colon and the sigmoid colon retain their mesocolons, which allows them greater mobility than the ascending colon and descending colon, which have fused with the posterior abdominal wall along with their mesocolons and the blood vessels that coursed through their meocolons. However, a gentle pulling of the ascending or descending colon will free them from the posterior abdominal wall along with their mesocolons and contained blood vessels with no breakage of the vessels.

18 Descending colon (partly hidden)

19 Haustrum (Latin, a water wheel, so named because of its fancied resemblance to the buckets on a water wheel). These are the outpouchings or sacculations of the colon. Haustra are unique to the large intestine.†

20 Tenia coli (Latin, worm of the colon); there are 3 of these longitudinal tape-like bands of smooth muscle that make up the outer longitudinal layer of smooth muscle. Being shorter than the wall of the large intestine, they cause the characteristic outpouching or sacculations of the colon.

*The 10-inch long duodenum (not shown here) is retroperitoneal, having fused to the rear wall, rendering it immobile.

†The empty large intestine may at times appear narrower than the small intestine should the latter be distended. The teniae, the appendices epiploica, and the haustra are helpful in distinguishing the large intestine from the small intestine.

Ab-25 Distribution of the superior mesenteric artery and vein

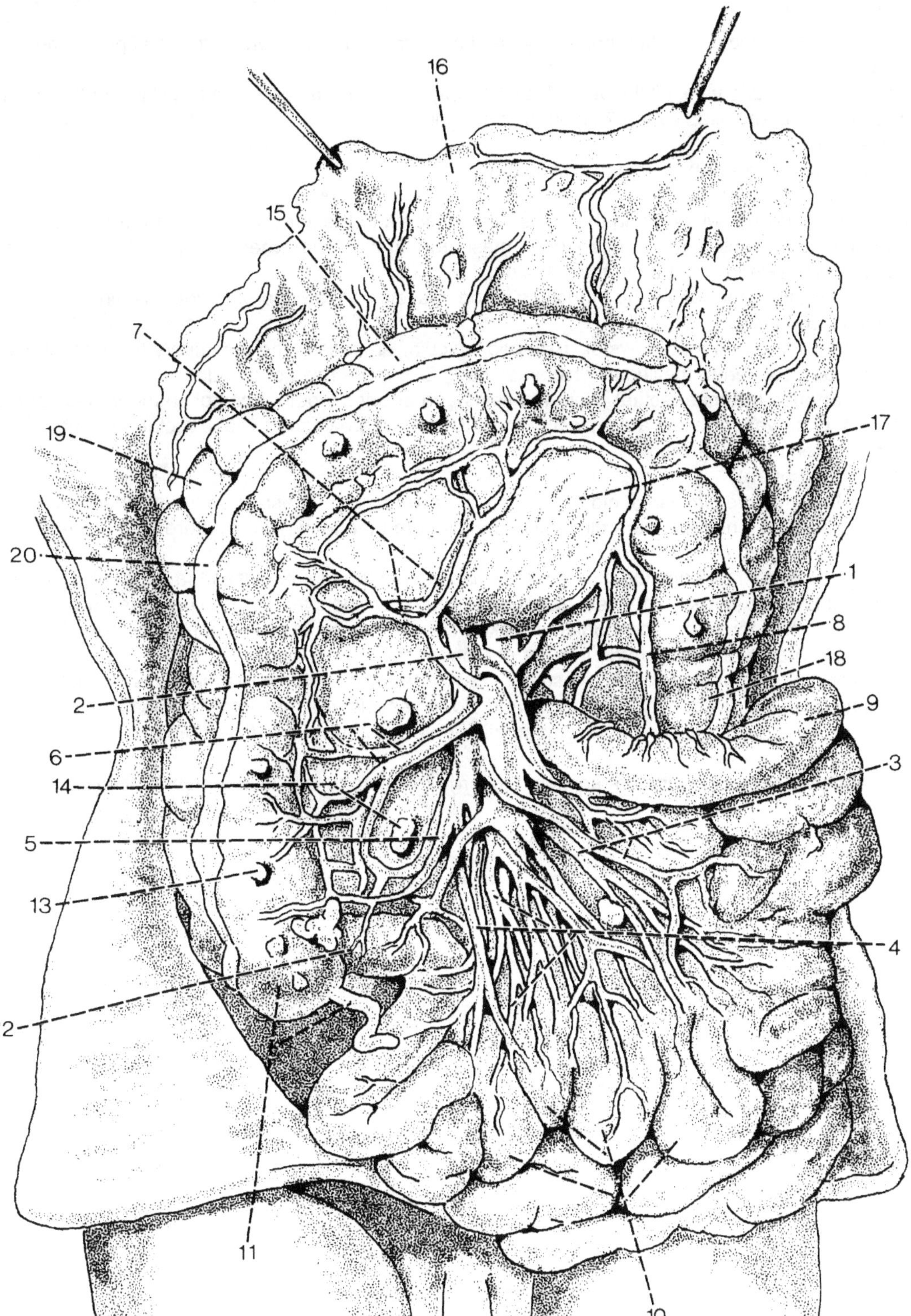

Redrawn and modified from Eycleshymer and Jones

Ab-26 Blood supply of the jejunum

(opposite page)

Color and label

1 Superior mesenteric artery; the mesentery has been stripped away from both the superior mesenteric artery and vein.
2 Superior mesenteric vein; all the vessels that supply the jejunum and ileum travel within the mesentery where they are enclosed by the 2 layers of peritoneum.
3 Jejunal arteries
4 Jejunal arteries and veins within the mesentery
5 Fat within mesentery
6 Translucent fat-free "windows" in the mesentery adjacent to the intestine; these are a distinguishing feature of the jejunal mesentery as opposed to the mesentery in the ileum where these "windows" are absent and where the fat extends right up to the intestine.
7 Arcades (1st tier); formed by the branching blood vessels as they approach the intestine.
8 Arcades (2nd tier)
9 Arcades (3rd tier); 3 tiers or rows of U-shaped vascular arcades in the mesentery is characteristic of the jejunum, as opposed to the ileum, which may have 5 or more rows of arcades.
10 Straight arteries (arteriae rectae). Here the veins and arteries together comprise the **vasae rectae** (straight vessels). Long vasae rectae are typical of the jejunum, whereas short vasae rectae and more arcades are characteristic of the ileum.
11 Jejunum (cut open)
12 Circular folds (*plicae circulares*; old name: valves of Kerckring). These folds greatly increase the internal (luminal) surface. They are more plentiful in the jejunum than in the ileum where they are fewer and farther between.
13 Cut edge of the peritoneum. On the right (13) *visceral* peritoneum encloses the intestine, forming its outermost layer or serosa. The mesenteric peritoneum connects the *visceral* peritoneum with the *parietal* peritoneum, thus forming a continuous unbroken sheet of peritoneum that lines the abdominal cavity and covers all the organs that protrude into the peritoneal cavity.
14 Two layers of peritoneum form the mesentery* and enclose the structures that pass through it. Part of one layer has been removed. In addition to fat and blood vessels, the mesentery carries lymphatic vessels, lymph nodes, sympathetic and parasympathetic nerves, and visceral afferent fibers.

* The double layer of peritoneum that anchors the large intestine to the posterior abdominal wall is called **mesocolon.**

Ab-26 Blood supply of the jejunum

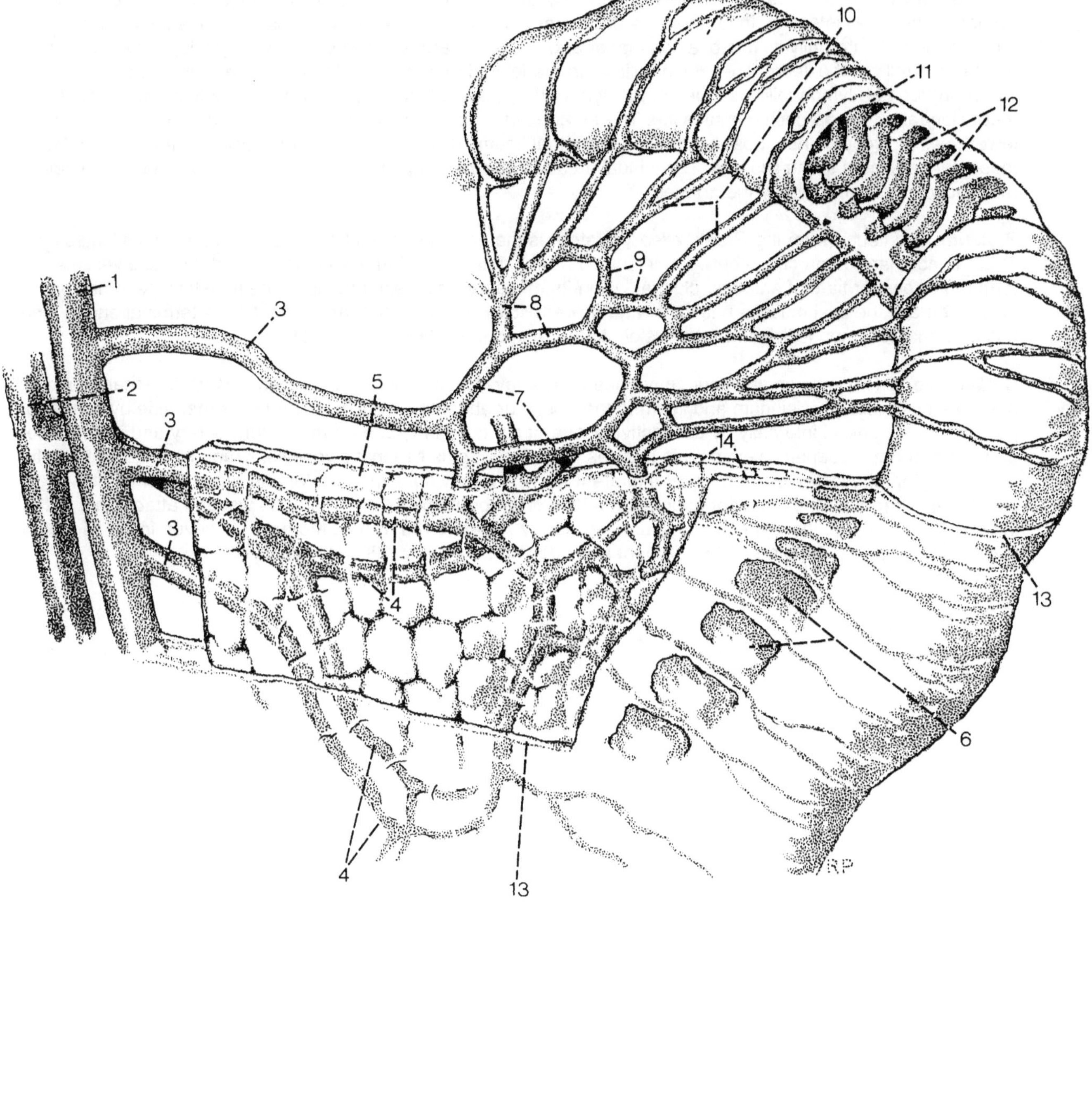

Ab-27 Blood supply to the small intestine

(opposite page)

A. Jejunum. The second part of the small intestine is the jejunum. It is the cranial two-fifths of the *mesenteric portion* of the small intestine. In general it is of greater diameter, has thicker walls, is more vascular and therefore redder, and internally its mucosa has higher and more numerous plicae circulares (circular folds) than the caudal three-fifths, the ileum. The lymph follicles in the jejunal mucosa tend to be small and scattered, unlike the larger aggregated lymph follicles found in the ileum.The jejunal blood vessels form branching arcades within the mesentery as they approach the intestine. The arcades of the jejunum tend to divide less and therefore have fewer rows of arcades than those found in the terminal ileum. There are fat-free translucent "windows" in the mesentery adjacent to the jejunum. The jejunal arcades give off long vasae rectae (straight vessels). The veins (not shown here) accompany the arteries.

B. Ileum. The ileum (from the Greek, *eileos*, twisted) is the caudal three-fifths of the mesenteric small intestine. There is no sharp demarcation between jejunum and the ileum. The ileum is characterized by blood vessels that form more rows or tiers of arcades, plus fat within its mesentery that extends up to the intestine ("encroaching fat"). Internally the ileal mucosa has lower and fewer plicae circulares that are absent at its terminal end. It also has aggregated lymph follicles that are visible to the naked eye (Peyer's patches).

C. Mesentery. The jejunum and ileum have been cut away. The mesentery is a highly folded, fan-shaped membrane that connects the jejunum and ileum to the posterior abdominal wall. It is lined on either side by a layer of peritoneum supported internally by connective tissue. It contains the superior mesenteric artery and its branches and the superior mesenteric vein and its radicles (little roots), plus lymphatic vessels, lymph nodes, sympathetic and parasympathetic nerves, and visceral afferent nerves. It may contain considerable amounts of fat. Its attachment or root on the posterior abdominal wall is only about 15 cm long (6 in). Its visceral attachment to the intestine is as long as the jejunum and ileum are, nearly 7 meters (23 ft) post mortem. However, in life its length is probably nearer to 4 meters (13 ft). (Blount and Lachman in Anson, 1966.)

Ab-27 Blood supply to the small intestine

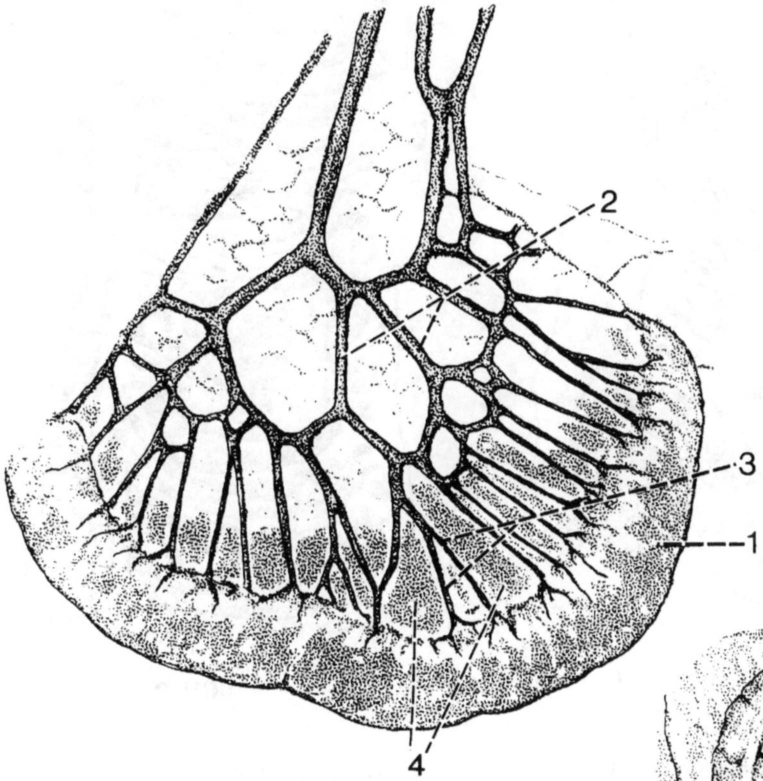

A. Jejunum

Color and label

1 Jejunum
2 Arcades in mesentery
3 Vasae rectae
4 Fat-free "windows"

B. Ileum

5 Ileum
6 Arcades in mesentery
7 Mesenteric fat extending to ileum; no "windows"

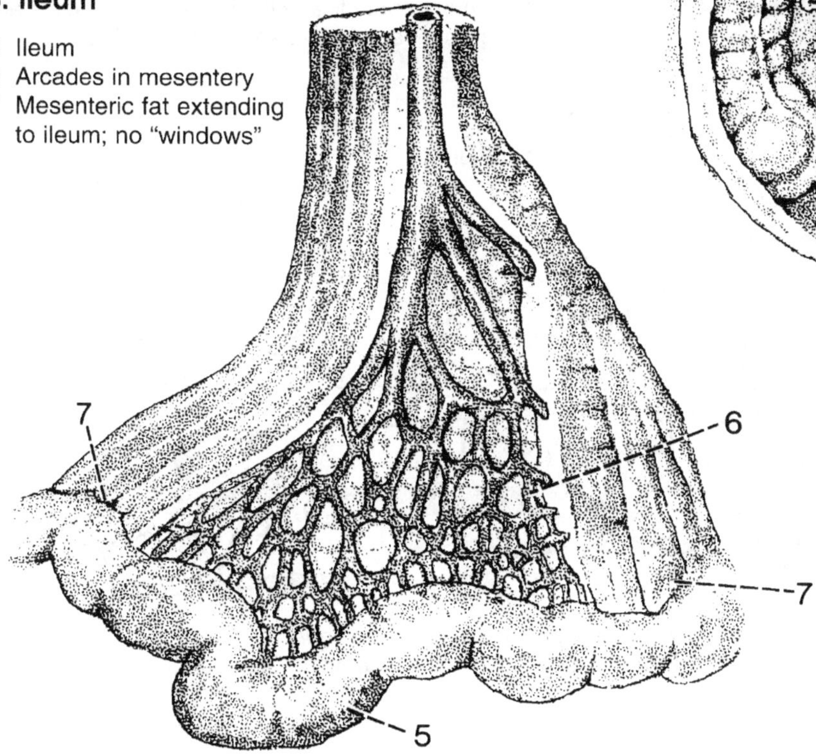

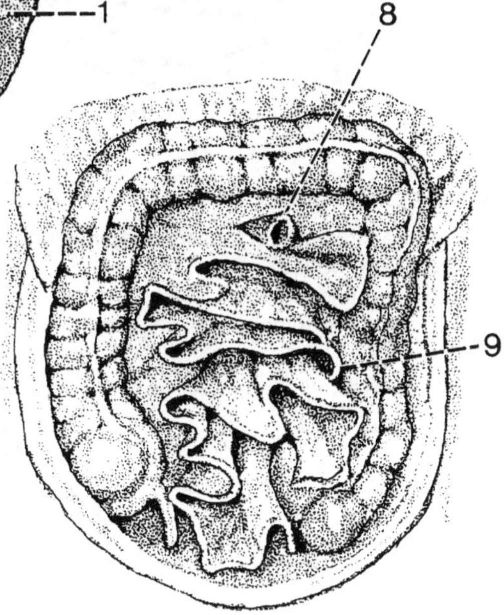

C. Mesentery

8 Duodeno-jejunal junction
9 Cut edge of mesentery

Ab-28 Mucosa of jejunum and ileum

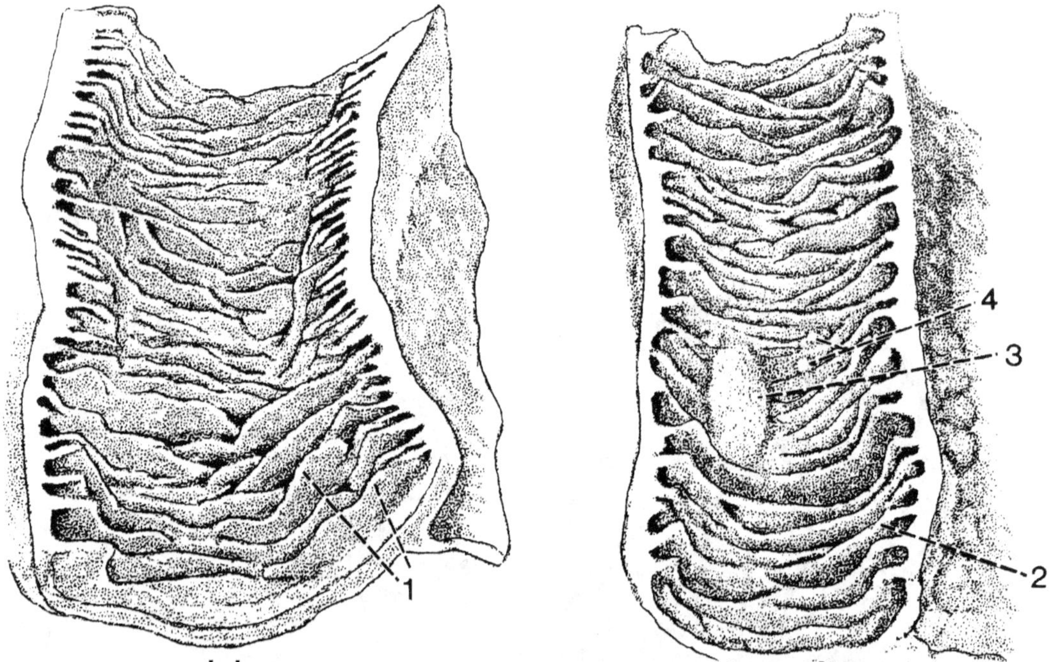

Jejunum

Redrawn from Anson

Ileum

Color and label

1 Plicae circulares (circular folds) in jejunum; tall and numerous
2 Circular folds in ileum; fewer and less prominent; absent at terminal portion of ileum
3 Aggregated lymph follicles
4 Isolated lymph follicles

Total number of plicae circulares in the adult is about 800 (Blount and Lachman in Anson, 1966).

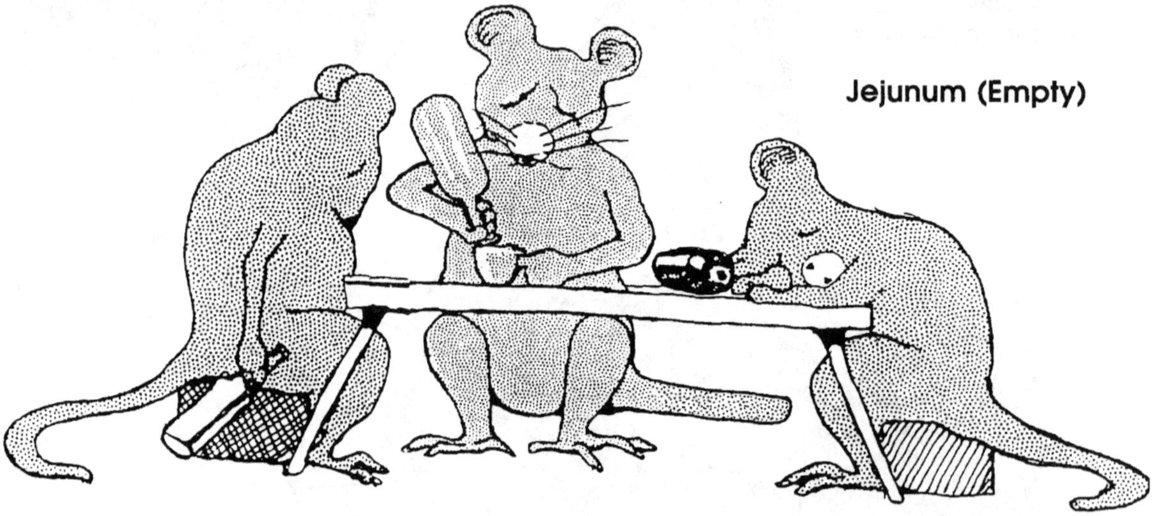

The ancient anatomists named the second part of the small intestine the *jejunum,* or empty part, because after death they found it to be devoid of contents. Besides meaning "empty or wanting," jejunum also meant "hungry or fasting."

Ab-29 Blood supply of large intestine

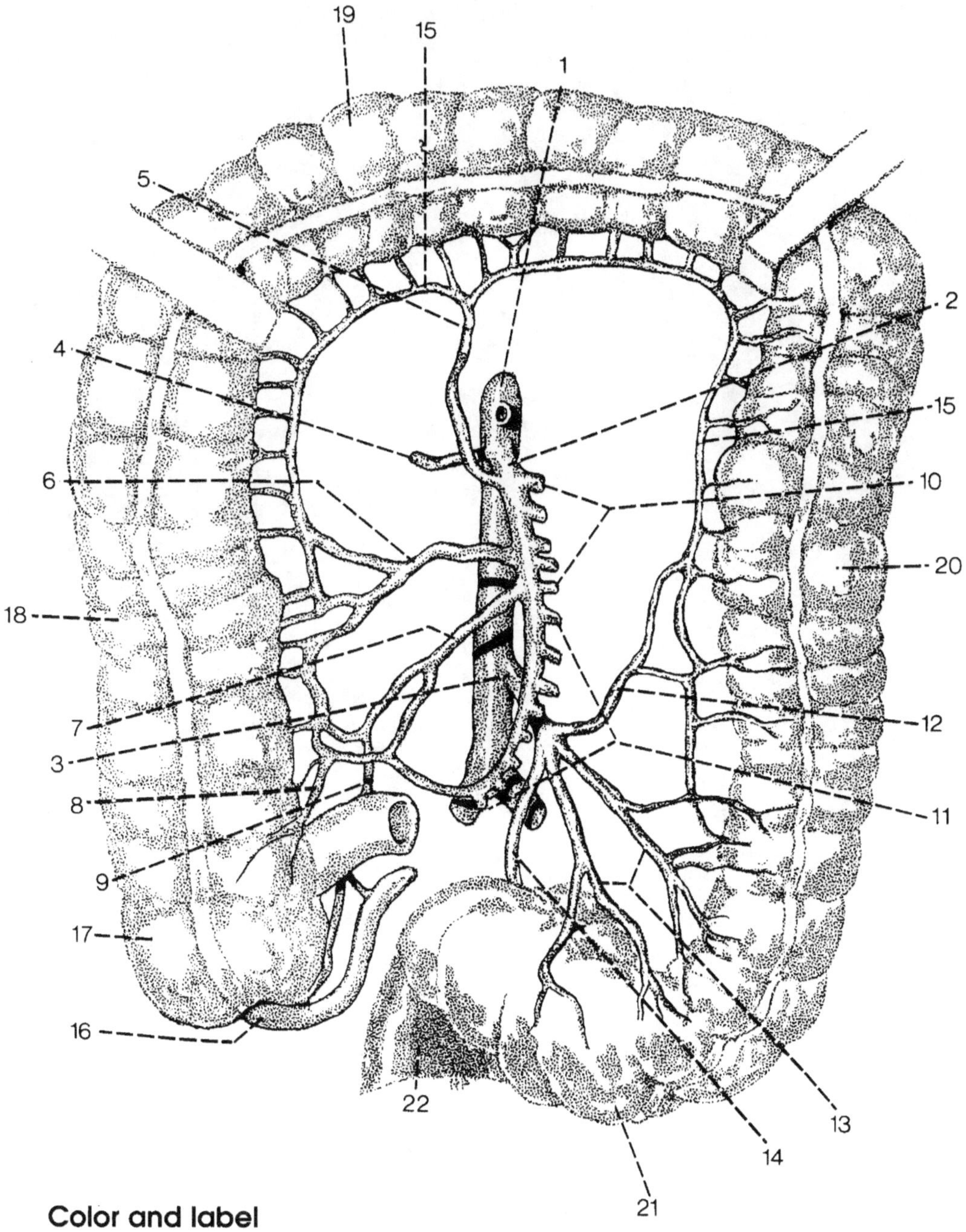

Color and label

1 Aorta
2 Superior mesenteric artery
3 Inferior mesenteric artery
4 Inferior pancreaticoduodenal artery
5 Middle colic artery
6 Right colic artery
7 Ileocolic artery
8 Anterior cecal branch
9 Posterior cecal branch
10 Jejunal arteries
11 Ileal arteries
12 Left colic artery
13 Sigmoid arteries
14 Superior rectal artery
15 Marginal artery
16 Vermiform appendix
17 Cecum
18 Ascending colon
19 Transverse colon
20 Descending colon
21 Sigmoid colon
22 Rectum

Ab-30 Ileocecal valve, vermiform appendix, terminal ileum, and cecum

(viewed from the front)

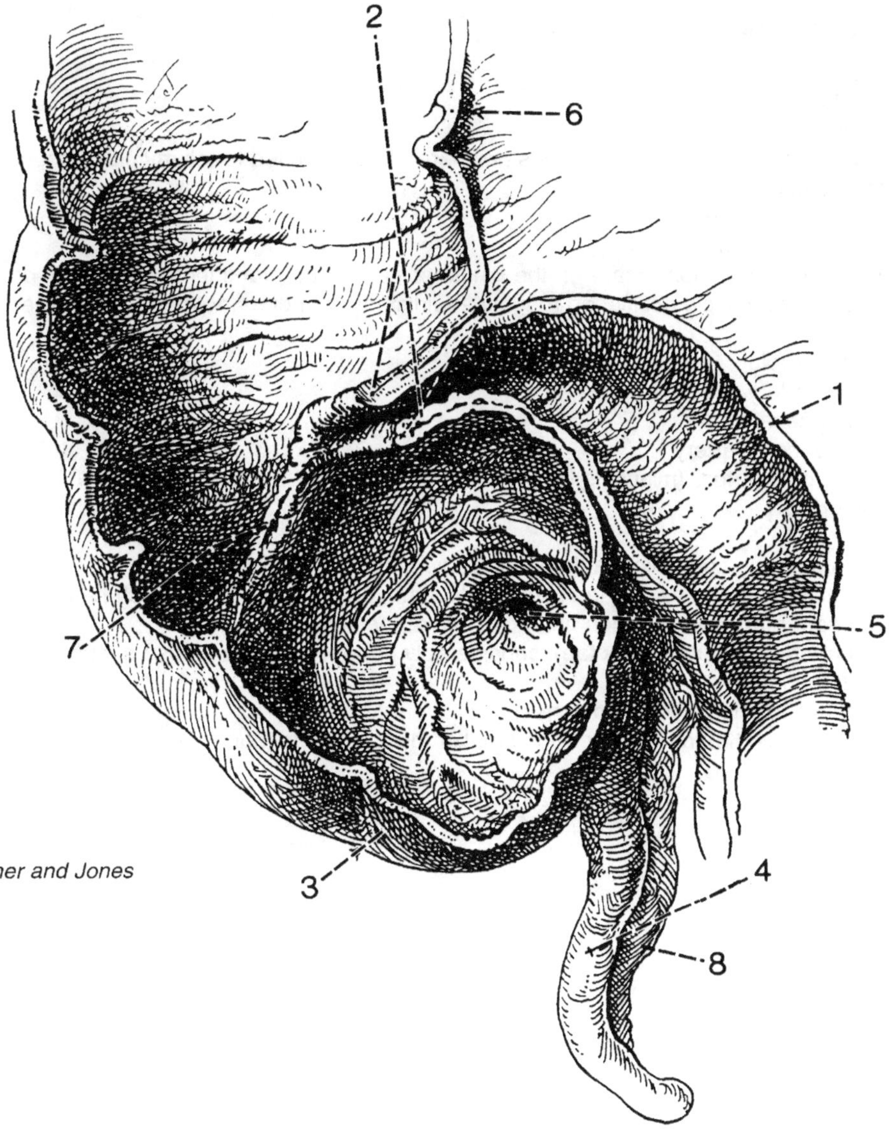

Eycleshymer and Jones

Color and label

1 Terminal ileum; note an absence of mucosal circular folds (plicae circulares)
2 Ileocecal valve; note that it is formed by 2 lips that project into the large intestine.
3 Cecum
4 Vermiform (*vermis*, Latin, worm) appendix. It has a small lumen that extends its entire length.
5 Orifice of vermiform appendix; occasionally guarded by a semilunar fold of mucous membrane.
6 Ascending colon
7 Frenulum of the ileocecal valve (Latin, diminutive of *frenum*, a bridle, bit, reins); a ridge that is formed by the fused lips of the the ileocecal valve. It runs downward and laterally, demarcating the cecum from the ascending colon.*
8 Flap of mesentery containing appendicular artery

*Churchill's Medical Dictionary, 1989

Ab-31 Arterial supply of vermiform appendix, terminal ileum, and cecum

(opposite page)

Color and label

1 Ileocecal valve
2 Frenulum
3 Terminal ileum
4 Cecum (Latin, blind; its lumen leads nowhere). But as I used to tell my class, "cecum and ye shall find."
5 Ascending colon
6 Vermiform appendix
7 Orifice of appendix
8 Tenia (Latin, "a ribbon or tape"); the teniae coli are three prominent longitudinal bands of smooth (nonstriated) muscle positioned roughly equidistant from one another (120 degrees) in the wall of the large intestine.
9 Semilunar fold
10 Ileocolic artery
11 Anterior cecal artery
12 Posterior cecal artery
13 Appendicular artery (minus its flap of mesentery)
14 Colic branch
15 Ileal branch
16 Mesentery (cut; containing fat between its two layers of peritoneum)
17 Encroaching fat (fat next to the ileum; unlike the jejunal mesentery, which has "clear windows")
18 Arcades (an arterial formation characteristic of the ileal arteries)
19 Straight arteries (arteriae rectae); considerably shorter here than those supplying the jejunum, which tend to be long
20 Lymphatic follicles (Peyer's patches)
21 Mucosal folds. Ileum has fewer and smaller mucosal folds than those in the jejunum.

Ab-31 Arterial supply of vermiform appendix, terminal ileum, and cecum

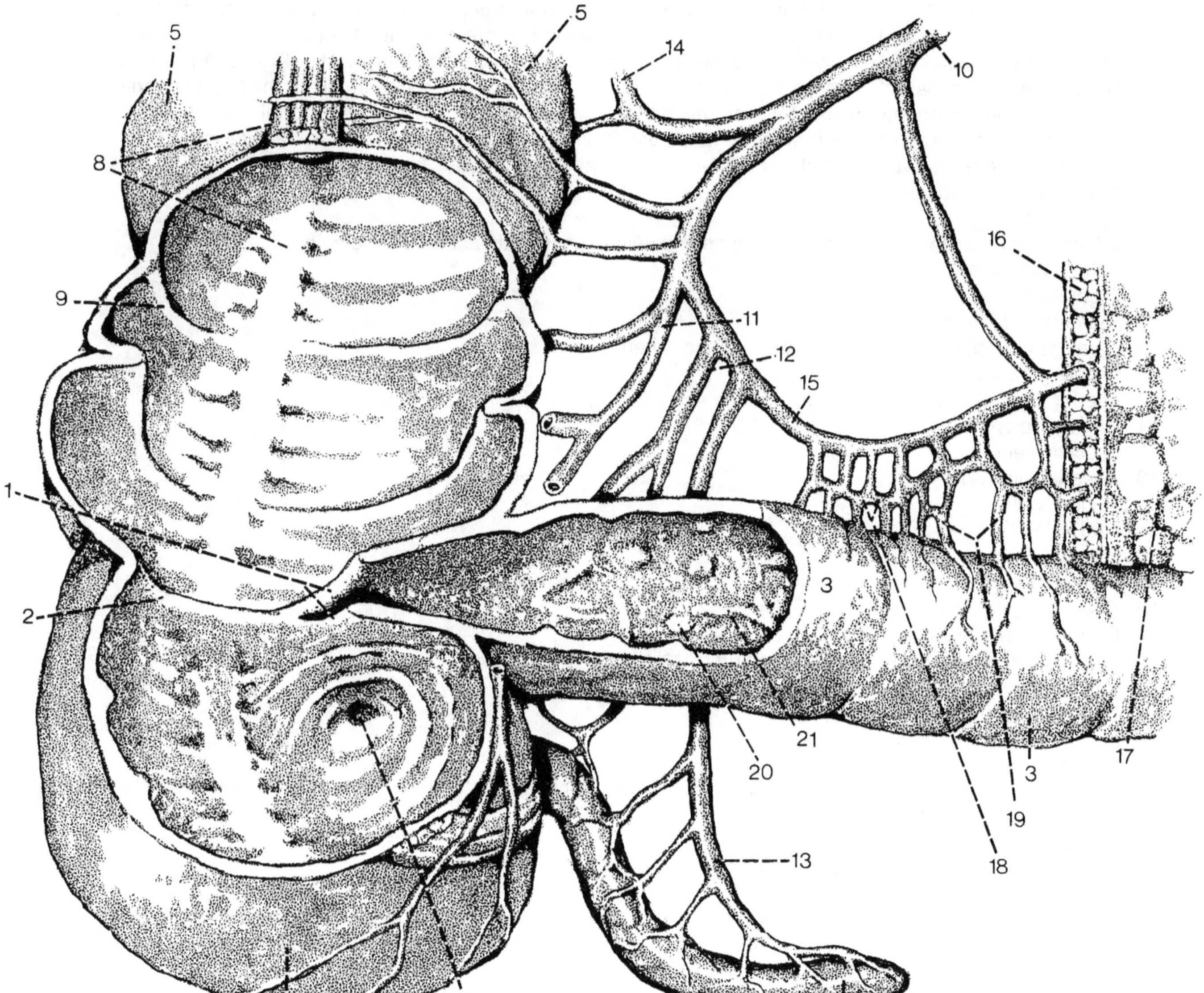

Ab-32 The hepatic portal system

(opposite page)

Color and label

1 Portal vein (also hepatic portal vein); this thick but rather short vein is formed by the convergence of the splenic vein and the superior mesenteric vein. The portal vein itself is only 7 or 8 cm long. The hepatic portal system conveys all the blood and absorbed carbohydrates and proteins from the stomach and intestines to the liver. The hepatic portal system begins with capillaries in the intestinal mucosa that feed into tiny venous tributaries or radicles. These drain into larger and larger coalescing veins that eventually end in the portal vein. However, instead of draining into the inferior vena cava, once it reaches the liver, the hepatic portal vein divides into branches inside the liver, much like an artery. The branches of the portal vein repeatedly divide into smaller and smaller branches, which end in irregular-shaped capillaries in the liver called sinusoids where the liver metabolizes the blood-borne absorbed food.
2 Superior mesenteric vein
3 Splenic vein
4 Inferior mesenteric vein. The inferior mesenteric vein usually ends in the splenic vein.
5 Left gastric vein
6 Right gastric vein
7 Superior pancreaticoduodenal vein
8 Right gastro-epiploic* vein (new name, gastro-omental vein)
9 Middle colic vein
10 Inferior pancreaticoduodenal vein
11 Right colic vein
12 Ileocolic vein
13 Appendicular vein
14 Jejunal veins
15 Ileal veins
16 Left colic vein
17 Sigmoid veins
18 Superior rectal vein
19 Dorsal pancreatic vein
20 Round ligament of the liver (obliterated umbilical vein)
21 Falciform ligament
22 Coronary ligament
23 Duodenum
24 Stomach (cut)
25 Spleen. The spleen removes old red blood cells from the circulation and sends the breakdown products to the liver via the splenic vein.
26 Right lobe of liver
27 Left gastro-epiploic (gastro-omental) vein

*Epiploic is from the Greek *epiploon*, the name used by Hippocrates for the omentum. This, in turn, came from the Greek *epipleo*, "I sail upon or float upon." The allusion, presumably, is to the omentum "floating upon" the abdominal viscera. (Haubrich, 1984)

Ab-32 The hepatic portal system

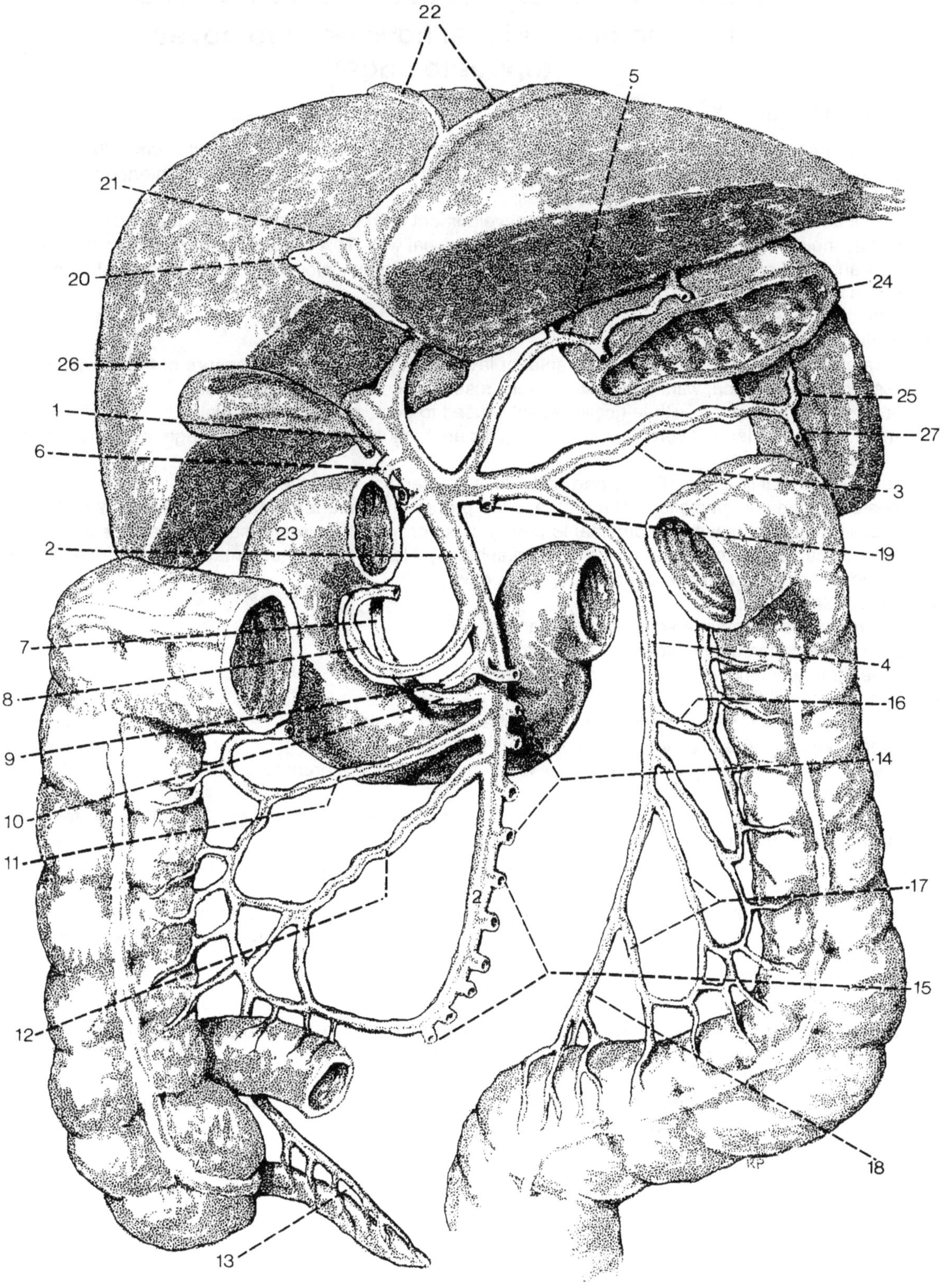

Ab-33 Posterior abdominal wall, peritoneal attachments

The stomach and liver have been removed.
(opposite page)

Color and label

1 Root of the mesentery. This is the posterior attachment of the whole jejunum and ileum. Whereas the root of the mesentery is only about about 15 cm long, its intestinal border is greatly lenghtened to about 4 meters due to its numerous folds and ruffles.
2 Site of ascending colon. During embryonic development both the ascending and descending colon as well as their mesocolons fuse to the posterior abdominal wall. This renders them relatively immobile, unlike the transverse colon and sigmoid colon, which retain their mesocolons and a fair amount of mobility.
3 Site of descending colon
4 Mesocolon of sigmoid colon
5 Transverse mesocolon
6 Greater omentum (posterior layer; the anterior layer arises from greater curvature of the stomach)
7 Ascending mesocolon, with right colic vessels, fused to posterior abdominal wall.
8 Descending mesocolon, with left colic vessels, fused to posterior abdominal wall.
9 Anterior layer (or leaf) of coronary ligament.* This anchors the liver to the diaphragm and encloses the bare area of the liver.
10 Hepatoduodenal ligament. This is part of the lesser omentum. Note the 3 cut vessels: the portal vein (posterior), the common bile duct (right), and the proper hepatic artery (left). The white arrow indicates the epiploic foramen (new name: omental foramen). It is here that the greater sac (the peritoneal cavity) communicates with the lesser sac (the omental bursa). Notice that the omental foramen lies *posterior* to the portal vein and *anterior* to the inferior vena cava.
11 Gastrosplenic ligament
12 Gastrophrenic (stomach-to-diaphragm) ligament
13 Left triangular ligament of coronary ligament
14 Superior mesenteric vein (left) and artery (right)
15 Duodenojejunal flexture
16 Area on underside of diaphragm occupied by bare area of liver
17 Hepatic veins (cut) ending in inferior vena cava
18 Inferior vena cava; this part of the inferior vena cava is firmly adherent to the liver.
19 Pancreas
20 Duodenum (first part). The 2nd, 3rd, and 4th parts of the duodenum become fused to the posterior wall, which renders the first immobile.†
21 Esophagus (thoracic part) with esophageal plexus (right and left vagus nerves).
22 Esophagus (abdominal part)
23 Posterior wall of omental bursa (lesser sac). This is a peritoneal-bound space in back of the stomach and liver. It communicates with the remainder of the peritoneal cavity by way of the omental (epiploic) foramen.
24 Rectum
25 Aorta

*Peritoneal ligaments consist of either a single layer of peritoneum (e.g., the coronary ligament) or a fused double layer (gastrosplenic ligament) reinforced with connective tissue.

†Structures such as the duodenum which lose their mesentery and become fused to the posterior abdominal wall are termed *secondarily retroperitoneal.*

Ab-33 Posterior abdominal wall, peritoneal attachments

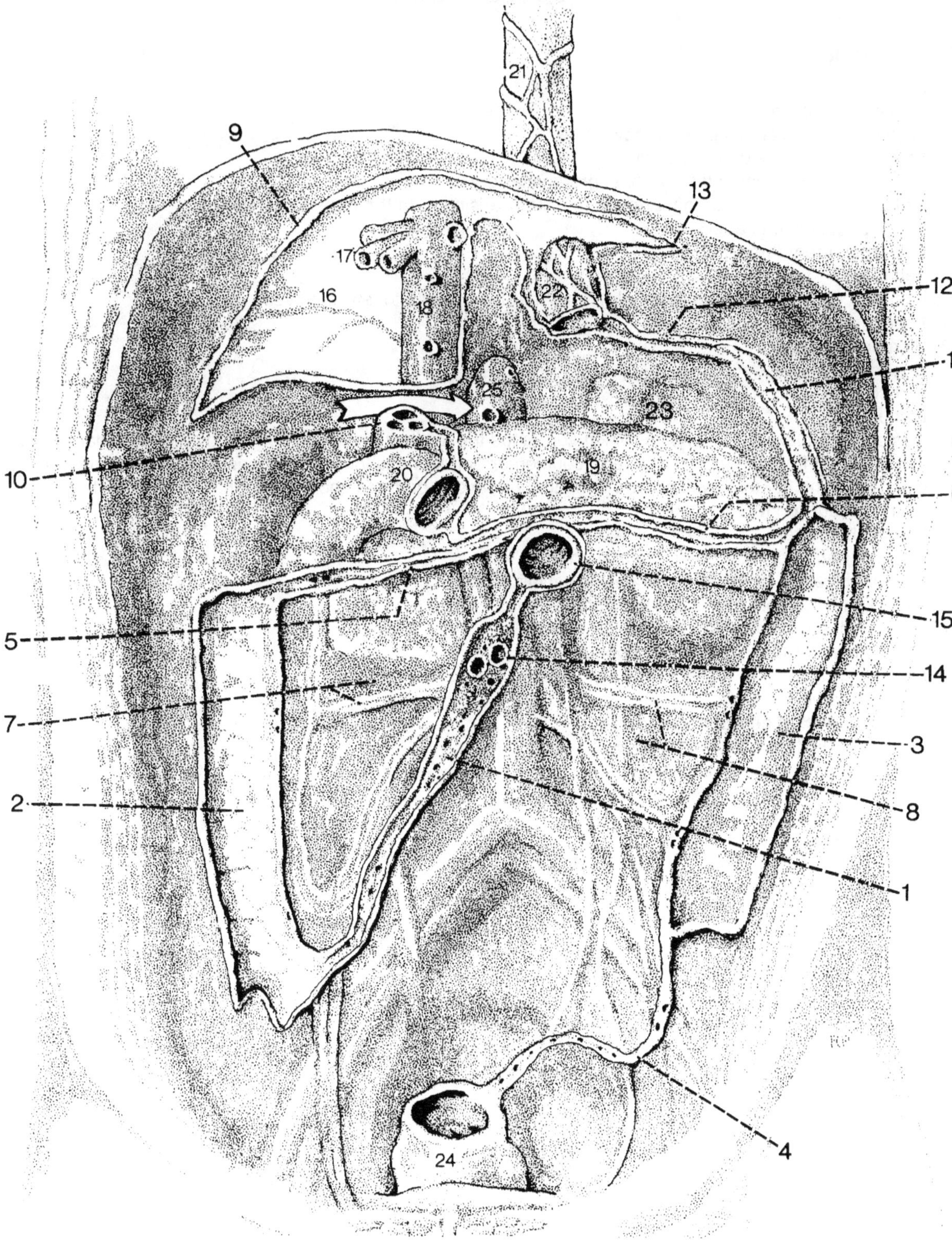

Ab-34 Posterior abdominal wall, kidneys and related structures

(opposite page)

Color and label

1 Aorta
2 Inferior vena cava
3 Hepatic veins (liver has been removed)
4 Esophagus with esophageal plexus
5 Inferior phrenic artery and superior suprarenal artery
6 Middle and inferior suprarenal arteries (the latter arising from the renal artery)
7 Superior mesenteric artery
8 Left renal artery (branches)
9 Left kidney
10 Left testicular vein (ovarian in female); note that it empties into left renal vein.
11 Inferior mesenteric artery
12 Sigmoid arteries
13 Superior rectal artery
14 Left common iliac artery and vein
15 Left ureter
16 Pampiniform plexus. This plexus, which surrounds the testicular artery, is formed by the testicular vein. It absorbs heat from the testicular artery (countercurrent heat exchange), thus ensuring that the arterial blood reaching the testis will be at a temperature several degrees cooler than 98.6, thus permitting sperm production to take place.
17 Internal iliac artery
18 External iliac artery (becomes femoral artery in leg)
19 Inferior epigastric artery and vein (lateral umbilical fold)
20 Medial umbilical fold (or plica); obliterated umbilical artery
21 Rectus abdominis muscle
22 Urinary bladder (covered with peritoneum)
23 Rectum
24 Femoral nerve
25 Genital branch of genitofemoral nerve
26 Femoral branch of genitofemoral nerve
27 Lateral femoral cutaneous nerve
28 Genitofemoral nerve
29 Ilioinguinal nerve
30 Iliohypogastric nerve
31 Right testicular vein. Note it forms the pampinform plexus on the right testcular artery more caudally
32 Right testicular artery arising from the aorta
33 Subcostal nerve (nerve T12)
34 Right ureter
35 Right renal vein
36 Right kidney
37 Celiac trunk
38 Right suprarenal gland

Ab-34 Posterior abdominal wall, kidneys and related structures

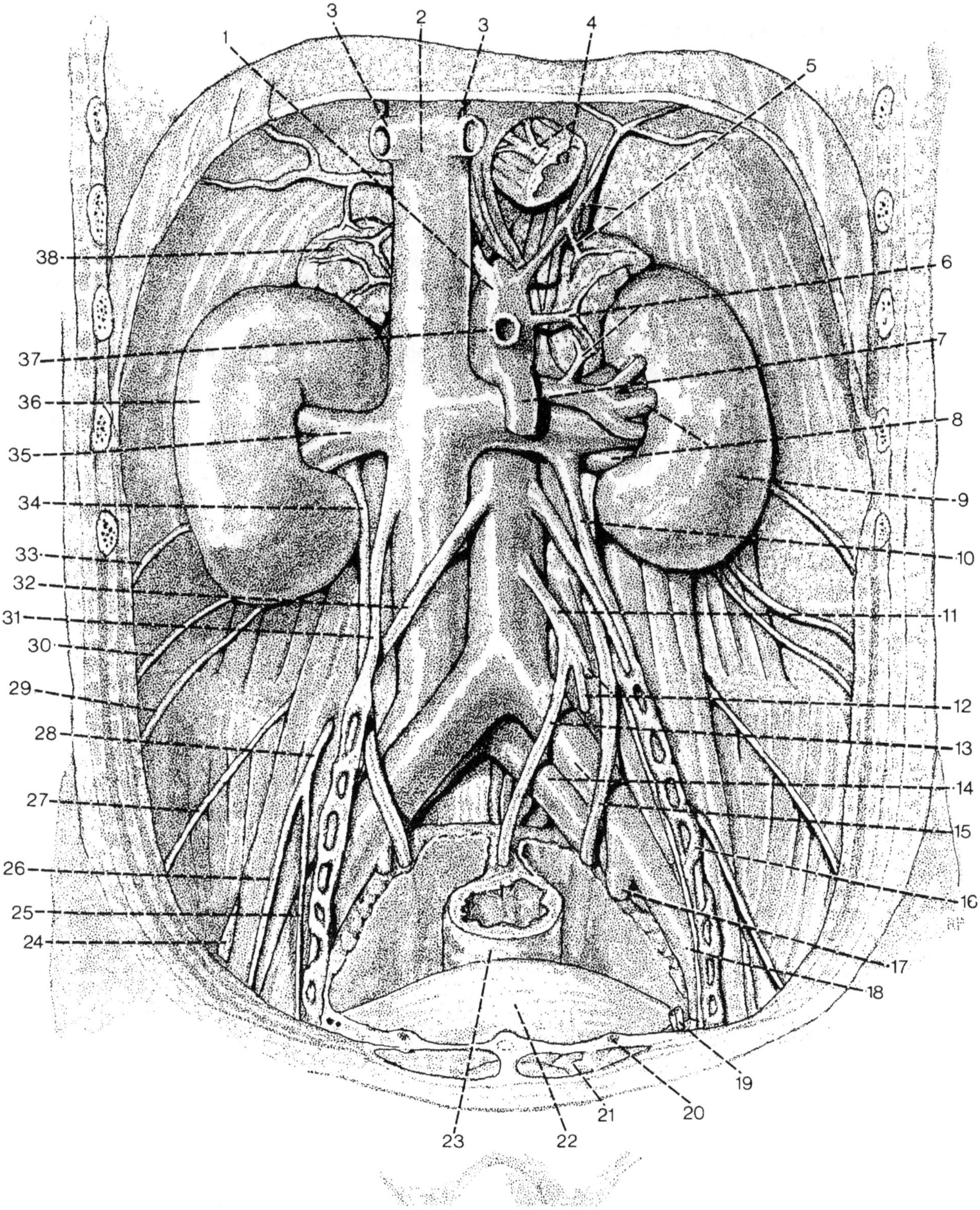

Ab-35 The kidney, I

(opposite page)

Color and label

Figure A. Right kidney (anterior view)

1 Renal artery
2 Renal vein
3 Ureter

Figure B. Left kidney (partially dissected; blood vessels have been removed)

1 Ureter
2 Renal pelvis (partially opened)
3 Major renal calix (also calyx); usually 2 or 3 in number. These branch off the renal pelvis.
4 Minor renal calices. Several of these branch off of each major calix. Each minor calix has 1 to 3 expanded and indented cuplike ends that fit tightly around 1 to 3 renal papillae (7). The apices of the papillae are pierced by the openings of the collecting tubules.
5 Two minor renal calices (cut open)
6 Renal pyramids (dissected free). These are the major component of the medulla of the kidney. Note their conical shape with their apices pointing toward the renal pelvis.
7 Renal papillae. These are the prominent conical apices of the renal pyramids that project into the minor calices and are perforated by the openings of the papillary (collecting) ducts of Bellini, forming the area cribrosa (*cribrum*, Latin, a sieve or strainer). (Papilla is the diminutive of *papula*, Latin, a nipple or teat.) (Churchill's Medical Dictionary,1989)
8 Renal papilla opening directly into a major calix.
9 Renal cortex (outer portion of the kidney)
10 Renal column. This is cortical tissue that lies in the medulla between the pyramids.
11 Renal sinus. This space actually lies outside the kidney in its medial central hollow. Blood vessels entering and leaving the kidney pass through it. Perirenal fat fills in all the interstices (small intervening spaces).

Figure C. A single pyramid

1 Base of pyramid (abuts renal cortex)
2 Apex of pyramid with papilla indenting minor calix (3)
3 Minor calix cuplike end around renal papilla
4 Plane of section (longitudinal) of figure D
5 Plane of section (transverse) of figure D

Figure D. Portion of pyramid in figure C enlarged and sectioned

1 Minor calix (expanded end surrounding papilla of pyramid)
2 Apical section of renal pyramid
3 Area cribrosa. So named because of the numerous tiny openings of the collecting ducts that give it a sievelike appearance.
4 Collecting ducts. (Also papillary ducts of Bellini)
5 Cross section of renal pyramid with collecting ducts (cut). The renal pyramid also contain the loops of Henle and the vasae rectae.

Ab-35 The kidney, I

The right kidney, anterior aspect

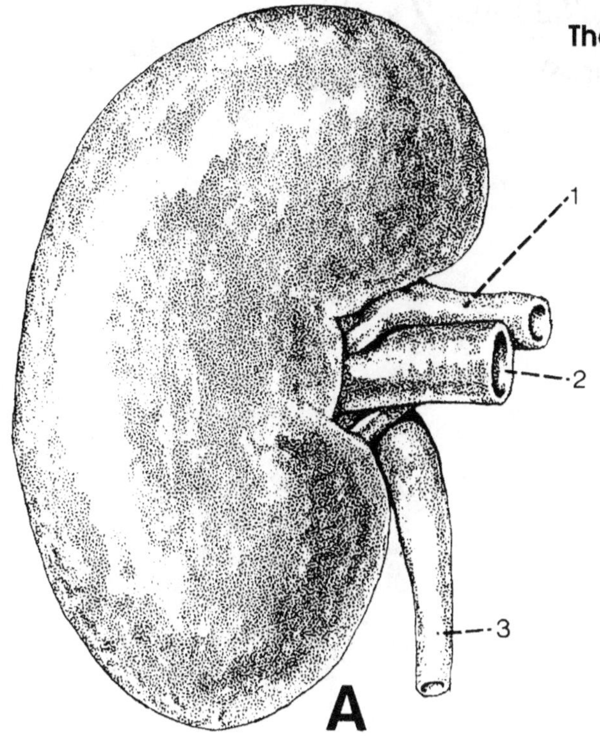

A

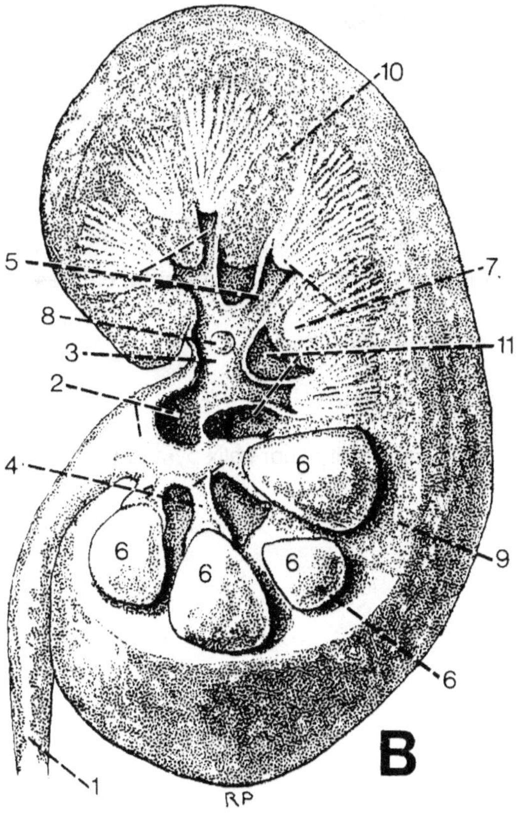

B

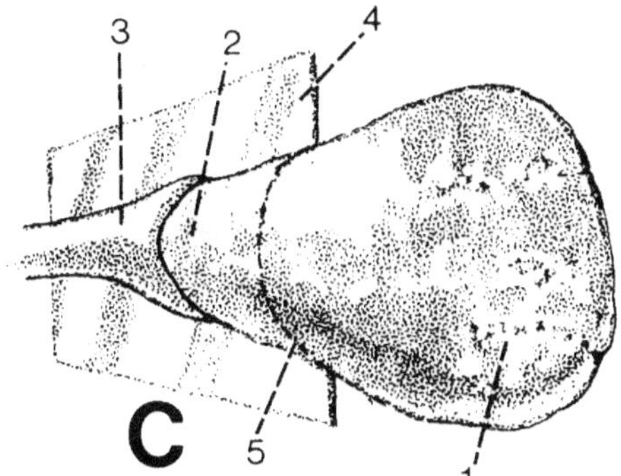

C

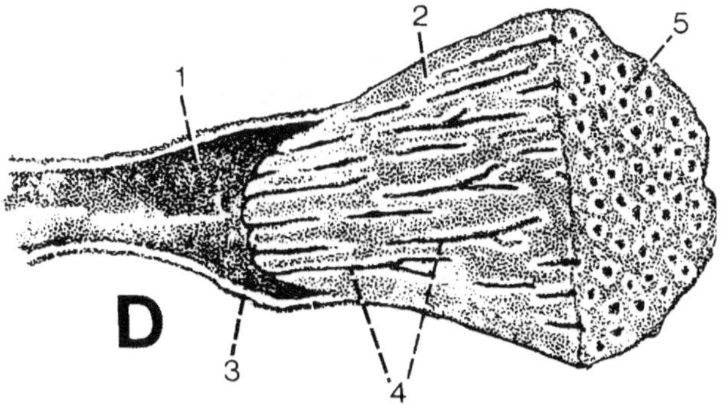

D

Ab-36 The kidney, II

(opposite page)

Color and label

Figure A. Left kidney. Sectioned coronally

1 Ureter
2 Renal pelvis
3 Major calix
4 Minor calix
5 Renal pyramid
6 Renal papillae
7 Renal column
8 Renal cortex
9 Fat in renal sinus
10 Capsule of kidney

Figure B. Left kidney. Pyramids, calices, pelvis, and ureter

1 Renal pyramids
2 Minor calices
3 Major calices
4 Renal pelvis
5 Ureter
6 Opening of minor calix pyramid removed)

Figure C. Detail of calix and papilla

1 Minor calix enclosing papilla
2 Minor calix with papilla missing
3 Minor calix cut open to expose papilla with openings of papillary ducts into minor calix
4 Cribriform area containing openings of papillary ducts. The latter are formed by the coalescing of the collecting tubules.
5 Renal papilla
6 Renal pyramid

Ab-36 The kidney, II

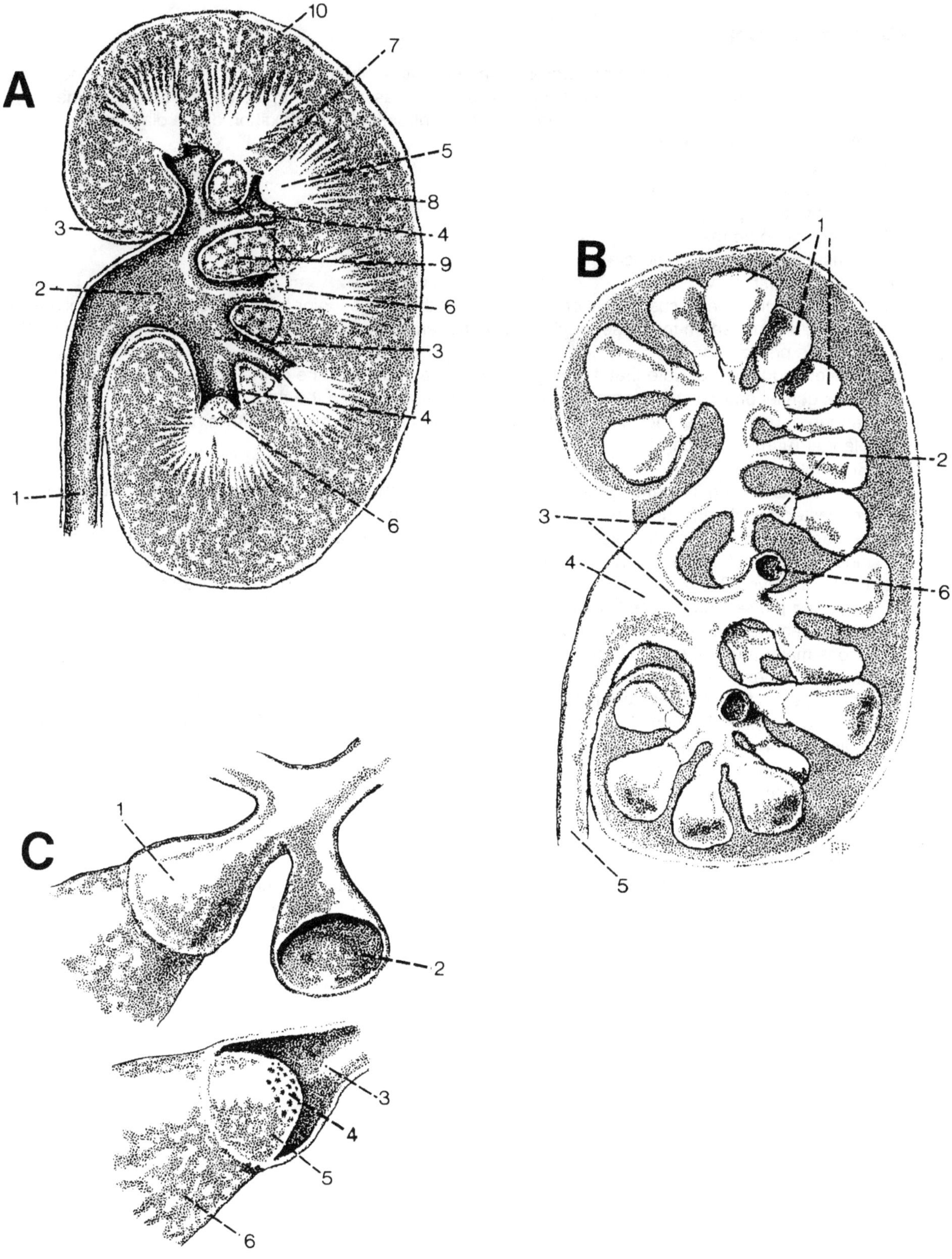

Ab-37 Posterior abdominal wall, showing principal muscles and nerves

(opposite page)

Color and label

1 Aortic hiatus and median (central) arcuate ligament. Note that the aorta passes posterior to the diaphragm so that, unlike the inferior vena cava which passes through the central tendon of the diaphragm, the aorta will be least affected by the contraction and relaxation of the diaphragm.
2 Inferior vena cava with hepatic veins
3 Esophagus
4 Diaphragm (muscular part)
5 Left crus of diaphragm
6 Subcostal nerve (nerve T12)
7 Transversus abdominis muscle
8 Iliohypogastric nerve
9 Iliacus muscle. The iliacus inserts on the tendon of the psoas major muscle. Together, as the iliopsoas muscle, they insert on the lesser trochanter of the femur where they act as a powerful flexor of the thigh upon the pelvis.
10 Genitofemoral nerve. Note that it emerges from the anterior surface of the psoas major muscle and splits into a genital branch and a femoral branch (labels 14 and 15 on the right side).
11 Tendon of psoas minor muscle. This thin shiny tendon is easily mistaken for a nerve.
12 Bladder (urinary bladder)
13 Rectum
14 Genital branch of genitofemoral nerve. The genital branch traverses the inguinal canal and supplies the cremaster muscle and the skin of the scrotum in males or the labium majus in females.
15 Femoral branch of genitofemoral nerve. The femoral branch passes into the thigh beneath the inguinal ligament, supplying the skin of the middle and upper anterior part of the thigh.
16 Femoral nerve. This large mixed (sensorimotor) nerve supplies the skin and muscles of the anterior thigh and the skin on the medial lower leg.
17 Lateral femoral cutaneous nerve. Supplies skin of lateral thigh.
18 Psoas major muscle. A major flexor of the thigh.
19 Ilioinguinal nerve. A mixed nerve supplying the lower anterolateral abdominal muscles. It accompanies the spermatic cord through the superficial inguinal ring and distibutes cutaneous fibers to the skin of the proximal and medial part of the thigh, the root of the penis, and the scrotum in males, or the mons pubis and labium majus in the female.
20 Iliohypogastric nerve. A mixed nerve supplying the skin of the gluteal region and lower anterior abdomen and motor fibers to the lower transversus abdominis, internal oblique, and external oblique muscles
21 Quadratus lumborum muscle
22 Psoas minor muscle
23 Medial and lateral arcuate ligaments. Anatomists agree that these are not ligaments in the true sense of the word, but the names will have to do until better ones come along.
24 Aorta and right crus of diaphragm

Ab-37 Posterior abdominal wall, showing principal muscles and nerves

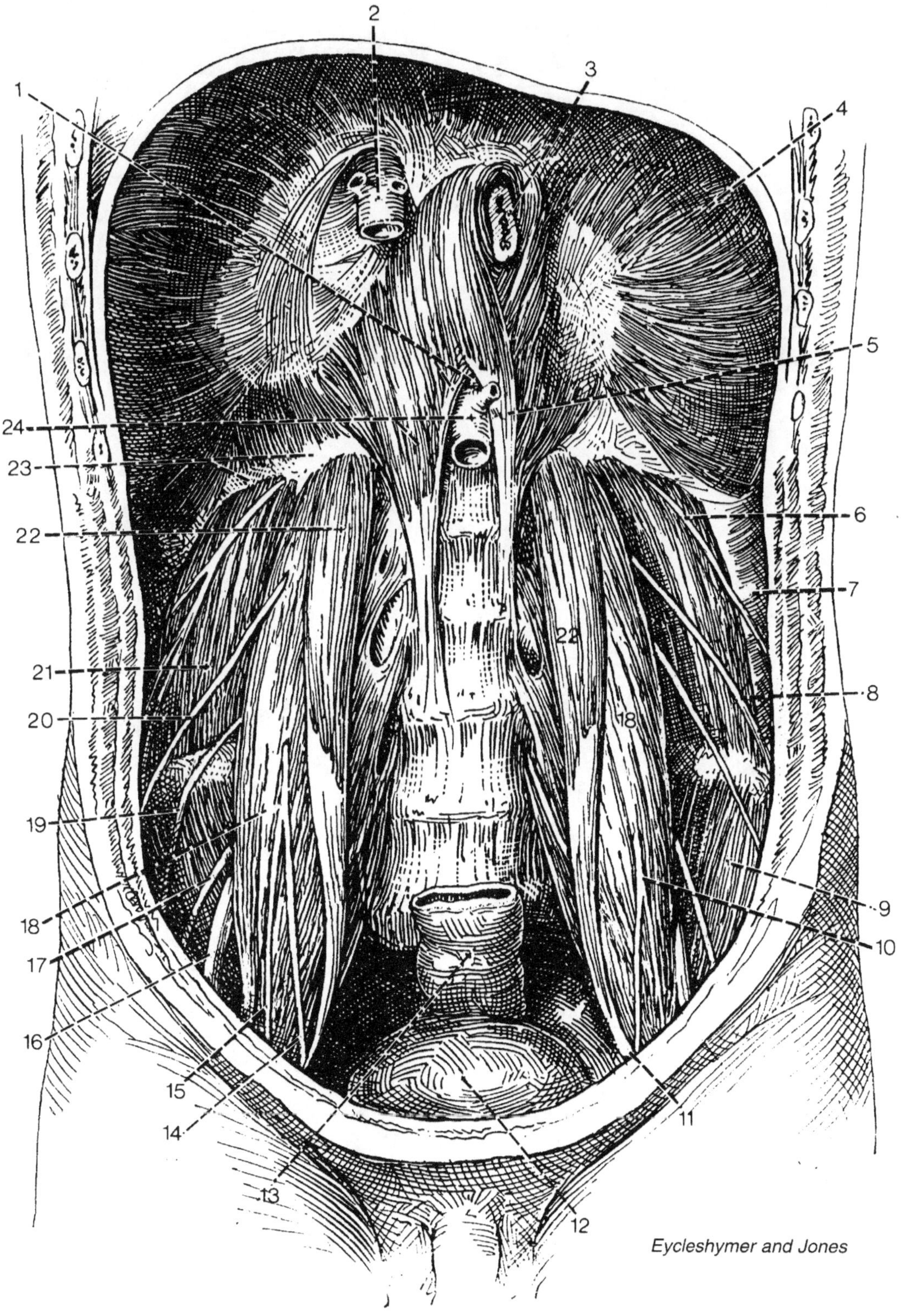

Eycleshymer and Jones

Part III: Pelvis and Perineum

Testicle, Latin, little witness

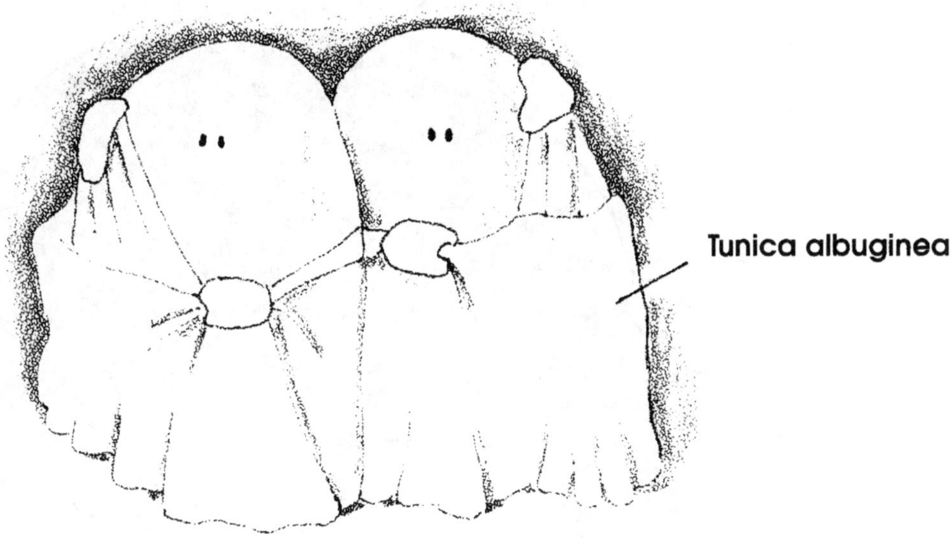

Normal testes

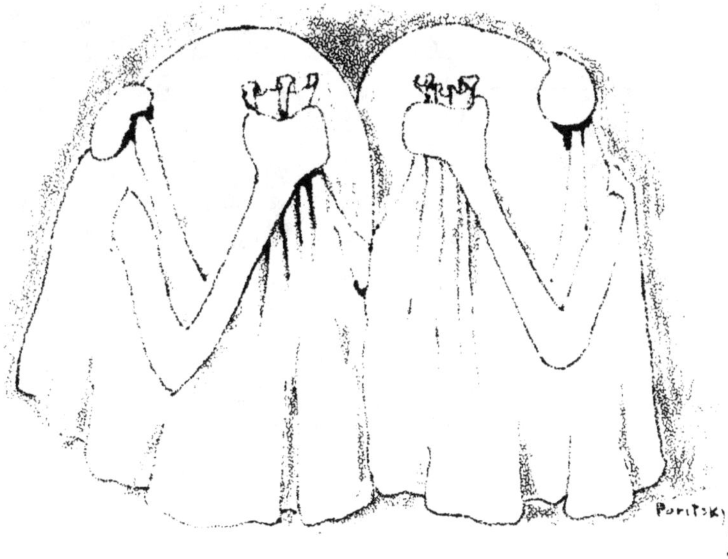

Embarrassed testes

Testis means "witness" in Latin and ***testicle*** means "little witness." There seem to be several theories to account for the word's origin. For one thing, the testes *testify* to one's manhood, and only men could give witness or *testify* in an ancient Roman court of law, or *forum*. Professor William Haubrich suggested that, in certain ancient cultures, when giving *testimony* the witness or *testifier* grasped the scrotum, presumably his own, but on occasion someone else's. In Genesis 24:9 there is a passage in which Abraham's servant places his hand on his master's scrotum while swearing an oath. An additional explanation is that the Romans used the term in the sense of "lookers-on" or "peepers," since the testes would be in a position to observe the sexual act close up.

Tunica albuginea, white tunic, the dense, white, collagenous tunic covering the testes.

P-1 Hip (coxal) bone

Right hip bone, lateral aspect

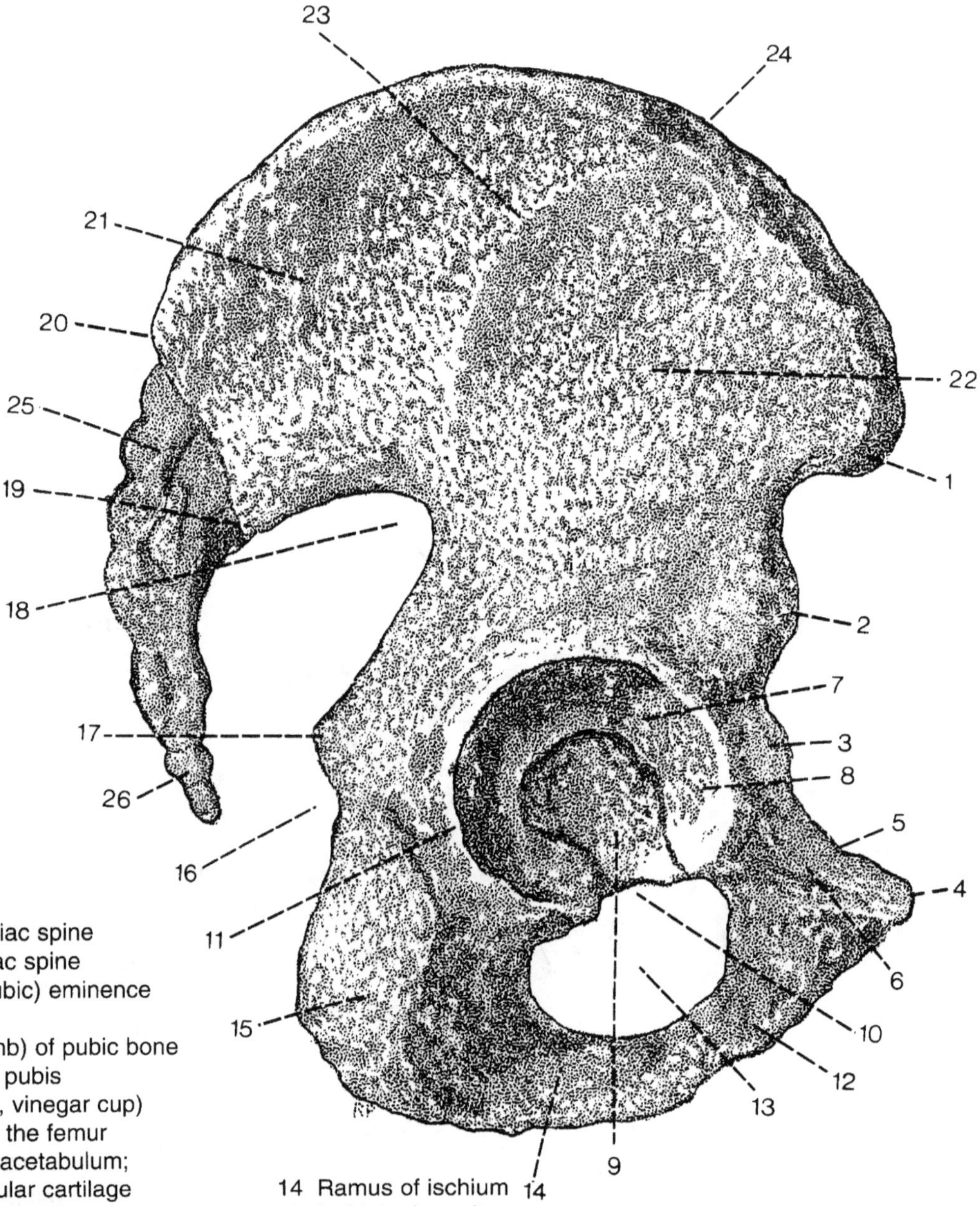

Color and label

1 Anterior superior iliac spine
2 Anterior inferior iliac spine
3 Iliopectineal (iliopubic) eminence
4 Pubic tubercle
5 Pecten (Latin, comb) of pubic bone
6 Superior ramus of pubis
7 Acetabulum (Latin, vinegar cup) socket for head of the femur
8 Lunate surface of acetabulum; covered with articular cartilage
9 Acetabular fossa; the depressed area in the floor of the acetabulum above the acetabular notch.
10 Acetabular notch
11 Border (limbus) of acetabulum
12 Inferior ramus of pubis; this fuses with the ramus of the ischium to form the ischiopubic ramus.
13 Obturator foramen (Latin, *obturo,* to stop up or block)
14 Ramus of ischium
15 Ischial tuberosity
16 Lesser sciatic notch
17 Ischial spine
18 Greater sciatic notch
19 Posterior inferior iliac spine
20 Posterior superior iliac spine
21 Posterior gluteal line
22 Ala (Latin, wing) of ilium
23 Anterior gluteal line
24 Iliac crest
25 Sacrum
26 Coccyx

P-2 Hip bone

Right hip bone, medial aspect

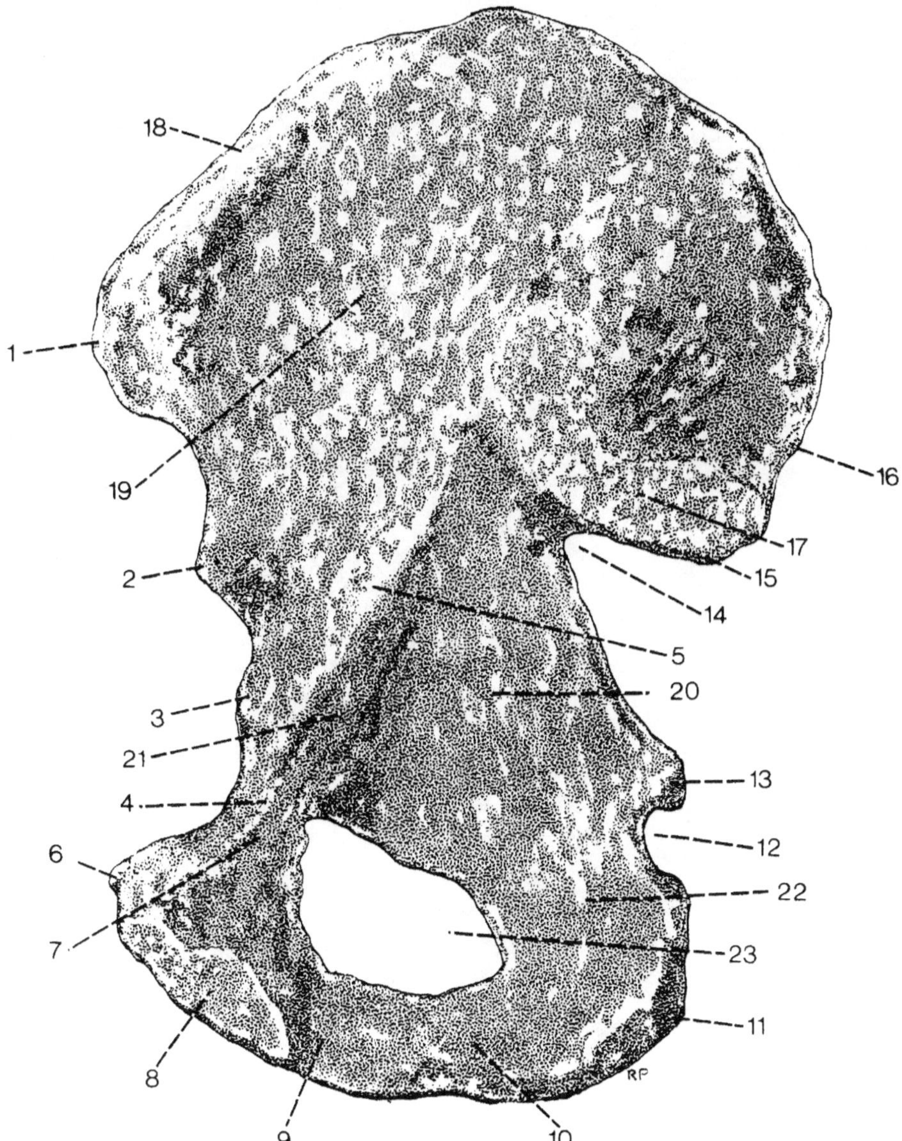

Color and label

1 Anterior superior iliac spine
2 Anterior inferior iliac spine
3 Iliopectineal eminence
4 Pecten of pubis
5 Arcuate line
6 Pubic tubercle
7 Superior ramus of pubic bone
8 Symphysis surface
9 Inferior ramus of pubic bone
10 Ramus of ischium; fusion of 9+10 = ischiopubic ramus.
11 Ischial tuberosity
12 Lesser sciatic notch
13 Ischial spine
14 Greater sciatic notch
15 Posterior inferior iliac spine
16 Posterior superior iliac spine
17 Auricular surface for sacroiliac joint
18 Iliac crest
19 Iliac fossa
20 Body of ilium
21 Body of pubis
22 Body of ischium
23 Obturator foramen

P-3 Hip bone lines of fusion

Color and label

1 Ilium
2 Ischium
3 Pubis
4 Acetabulum (fuses at 15 years)
5 Iliac crest (appears at 16 years; fuses at 25 years)
6 Anterior inferior iliac spine (appears at 16 years; fuses at 25)
7 Pubic tubercle (appears at 16; fuses at 25)
8 Ischial tuberosity (appears at 16; fuses at 25 years)
9 Sacrum

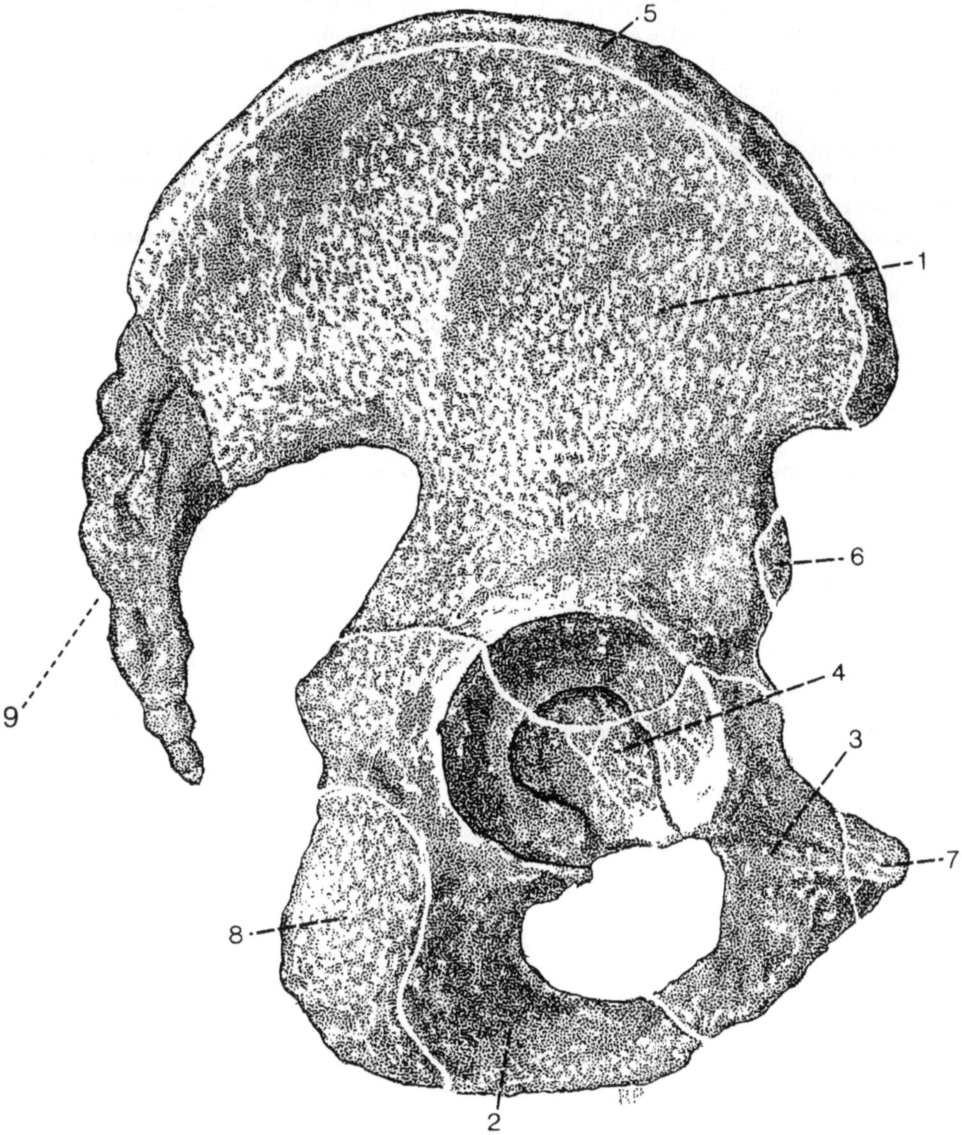

The hip bone consists of the ilium, ischium, and pubis. At birth these bones are separated and joined to one another by cartilage. They do not coalesce into the bony hip bone until the age of 15. Notice how the socket-like acetabulum is formed by each of the three bones. Peripheral parts of the hip bone such as the iliac crest, anterior inferior iliac spine, pubic tubercle, and ischial tuberosity remain as cartilage longer. Bone formation in these peripheral parts first appears at 16 years and fuses with the main bone mass at 25-30 years. The presence of cartilage between the three main bones and the extent of bone fusion are useful clues in estimating the age of the skeleton.

P-4 Male pelvis dissection

(opposite page)

Color and label

1 Skin
2 Superficial (fatty) layer of superficial fascia (Camper's)
3 Deep (membranous) layer of superficial fascia (Scarpa's)
4 Skin of scrotum
5 Dartos tunic; the layer of subcutaneous areolar connective tissues of the scrotum that contains fibers of smooth muscle (dartos muscle, responsible for the deep wrinkles in the skin of the scrotum).
6 Tunica vaginalis (parietal layer). This thin, moist layer which covers most of the testis is reflected posteriorly to form a surrounding parietal layer. The tunica vaginalis is derived in the embryo from a tubular extension of peritoneum (processus vaginalis) that descended with the testis into the developing scrotum. It is usually closed off at the deep inguinal ring at birth.
7 Testis; covered with tunica vaginalis (visceral layer)
8 Epididymis (head); this contains the beginning of the convoluted ductus epididymis that conveys the spermatozoa from the testis to the ductus (vas) deferens which carries them, within the spermatic cord, into the abdomen to the prostate gland where they enter the prostatic urethra.
9 Pampiniform plexus (cut); formed by the intertwining radicles of the testicular vein that surround the testicular artery. This plexus of vine-like venules absorbs heat from the testicular artery so that the arterial blood reaching the testis has cooled enough for spermatogenesis to take place. Undescended testes that remain in the abdomen will not produce viable sperm.
10 Ductus deferens (vas deferens)
11 Superior ramus of pubic bone (cut)
12 Ramus of ischium (cut); this has fused with the more medial inferior ramus of pubis to form the ischiopubic ramus.
13 Colles' fascia (superficial perineal fascia continuous with Scarpa's fascia)
14 Testicular artery (cut)
15 Levator ani muscle
16 Rectum
17 Peritoneum (cut); on superior surface of bladder
18 Prostate gland
19 Bladder (urinary bladder)
20 Seminal vesicle
21 Ureter
22 Superficial fascia of penis (loose areolar connective tissue)
23 Corpus cavernosus penis
24 Corpus spongiosum penis
25 Prepuce of penis (foreskin)
26 Glans of penis
27 External anal sphincter

P-4 Male pelvis dissection

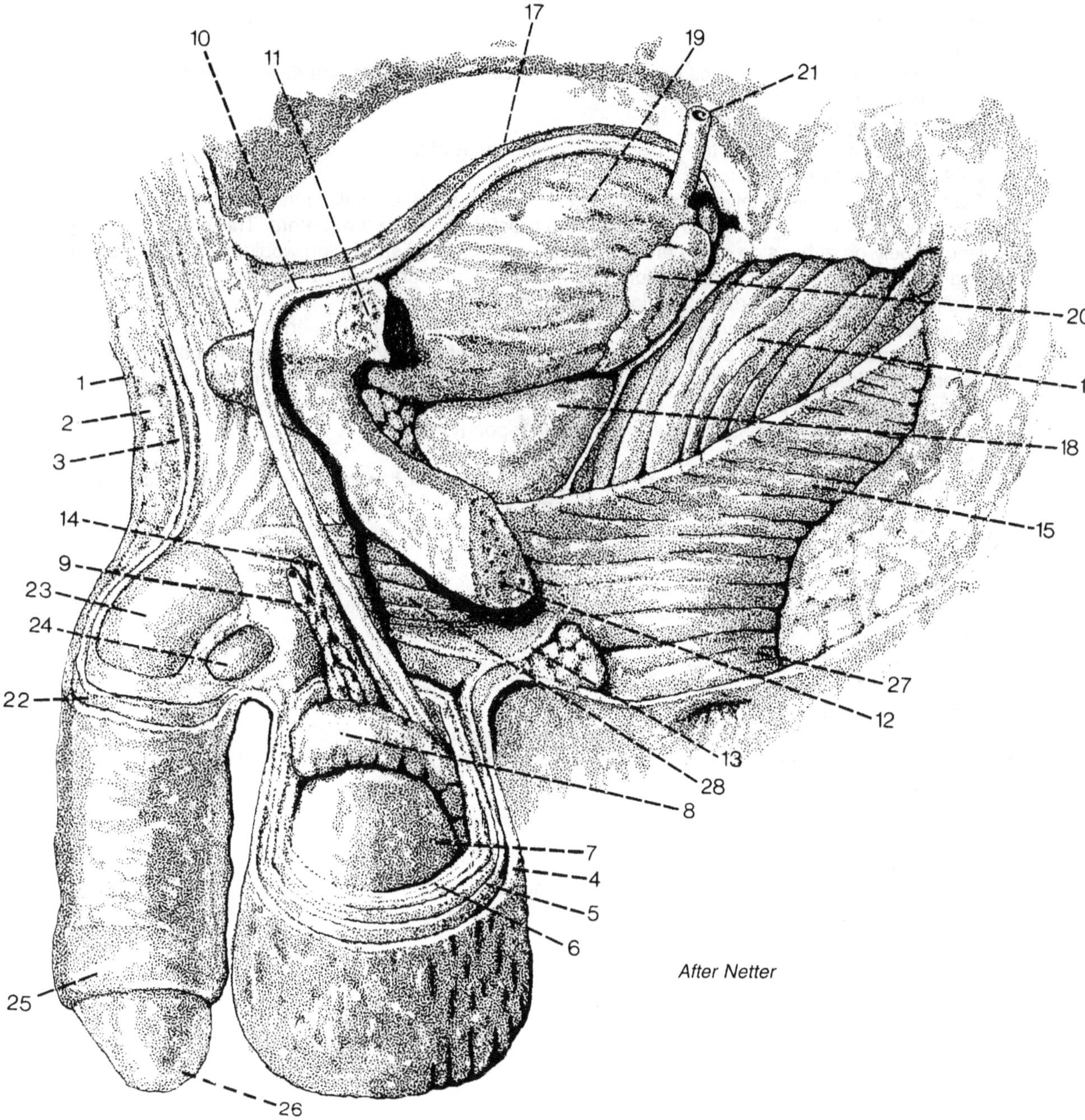

After Netter

P-5 Male pelvis median section

(opposite page)

Color and label

1 Pubic symphysis
2 Bladder
3 Peritoneum on superior surface of bladder; its vertical displacement will depend upon the fullness of the bladder.
4 Suspensory ligament of penis
5 Prostate gland; it surrounds the proximal (upper) portion of the male urethra; its secretion contributes to the seminal fluid.
6 Ejaculatory duct; this receives both the semen from the testis as well as the seminal vesicle secretion, both of which it conveys through the prostate gland to the urethra. The 2 ducts actually lie obliquely on either side of the median plane so that a median section would most likely not pass totally through either of them as pictured here passing through the right ejaculatory duct.
7 Vas (ductus) deferens (terminal portion)
8 Urethra; note that the urethra passes first through the prostate gland, then the urethral sphincter muscle, and then through the length of the corpus spongiosum of the penis; recent investigations list many more subdivisions and parts of the male urethra.*
9 Corpus cavernosum penis
10 Corpus spongiosum penis; it contains the penile (spongy) urethra
11 Bulbospongiosus muscle
12 Urethral sphincter muscle; note that it is more vertical than horizontal as sometimes described. It extends from the bladder to the perineal membrane.†
13 Seminal vesicle; this convoluted tubular structure joins the vas deferens to form the ejaculatory duct. It produces part of the seminal fluid.
14 Perineal membrane
15 Bulbo-urethral gland and duct (left)
16 Superficial perineal fascia (Colles' fascia)
17 Deep fascia of penis (Buck's fascia)
18 Dartos tunic (membranous/smooth muscle layer of superficial fascia of testes; devoid of fat)
19 Septum of scrotum
20 Glans penis; this is the expanded end of the corpus spongiosum penis.
21 Prepuce of penis (foreskin); a fold of skin that covers the glans; removed in circumcision.
22 Navicular fossa of the urethra
23 External anal sphincter
24 Rectum

*The Terminologia Anatomica lists 31 successive parts of the male urethra.
† Oelrich, American Journal of Anatomy, Vol. 158, 1980.

P-5 Male pelvis median section

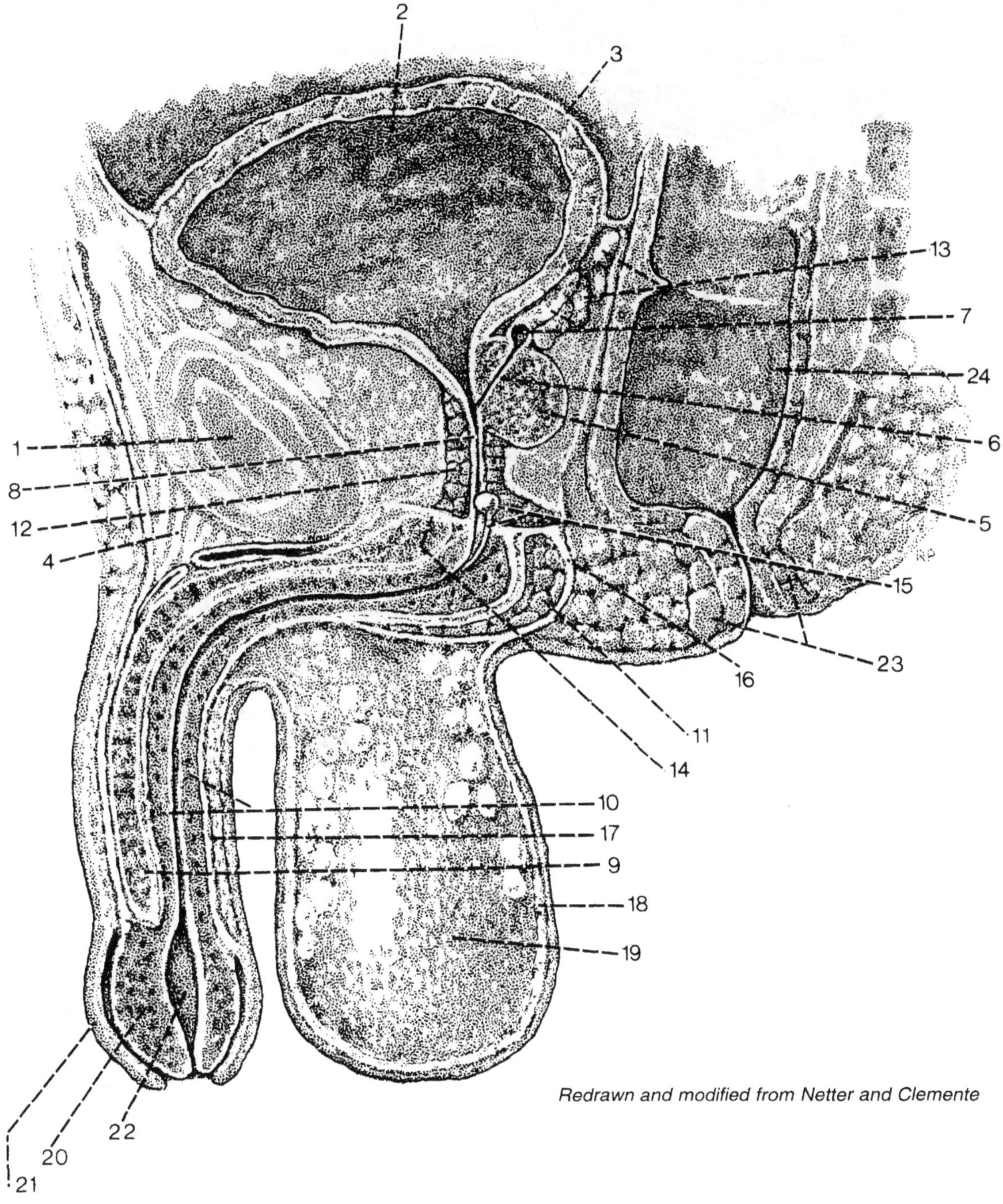

Redrawn and modified from Netter and Clemente

P-6 Male reproductive organs

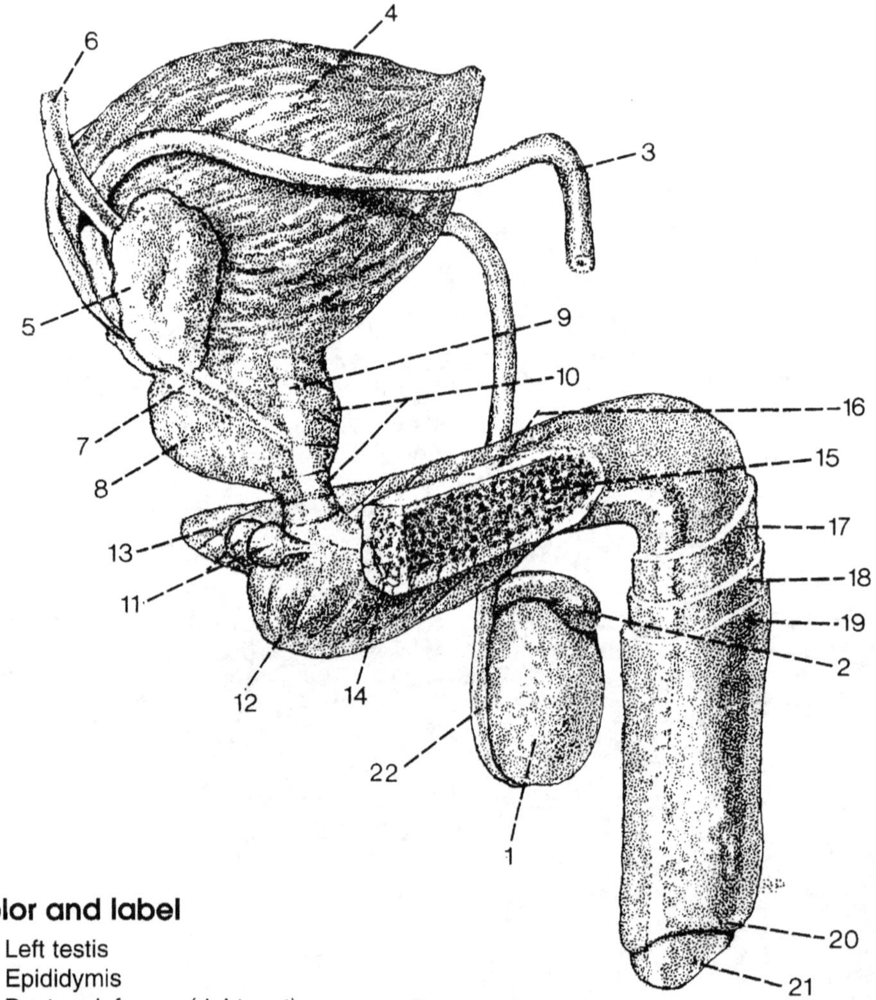

Color and label

1 Left testis
2 Epididymis
3 Ductus deferens (right; cut)
4 Bladder
5 Seminal vesicle (right)
6 Right ureter
7 Ejaculatory duct; this receives the semen from the testis plus the secretion from the seminal vesicle and conveys them through the prostate to the urethra.
8 Prostate gland
9 Prostatic urethra
10 Urethral sphincter muscle; its individual muscle fibers are smaller than those in associated muscles and are embedded in connective tissue, which obscures the visibility of the whole muscle (Oelrich, 1980).
11 Bulborethral glands; these lie within the basal posterolateral portions of the urethral sphincter muscle (not shown); this portion corresponds to the deep transverse perineus muscle in the male.
12 Bulb of penis and bulbospongiosus muscle
13 Left crus of penis and ischiocavernosus muscle
14 Right crus of penis; cut both on superior surface (16) and lateral surface (15).
15 Site of attachment to ischiopubic ramus
16 Site of attachment to overlying perineal membrane (not shown)
17 Deep fascia of penis
18 Superficial fascia of penis
19 Skin of penis
20 Prepuce (foreskin)
21 Glans
22 Left ductus deferens

P-7 The penis

Anterior aspect

Color and label

Figure A. Three erectile bodies

The skin, superficial fascia, and attached muscles (ischiocavernosus and bulbospongiosus) have been removed.

1 Corpus spongiosum penis; contains the penile (spongy) urethra. Proximally its enlarged bulb is firmly attached to the underside of the perineal membrane.
2 Glans of penis. This is the expanded, acorn-shaped end of the corpus spongiosum (whence its name). The glans and distal corpus spongiosum have been separated from the two corpora cavernosa. (Glans is Latin for acorn)
3 Corpus cavernosum penis. Proximally the two crura of the corpora cavernosa are firmly attached to the perineal membrane and the ischiopubic ramus. The two overlying ischiocavernosus muscles have been removed. The conical end of the two united corpora fit into the concavity of the glans
4 Bulb of the penis; the overlying bulbospongiosus muscle has been removed.
5 Crus of penis; the two immobile crura and the bulb comprise the root of the penis. The pendulous free portion is the body of the penis.
6 Perineal membrane (formerly called inferior fascial layer of the urogenital diaphragm; there is no urogenital diaphragm as such).

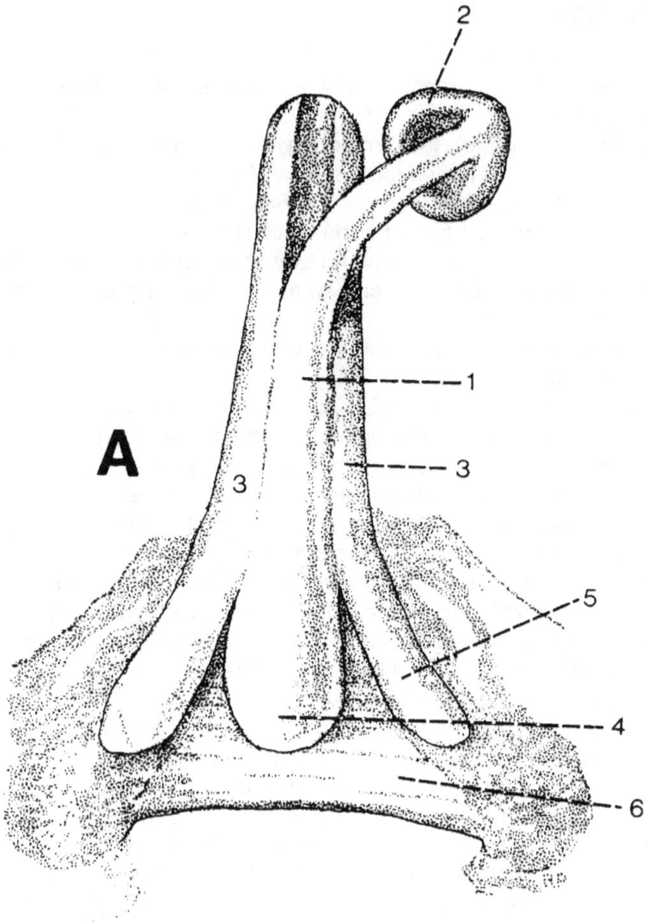

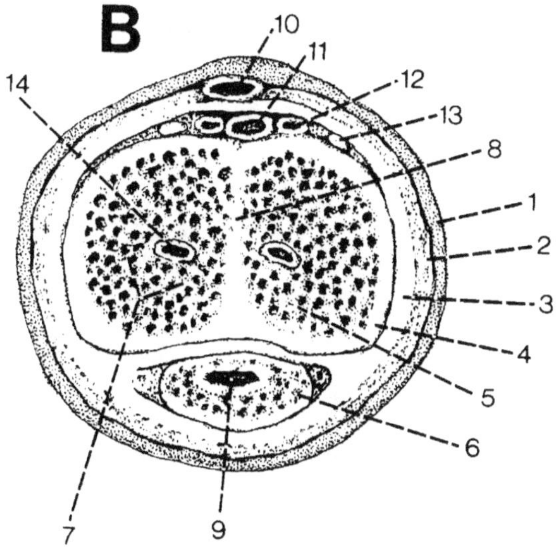

Figure B. Body of penis in cross section

1 Skin
2 Loose connective tissue (superficial fascia)
3 Deep fascia of penis (Buck's fascia)
4 Tunica albuginea
5 Corpus cavernosum penis
6 Corpus spongiosum penis
7 Erectile tissue with cavernous spaces
8 Septum of penis
9 Spongy (penile) part of urethra
10 Superficial dorsal vein of penis
11 Deep dorsal vein of penis
12 Dorsal artery of penis
13 Dorsal nerve of penis
14 Deep artery of penis

The penis becomes erect and enlarged by blood filling the cavernous spaces in the erectile tissue.

P-8 Scrotum and spermatic cord

(opposite page)

Color and label

1 Spermatic cord
2 Ductus (vas) deferens; this is the only structure in the spermatic cord solid enough be identified by palpation.
3 Epididymis (head); the Greek *didymos* actually meant "double, twofold, or twins" but was also used to refer to the paired testes and ovaries.*
4 Pampiniform plexus; this intertwining plexus of small veins which surrounds the testicular artery drains into the testicular vein. It acts as a countercurrent heat exchanger with the testicular artery, thus cooling the arterial blood and allowing the testes to maintain a temperature several degrees below body temperature.
5 Testicular artery
6 Ductus deferens artery; this lies on the ductus deferens. It arises from the patent (open) part of the umbilical artery.
7 Testis; covered with the visceral layer of the tunica vaginalis
8 Superficial inguinal ring; opening in the aponeurosis of the external abdominal oblique muscle
9 Ilioinguinal nerve; this is the major continuation of the first lumbar nerve; in the abdomen this nerve supplies the abdominal muscles and the skin over the pubic symphysis; it then passes through the deep inguinal ring and spermatic cord to supply the skin of the anterior scrotum in the male and anterior labia in the female.
10 Genitofemoral nerve; this nerve derived mainly from nerves L1 and L2 divides into a femoral branch, which supplies the skin of the medial thigh, and a genital branch, which enters the deep inguinal ring and supplies the cremaster muscle. Scratching of the medial thigh will cause the cremaster muscle to contract and the testis to rise (cremasteric reflex).
11 Tunica vaginalis (parietal layer)
12 External spermatic fascia; a tubular layer of fibrous tissue that forms the outermost covering of the spermatic cord and testis; it extends downward from the margins of the superficial inguinal ring.
13 Cremasteric fascia and cremaster muscle
14 Internal spermatic fascia; innermost sheath surrounding the spermatic cord and the testis; it is a tubular prolongation of the transversalis fascia at the deep inguinal ring.
15 Epididymis (Greek, "upon the testis"); shown here isolated with efferent ductules; it receives the immature spermatozoa from the efferent ductules; its elongated coiled duct provides for the storage, transit, and maturation of spermatozoa and is continuous with the ductus deferens at the inferior pole of the testis. It consists of a head, body, and tail.
16 Testis; sectioned with lobules visible; each lobule contains a convoluted seminiferous tubule from whose lining the spermatozoa develop.
17 Skin of scrotum; the underlying smooth muscle (dartos tunic) gives the skin the characteristic corrugated appearance.
18 Dartos tunic
19 Septum of scrotum

*Haubrich, Medical Meanings, 1984.

P-8 Scrotum and spermatic cord

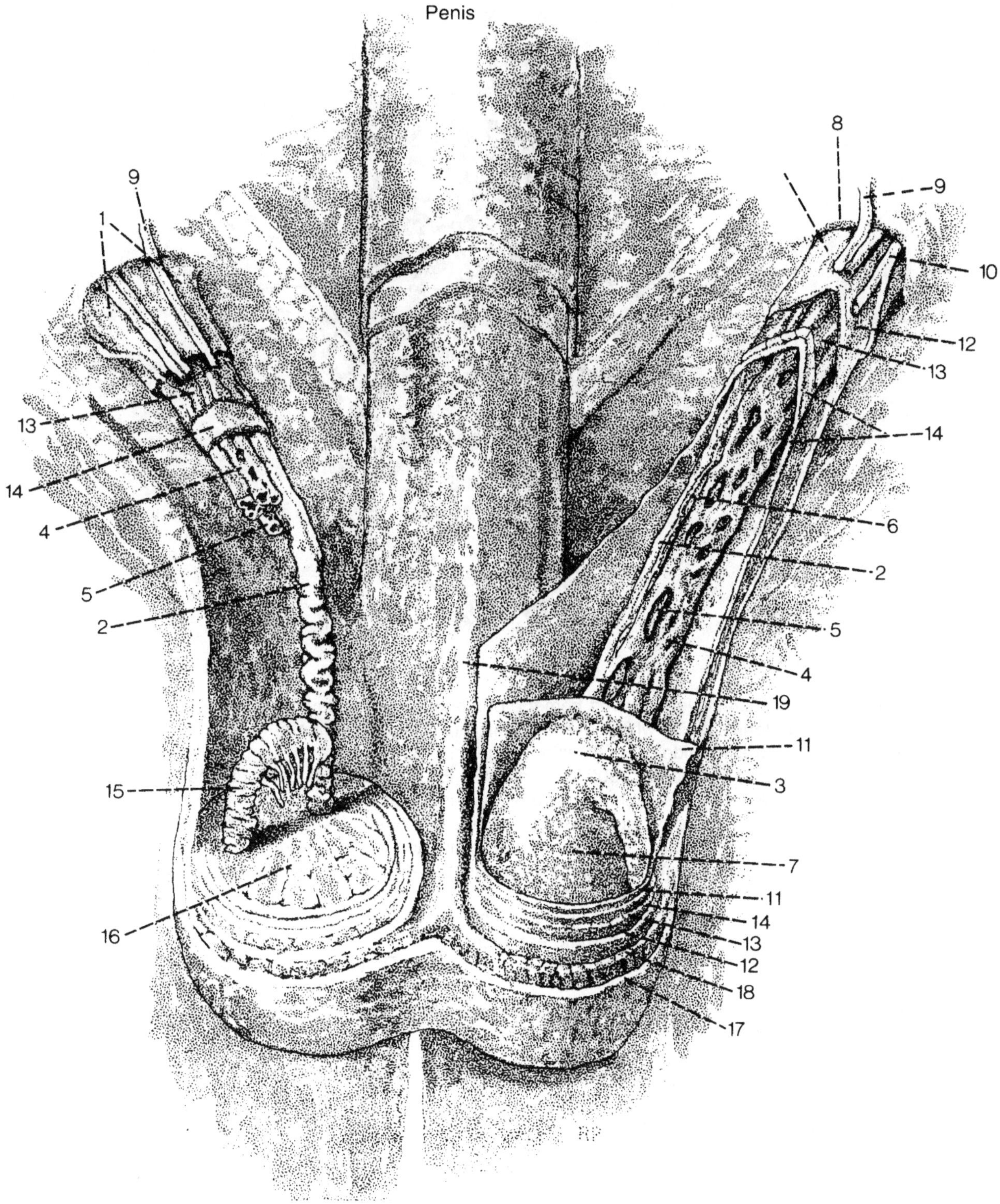

P-9 The testis

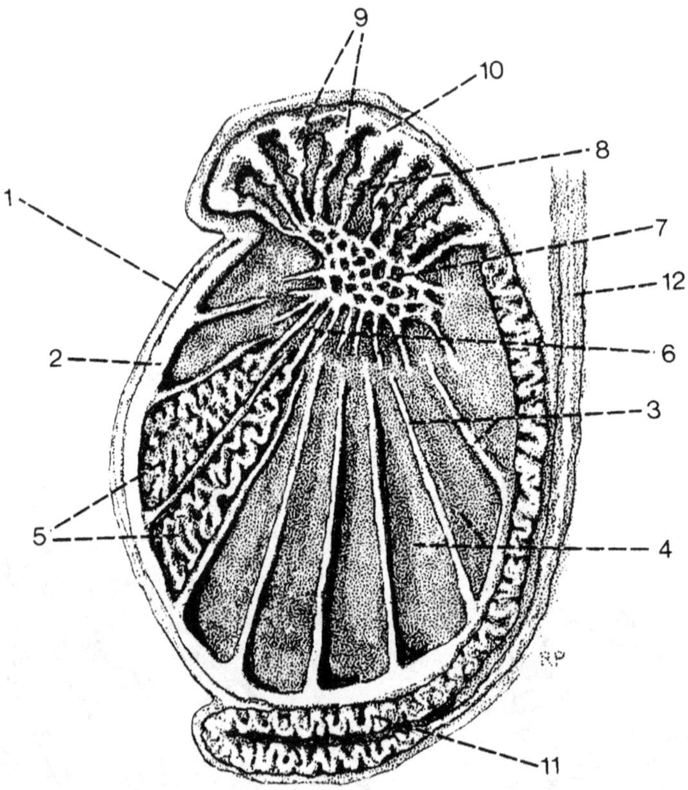

Color and label

1 Tunica vaginalis (visceral layer); derived from the peritoneum during development
2 Tunica albuginea; dense, bluish-white covering consisting of collagen fibers
3 Septula (septums); these divide the testis into wedge-shaped lobules.
4 Lobules of testis; these number 200-300 in each testis. Each contains 1-3 seminiferous tubules Only two lobules are shown here containing seminiferous tubules.
5 Seminiferous tubules (convoluted part); these are highly contorted closed loops that open at both ends into straight tubules (tubuli recti). There are an estimated 400-600 seminiferous tubules in each testis. Each seminiferous tubule is about 70-80 cm long.
6 Seminiferous tubules (tubuli recti, straight part)
7 Rete testis; network of channels formed by the straight seminiferous tubules, traversing the mediastinum testis and draining into the efferent ductules.
8 Efferent ductules of testis; these number between 12 and 20. They become the conical lobules of the epididymis.
9 Lobules of epididymis; each contains a highly contorted efferent ductule. Together they comprise the head of the epididymis.
10 Head of epididymis
11 Tail of epididymis; the epididymis is extremely coiled; unraveled, its total length is about 3 meters.

Bannister and Dyson in Gray's Anatomy, 1995.

P-10 Urethral sphincter in the male

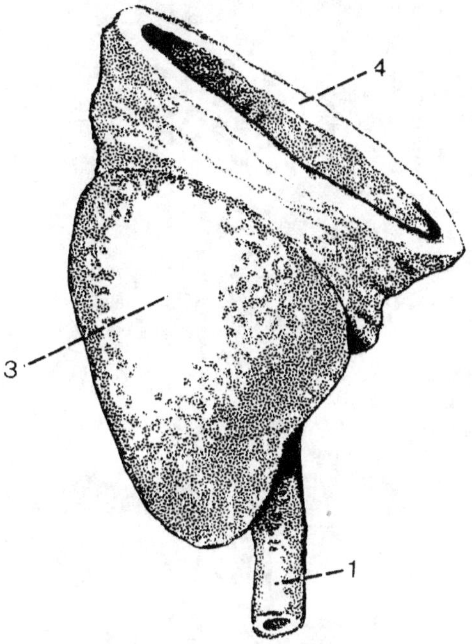

Lateral view with urethral sphincter muscle removed

Color and label

1 Urethra (membranous part)
2 Urethral sphincter muscle
3 Prostate gland
4 Bladder (lower part)
5 Lateral part of urethral sphincter muscle (this part corresponds to deep transverse perineus muscle)

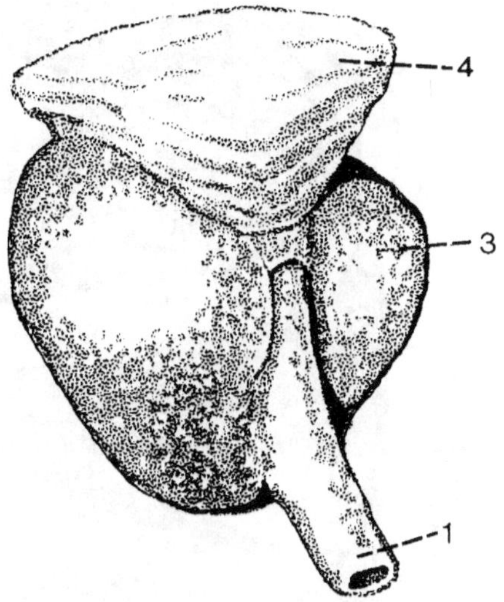

Oblique view with urethral sphincter muscle removed

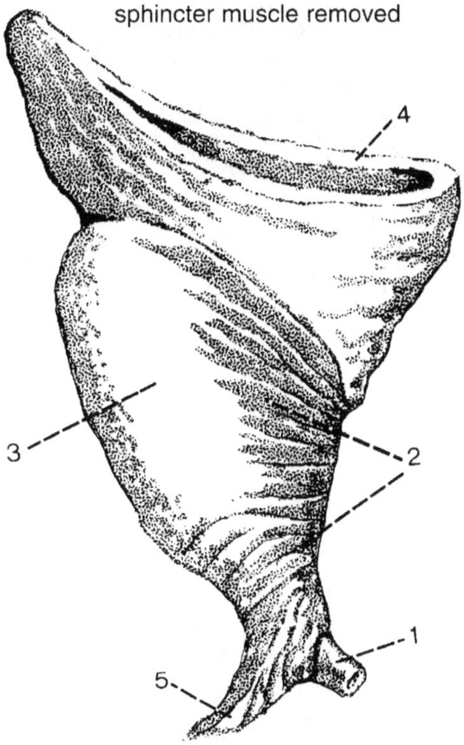

Lateral view from the right

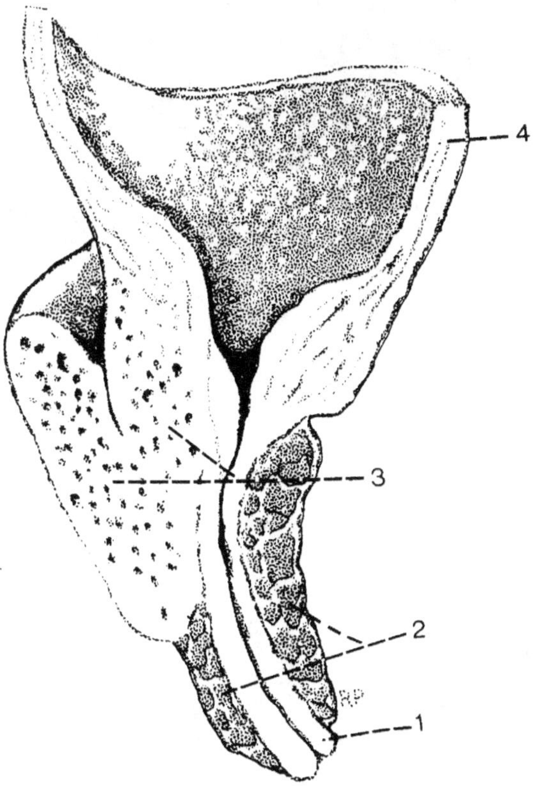

Median section showing extent of contact between urethra and urethral sphincter muscle

There is no distinct superior fascia of the so-called urogenital diaphragm separating the sphincter muscle from the prostate. The fascia of the sphincter muscle is inseparable from the prostatic sheath, is oriented vertically, and passes through the urogenital hiatus to unite with the fascia of the pudendal canals at the ischiopubic rami. Thus the sphincter muscle is a component of the bladder-urethra-prostate-shincter unit which lies within the pelvis, in the urogenital hiatus, and rests upon the perineal membrane. The concept of a urogenital diaphragm is not borne out by this study (Oelrich, 1980, Am J Anat 158).

P-11 Male pelvis, frontal section I

Viewed from behind

Color and label

1 Ductus deferens
2 Ampulla* of ductus deferens
3 Seminal vesicle
4 Ejaculatory duct
5 Urethra (prostatic part)
6 Prostate gland (a wedge has been cut out)
7 Urethral sphincter muscle
8 Bulbourethral glands (also called Cowper's glands); these two small glands lie in the urethral sphincter; their small ducts discharge a mucoid secretion into the spongy (penile) urethra.
9 Urethral sphincter muscle (lateral part)
10 Bladder
11 Pudendal canal; containing pudendal nerve and internal pudendal artery and vein.
12 Ischiopubic ramus
13 Perineal membrane
14 Levator ani muscle
15 Obturator internus muscle
16 Obturator membrane
17 Ischiocavernosus muscle covering crus of penis
18 Bulbospongiosus muscle
19 Superficial perineal fascia (Colles' fascia)
20 Fascia lata (deep fascia of thigh)
21 Superficial perineal pouch
22 Ureter

*A saccular dilation of a canal or duct.

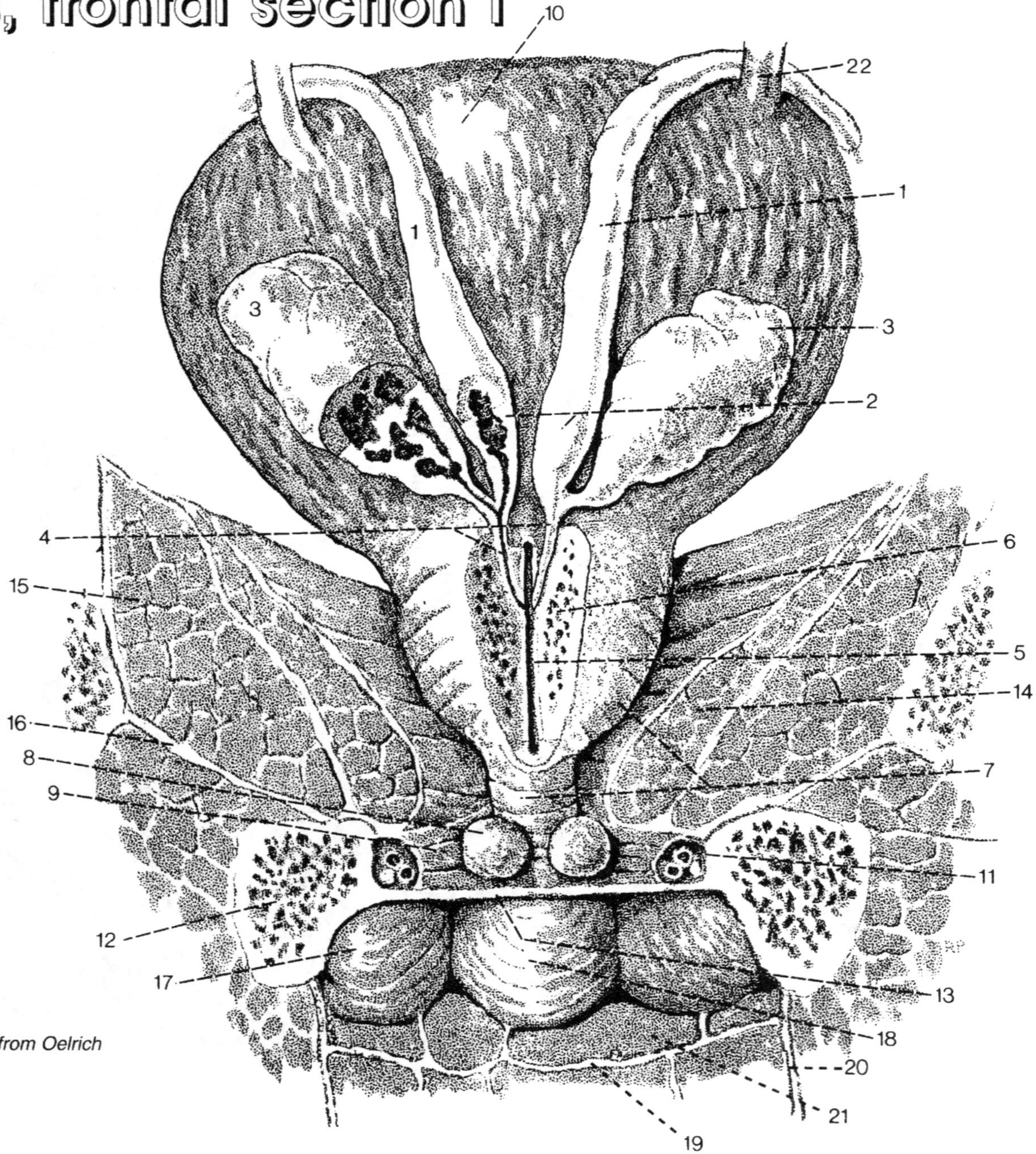

Redrawn from Oelrich

P-12 Male pelvis, frontal section II

Posterior aspect - viewed from behind

Color and label

1 Perineal membrane
2 Urethra (membranous part)
3 Urethral sphincter muscle
4 Deep transverse perineus muscle
5 Prostate gland
6 Ductus deferens
7 Seminal vesicle
8 Levator ani muscle; note the thickening of its inferior border
9 Obturator internus muscle
10 Inferior pubic ramus
11 Corpus cavernosus penis
12 Ischiocavernosus muscle
13 Corpus spongiosus penis
14 Bulbospongiosus muscle
15 Superficial perineal fascia (Colles')
16 Deep fascia of penis (Buck's)
17 Obturator membrane
18 Pudendal canal with internal pudendal artery, vein, and pudendal nerve
19 Fascia lata (deep fascia of thigh)
20 Ilium
21 Sheath of prostate
22 Transversalis fascia
23 Puboprostatic ligament
24 Ejaculatory duct

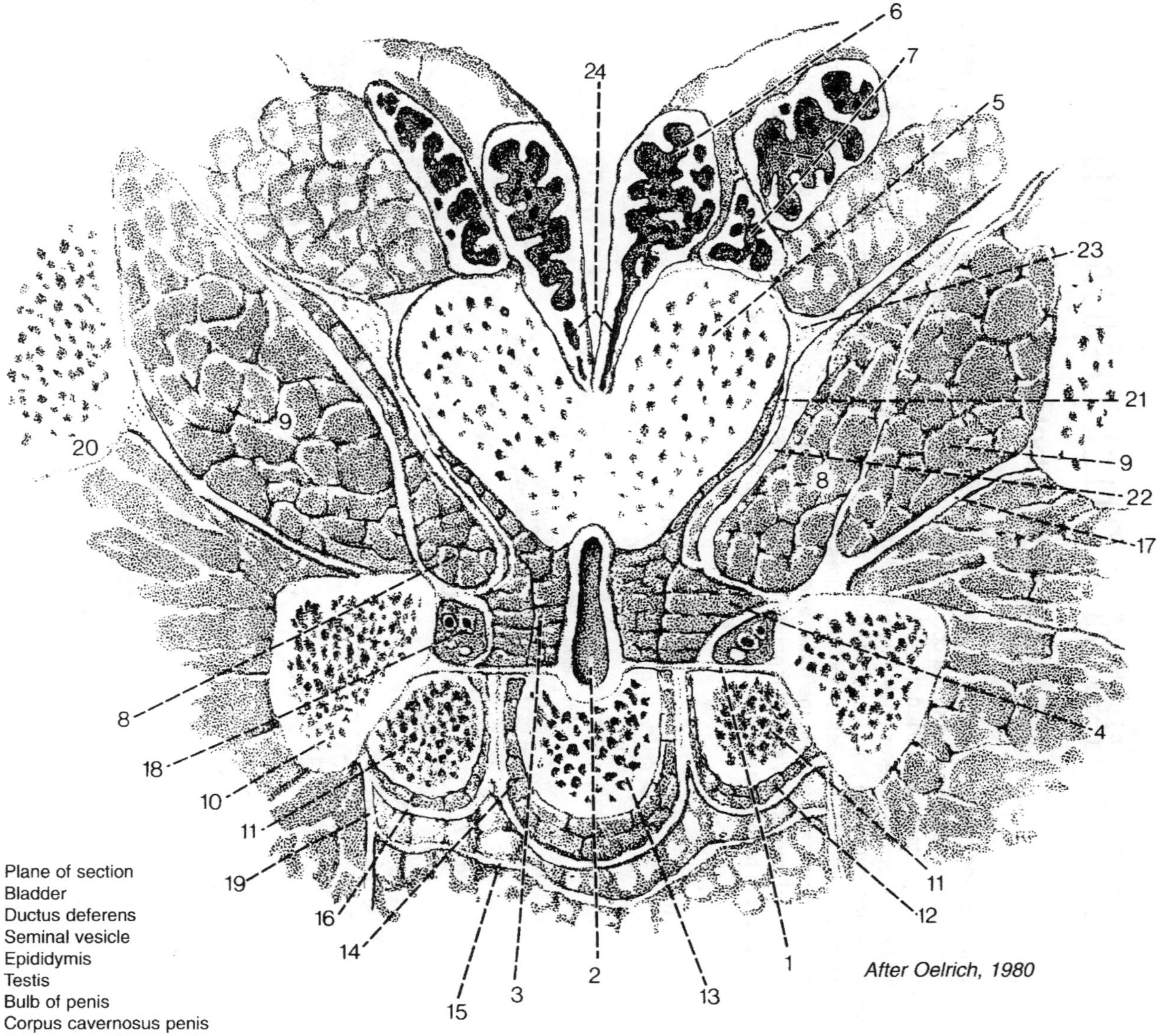

After Oelrich, 1980

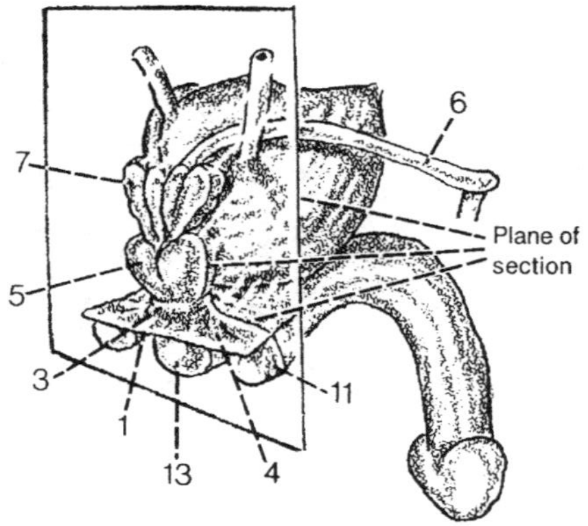

1 Plane of section
2 Bladder
3 Ductus deferens
4 Seminal vesicle
5 Epididymis
6 Testis
7 Bulb of penis
8 Corpus cavernosus penis
9 Corpus spongiosus penis
10 Urethra
11 Perineal membrane
12 Urethral sphincter muscle

P-13 Pelvis and perineum

Viewed from below

The perineum is a diamond-shaped area defined by four landmarks that border the pelvic outlet. These are the pubic symphysis, the two ischial tuberosities, and the coccyx. It is divided into two regions or triangles: the anterior **urogenital triangle** (UGT) and the posterior **anal triangle** (AT). The anterior urogenital triangle is outlined by lines drawn from the pubic symphysis to each ischial tuberosity, and by a third line connecting the tuberosities. The posterior anal triangle is defined anteriorly by the same line between the two ischial tuberosities and two lines connecting them posteriorly to the coccyx. The term perineum also includes all the structures superficial to (below) the diamond shape shown here; these include the bulb of the penis and anus in the male, and the lower vagina, external genital organs, and anus in the female. In obstetrics and gynecology the term perineum is usually restricted to the region between the anal and vaginal orifices. More loosely, the term refers to that part of the lower trunk that lies between the thighs.

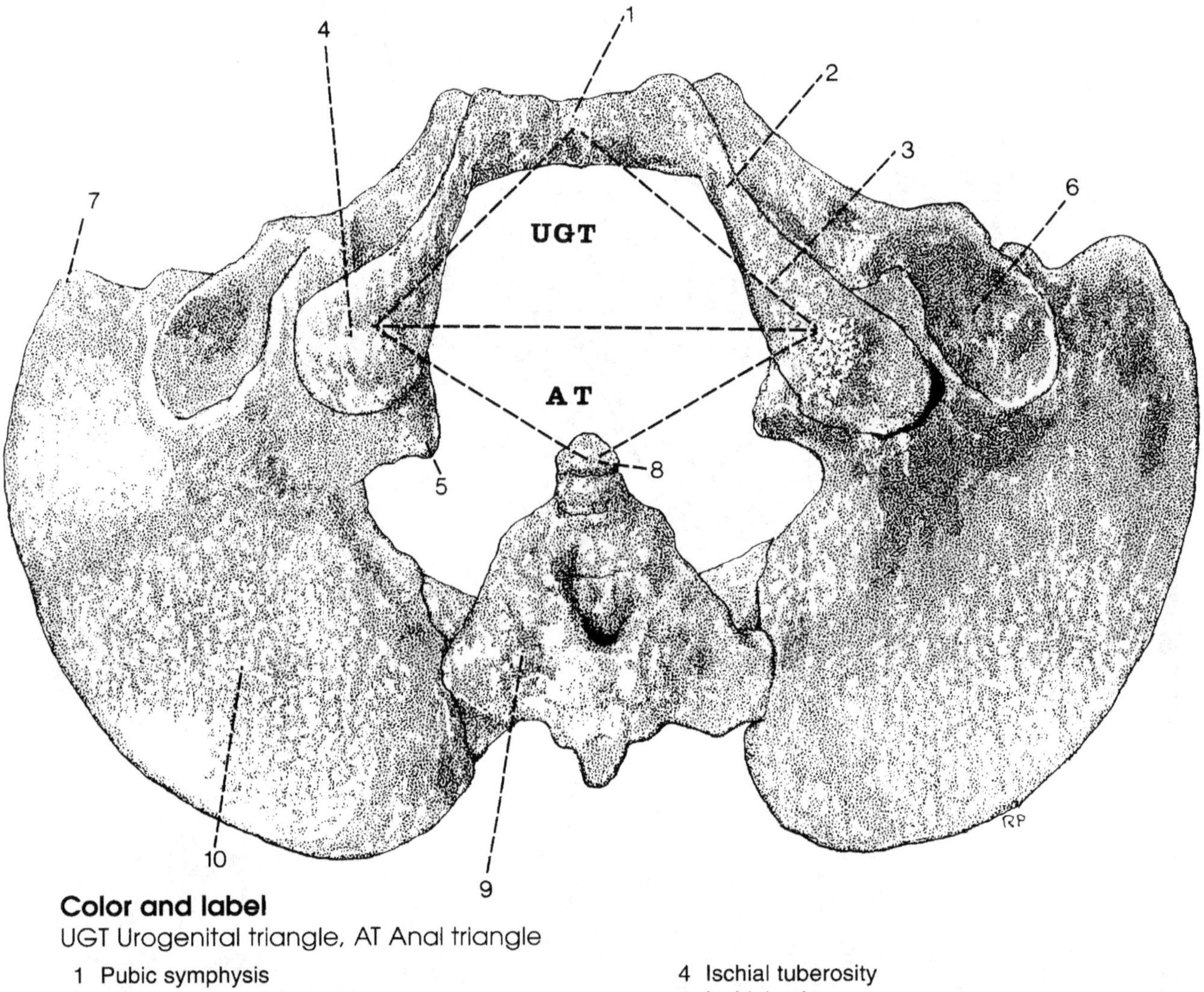

Color and label

UGT Urogenital triangle, AT Anal triangle

1 Pubic symphysis
2 Inferior ramus of the pubic bone
3 Ramus of the ischial bone; this fuses with the inferior pubic ramus by the 3rd decade, forming the ischiopubic ramus
4 Ischial tuberosity
5 Ischial spine
6 Acetabulum
7 Anterior superior iliac spine
8 Coccyx
9 Ala of sacrum
10 Ala of ilium

P-14 Muscles of male perineum

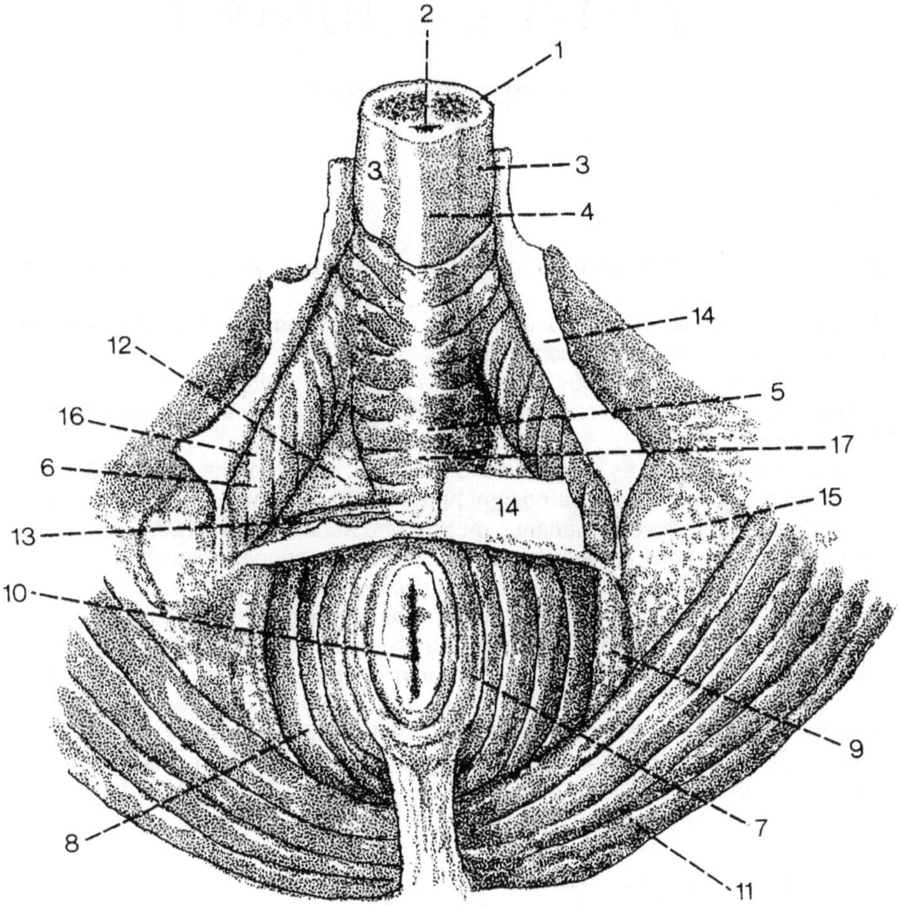

Color and label

1 Penis (cut)
2 Urethra
3 Corpus cavernosum penis; these separate posteriorly and form the two crura.
4 Corpus spongiosum penis; posteriorly this expands into the bulb of the penis.
5 Bulbospongiosus muscle; this covers the bulb of the penis
6 Ischiocavernosus muscle; this covers the crus and anchors it to the ischiopubic ramus and the perineal membrane.
7 External anal sphincter
8 Levator ani muscle; this funnel-shaped muscle is surrounded externally by a wedge of fat that fills the space, the ischiorectal fossa; here shown empty.
9 Pudendal canal
10 Anus
11 Gluteus maximus muscle
12 Perineal membrane
13 Superficial transverse perineus muscle
14 Superficial perineal fascia (Colles', cut and partially reflected)
15 Ischial tuberosity
16 Crus of penis (covered by ischiocavernosus muscle)
17 Bulb of penis (enlarged proximal part; covered by bulbospongiosus muscle)

P-15 Nerves and arteries of the male perineum

(opposite page)

Color and label

1 Pudendal canal; this conveys the internal pudendal artery and vein, and pudendal nerve (the veins are not shown).
2 Inferior rectal artery (branch of internal pudendal); fat has been removed from the ischiorectal fossa.
3 Perineal artery (branch of internal pudendal artery)
4 Branch to superficial transverse perineus muscle
5 Perineal artery in superficial perineal space; this space lies between the deep perineal membrane and the superficial Colles' fascia.
6 Dorsal artery of the penis; this gives off a medial branch to the bulb of the penis and a lateral deep artery of the penis that supplies each corpus cavernosum; here it courses deep to the perineal membrane within the substance of the deep transverse perineus muscle and sphincter urethra muscle.
7 Posterior scrotal branches; these are terminal branches of the perineal artery.
8 Pudendal nerve within pudendal canal; derived from sacral nerves S2, S3, S4.
9 Inferior rectal nerves; these supply the external anal sphincter and skin of the anal region
10 Dorsal nerve of the penis; this supplies the glans and prepuce of the penis; here it travels deep to the perineal membrane within the substance of the sphincter urethra and deep transverse perineus muscles.*
11 Perineal nerve; this supplies the muscles in the superficial perineal space (or pouch) (bulbospongiosus, ischiocavernosus, and superficial transverse perineus muscles).
12 Perineal membrane (partially removed)
13 Perineal nerve on left crus of penis.
14 Posterior scrotal nerves (terminal branches of perineal nerve)
15 Left superficial transverse perineus muscle (cut and reflected)
16 Ischiocavernosus muscle on left crus of penis (pulled laterally)
17 Right crus of penis (covered with ischiocavernosus muscle)
18 Bulb of penis (covered by bulbospongiosus muscle)
19 Penis (corpus spongiosum with urethra)
20 Testes
21 Central perineal tendon (or perineal body)
22 Anus
23 Anococcygeal ligament
24 Coccyx
25 External anal sphincter
26 Levator ani muscle (pelvic diaphragm); this marks the superior extent of the perineum; structures inferior to this muscle are considered within the perineum.
27 Gluteus maximus muscle
28 Colles' fascia (membranous layer of superficial perineal fascia; external or inferior layer of superficial perineal space)

* These muscles and enclosing fascial membranes were formerly believed to form a flat "urogenital diaphragm." The space occupied by the two muscles was called the "deep perineal pouch"; however, because the sphincter urethra in the male appears to be more cylindrical than flat and extends from the perineal membrane to the bladder with no intervening superior fascial layer, the use of the term "urogenital diaphragm" remains questionable.

P-15 Nerves and arteries of the male perineum

Inferior aspect; nerves on the left; arteries on the right

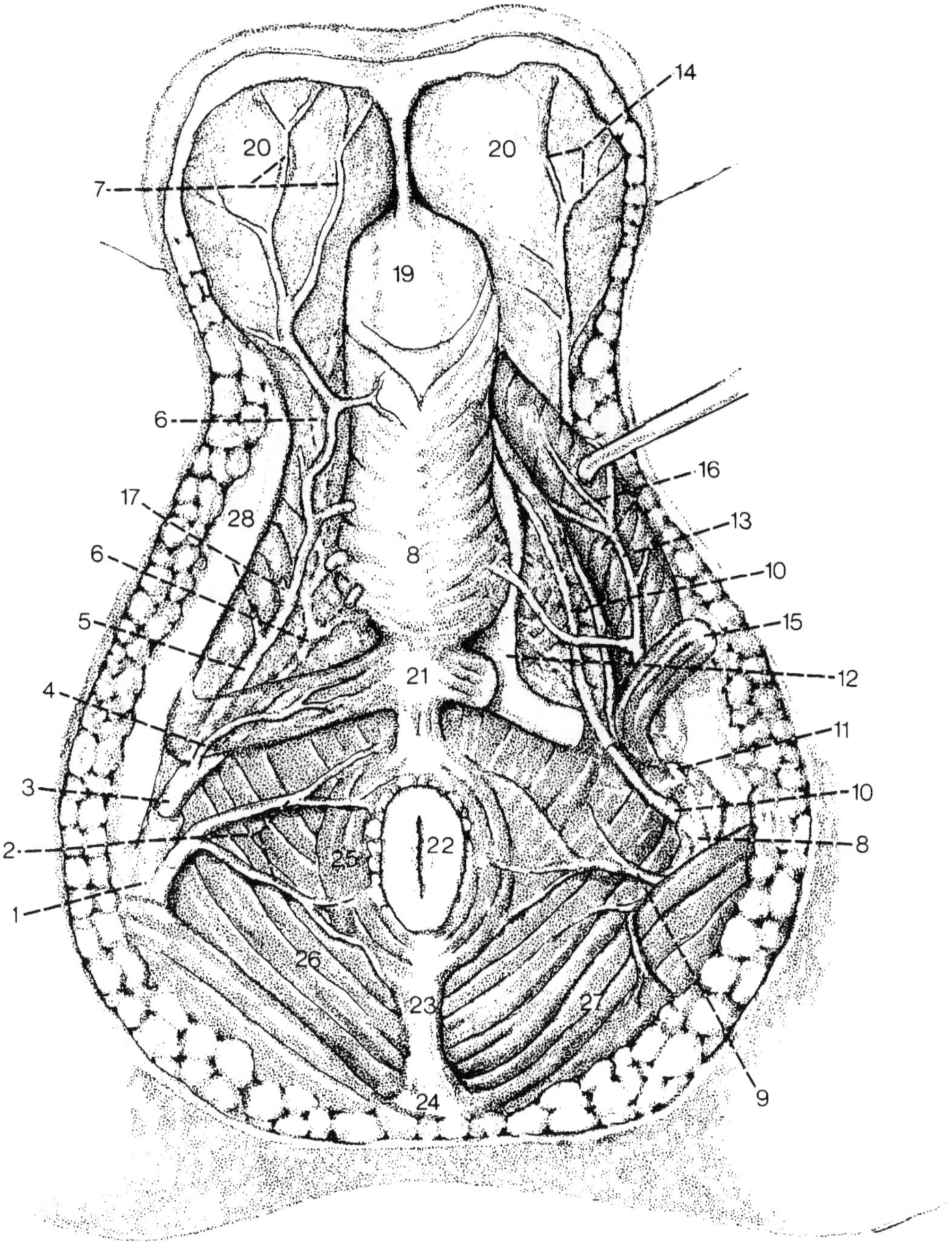

Redrawn from Brooks, JD: Anatomy of the lower urinary tract and male genitalia. In Campbell's Urology, 7th ed., Philadelphia, W.B. Saunders, 1998.

P-16 Male pelvis and perineal muscles

Viewed from the left; sectioned sagittally to the left of the rectum and penis

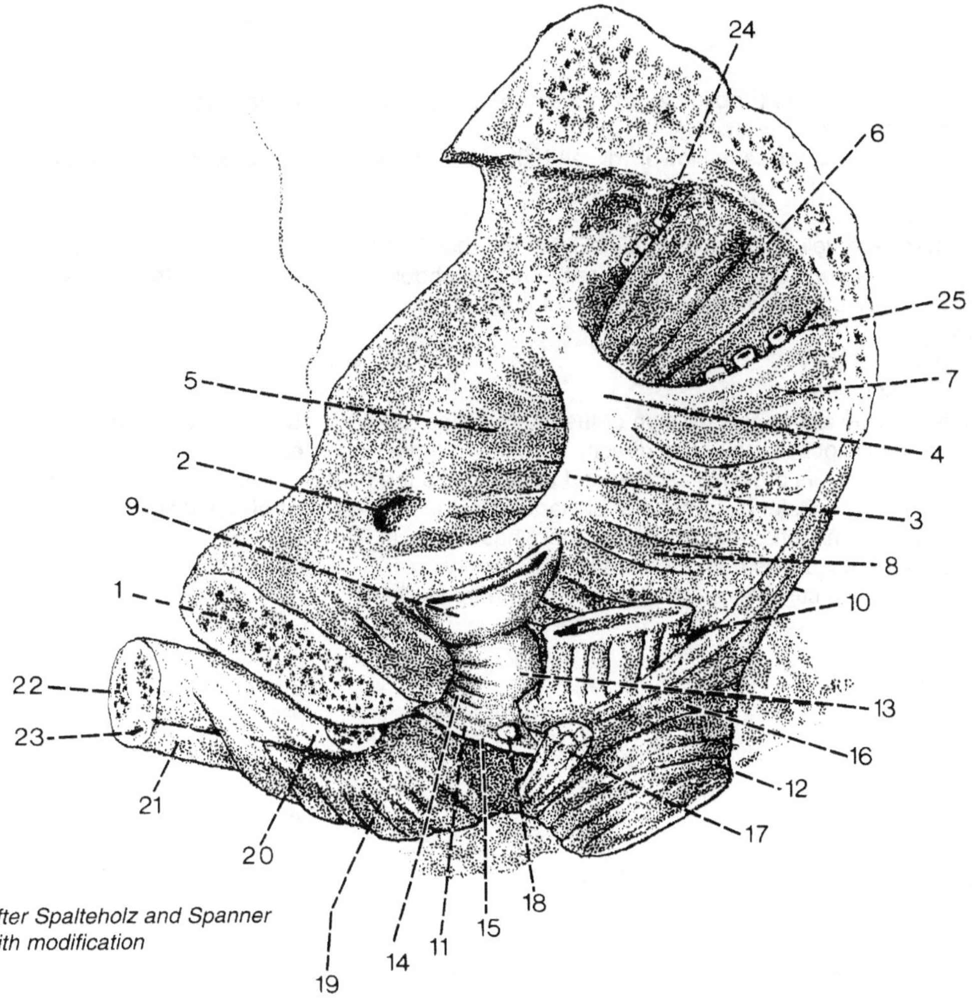

After Spalteholz and Spanner with modification

Color and label

1 Pubic bone (sectioned)
2 Obturator canal
3 Tendinous arch of levator ani muscle
4 Ischial spine
5 Obturator internus muscle
6 Piriformis muscle
7 Coccygeus muscle
8 Levator ani muscle
9 Bladder (cut, lower portion)
10 Rectum (cut)
11 Deep transverse perineus muscle
12 External anal sphincter
13 Prostate gland
14 Urethral sphincter muscle (sphincter urethrae)
15 Perineal membrane
16 Puborectalis muscle (part of the levator ani muscle)
17 Superficial transverse perineus muscle
18 Bulbo-urethral gland
19 Bulbospongiosus muscle
20 Ischiocavernosus muscle (left, covering the left crus of penis)
21 Penis (cut)
22 Urethra (spongy, in corpus spongiosum penis)
23 Superior gluteal artery, vein, and nerve
24 Inferior gluteal artery, vein, and nerve

P-17 Arterial supply of male pelvis

Mainly arteries on right side (opposite page)

Color and label

1 Abdominal aorta; note that it divides (or bifurcates) into a right and a left common iliac artery.
2 Left common iliac artery and vein (both cut)
3 Inferior mesenteric artery; this supplies the lower (distal) half of the large intestine (or colon) and the upper two-thirds of the rectum.
4 Right common iliac artery
5 Right external iliac artery and vein; below the inguinal ligament they become the femoral artery and vein.
6 Inferior epigastric artery; this supplies the lower half of the rectus abdominis muscle. It anastomoses with the superior epigastric artery at approximately the level of the umbilicus.
7 Deep circumflex artery
8 Right internal iliac artery
9 Anterior trunk of internal iliac artery
10 Posterior trunk of internal iliac artery; this division of the internal iliac artery into two trunks is often not present; rather its terminal branches may arise directly from the internal iliac artery.
11 Umbilical artery; after birth only its proximal section and its branch to the bladder (superior vesical artery) remain open or patent; the remainder becomes the obliterated cord-like medial umbilical ligament.
12 Right superior vesical artery; the left superior vesical artery has been cut.
13 Obturator artery; this frequently arises from the external iliac artery.
14 Inferior vesical artery (right; left cut); *vesica* is Latin for the urinary bladder.
15 Middle rectal artery
16 Inferior gluteal artery
17 Internal pudendal artery
18 Iliolumbar artery
19 Lateral sacral artery
20 Superior gluteal artery
21 Middle sacral artery
22 Inferior rectal artery
23 Perineal artery
24 Dorsal artery of penis
25 Deep artery of penis
26 Obturator nerve
27 Lumbosacral trunk; this supplies nerve fibers from lumbar nerves L4 and L5 to the sacral plexus, which supplies the leg.
28 First sacral nerve S1
29 Obturator internus muscle
30 Coccygeus muscle
31 Ductus (vas) deferens (right; left cut and unlabelled)
32 Bladder
33 Prostate gland
34 Ureter (right; left cut and unlabelled)

After Spalteholz and Spanner with modification.

P-17 Arterial supply of male pelvis

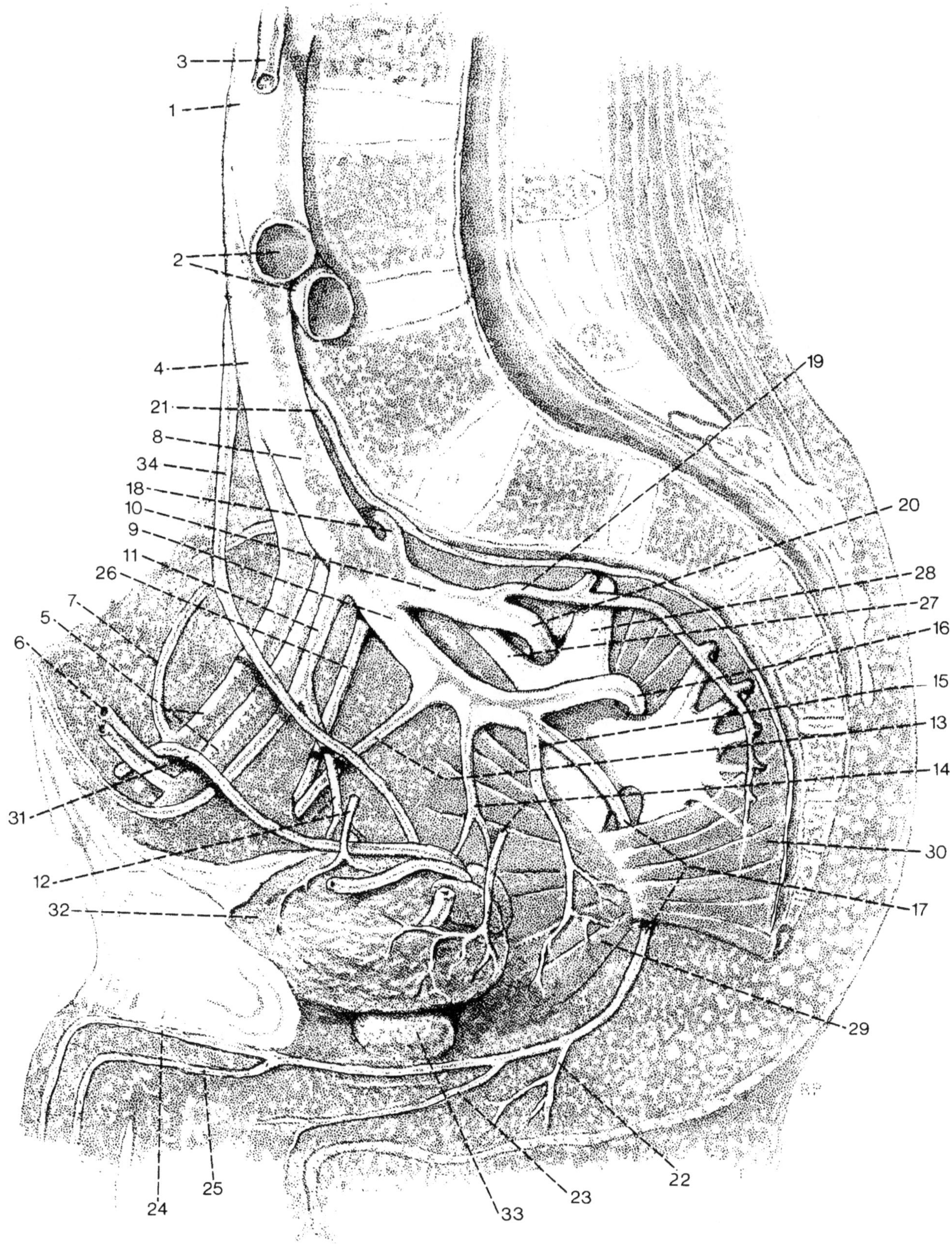

P-18 Male urogenital tract

Bladder, prostate, and penis have been cut open ventrally
Viewed from the front

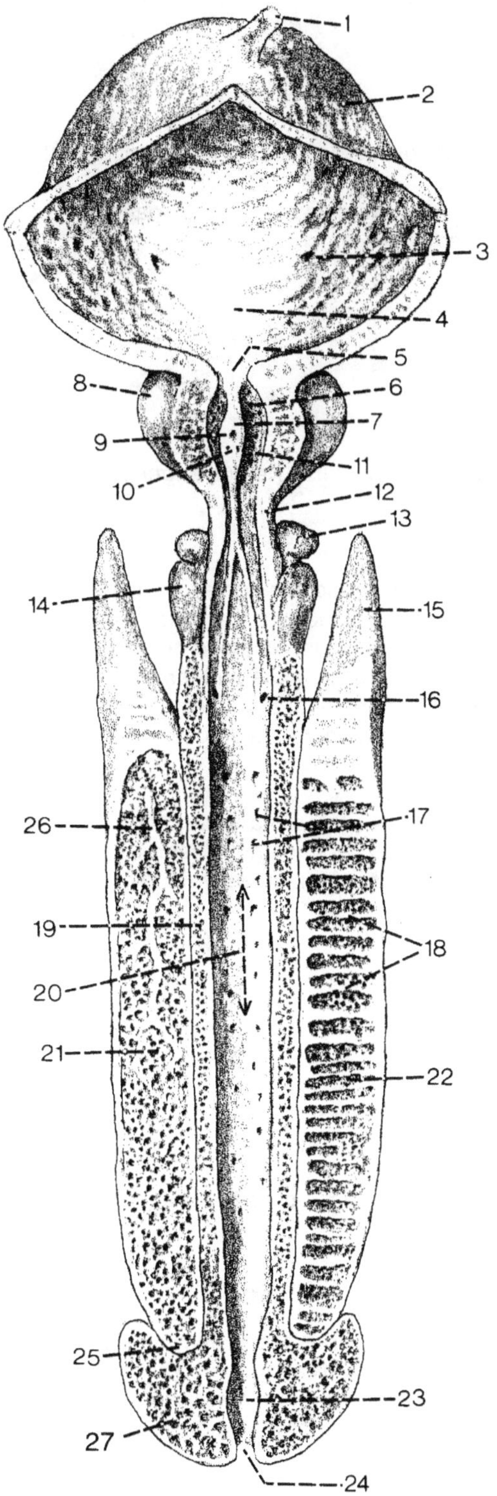

Color and label

1 Urachal cord or ligament; remnant of the the fetal urachus; it persists as a midline fibrous cord between the apex of the bladder and the umbilicus; it forms the median umbilical fold (or plica).
2 Urinary bladder
3 Opening (ostium) of the left ureter into the bladder
4 Trigone of bladder (trigonum vesicae)
5 Internal urethral opening (ostium)
6 Openings of prostatic ductules
7 Seminal colliculus
8 Prostate gland
9 Prostatic utricle; a minute saccular depression in the seminal colliculus; it is the remnant of the embryonic paramesonephric (Mullerian) ducts, which in the male largely disappear; in the female the lower parts form the uterus and upper vagina.
10 Openings of right and left ejaculatory ducts
11 Prostatic sinus
12 Membranous part of urethra; narrowest part of urethra; here the urethra is surrounded by striated muscle.
13 Bulbo-urethral gland
14 Bulb of penis
15 Left crus of penis; the two crura of the penis are firmly attached to the two ischiopubic rami.
16 Opening of bulbourethral glands
17 Urethral lacunae; small recesses in the urethral wall into which the ducts of the urethral glands empty
18 Septum of penis; the penis is divided here slightly to the right of the midline septum, thus causing the midline septa to lie with the left corpus cavernosum.
19 Corpus spongiosum; note that the urethra passes through the corpus spongiosum
20 Penile (spongy) portion of urethra
21 Erectile tissue in right corpus cavernosum
22 Erectile tissue in left corpus cavernosum
23 Navicular fossa
24 External urethral opening
25 Apex of right corpus cavernosum
26 Deep artery of penis
27 Glans of penis

Redrawn from Pernkopf

P-19 Autonomic ganglia and nerves in the male abdomen and pelvis

Viewed from the left
(opposite page)

Color and label

1 Diaphragm (a small portion arising from the posterior wall)
2 12th thoracic nerve (subcostal nerve)
3 Lesser (or minor) splanchnic nerve; arises from the last two thoracic ganglia and passes to the aorticorenal ganglion. It carries preganglionic sympathetic fibers.
4 Greater splanchnic nerve: contains preganglionic sympathetic nerves from thoracic sympathetic ganglia T5 to T9, which end in the celiac ganglion, celiac plexus, and adrenal medulla.
5 Second lumbar sympathetic ganglion with communicating rami
6 Iliohypogastric nerve; notice its origin from 1st lumbar nerve.
7 Ilioinguinal nerve; it also contains nerve fibers from lumbar nerve L1.
8 Obturator nerve; it carries fibers from lumbar nerves L2, L3, L4.
9 Fifth lumbar nerve (L5)
10 Femoral nerve; notice its fibers also come from lumbar nerves L2, L3,L4.
11 Sacral nerve S2; notice its communicating rami.
12 Communicating ramus from sacral nerves S2, S3, and S4; named pelvic nerve (also *nervus erigens*, because of its reported role in penile erection).
13 Pelvic plexus
14 Vesical (bladder) plexus
15 Prostatic plexus on the side of prostate gland; this plexus contains largely microscopic nerves destined for the corpus spongiosum, the dorsal, deep, and urethral arteries. The nerves destined for the corpora cavernosa of the penis (cavernous nerves) are responsible for erection of the penis. As these nerves pass downward and forward they intermingle with the extensive prostatic venous plexus and form a neurovascular bundle (not shown here) (Lepor et al, J Urol, 133, 1985). The terminal branches of these nerves innervate the helicine arteries and the erectile tissue within the corpora cavernosa. (Lue et al, J Urol, 131, 1984).
16 Aortic plexus
17 Celiac gangion (left); note its relation to the celiac arterial trunk and the latter's three branches, the common hepatic artery, the left gastric artery, and the splenic artery. It contains sympathetic neurons whose unmyelinated postganglionic axons* innervate the stomach, liver, gallbladder, spleen, kidney, small intestine, and ascending and transverse colon.
18 Aorticorenal ganglion. It innervates the vasculature of the kidney.
19 Superior mesenteric plexus on superior mesenteric artery
20 Renal plexus on left renal artery
21 Abdominal aortic plexus
22 Inferior aortic plexus
23 Inferior mesenteric artery
24 External iliac plexus on right common iliac artery; left common iliac artery has been cut.
25 Hypogastric plexus
26 Branches of vesical plexus on side of bladder
27 Dorsal nerve of penis; this is the deep terminal branch of the pudendal nerve. It supplies the skin of the penis, the prepuce, and the glans.

g, sympathetic chain ganglia; B, urinary bladder; ur, ureter; A, abdominal aorta; dd, ductus deferens.

* Preganglionic (myelinated) fibers exit the spinal cord with spinal nerves that they then leave by way of *white communicating rami.* Postganglionic (unmyelinated) axons travel within *gray communicating rami.* The distinction between white and gray is attributed to the presence or absence of myelin. However, in the dissecting laboratory it is impossible to distinguish between the two types of fibers, white or gray, with the naked eye.

Redrawn from Francis and Voneida in Morris' Anatomy, 1966.

P-19 Autonomic ganglia and nerves in the male abdomen and pelvis

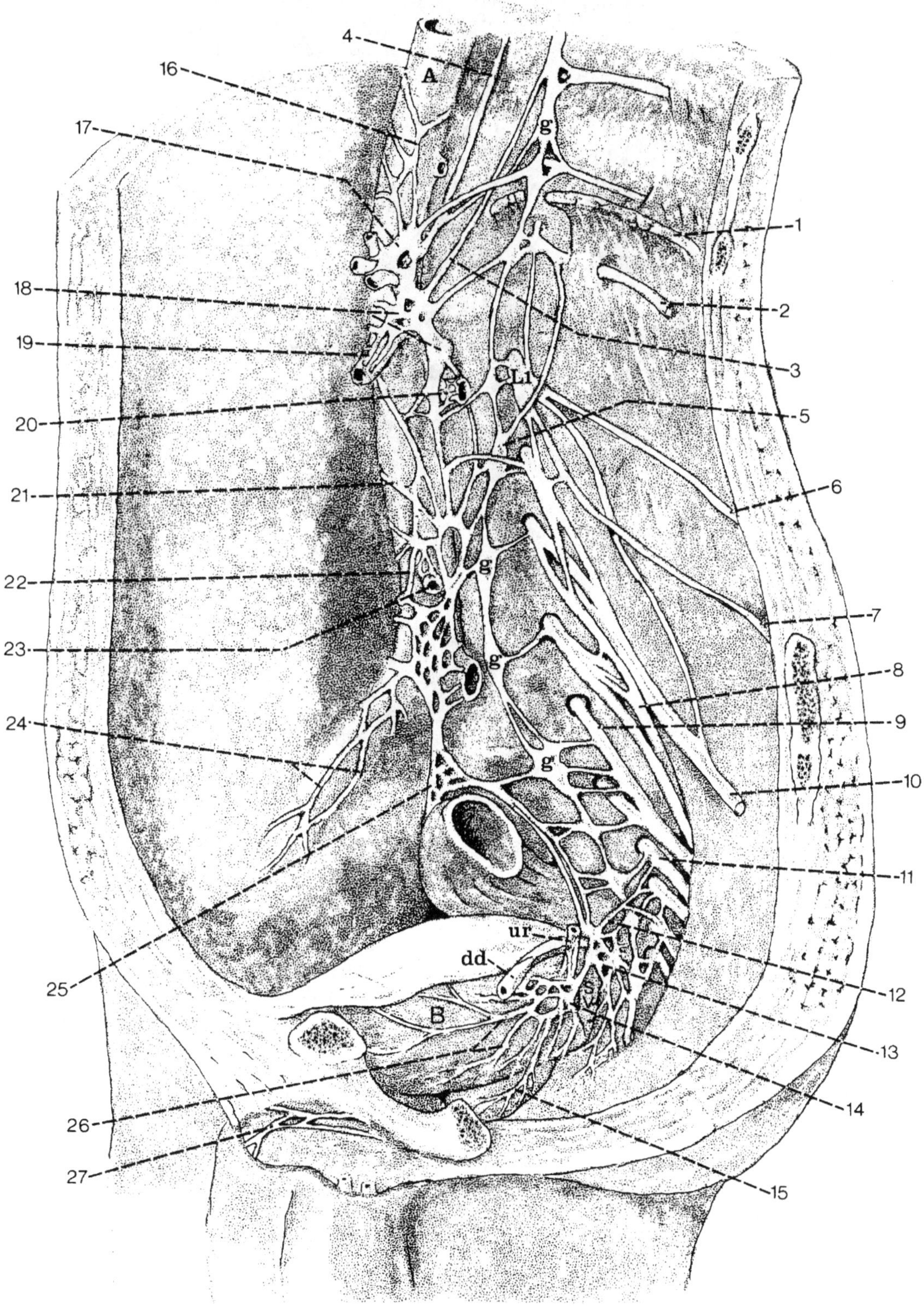

P-20 Female perineum

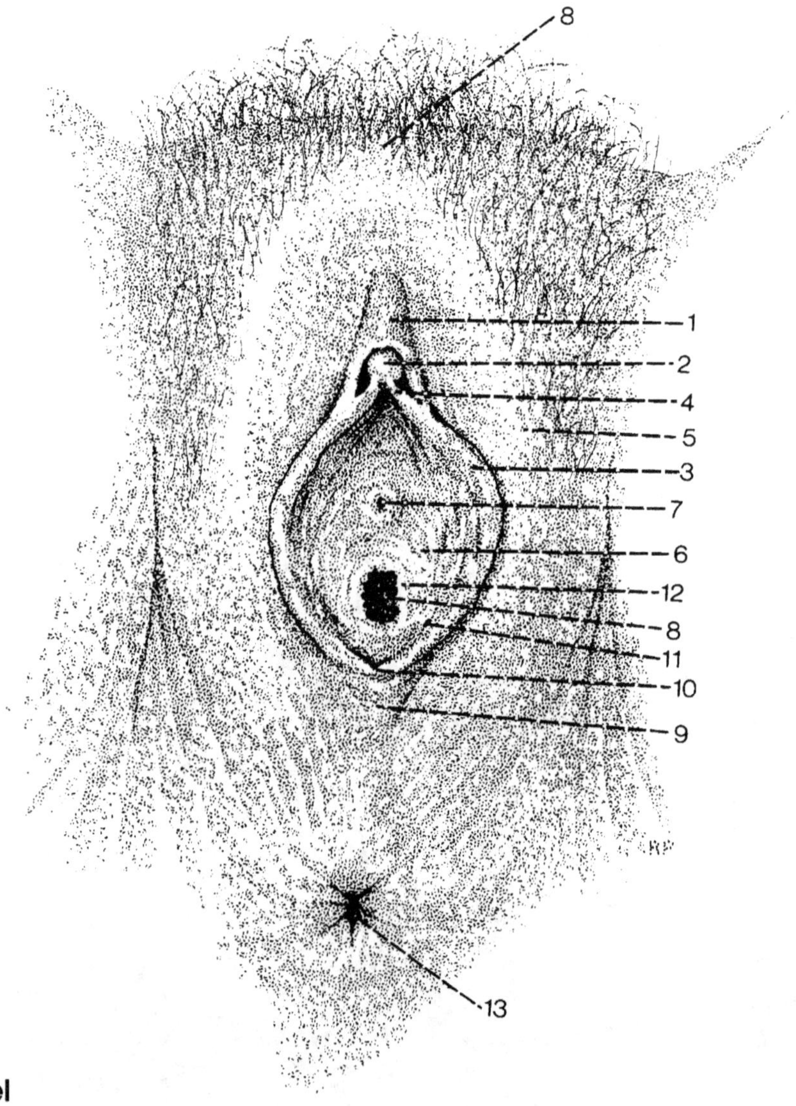

Color and label

1 Prepuce of clitoris; a fold of skin that covers the body of the clitoris; formed by the anterior union of the labia minora.
2 Glans of clitoris; erectile tissue at the end of the clitoris; richly supplied with nerve endings making it extremely sensitive.
3 Labium minus (singular; plural is *labia minora*, minor lips); a fold of skin bordering the vestibule of the vagina. Anteriorly the two labia minora split into a medial and lateral fold; the lateral folds unite anteriorly over the clitoris and form its prepuce; the medial folds insert on the deep surface of the clitoris and form the frenulum of the clitoris.
4 Frenulum of clitoris (Latin *frenum*, rein); attached to the under surface of the clitoris; formed by the insertion of the two medial folds of the labia minora.
5 Labium majus (singular; plural is *labia majora*, major lips)
6 Vestibule of vagina; almond-shaped space opening between the labia minora containing the openings of the vagina, urethra, and the two ducts of the greater vestibular glands.
7 External urethral opening
8 Mons pubis; the rounded fleshy prominence over the pubic symphysis
9 Posterior labial commissure; a slight fold uniting the labia majora posteriorly in front of the anus
10 Frenulum of labia minora; posterior union of the labia minora (also called the fourchette, French, diminutive of *fourche,* pitchfork).
11 Opening (left) of greater vestibular gland
12 Hymen (remains of); the membranous fold that partially or wholly occludes the external opening of the vagina.
13 Anus

P-21 Female erectile tissue

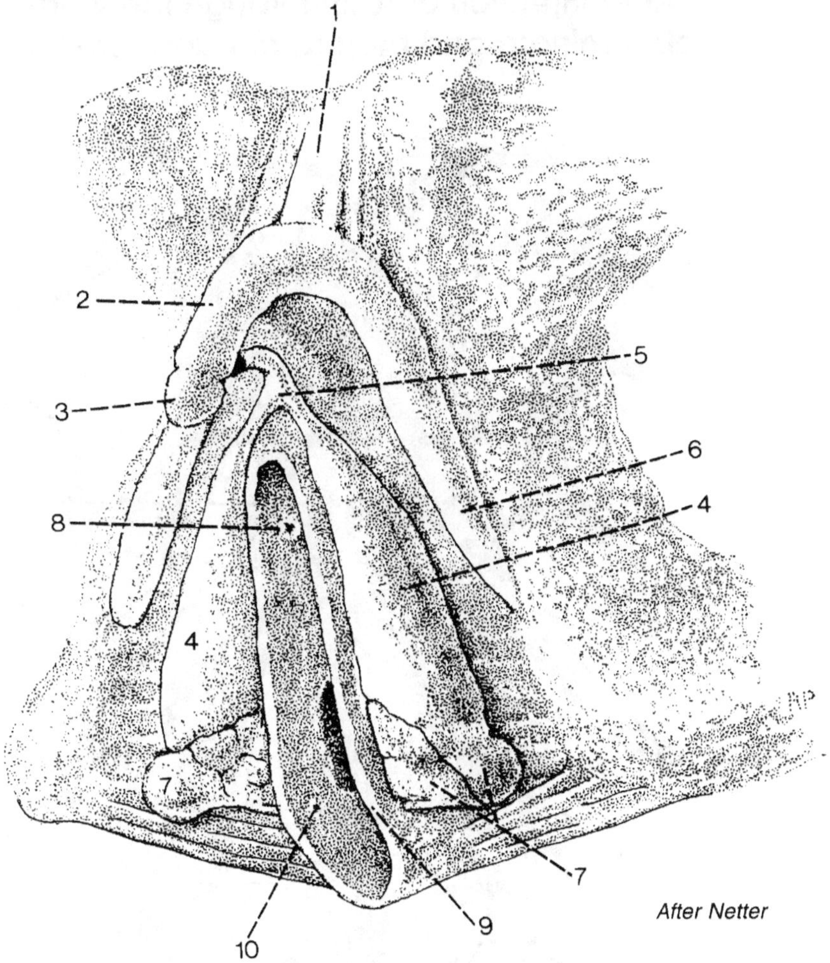

After Netter

Color and label

1 Suspensory ligament of clitoris; this suspends the body of the clitoris from the pubic symphysis.
2 Body of the clitoris. The clitoris is homologous to the male penis. Like the penis, it is an erectile organ. It consists of a body, two crura, and a glans. The body, about 2 cm (1 inch) long, consists of two fused corpora cavernosa. It is covered by the prepuce of the clitoris.
3 Glans of clitoris; the glans is a small rounded tubercle located at the free distal end of the body. It is partly covered by the hood-like prepuce of the clitoris. It is highly sensitive.
4 Vestibular bulb; these are two oval masses of erectile tissue on either side of the opening of the vagina. They are situated on the inferior surface of the perineal membrane and each is covered by the bulbospongiosus muscle (not shown).They are homologous to the corpus spongiosus of the male penis. They differ from the male, however, in that they are not fused but remain separate and do not contain the urethra, as does the male corpus spongiosum. Each is connected to the other anteriorly by a narrow pars intermedia bulborum, which together form the commissure of the vestibular bulb. The commissure is also continuous with the glans of the clitoris by a short narrow extension.
5 Commissure of vestibular bulb; formed by the joining of the two pars intermedia bulborum (two intermediate parts of the bulbs).
6 Left crus of clitoris; The two crura are continuous with the corpora cavernosa and serve to attach them to the inferior rami of the pubic bone. They are both covered by the ischiocavernosa muscles (not shown here).
7 Greater vestibular gland and duct (also called Bartholin's gland); these lie posterior to the bulb of the vestibule and discharge their mucoid secretion into the vestibule of the vagina. They correspond to the bulbo-urethral glands in the male.
8 External urethral orifice
9 Labium minus
10 Orifice of duct of greater vestibular gland

P-22 Clitoris and vestibular bulb

After injection of resin through the veins
Labia minora and majora cut and removed

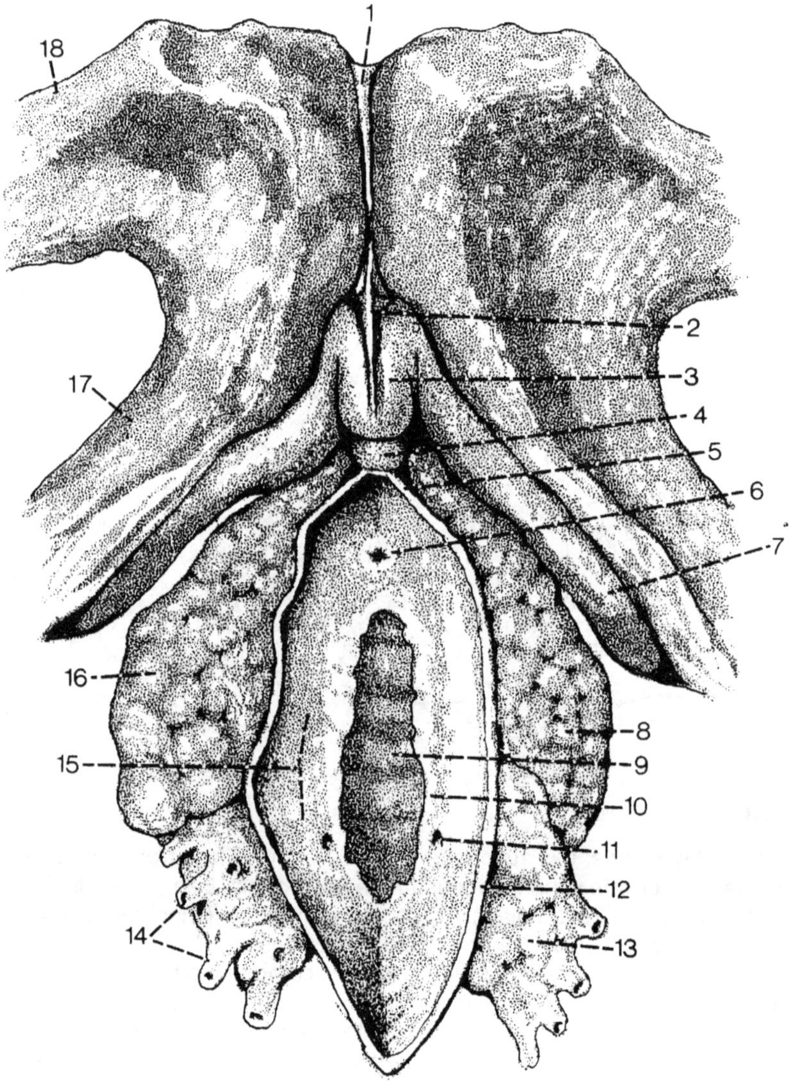

Color and label

1 Pubic symphysis
2 Suspensory ligament of clitoris
3 Body of clitoris
4 Glans of clitoris
5 Frenulum of clitoris
6 Urethral external orifice
7 Crus (left) of clitoris
8 Vestibular bulb (left)
9 Vagina
10 Opening of vagina (vaginal orifice)

11 Opening of duct of greater vestibular gland
12 Line of excision of labia minora
13 Greater vestibular gland
14 Venous plexus
15 Vestibule of the vagina
16 Right vestibular bulb
17 Inferior ramus of pubis
18 Superior ramus of pubis

Redrawn from Toldt

P-23 Female pelvis, median section

Ileum and colon removed except for terminal portion of large intestine

Color and label

1 Uterus (body)
2 Cervix of uterus
3 Fundus of uterus
4 Ovary
5 Bladder
6 Urethra
7 Vagina
8 Anus
9 Rectum
10 Uterine tube (also oviduct, fallopian tube, salpinx)
11 Ampulla (dilation) of oviduct
12 Infundibulum (funnel-like) of fallopian tube
13 Fimbria (Latin, fringe) of fallopian tube
14 Proper ovarian ligament
15 Ovarian suspensory ligament
16 Rectouterine pouch

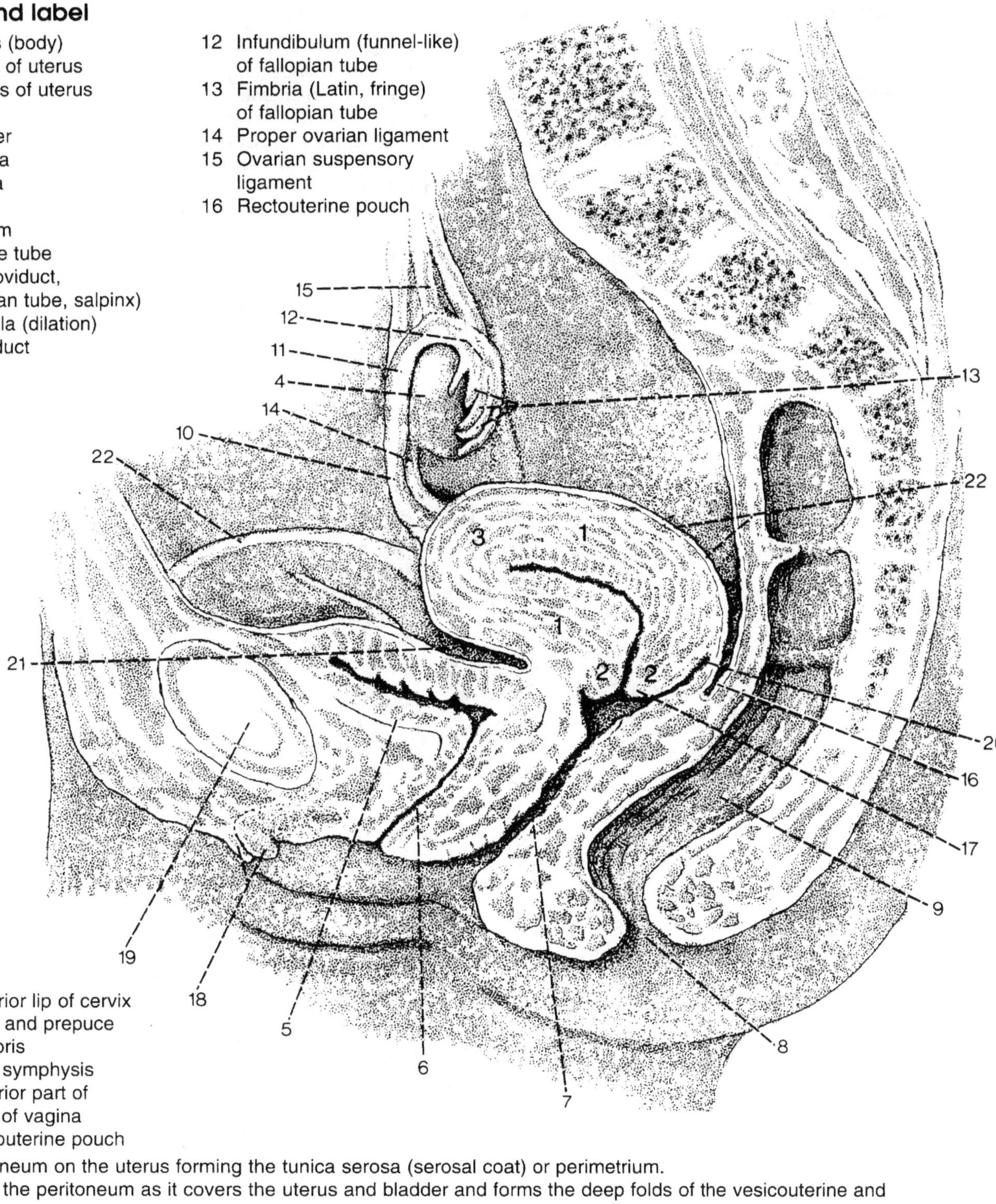

17 Posterior lip of cervix
18 Glans and prepuce of clitoris
19 Pubic symphysis
20 Posterior part of fornix of vagina
21 Vesicouterine pouch
22 Peritoneum on the uterus forming the tunica serosa (serosal coat) or perimetrium.
Trace the peritoneum as it covers the uterus and bladder and forms the deep folds of the vesicouterine and rectouterine pouches.

P-24 Female superficial perineal muscles

Color and label

1 Suspensory ligament of clitoris
2 Prepuce covering body of clitoris
3 Bulbospongiosus muscle* (covering bulb of vestibule and greater vestibular gland)
4 Ischiocavernosus muscle* (covering the left crus of the clitoris)
5 Glans of the clitoris
6 External urethral opening (orifice)
7 Vagina
8 Labium minus (cut)
9 Perineal membrane
10 Superficial transverse perineus muscle
11 Levator ani muscle
12 External anal sphincter muscle
13 Anus
14 Gluteus maximus muscle

*These muscles are thinner and more delicate than those in the male.

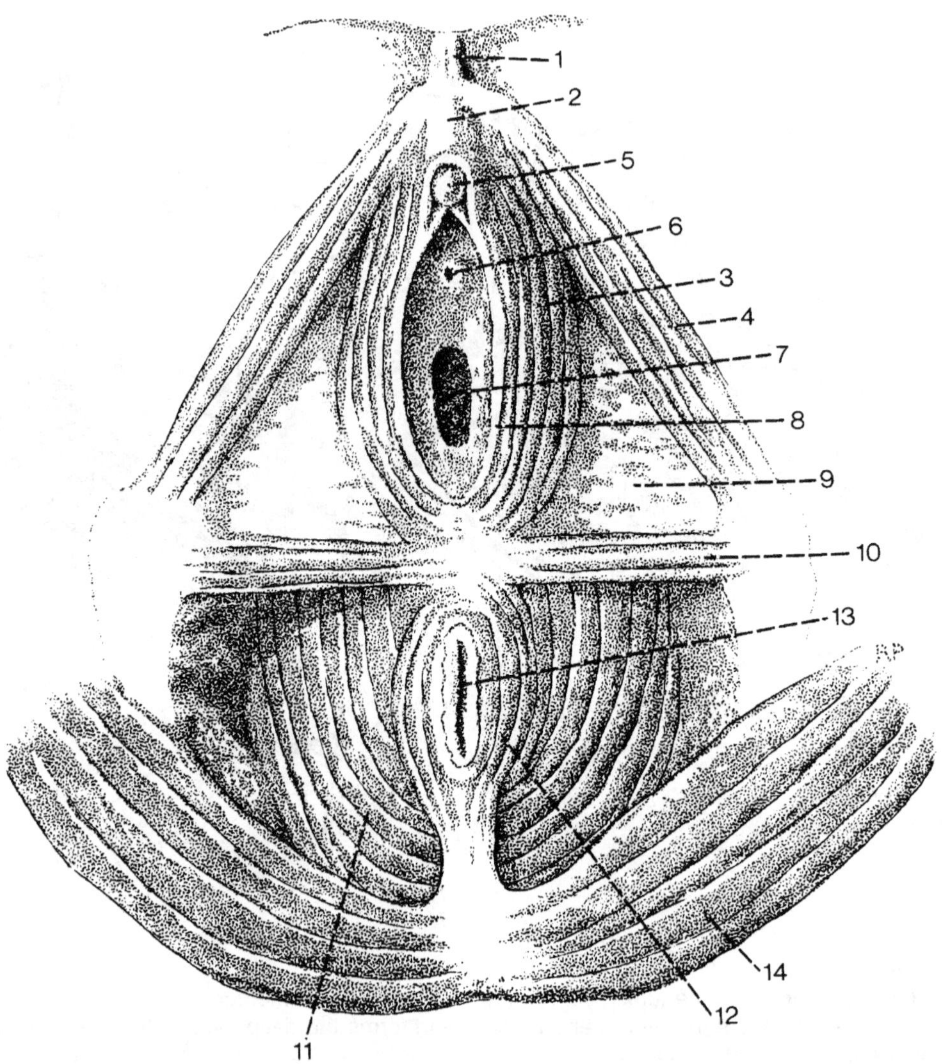

P-25 Nerves of the female perineum

Color and label

1 Clitoris (prepuce removed)
2 Vestibule of vagina
3 Anus
4 Superficial transverse perineus muscle (cut on left side)
5 Gluteus maximus muscle
6 Labium majus pudendi (major pudendal lip) (cut)
7 Perineal nerve; this is a branch of the pudendal nerve; it gives off the posterior labial nerves and supplies the bulbospongiosus and ischiocavernosus muscles and the vestibular bulb.
8 Posterior labial nerves
9 Inferior rectal nerves
10 Dorsal nerve of clitoris; note that it becomes more superficial by penetrating the perineal membrane
11 Posterior femoral cutaneous nerve
12 Perineal branch of posterior femoral cutaneous nerve
13 Inferior clunial nerve
14 Perineal membrane

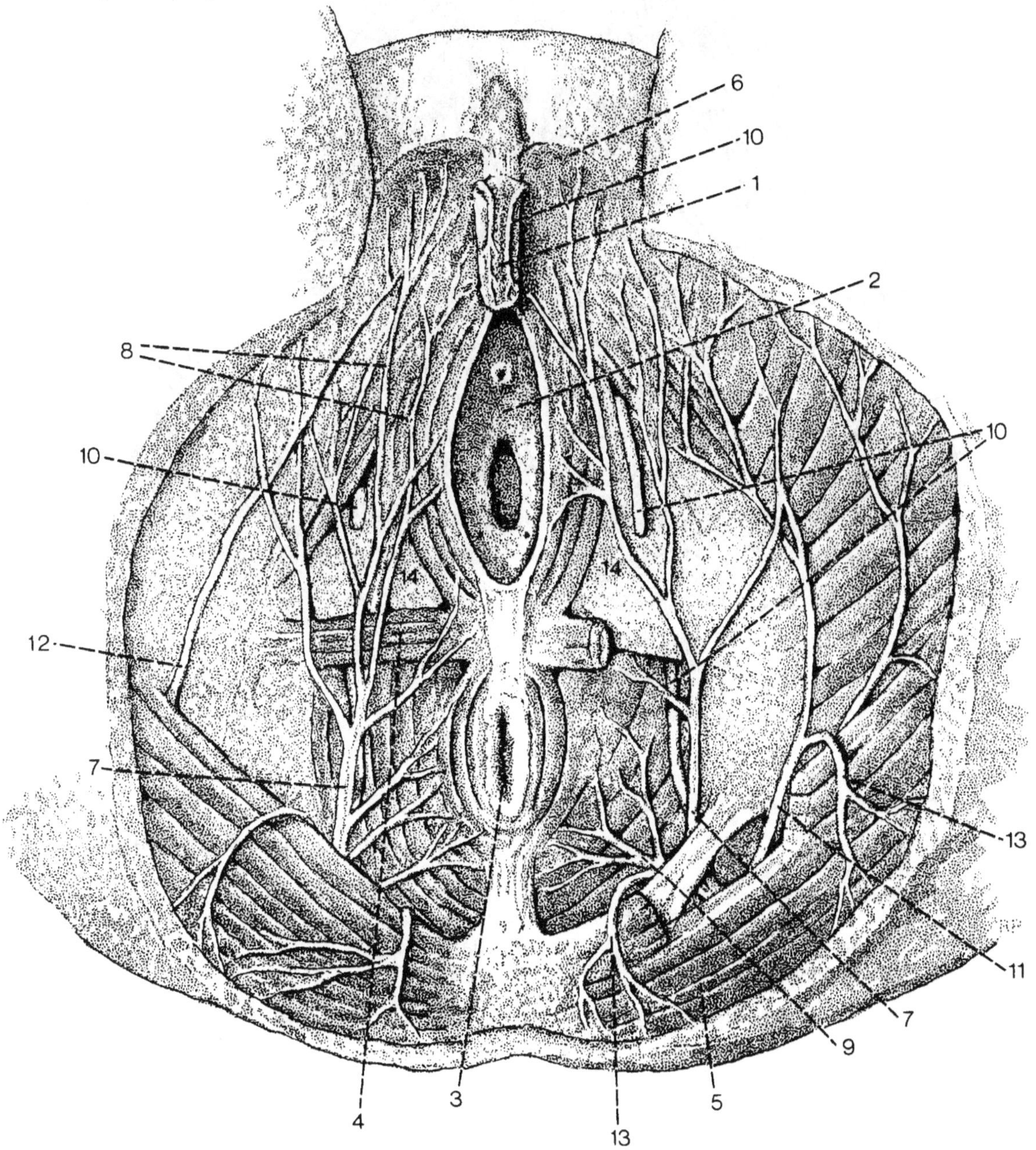

P-26 Arteries of female perineum

Veins (not shown) would accompany arteries

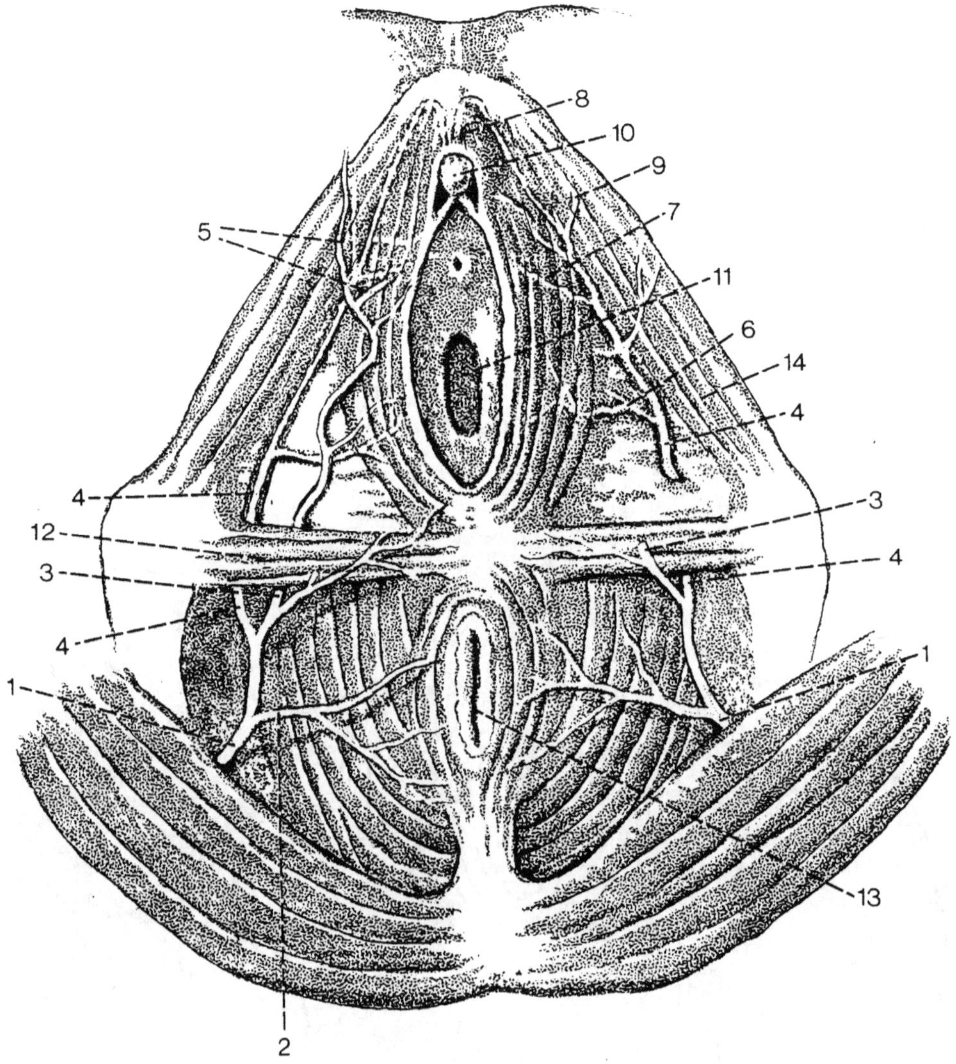

Color and label

1 Internal pudendal artery
2 Inferior rectal artery and branches
3 Perineal artery (cut on left)
4 Artery of clitoris
5 Posterior labial arteries;
terminal branches of perineal artery
6 Artery of vestibular bulb; off clitoral artery
7 Urethral artery
8 Dorsal artery of clitoris
9 Deep artery of clitoris; to crus of clitoris
10 Glans of clitoris
11 Vagina
12 Superficial transverse perineus muscle
14 Ischiocavernosus muscle

P-27 The uterus

Viewed from the left
Parasagittal section to the left of the uterus

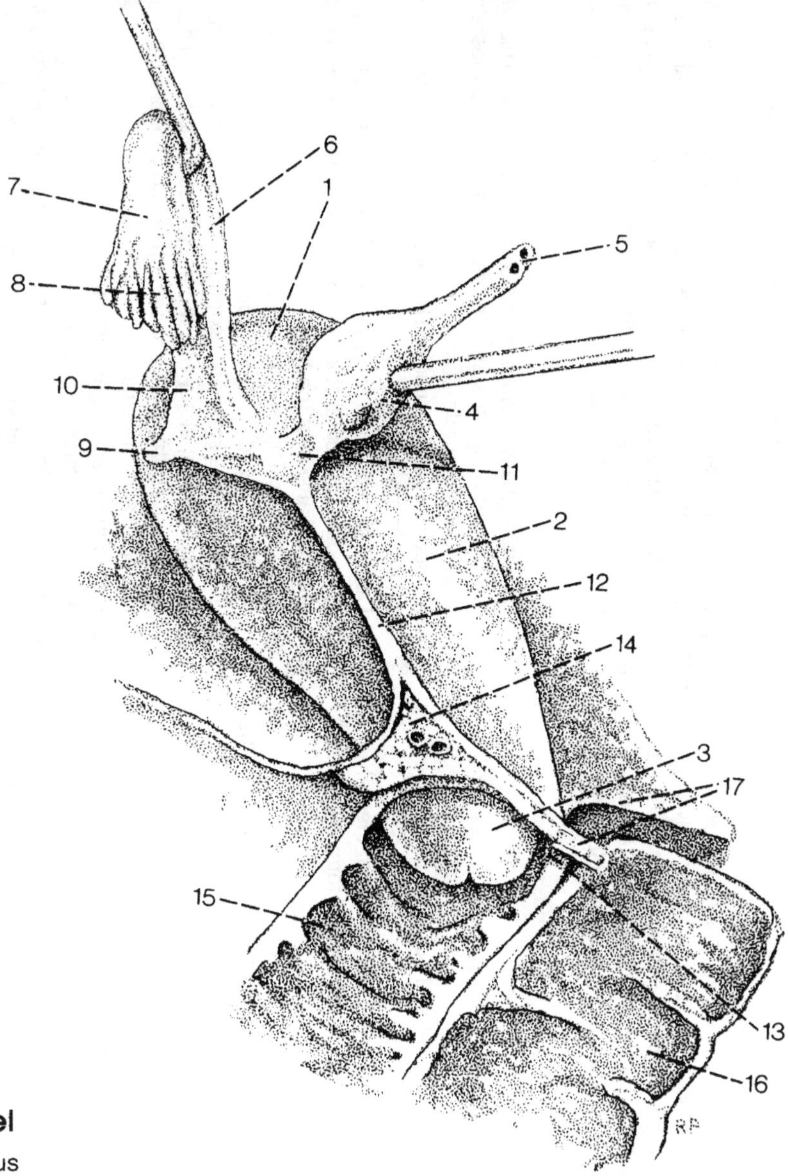

Color and label

1 Fundus of uterus
2 Body of uterus
3 Cervix of uterus (intravaginal part)
4 Ovary
5 Suspensory ligament of ovary with ovarian artery and vein (cut)
6 Uterine tube (oviduct)
7 Infundibulum of uterine tube
8 Fimbria of uterine tube
9 Round ligament of uterus (cut)
10 Mesosalpinx; fold of broad ligament attached to uterine tube (*salpinx* is Greek for trumpet or tube)
11 Mesovarium; fold of broad ligament attached to ovary
12 Mesometrium; major part of broad ligament; attached to sides of uterus
13 Posterior fornix of vagina; the vaginal fornix is actually a circular cleft around the intravaginal cervix; for descriptive purposes it is divided into an anterior part, right and left lateral parts, and a posterior part.
14 Lateral cervical ligament with uterine artery and vein(s)
15 Vagina (cut midsagittally)
16 Rectum (midsagittal cut)
17 Uterosacral ligament and fold

P-28 Female pelvic diaphragm and related structures (viewed from below and from the right) (opposite page)

The fat in the **ischiorectal fossa** (the wedge-shaped space between the obturator internus muscle and the pelvic diaphragm) has been removed.

The **pelvic diaphragm** consists of two paired muscles, the **levator ani** and the **coccygeus,** which meet in the midline and together form the hammock-like muscle. The pelvic diaphragm forms the floor of the pelvis. It supports the pelvic viscera and raises the pelvic floor. It resists increased intra-abdominal pressure and constricts the anorectal junction and the vagina. It is pierced by the anal canal, the urethra, and the vagina. Each levator ani consists of three muscles: the pubococcygeus, the puborectalis, and the iliococcygeus. The puborectalis lies internal to the pubococcygeus and cannot be seen from below. In addition to the three muscles named above, two additional muscles are sometimes considered part of the levator ani: the levator prostate in the male and the pubovaginalis in the female (not shown here).

Color and label

1 Anus
2 External anal sphincter (superficial layer)
3 Pubococcygeus muscle.
4 Iliococcygeus muscle. This forms the lateral and posterior part of the levator ani muscle.
5 Coccygeus muscle. This forms the posterior superior part of the pelvic diaphragm. The levator ani and the coccygeus together form the pelvic diaphragm.
6 Coccyx (the tail bone)
7 Anococcygeal ligament. This is a fibromuscular band extending from the external anal sphincter to the coccyx. Some of the fibers from the two sides of the levator ani interdigitate across this ligament while other fibers terminate on the ligament.
8 Obturator internus muscle. This leg muscle along with the obturator membrane and the obturator externus muscle largely block off the obturator foramen.
9 Superficial transverse perineal muscle
10 Perineal body (also central tendon of perineum). A fibromuscular mass between the anus and bulb of the penis in the male, and between the vagina and anus in the female. It serves as an anchor and attachment for the muscles in the region.
11 Perineal membrane (formerly called inferior fascia of urogenital membrane)
12 Greater vestibular gland and its opening in the vestibule of the vagina
13 Vestibular bulb. This is female erectile tissue. It is homologous to the corpus spongiosus penis in the male.
14 Vagina
15 Bulbospongiosus muscle. This thin, delicate muscle overlies the vestibular bulb in the female. It is partly removed on the left side.
16 Glans and prepuce of the clitoris
17 Obturator (Latin, *obturare*, to stop up) membrane. This membrane and the obturator internus and obturator externus muscles almost completely seal off the obturator foramen.
18 Ischiocavernosus muscle. This delicate muscle covers the crus of the clitoris in the female.
19 Obturator nerve, artery, and vein. These exit the pelvis through a small opening in the obturator membrane and supply the medial thigh muscles and medial skin of the thigh.
20 Acetabulum. This cup-shaped socket fits over the head of the femur. Together they form the hip joint.
21 Sacrotuberous ligament (extends from sacrum to ischial tuberosity). This strong ligament along with the deeper sacrospinous ligament (not seen here) convert the two sciatic notches into two foramina, the greater and lesser sciatic foramina.
22 Ischial tuberosity (right and left)
23 Anterior superior iliac spine
24 Right obturator internus. This leg muscle arises mainly from the internal surface of the obturator membrane. It leaves the pelvis through the lesser sciatic foramen and inserts on the greater trochanter of the femur.
25 Sciatic nerve. This is the largest nerve in the body. It is actually a double nerve that divides lower in the thigh into its two component parts: the common peroneal nerve and the tibial nerve.
26 Pudendal nerve and internal pudendal artery and vein. These exit the pelvis through the greater sciatic foramen and re-enter the pelvis through the lesser sciatic foramen. They supply the anus and external genitalia.
27 Piriformis muscle. This leg muscle leaves the pelvis through the greater sciatic foramen, which it largely fills, and inserts on the greater trochanter of the femur.
28 Supraspinal ligament

P-28 Female pelvic diaphragm and related structures

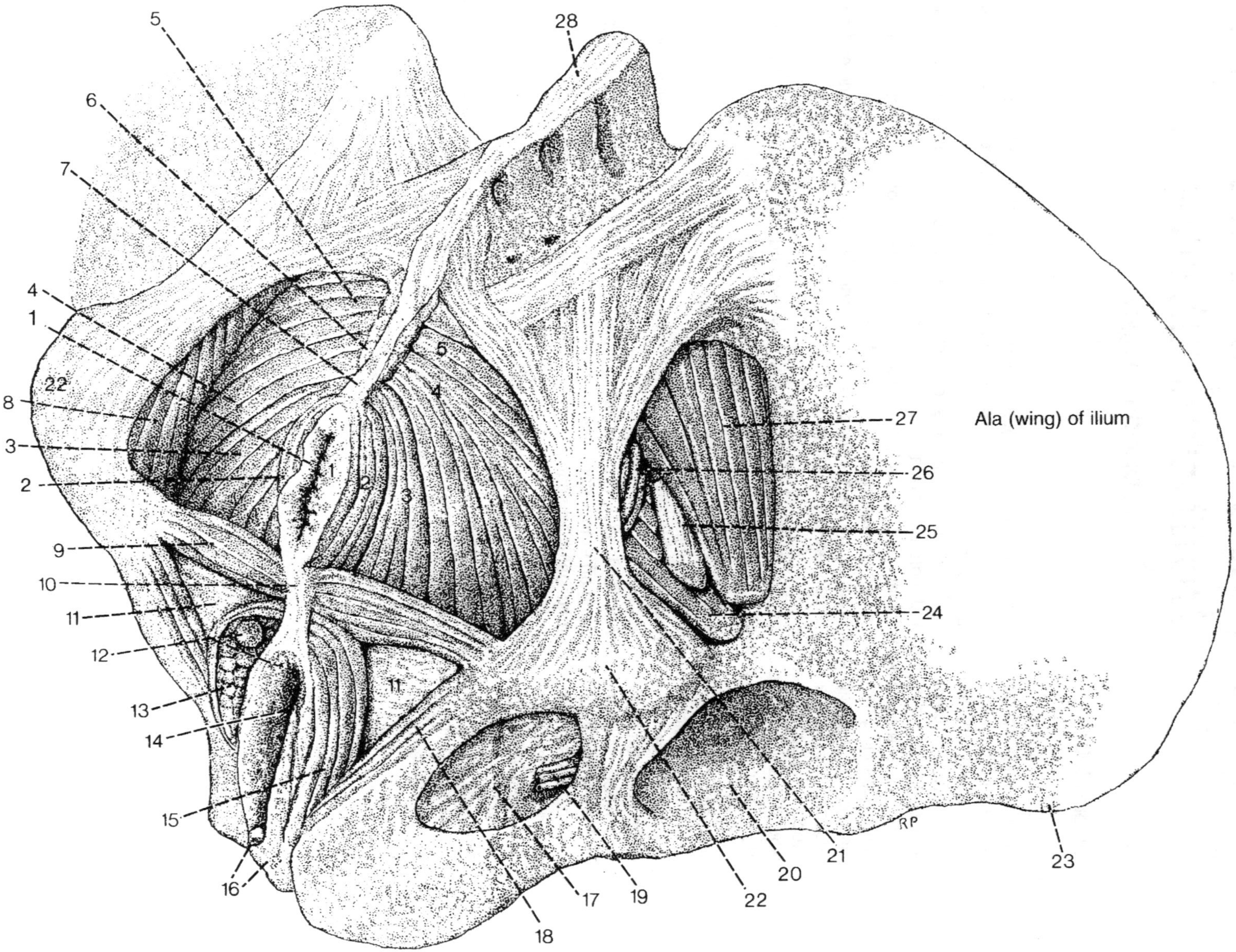

P-29 Female pelvis from the front and above

(opposite page)

Color and label

1 Fundus of uterus
2 Bladder (superior surface covered by peritoneum); all the intraperitoneal pelvic and abdominal organs are covered on their external surface by peritoneum, which forms the outer tunica serosa or serosal layer.
3 Right ovary; with developing follicles
4 Left ovary; with developing follicles. These rupture at ovulation and release their eggs into the oviduct. Only about 300 follicles mature and rupture at ovulation during a woman's reproductive life.
5 Uterine tube (also called fallopian tube, oviduct). Salpingitis is inflammation of the fallopian tube (salpingo- is the combining form from *salpinx,* Greek for a trumpet or tube)
6 Fimbriae (L. fringe, thread, fiber) of the uterine tube. They are finger-like processes extending from the circumference of the distal expanded end (infundibulum) of the uterine tube.
7 Proper ovarian ligament
8 Round ligament of the uterus. This is a narrow fibrous band that extends from the uterus to the deep inguinal ring where it passes through the inguinal canal to end in the labium majus.
9 Rectum
10 Suspensory ligament of the ovary with the ovarian artery and vein
11 Vermiform appendix (worm-like, L. *vermis*, worm)
12 Cecum of large intestine; this is the beginning of the large intestine. "Cecum and ye shall find."
13 Ileum (terminal portion)
14 Appendices epiploica (fatty appendages). These small globules of fat are found only on the large intestine and are an aid in distinguishing an empty, constricted colon from a full, small intestine.
15 Vesicouterine pouch; the peritoneal-lined space or recess between the bladder and uterus.
16 Broad ligament
17 Rectouterine fold; a crescentric fold of peritoneum extending from the rectum to the base of the broad ligament.
18 Tenia coli; there are three of these thickened, tapelike bands of smooth muscle arranged longitudinally on the surface of the large intestine. They are responsible for the bulging haustra of the large intestine.

P-29 Female pelvis from the front and above

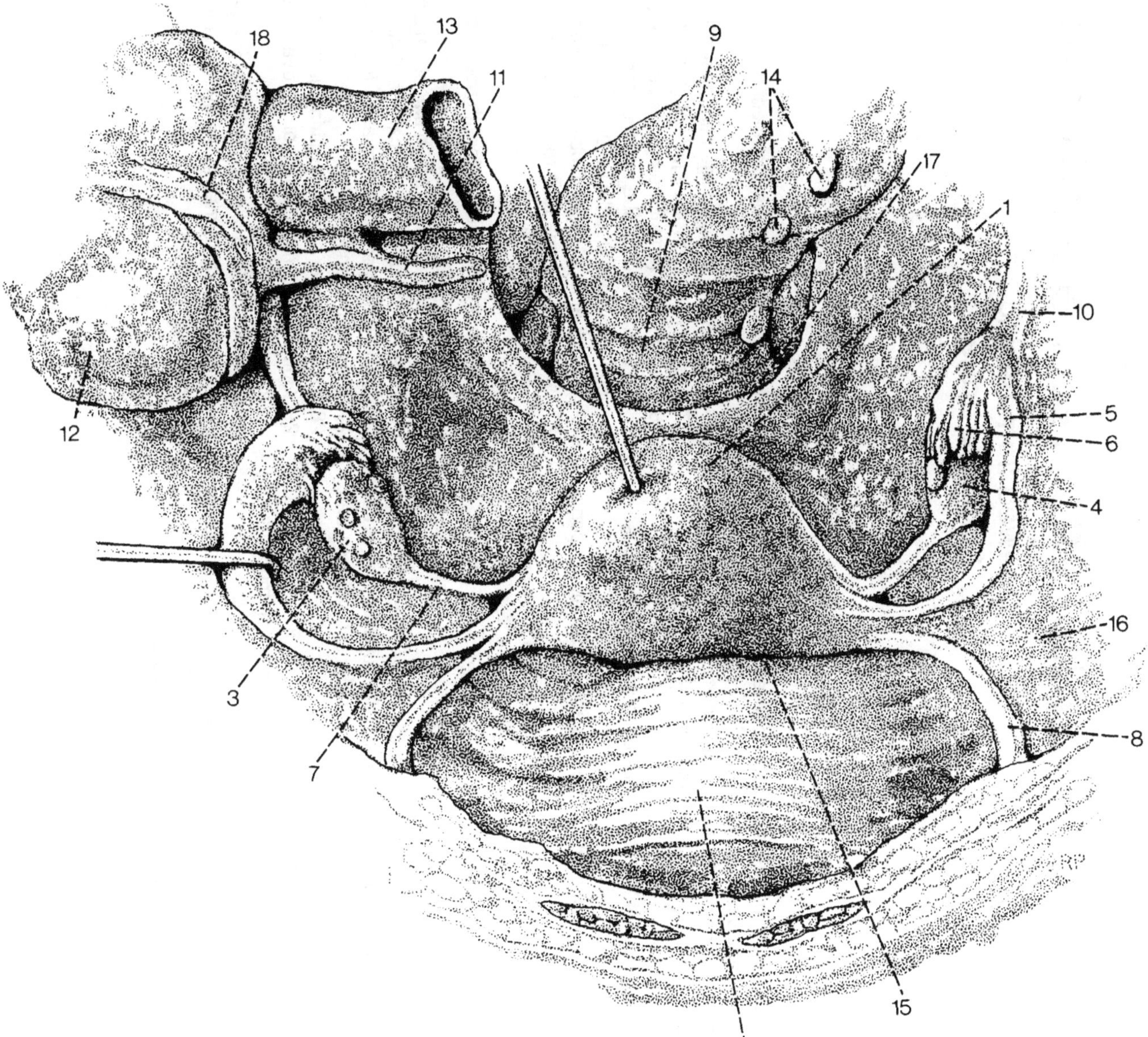

P-30 Uterus and related structures

Viewed from behind (opposite page)

Color and label

1 Fundus of uterus (the word *uterus* is probably derived from the Greek *hystera*, womb). Hysterectomy is surgical excision of the uterus. Hysteria was originally thought to be caused by the internal movements of an unrestrained uterus that had broken free of its moorings.
2 Cavity of uterus
3 Body of uterus (a segment of the uterus has been removed to expose its cavity and the layers of its wall)
4 Cervix of uterus (supravaginal part; that portion above the vagina; *cervix*, Latin, neck)
5 Cervix of uterus (vaginal part; that portion projecting into the vagina)
6 Cervical canal
7 Vagina (anterior wall)
8 Opening of the uterus (ostium uteri)
9 Anterior lip of the cervix
10 Lateral fornices of vagina (left and right); actually the vaginal fornix is a circular cleft between the intravaginal cervix and the superior wall of the vagina; for descriptive purposes, it is divided into right, left, anterior, and posterior fornix.
11 Isthmus of uterus (narrow portion)
12 Endometrium (mucosal lining); this is lost and restored each month during the menstrual cycle.
13 Myometrium (muscular layer, consisting of nonstriated or smooth muscle); this becomes greatly enlarged and thickened in pregnancy.
14 Perimetrium (outer covering of peritoneum, also tunica serosa)
15 Mesometrium of broad ligament (that part attached to the sides of the uterus)
16 Mesovarium of broad ligament (that part attached to the ovary)
17 Mesovarium of broad ligament (part attached to the uterine tube)
18 Uterine tube (opened on the left side) eggs released from the ovary travel down the uterine tube into the uterus. Fertilization of the egg by a spermatozoon usually occurs within the uterine tube.
19 Infundibulum of uterine tube (expanded end)
20 Ampulla of uterine tube (dilation of tube)
21 Fimbria of uterine tube
22 Ureter
23 Uterine artery; it connects with both the artery of the vagina and the ovarian artery.
24 Recto-uterine ligament with smooth muscle
25 Lateral cervical ligament (cardinal ligament, Mackenrodt's ligament)
26 Ovary (cut open on left); mature follicle on right ovary
27 Proper ovarian ligament
28 Ovarian artery and vein within suspensory ligament of the ovary
29 Corpus albicans; remnant of the ovarian corpus luteum weeks after ovulation.
30 Corpus luteum (yellow body of the ovary). The yellow progesterone-secreting body formed in the ovary at the site of a ruptured ovarian follicle.
31 Artery of the vagina

P-30 Uterus and related structures

Viewed from behind

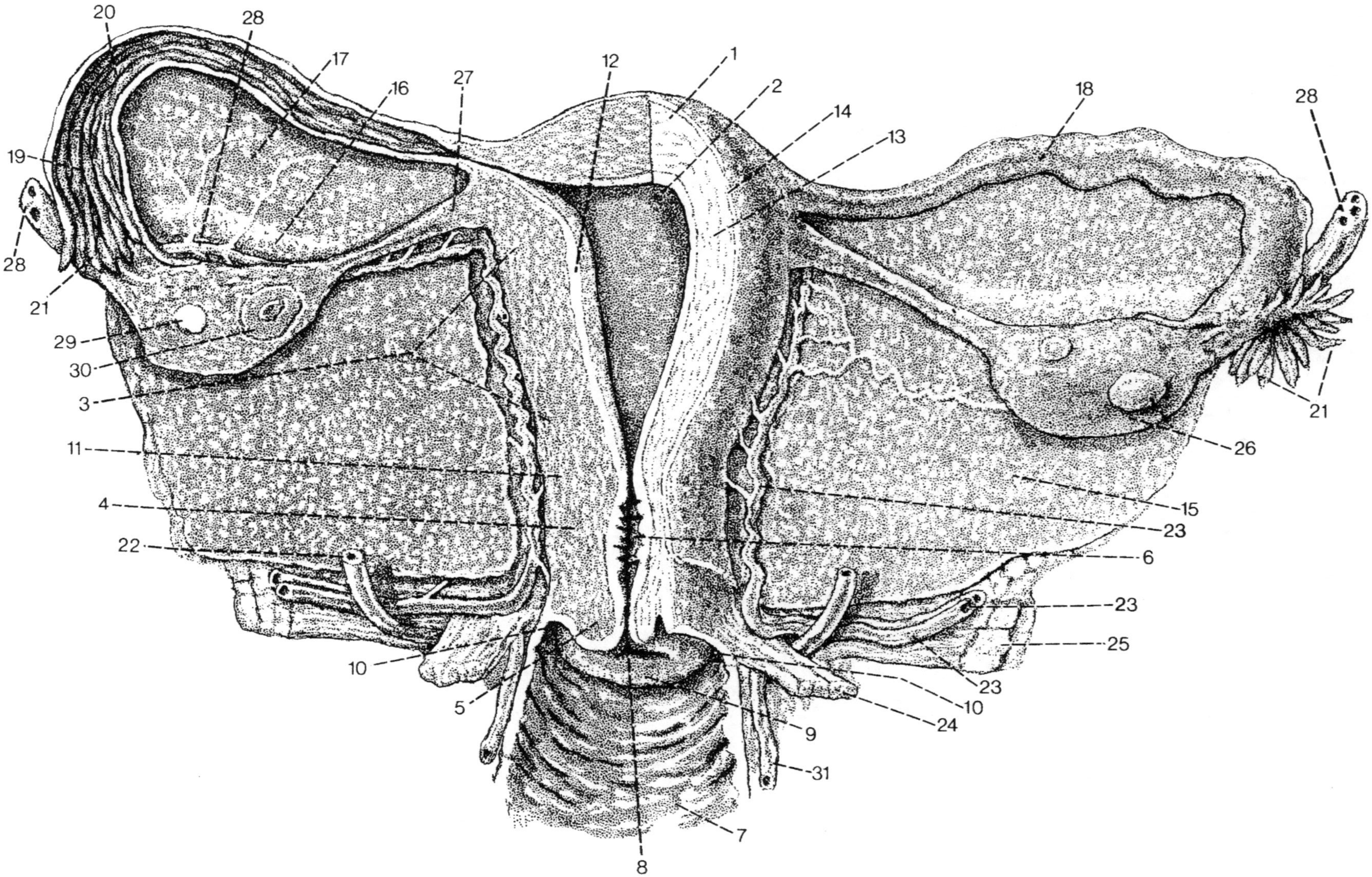

P-31 Female pelvic diaphragm from above

Color and label

1 Urethra
2 Vagina
3 Rectum
4 Puborectalis muscle (part of levator ani)
5 Pubococcygeus muscle (part of levator ani)
6 Iliococcygeus muscle (part of levator ani)
7 Coccygeus muscle (part of pelvic diaphragm) (coccygeus + levator ani = pelvic diaphragm)
8 Obturator internus muscle
9 Tendinous arch of levator ani
10 Pubovaginalis (part of levator ani)
11 Ischial spine
12 Obturator canal
13 Dorsal vein of clitoris
14 Pubic symphysis
15 Piriformis muscle

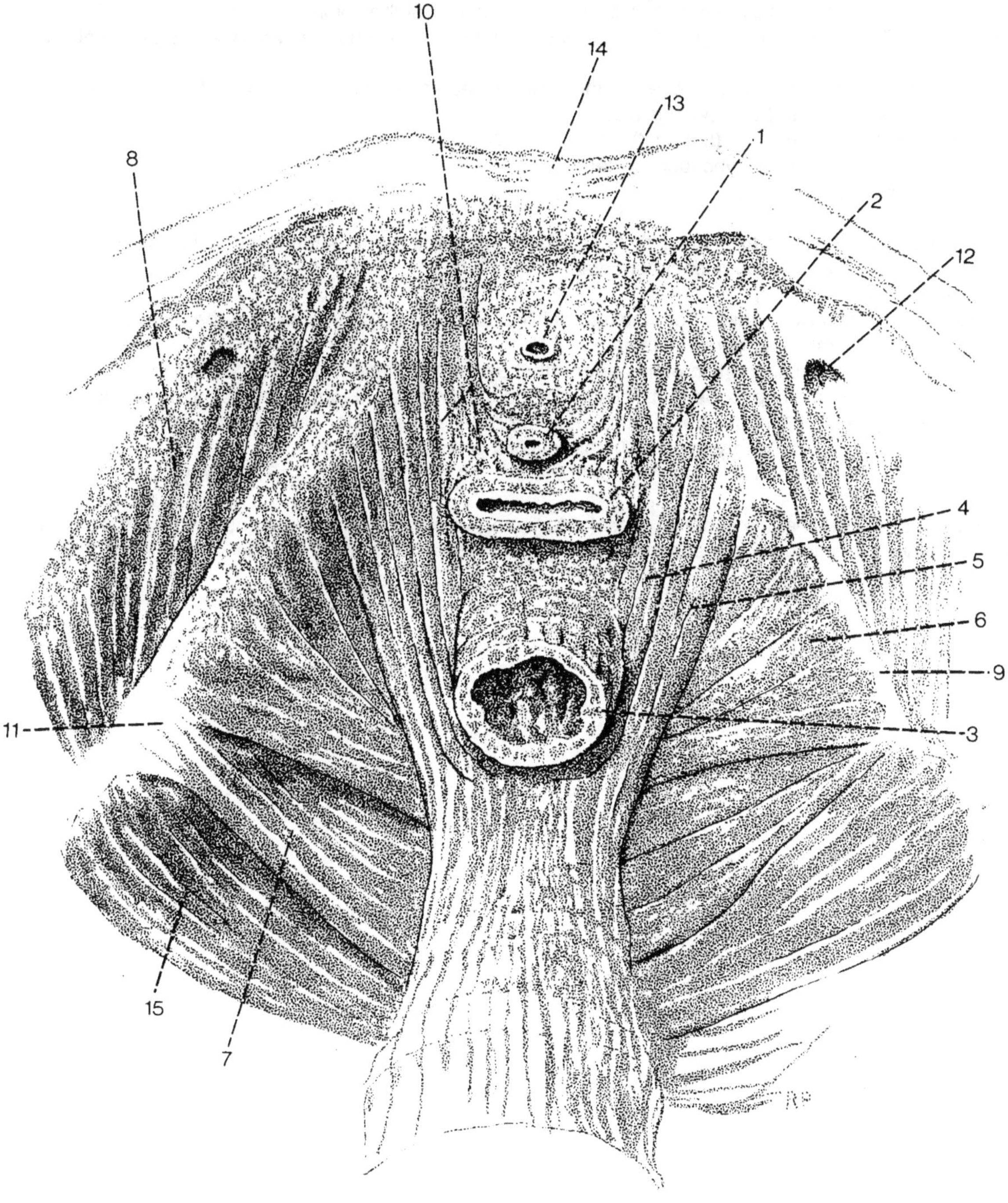

P-32 Arterial supply of the female pelvis

Viewed from the left; part of the left hip bone has been removed; veins (not shown) accompany artery (opposite page)

Color and label

1 Aorta; the aorta bifurcates (divides) into the right and left common iliac arteries
2 Inferior mesenteric artery; this artery supplies the lower one half of the colon
3 Right common iliac artery; the common iliac artery divides into an external iliac artery and an internal iliac artery .
4 Right external iliac artery and vein; these continue into the leg as the femoral artery and vein.
5 Left common iliac artery and vein (vein is cut)
6 Left external iliac artery and vein (both cut)
7 Internal iliac artery (old name, hypogastric artery)
8 Superior gluteal artery
9 Inferior gluteal artery
10 Internal pudendal artery; this exits the greater sciatic foramen and reenters the lesser sciatic foramen (accompanied with the vein and pudendal nerve)
11 Inferior rectal artery
12 Obturator artery; this usually arises from the internal iliac artery, but it may arise from the external iliac artery and complicate exploratory surgery in this area.
13 Umbilical artery; the proximal portion of this artery (that part to the bladder) remains patent (open), whereas after birth the distal portion up to the umbilicus becomes obliterated and forms the medial umbilical plica.
14 Superior vesical (*vesica* Latin, bladder, blister) artery; supplies the superior portion of the bladder.
15 Obliterated part of umbilical artery (median umbilical plica or fold)
16 Uterine artery; note that it anastomoses with both the ovarian artery and the vaginal artery.
17 Vaginal artery
18 Piriformis muscle; note that the superior gluteal artery (and vein and nerve) comes out of the greater sciatic foramen **above** the piriformis, whereas the inferior gluteal vessels and nerve exit the same foramen **below** the piriformis muscle.
19 Coccygeus muscle (part of the pelvic diaphragm)
20 Levator ani muscle
21 Obturator internus muscle
22 External anal sphincter
23 Labia minora
24 Glans of clitoris
25 Left ureter
26 Fundus of uterus
27 Bladder
28 Inferior vena cava
29 Branch of uterine artery to ovarian artery

P-32 Arterial supply of the female pelvis

Viewed from the left; part of the left hip bone has been removed; veins (not shown) accompany artery

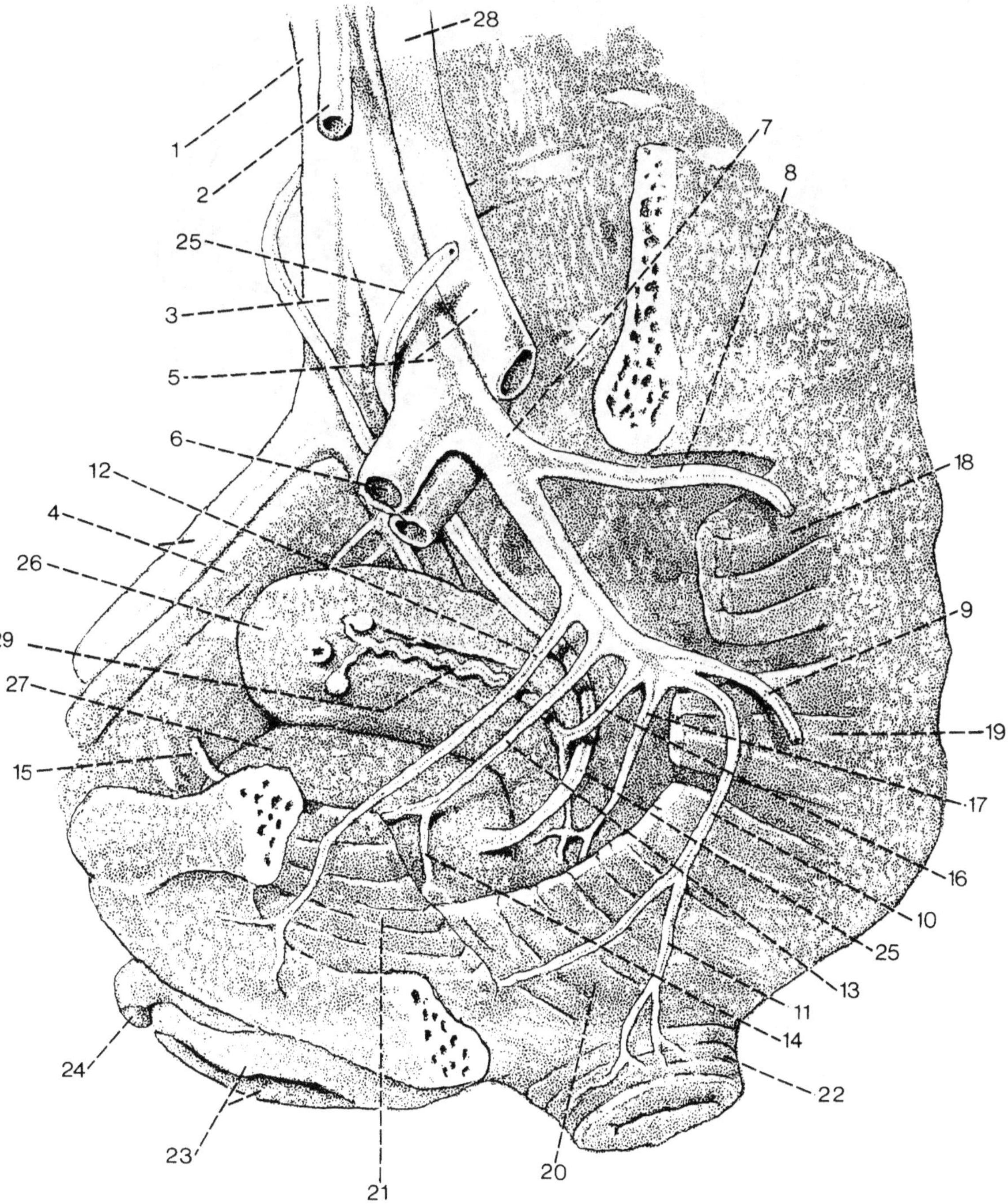

P-33 Muscles on medial surface of pelvis

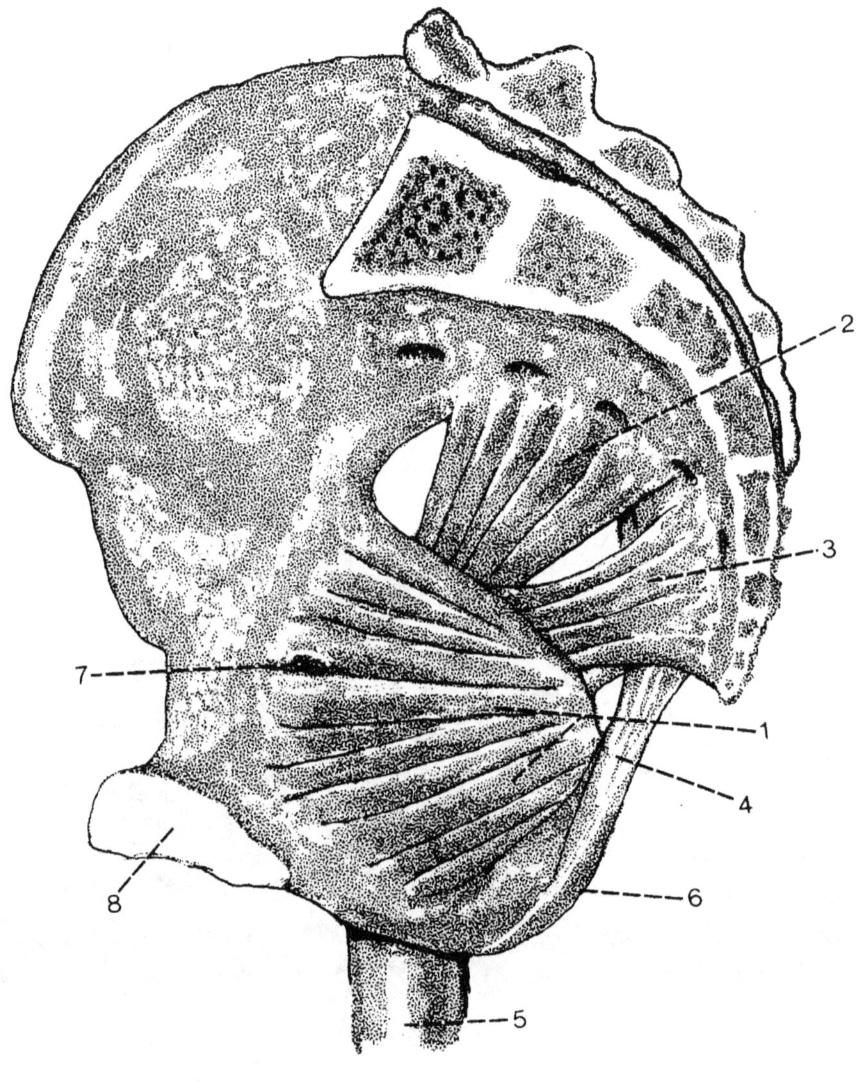

Color and label

1 Obturator internus muscle; note how it covers the obturator foramen internally; it exits the pelvis through the lesser sciatic foramen and inserts on the femur.
2 Piriformis muscle. This muscle exits the pelvis via, the greater sciatic foramen, which it largely fills; it also inserts on the femur.
3 Coccygeus muscle; in tailed mammals this muscle pulls the tail between the legs.
4 Sacrotuberous ligament; this extends from the sacrum to the ischial tuberosity.
5 Femur
6 Ischial tuberosity
7 Obturator canal; this small opening transmits the obturator nerve, artery, and vein.
8 Pubic symphysis

P-34 Female urogenital sphincter I

Viewed from below

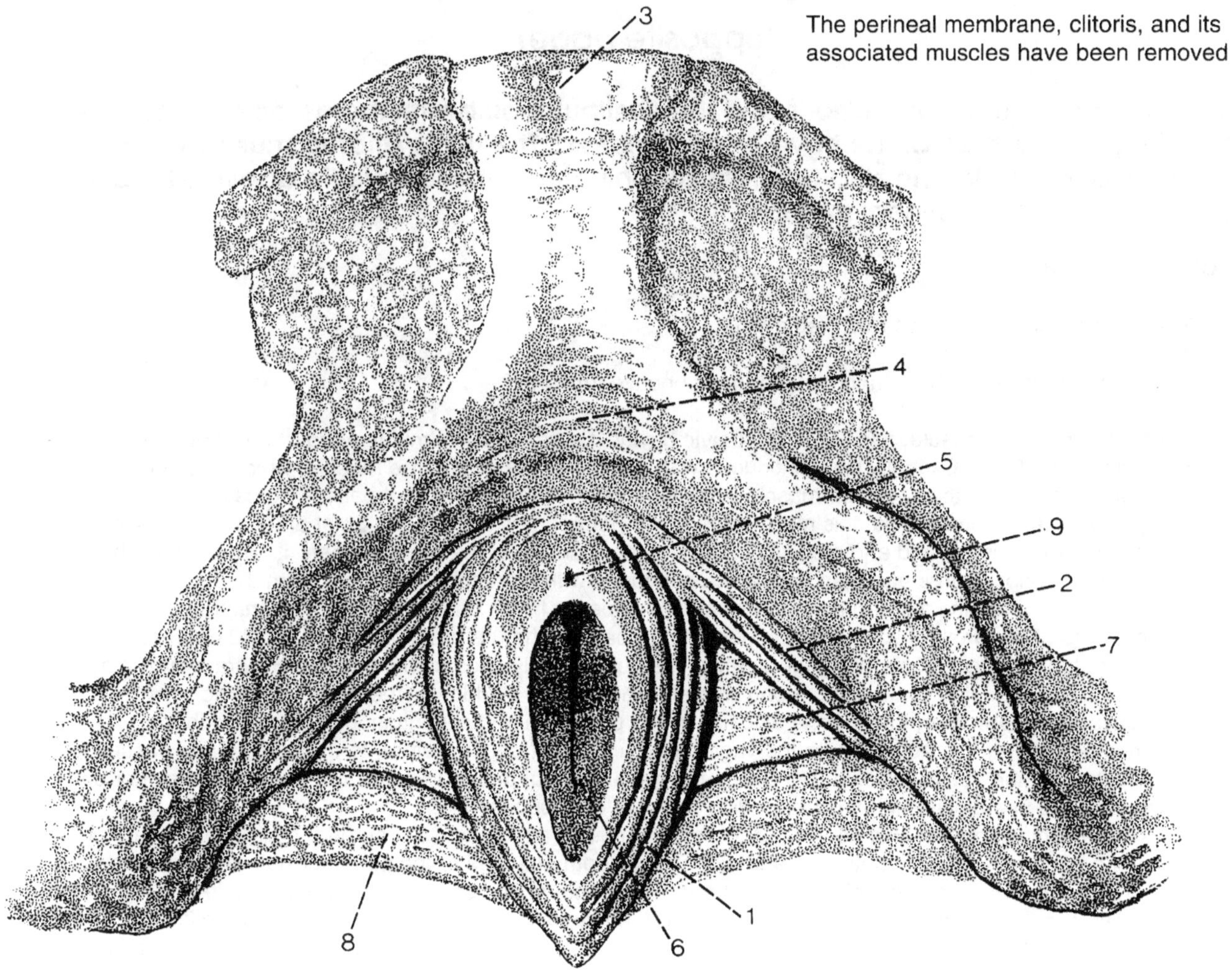

The striated urogenital sphincter muscle of the female consists of:

The **urethrovaginal sphincter** surrounding the urethra and the vaginal vestibule (1)
The **compressor of the urethra** arching across the ventral side of the urethra (2)
The **sphincter** surrounding the middle third of the urethra (see figure P-35)

Color and label

1 Urethrovaginal sphincter muscle
2 Urethral compressor muscle: this arches across the ventral side of the uretha
3 Pubic symphysis
4 Arcuate pubic ligament
5 Urethra
6 Vagina
7 Transverse vaginal muscle; this is a variable striated muscle
8 Smooth muscle of urethrovaginal compartment
9 Ischiopubic ramus

After Oelrich T, Anat Rec 205:223, 1983.

P-35 Female striated urethral sphincter II

(opposite page)

The body and crura of the clitoris and the vestibular bulb with the associated muscles plus the perineal membrane have been removed. The three striated muscles (5,6,7 below) that comprise the striated urethral sphincter in the female lie above (deep to or cephalic to) the perineal membrane.

Color and label

1 Bladder; cephalic portion has been removed
2 Vagina
3 Urethra; the urethra is not a straight tube but is concave forward.
4 Vaginal wall
5 **Urethral sphincter muscle**; this lies in the pelvic cavity. It surrounds the middle third of the urethra for approximately 1.5 cm. Caudally it is continuous with the compressor urethrae muscle, which lies in the perineum. In the adult the sphincter muscle is thickest ventrally and thins as it passes dorsally.
6 **Compressor urethrae muscle**; this muscle lies in the perineum. It begins at a point anterior to the ischial tuberosity. It extends forward and medially to the anterior surface of the urethra where it forms a thick bundle around the anterior urethra and then becomes continuous with corresponding fibers from the opposite side of the body, thus forming a broad arching muscle. Its superior fibers on the urethra are continuous with the inferior fibers of the urethral sphincter. Because it approaches the urethra at an angle of 130 degrees, it appears to have the action of pulling the urethral meatus caudally, thus elongating the urethra, which may be important in providing continence (along with elevation of the bladder by the pelvic diaphragm).
7 **Urethrovaginal sphincter**; this muscle also lies in the perineum and is continuous ventrally with the compressor urethra. It surrounds both the vagina and urethra. It begins ventral to the urethra and passes dorsally deep to the vestibular bulb (removed) along the sides of the vagina until it reaches its posterior point where its fibers interdigitate with corresponding fibers of the opposite side.
8 Transverse vaginal muscle; this very thin, fan-shaped muscle attaches to the anterior portion of the lateral wall of the vagina. It varies in both size and extent. It seldom attaches to the posterior half of the vagina.
9 Smooth muscle of the urethrovaginal compartment. The amount and density of smooth muscle and connective tissue tend to increase with age, making the identification of striated muscle more difficult in the adult. The smooth muscle is extensive throughout the perineal region from the ischiopubic rami to the lateral wall of the urethra.
10 Ischiopubic ramus (pubic symphysis and medial portion removed)
11 Uterus (cephalic portion removed)

After Oelrich: The striated urogenital sphincter in the female. Anat Rec 205:223-232, 1983.

Recent work has shown the striated muscle on the caudal third of the urethra is innervated by fibers of the pudendal nerve, whereas three layers of smooth muscle on the superior two-thirds of the urethra receive thin fibers from the pelvic plexus. (Colleselli et al: The female urethral sphincter. J Urol 160:49-54, 1998.)

P-35 Female striated urethral sphincter II

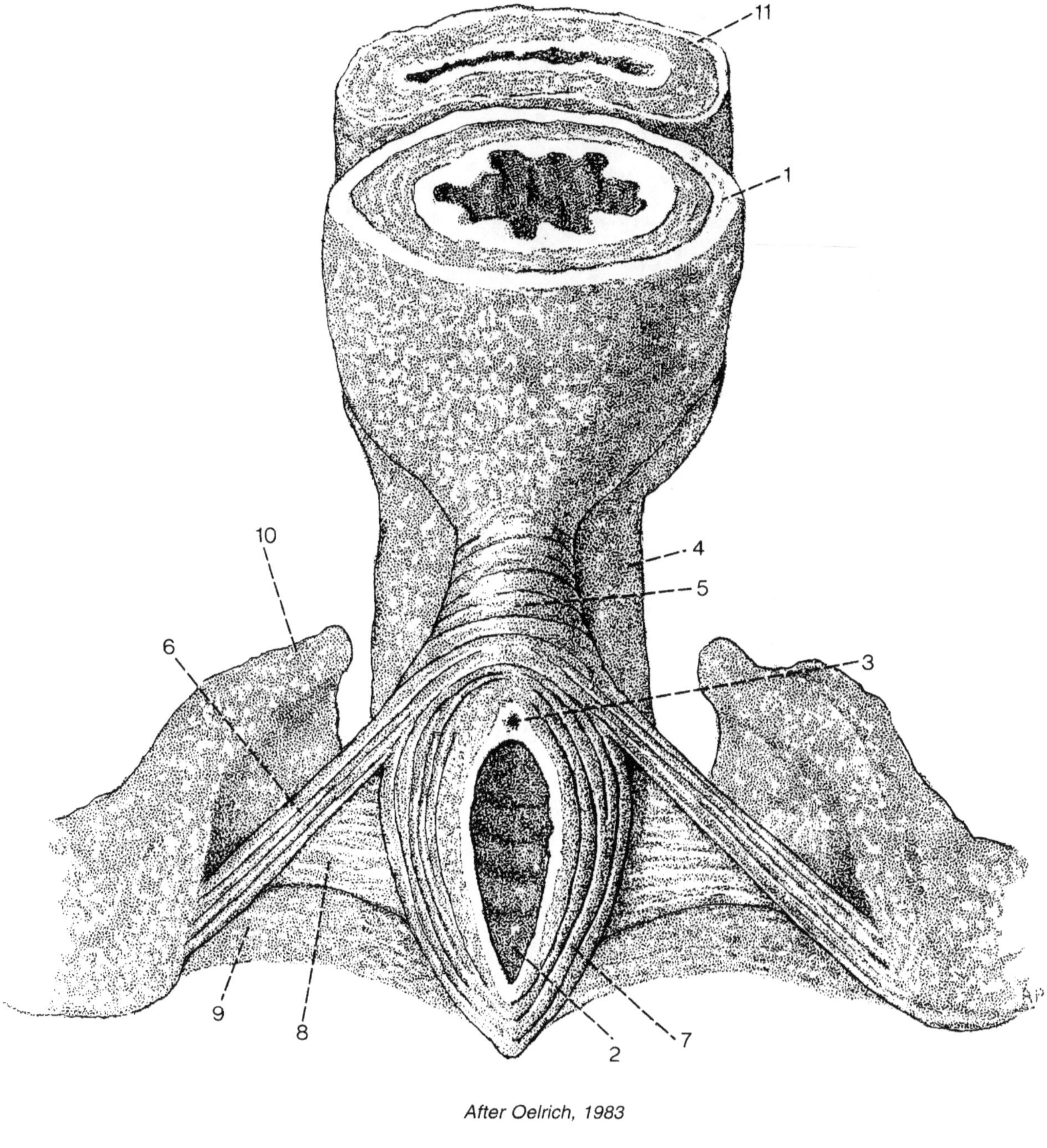

After Oelrich, 1983

P-36 Pelvis and ligaments

Anterior aspect

Color and label

1 Anterior superior iliac spine
2 Anterior inferior iliac spine
3 Iliopectineal eminence
4 Iliac fossa
5 Iliac crest
6 Ischial spine
7 Sacrospinous ligament
8 Sacrotuberous ligament
9 Greater sciatic foramen
10 Lesser sciatic foramen
11 Anterior longitudinal ligament
12 Anterior sacroiliac ligament
13 Iliolumbar ligament (superior band)
14 Iliolumbar ligament (inferior band)
15 Pectineal ligament
16 Superior pubic ligament
17 Interpubic disk (in pubic symphysis)

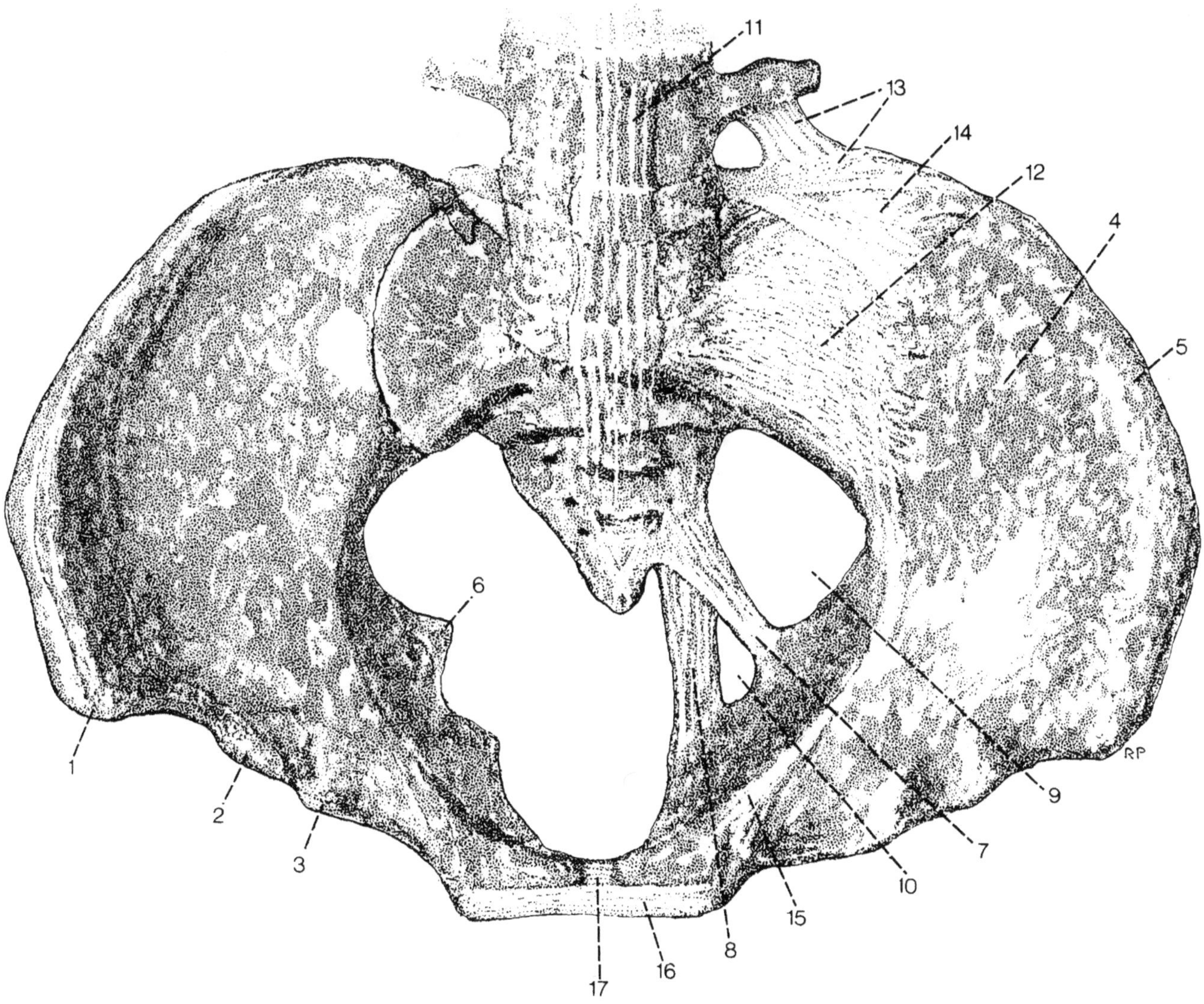

Part IV: The Upper Limb

Phalanx: Etymological cartoon

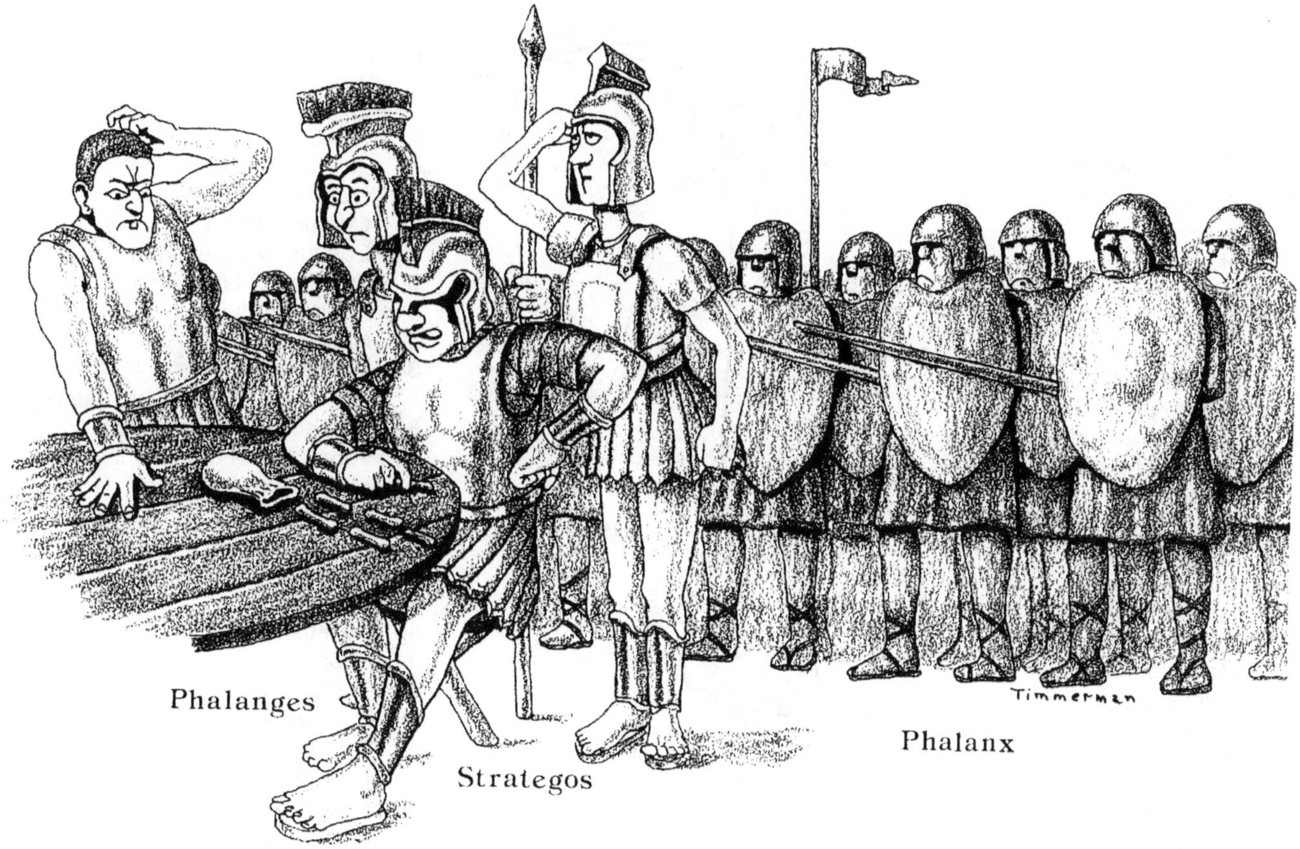

Phalanx (Greek) was a compact formation of infantry soldiers with overlapping shields and projecting spears. It was developed by Philip II of Macedon and later used extensively by Alexander the Great.

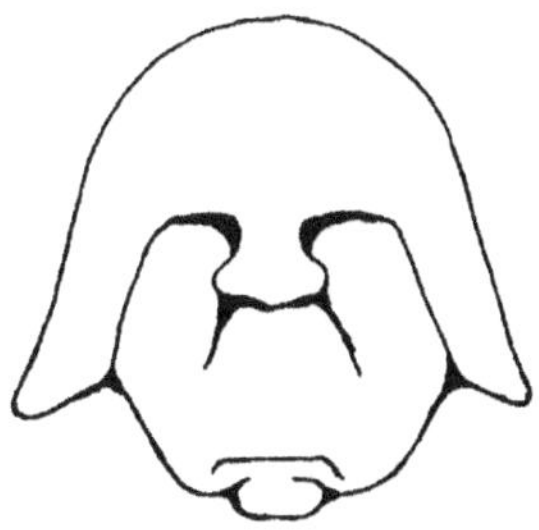

The ***phalanges*** (plural of *phalanx*) are the bones of the fingers and toes. Supposedly Aristotle gave them this name. He thought that the bones within the fingers resembled a formation of infantry phalanges drawn up for battle. The thumb (*pollex*, Latin) has only two phalanges, as does the big toe (*hallux*, Latin). The rest of the fingers (digits 2-5) each has three phalanges; thus each hand and each foot has fourteen phalanges (2+3+3+3+3=14). The wrist (*carpus*, Latin) consists of eight carpal bones in two rows of four. Within the palm of the hand are the five metacarpal (beyond the carpus) bones. These are the largest and strongest bones of the hand, especially the second and third metacarpal bones, which directly receive the force of impact when the fist strikes a blow. The foot has seven tarsal bones, five metatarsal bones, and fourteen phalanges. *Tarsos* is Greek for a flat surface, or sole of the foot, or edge of the eyelid. In anatomy the tarsus refers specifically to the instep of the foot or to that part of the foot containing the seven tarsal bones.

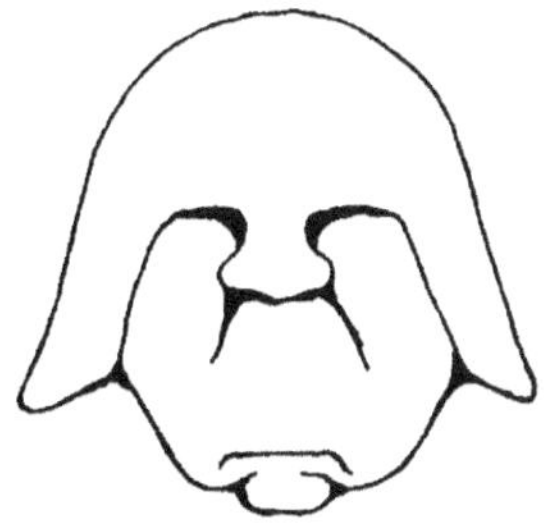

A Greek general was a ***strategos***, hence our word *strategy*. An army was a *stratos* and "to lead" was *agein*; thus to be a general or "to lead an army" was *stratos* + *agein* = *strategein,* which got shortened to *strategos.*

UL-1 Bones of the upper extremity

Anterior aspect

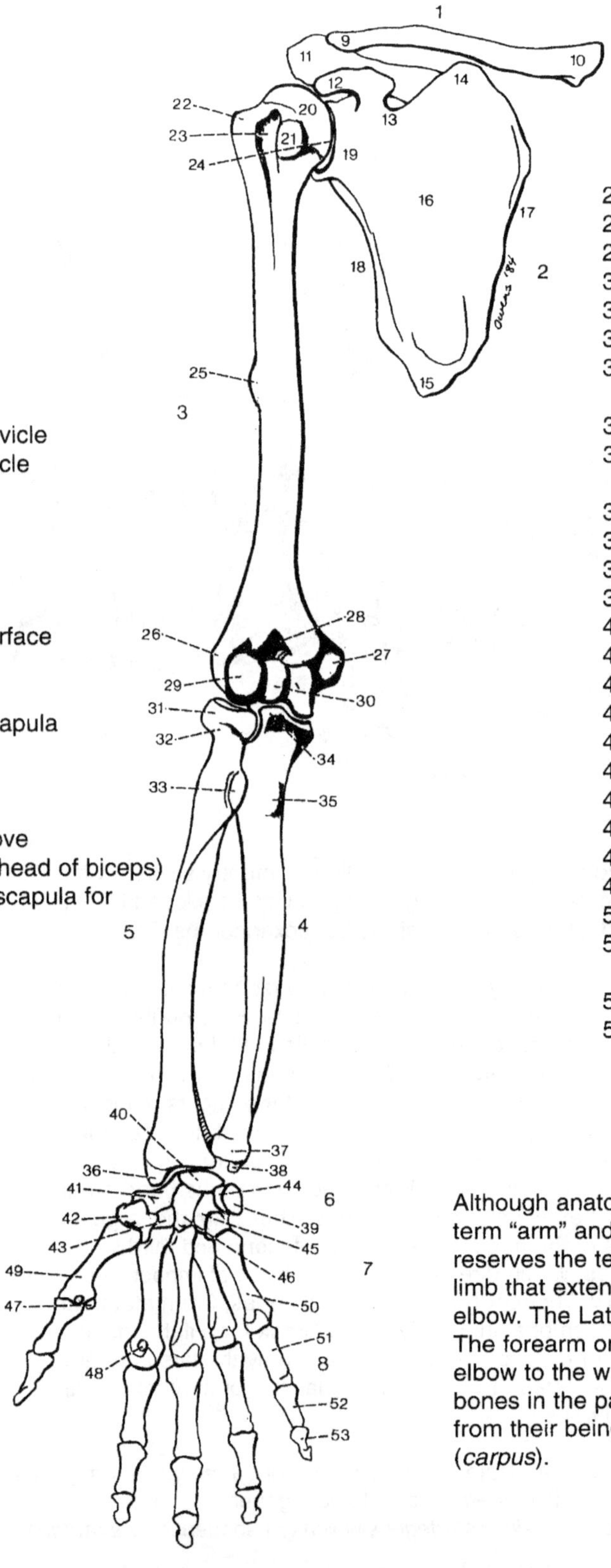

Color and label

1 Clavicle
2 Scapula
3 Humerus
4 Ulna
5 Radius
6 Carpal bones (8)
7 Metacarpals (5)
8 Phalanges (14)
9 Acromial end of clavicle
10 Sternal end of clavicle
11 Acromion
12 Coracoid process
13 Scapular notch
14 Superior angle
15 Inferior angle
16 Costal (anterior) surface
17 Medial border
18 Lateral border
19 Neck (collum) of scapula
20 Head of humerus
21 Lesser tubercle
22 Greater tubercle
23 Intertubercular groove (for tendon of long head of biceps)
24 Glenoid (socket in scapula for head of humerus)
25 Deltoid tuberosity
26 Lateral epicondyle
27 Medial epicondyle
28 Coronoid fossa
29 Capitulum of humerus
30 Trochlea of humerus
31 Head of radius
32 Neck of radius
33 Radial tuberosity (for insertion of biceps brachii)
34 Coronoid process of ulna
35 Tuberosity of ulna (for insertion of brachialis muscle)
36 Styloid process of radius
37 Head of ulna
38 Styloid process of ulna
39 Pisiform
40 Lunate
41 Scaphoid
42 Trapezium
43 Trapezoid
44 Triquetral
45 Hamate
46 Capitate
47 Sesamoid bones of thumb
48 Sesamoid bone of index finger
49 First metacarpal
50 Fifth metacarpal
51 Proximal phalanx of little finger (digiti minimi)
52 Middle phalanx
53 Terminal phalanx

Although anatomists would prefer to use the term "arm" and so forth, anatomical terminology reserves the term **arm** for that part of the upper limb that extends only from the shoulder to the elbow. The Latin term for this part is *brachium*. The forearm or antebrachium extends from the elbow to the wrist or the carpus. The *metacarpal* bones in the palm of the hand take their name from their being beyond (*meta*, beyond) the wrist (*carpus*).

UL-2 Bones of the upper extremity

Color and label

1 Clavicle (collar bone)
2 Scapula (shoulder blade)
3 Humerus
4 Ulna
5 Radius
6 Medial border of scapula
7 Lateral border of scapula
8 Superior border of scapula
9 Superior angle of scapula
10 Inferior angle of scapula
11 Lateral angle (glenoid cavity)
12 Spine of scapula
13 Acromion
14 Scapular notch
15 Coracoid process
16 Supraspinous fossa
17 Infraspinous fossa
18 Infraglenoid tubercle
19 Neck of scapula
20 Head of humerus
21 Anatomical neck of humerus
22 Surgical neck of humerus (usual site of proximal humerus fracture
23 Deltoid tuberosity
24 Medial epicondyle of humerus
25 Lateral epicondyle of humerus
26 Radial groove for radial nerve
27 Olecranon fossa
28 Sulcus for ulnar nerve
29 Olecranon of ulna
30 Head of radius
31 Neck of radius
32 Styloid process of ulna
33 Styloid process of radius
34 Pisiform (carpal) bone
35 Triquetral (carpal) bone
36 Lunate bone (most frequently dislocated wrist bone)
37 Scaphoid bone (most frequently fractured wrist bone)
38 Hamate (carpal) bone
39 Capitate (carpal) bone
40 Trapezoid (carpal) bone
41 Trapezium (carpal) bone
42 Metacarpal bones
43 Proximal phalanges
44 Middle phalanges
45 Distal phalanges

*Most frequent site of fracture of the clavicle (which is the most frequently broken bone)

Posterior aspect

Shoulder girdle, clavicle, and scapula

(upper) Arm (brachium)

Forearm (antebrachium)

Wrist (carpus)

Fingers (digits)

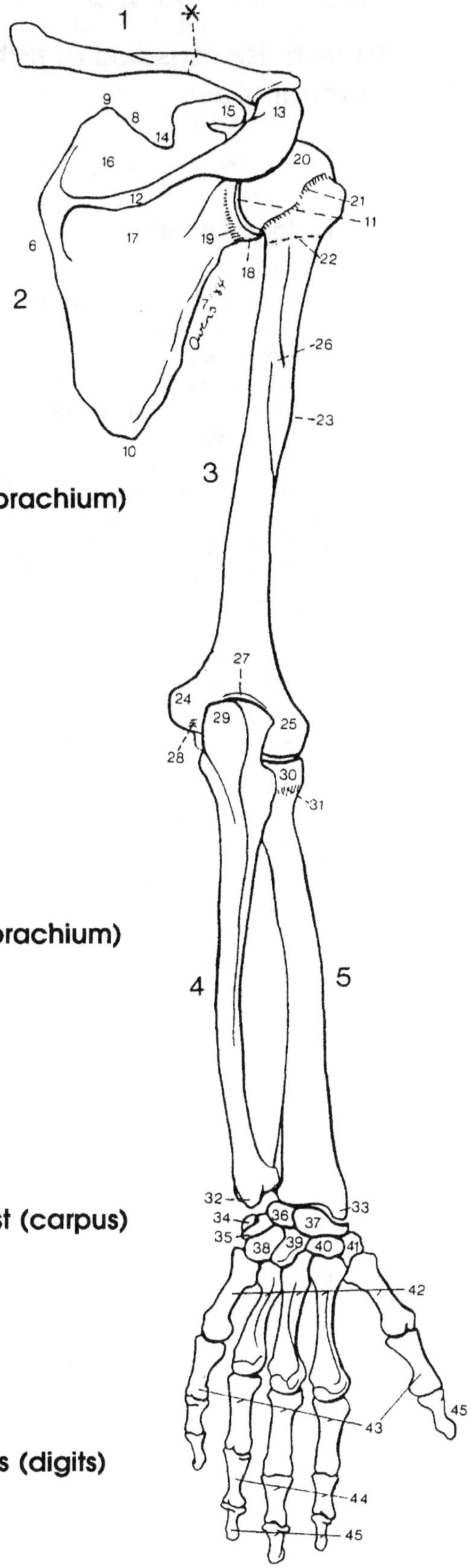

UL-3 Muscles of upper extremity I

Superficial muscles of right arm
Anterior view

Color and label

1 Clavicle
2 Trapezius (a small portion)
3 Pectoralis major
4 Coracobrachialis
5 Triceps brachii (long head)
6 Triceps brachii (medial head)
7 Brachialis
8 Pronator teres
9 Bicepital aponeurosis
10 Flexor carpi radialis
11 Palmaris longus
12 Flexor digitorum superficialis
13 Flexor carpi ulnaris
14 Pisiform bone
15 Flexor retinaculum
16 Palmaris brevis
17 Flexor pollicis brevis
18 Abductor pollicis brevis
19 Flexor pollicis longus
20 Flexor digitorum superficialis
21 Extensor carpi radialis longus
22 Extensor carpi radialis brevis
23 Brachioradialis
24 Biceps brachii tendon
25 Brachialis
26 Biceps brachii
27 Triceps brachii (lateral head)
28 Deltoid

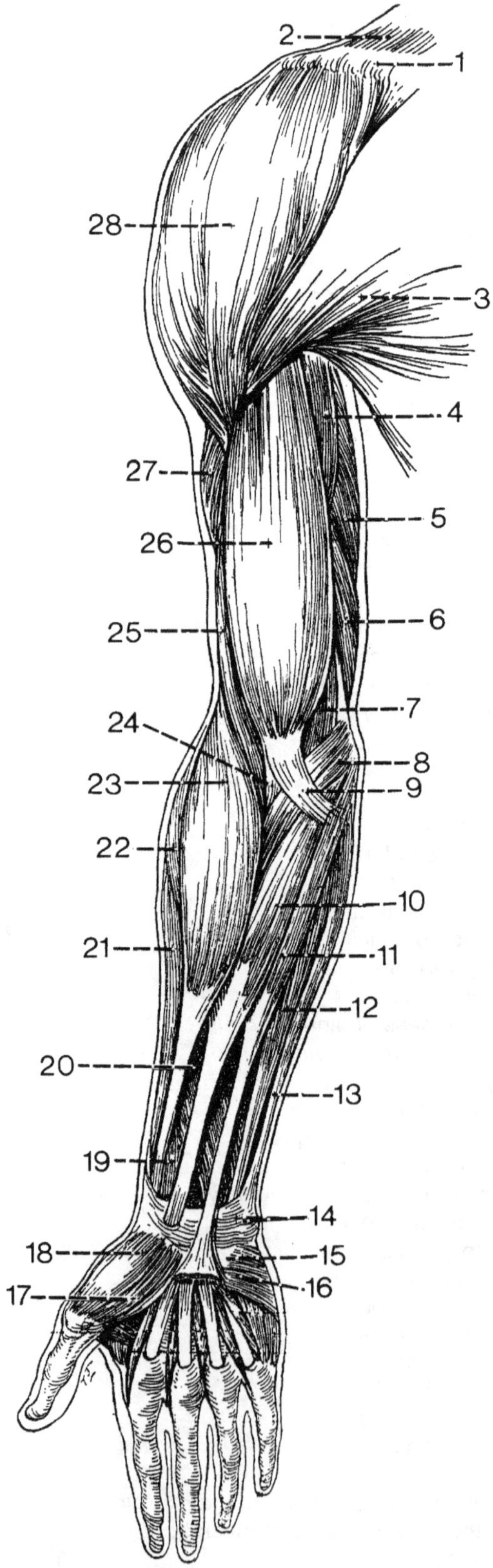

Eycleshymer and Jones

UL-4 Muscles of upper extremity II

Superficial muscles of right arm
Posterior view

Color and label

1 Clavicle
2 Deltoid
3 Triceps brachii (lateral head)
4 Brachialis
5 Tendon of triceps brachii
6 Brachioradialis
7 Lateral epicondyle of humerus
8 Extensor carpi radialis longus
9 Extensor carpi radialis brevis
10 Abductor pollicis longus
11 Extensor pollicis brevis
12 Extensor pollicis longus
13 Tendon of extensor pollicis longus
14 Tendon of extensor pollicis brevis
15 Tendons of extensor digitorum
16 Extensor retinaculum
17 Extensor digiti minimi
18 Extensor digitorum
19 Extensor carpi ulnaris
20 Flexor carpi ulnaris
21 Anconeus
22 Olecranon
23 Medial epicondyle of humerus
24 Triceps brachii (medial head)
25 Triceps brachii (long head)

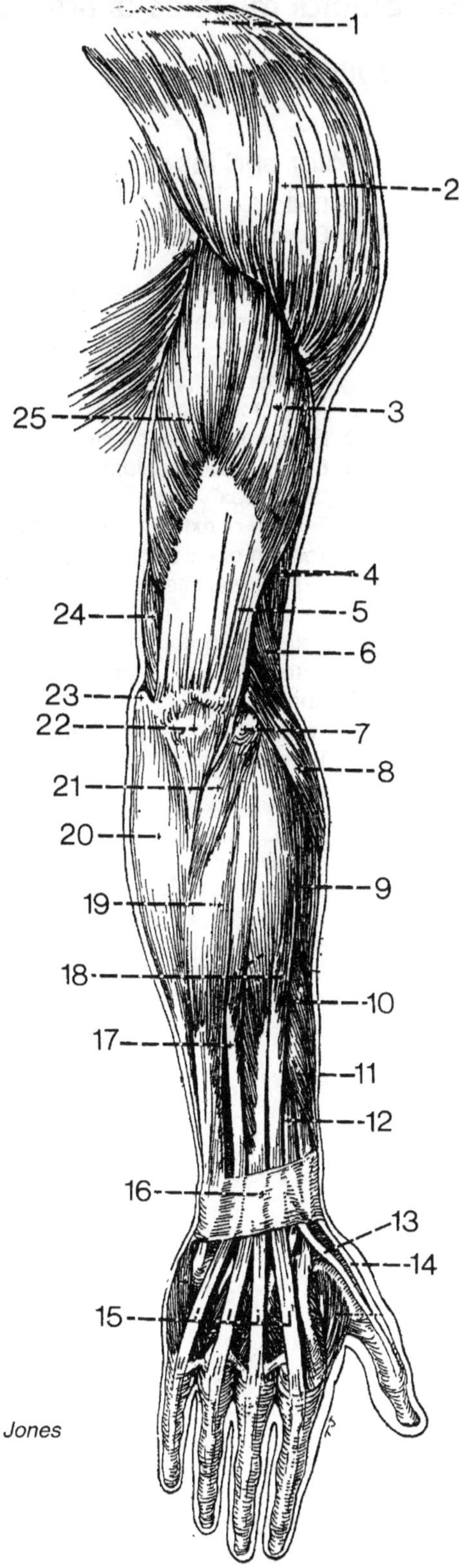

Eycleshymer and Jones

UL-5 Muscles of upper extremity III

Superficial muscles of right arm

Lateral aspect

Color and label

1 Deltoid
2 Biceps brachii
3 Brachialis
4 Lateral intermuscular septum
5 Brachioradialis
6 Extensor carpi radialis longus
7 Extensor carpi radialis brevis
8 Abductor pollicis longus
9 Extensor pollicis brevis
10 Extensor retinaculum
11 "Snuff box"
12 Tendon of extensor pollicis longus
13 Tendon of extensor pollicis brevis
14 First dorsal interosseous
15 Tendons of extensor digitorum
16 Extensor digitorum
17 Extensor carpi ulnaris
18 Anconeus
19 Triceps brachii (lateral head)
20 Triceps brachii (long head)

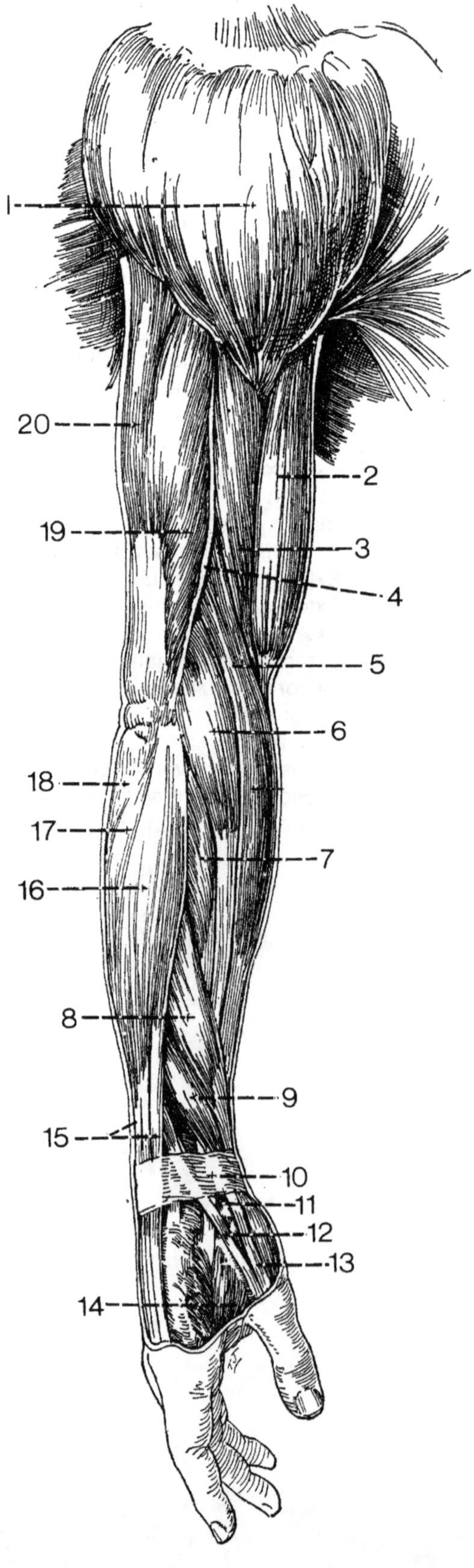

Eycleshymer and Jones

UL-6 Right scapula (shoulder blade)

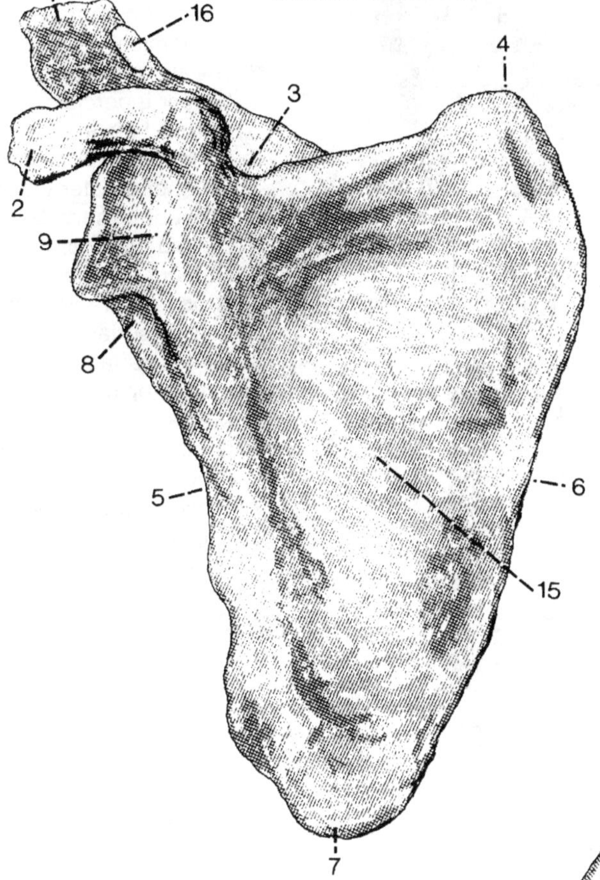

Costal surface

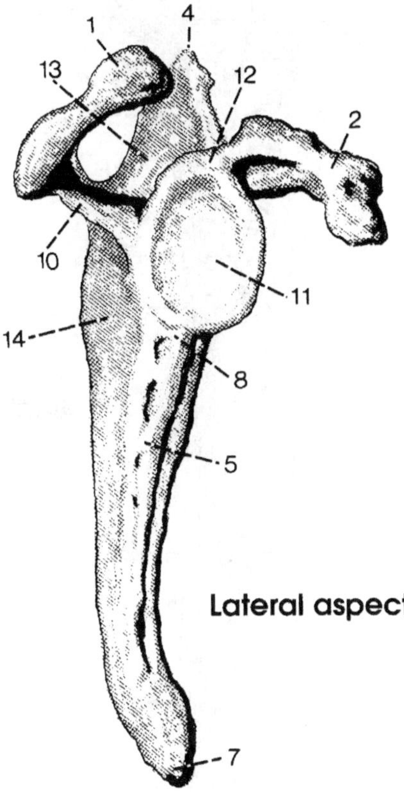

Lateral aspect

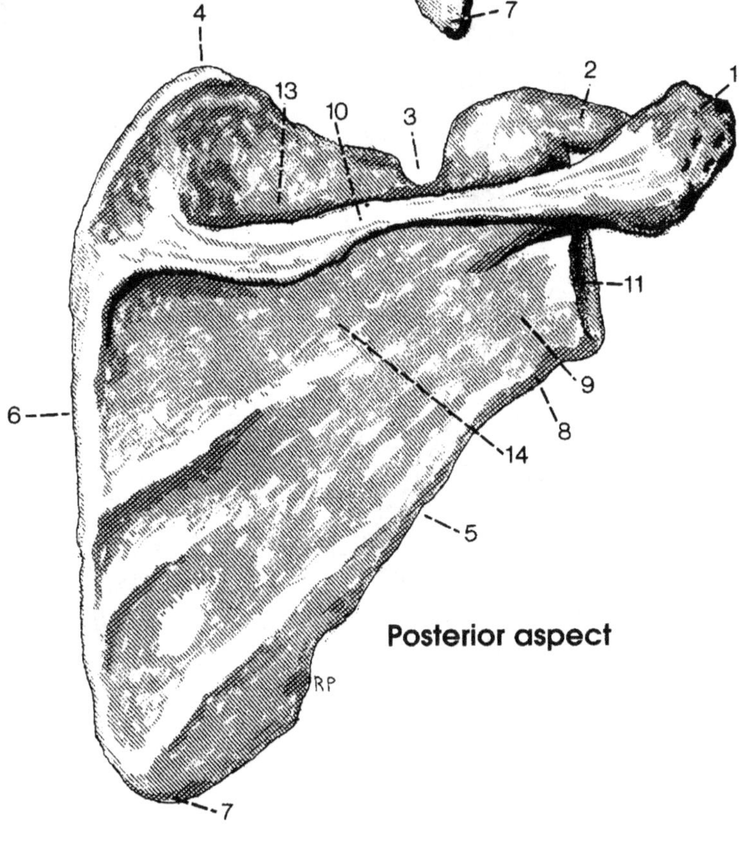

Posterior aspect

Color and label

1 Acromion
2 Coracoid process
3 Scapular notch
4 Superior angle
5 Lateral border
6 Medial (vertebral) border
7 Inferior angle
8 Infraglenoid tubercle
9 Neck (collum) of scapula
10 Spine of scapula
11 Glenoid cavity (lined with articular cartilage)
12 Supraglenoid tubercle
13 Supraspinous fossa
14 Infraspinous fossa
15 Costal surface (covered by subscapularis muscle)
16 Articular surface of acromion (articulates with clavicle)

UL-7 The humerus

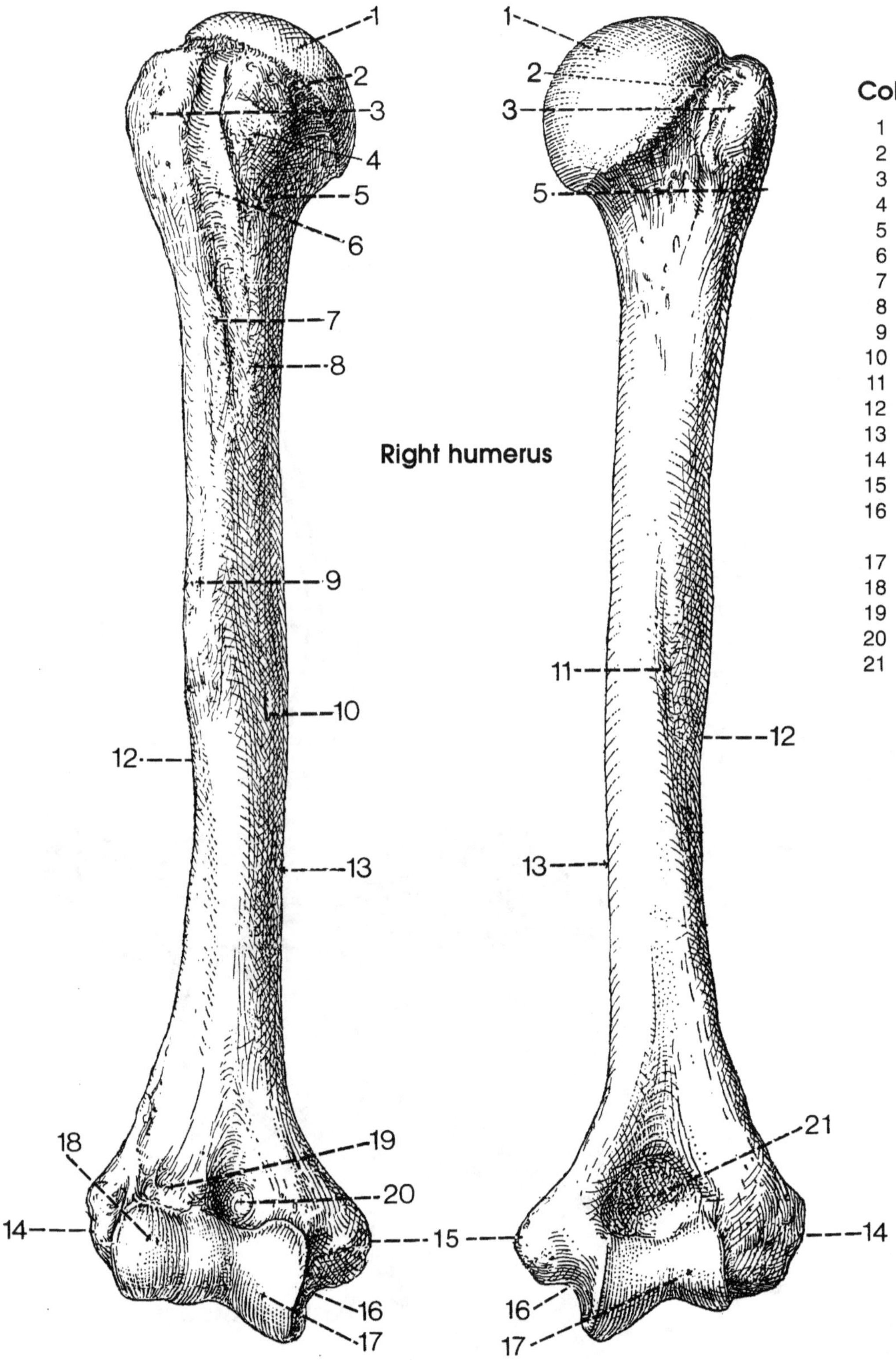

Anterior **Posterior**

Eycleshymer and Jones

Color and label

1. Head of humerus
2. Anatomical neck
3. Greater tubercle
4. Lesser tubercle
5. Surgical neck
6. Intertubercular groove
7. Crest of greater tubercle
8. Crest of lesser tubercle
9. Deltoid tuberosity
10. Nutrient foramen
11. Groove for radial nerve
12. Lateral surface
13. Medial surface
14. Lateral epicondyle
15. Medial epicondyle
16. Groove for ulnar nerve ("funny bone")
17. Trochlea (L. pulley)
18. Capitulum
19. Radial fossa
20. Coronoid fossa
21. Olecranon fossa

UL-8 The radius and ulna

Right ulna and radius

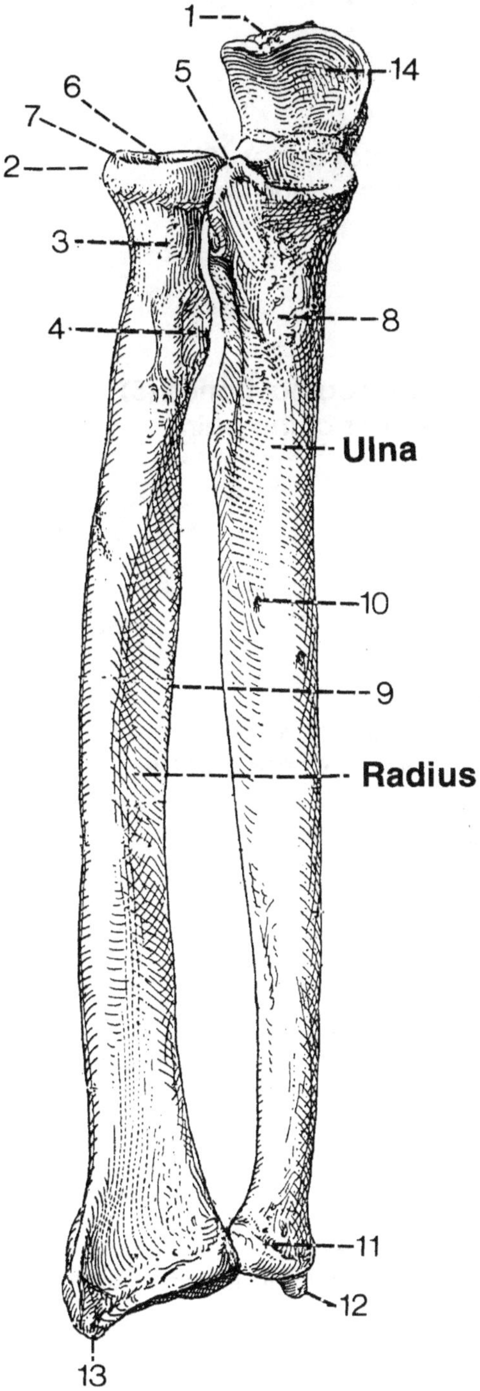

Anterior

Color and label

1 Olecranon
2 Head of radius
3 Neck of radius
4 Radial tuberosity
5 Coronoid process of ulna
6 Articular fovea in head of radius
7 Articular circumference of radial head
8 Ulnar tuberosity
9 Interosseous margin of radius
10 Nutrient foramen
11 Head of ulna
12 Styloid process of ulna
13 Styloid process of radius
14 Trochlear notch

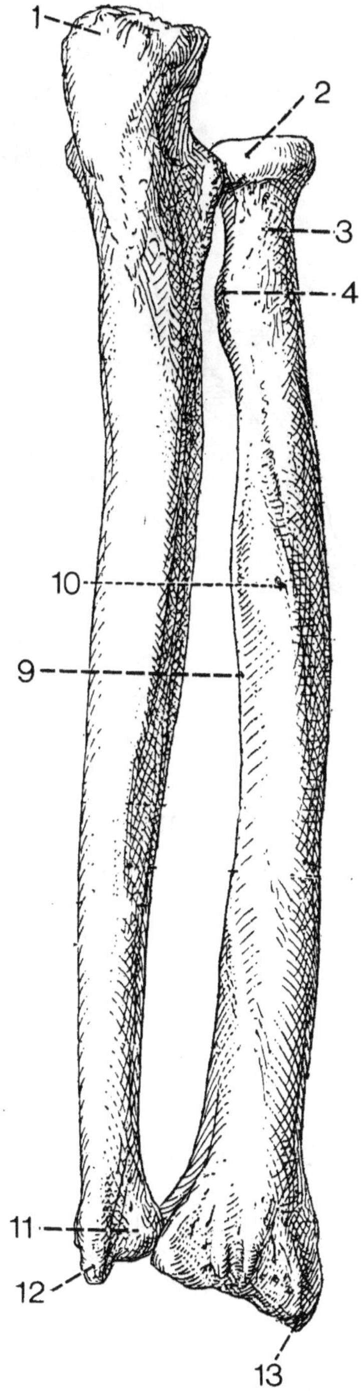

Posterior

Eycleshymer and Jones

UL-9 Bones of the hand (manus)

Palmar aspect, right hand

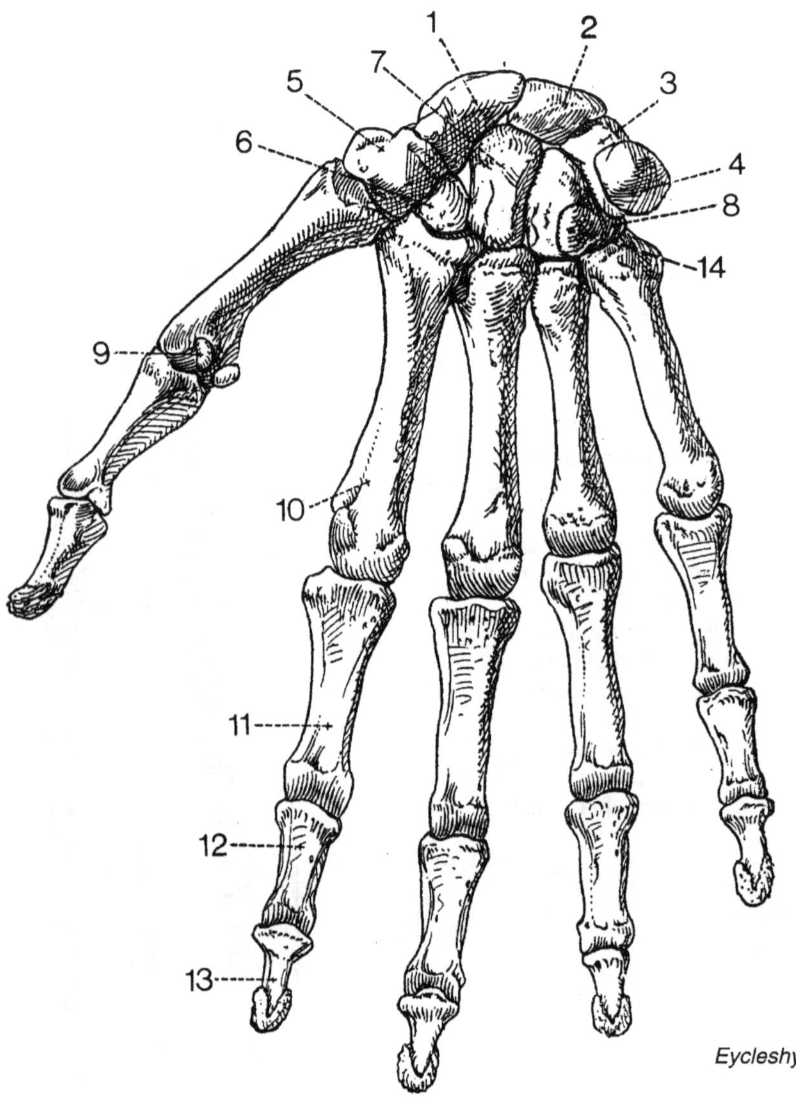

Eycleshymer and Jones

Color and label

1 Scaphoid (Gr. *scapha*, a hollowed-out, small, light boat)
2 Lunate (L. *luna*, the moon, moon-shaped)
3 Triquetral (three-sided)
4 Pisiform (L. *pisum*, a pea)
5 Trapezium (Gr. *trapeza*, a table)
6 Trapezoid (table-shaped)
7 Capitate (L. *caput*, head-shaped)
8 Hamate (hooked)
9 Sesamoid bones (resembling a sesame seed)
10 Second metacarpal bone
11 Proximal phalanx (of index finger, second digit) (second digit)
12 Middle phalanx
13 Distal phalanx
14 Hamulus of hamate (L. little hook, hook of hamate)

UL-10 Bones of the hand (manus)

Dorsal aspect, right hand

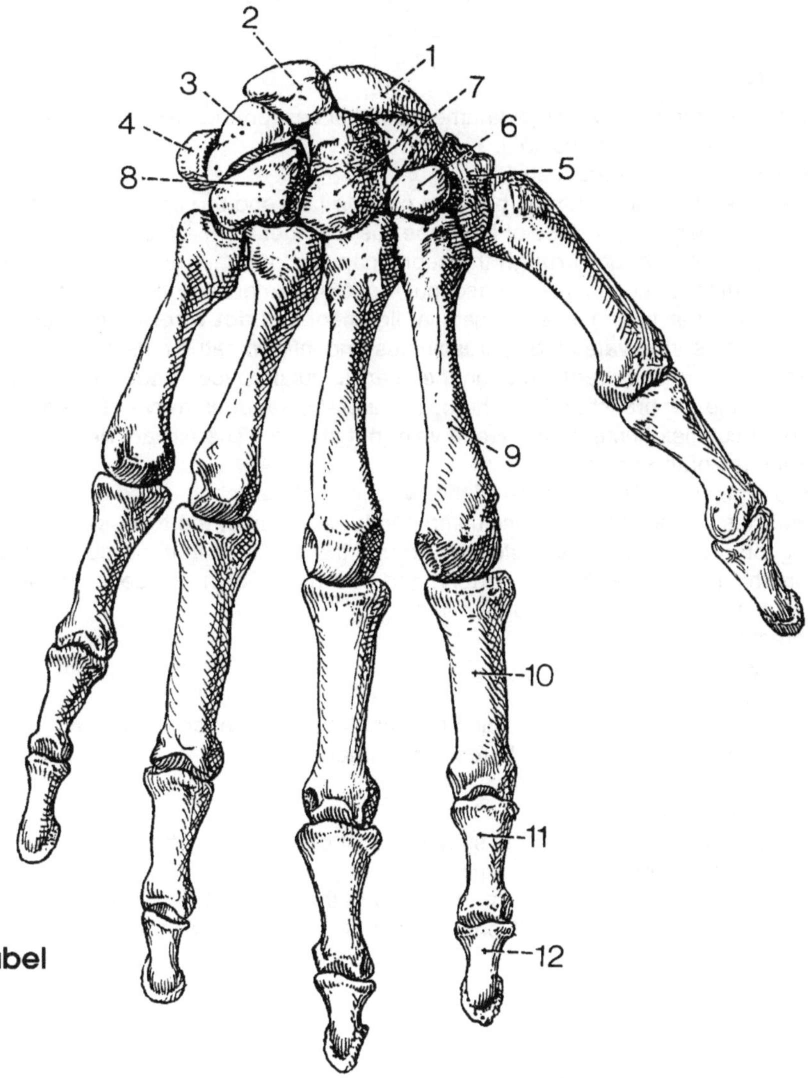

Eycleshymer and Jones

Color and label

1 Scaphoid
2 Lunate
3 Triquetral
4 Pisiform
5 Trapezium
6 Trapezoid
7 Capitate
8 Hamate
9 Second metacarpal
10 Proximal phalanx of index finger
11 Middle phalanx
12 Distal phalanx

Note that the thumb (L. *pollex*; combining form, *pollicis*), the most movable of the fingers, has only two phalanges, unlike the other four digits, which each have three phalanges.

UL-11 Dissection of posterior shoulder and arm

(opposite page)

Color and label

1 Accessory nerve; cranial nerve XI (old name, spinal accessory nerve). This nerve supplies two muscles, the trapezius and the sternocleidomastoid.
2 Trapezius muscle (upper fibers; cut)
3 Trapezius muscle; its fibers insert on both the clavicle (26) and the spine of the scapula (10).
4 Trapezius (lower fibers); both sides of the trapezius together form a four-sided, kite-shaped muscle.
5 Suprascapular nerve passing **through** the suprascapular foramen (notch) and **under** the transverse scapular ligament that bridges the suprascapular notch. The accompanying suprascapular artery and vein (not shown) pass **over** the transverse scapular ligament and **not through** the suprascapular foramen. The suprascapular nerve innervates the supraspinatus and infraspinatus muscles.
6 Axillary nerve passing backwards through the quadrangular space. It supplies the deltoid muscle and the teres minor muscle. Its branches form the upper lateral cutaneous nerve of the arm. It is accompanied by the posterior circumflex humeral artery and vein (not shown). The axillary nerve is one of the five major terminal branches of the brachial plexus.
7 Radial nerve. This nerve is the largest of the five terminal branches of the brachial plexus. It supplies all the extensor muscles in the upper limb, including the three heads of the triceps, the brachioradialis, and the extensor digitorum. Here it winds posteriorly around the humerus in the radial groove accompanied by the profunda brachii artery (deep brachial artery) and vein (not shown). Its sensory fibers supply sensibility to most of the posterior surface of the upper limb.
8 Profunda brachii artery
9 Acromion process of scapula
10 Spine of scapula
11 Deltoid muscle (origin cut; arising on spine of scapula and acromion). It also arises from the lateral clavicle.
12 Deltoid muscle insertion on deltoid tuberosity of humerus
13 Deltoid muscle (cut in a coronal plane)
14 Supraspinatus muscle (cut)
15 Supraspinatus muscle (insertion on the superior facet of the greater tubercle of the humerus)
16 Infraspinatus muscle (cut)
17 infraspinatus muscle (insertion on the middle facet of the greater tubercle of the humerus)
18 Teres minor muscle. The **rotator cuff** is formed by the subscapularis muscle anteriorly, the supraspinatus superiorly, and the infraspinatus and teres minor posteriorly.
19 Teres major muscle
20 Levator scapuli muscle
21 Rhomboid minor muscle
22 Rhomboid major muscle
23 Superficial branch of transverse cervical artery
24 Descending branch of superficial branch of transverse cervical artery
25 Deep branch of transverse cervical artery
26 Clavicle
27 Long head of triceps brachii
28 Lateral head of triceps brachii
29 Ascending branch of superficial branch of transverse cervical artery

UL-11 Dissection of posterior shoulder and arm

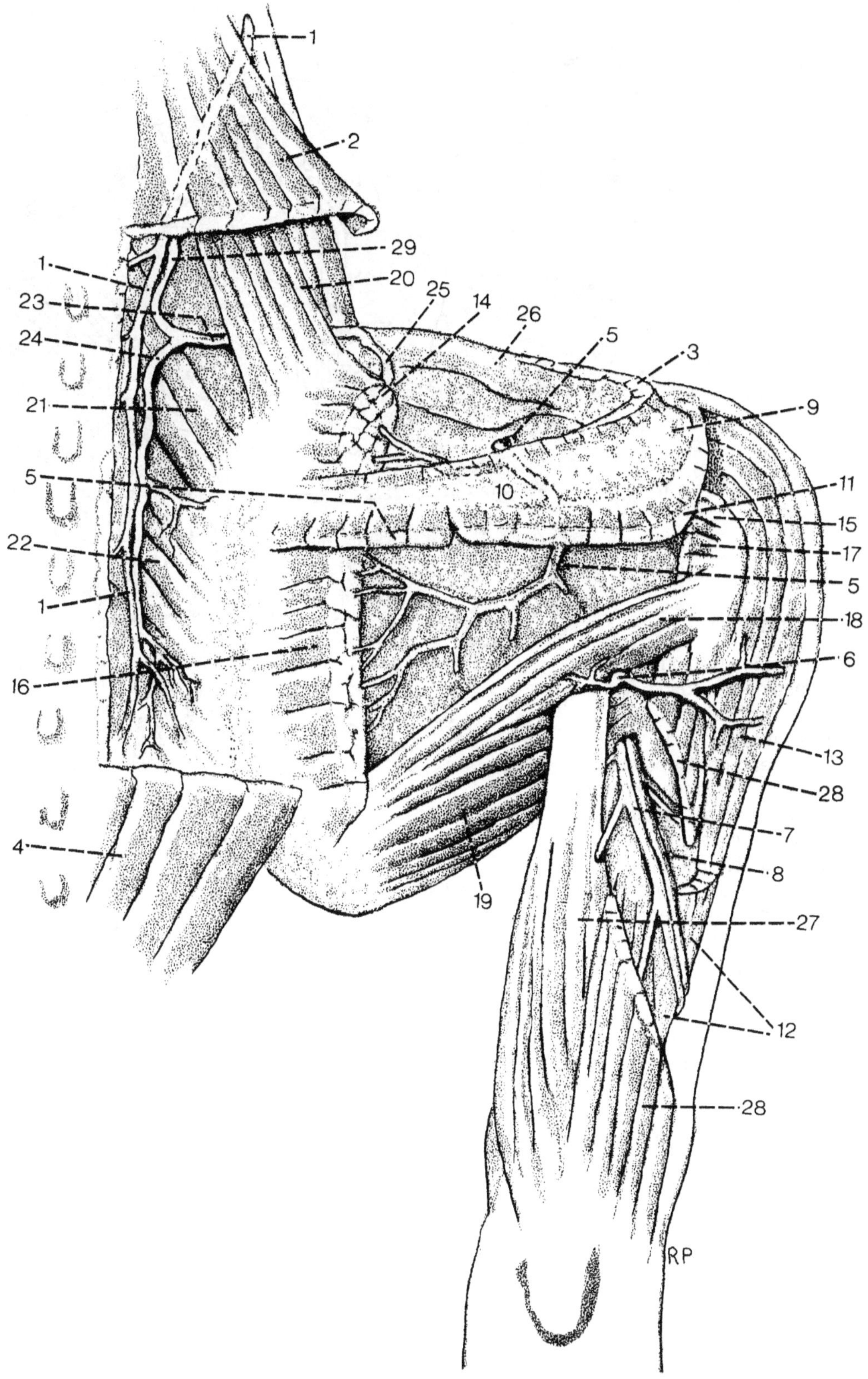

UL-12 Nerves and arteries of the posterior shoulder

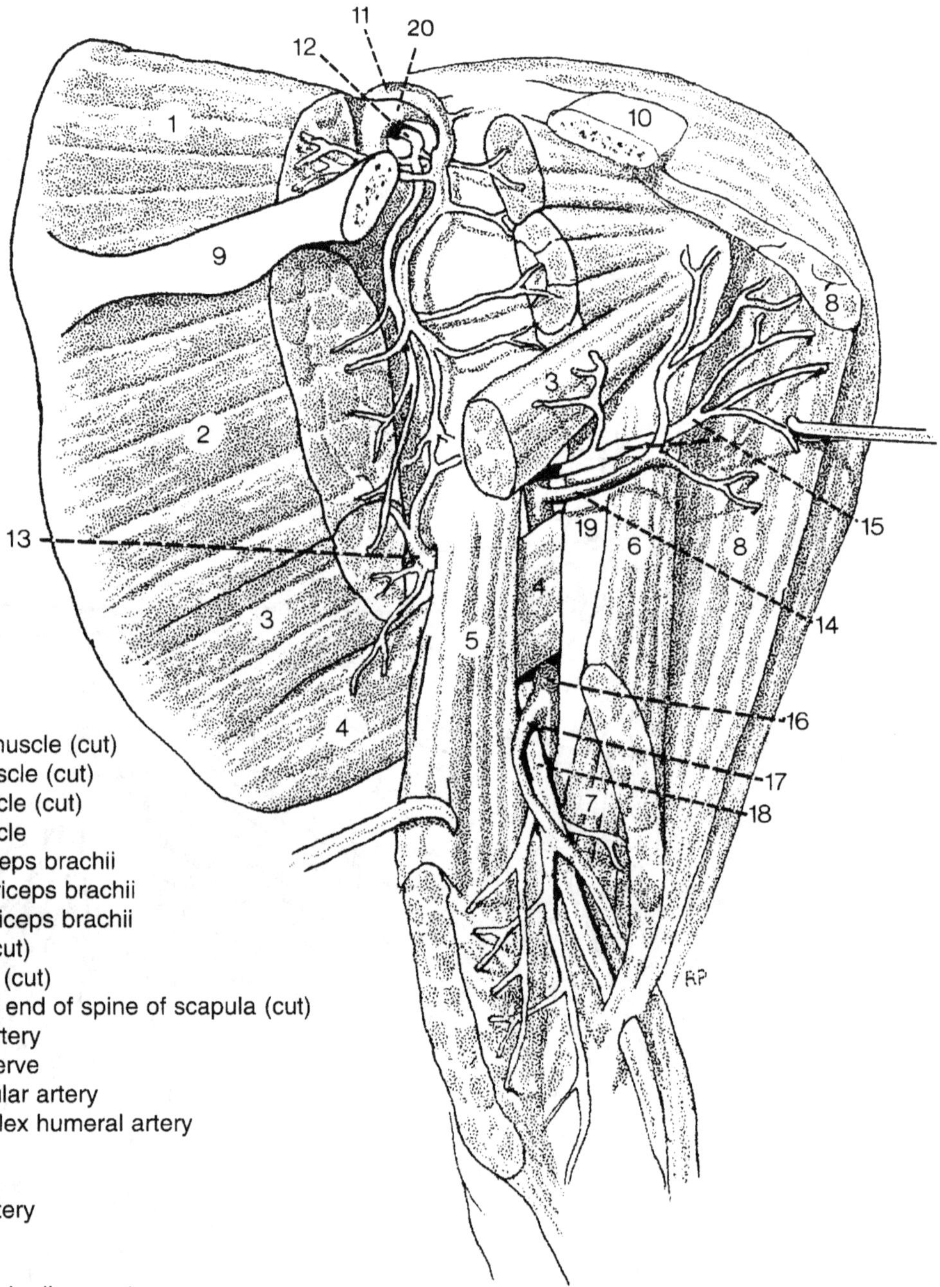

Color and label

1 Supraspinatus muscle (cut)
2 Infraspinatus muscle (cut)
3 Teres minor muscle (cut)
4 Teres major muscle
5 Long head of triceps brachii
6 Lateral head of triceps brachii
7 Medial head of triceps brachii
8 Deltoid muscle (cut)
9 Spine of scapula (cut)
10 Acromion; lateral end of spine of scapula (cut)
11 Suprascapular artery
12 Suprascapular nerve
13 Circumflex scapular artery
14 Posterior circumflex humeral artery
15 Axillary nerve
16 Brachial artery
17 Deep brachial artery
18 Radial nerve
19 Humerus
20 Transverse scapular ligament

After Wolf-Heidegger

UL-13 Quadrangular space

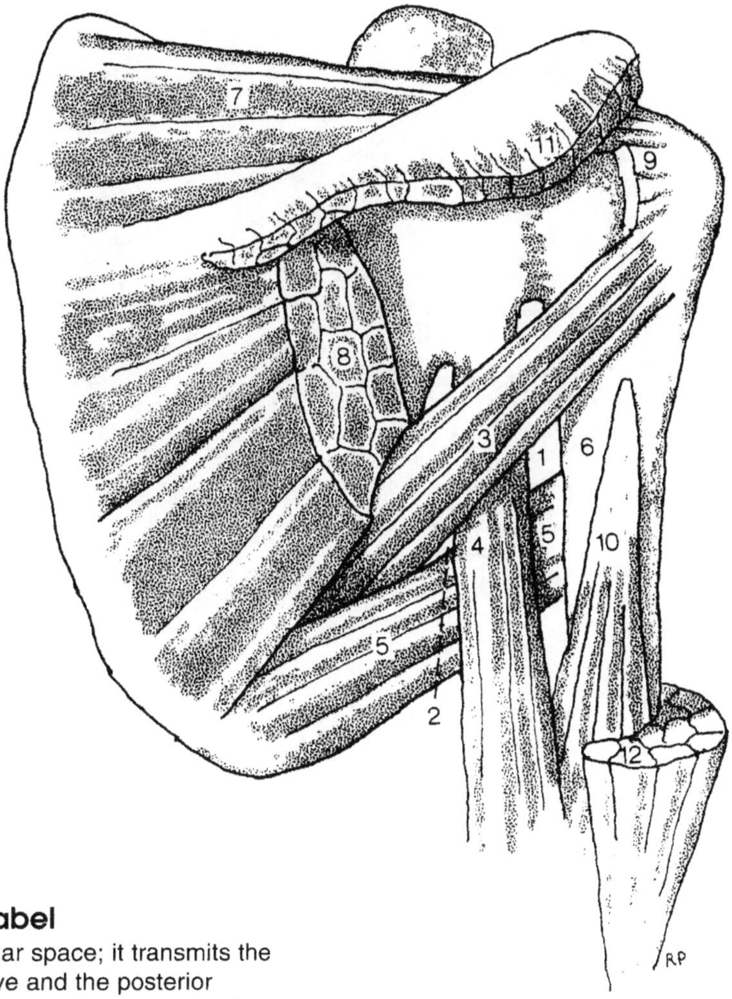

Color and label

1 Quadrangular space; it transmits the axillary nerve and the posterior circumflex humeral artery and vein.
2 Triangular space
3 Teres minor (superior border of quadrangular space)
4 Long head of triceps brachii (medial border of space)
5 Teres major (inferior border of space)
6 Surgical neck of humerus (lateral border of space)
7 Supraspinatus muscle
8 Infraspinatus muscle
9 Insertion of infraspinatus muscle
10 Lateral head of triceps brachii
11 Origin of deltoid on spine and acromion of scapula
12 Deltoid muscle

UL-14 The brachial plexus

General plan

The posterior cord and nerves that arise from it (radial and axillary) are shaded.

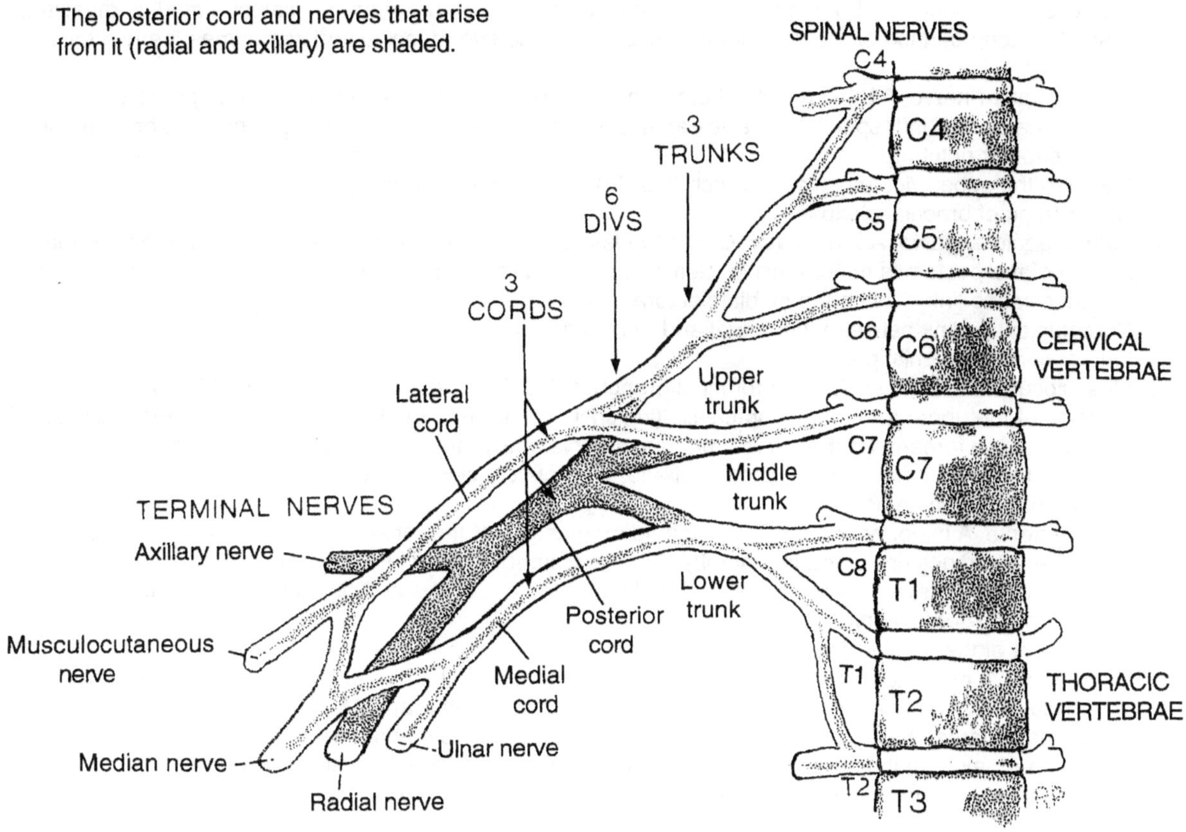

The **brachial plexus** supplies movement and sensation to the arm or upper extremity. It arises from spinal nerves in the neck. These nerves exchange nerve fibers (axons) by dividing and coalescing through five successive stages: nerves, trunks, divisions, cords, and terminal nerves. Beginning with cervical nerve C5 (with a contribution from cervical nerve C4) down to thoracic nerve T1 (with a contribution from T2), they fuse into three trunks (an upper, middle, and lower trunk); each trunk then divides into an anterior and a posterior division resulting in six divisions; the six divisions coalesce into three cords, which then give off five large terminal nerves, the radial nerve, the axillary nerve, the median nerve, the musculocutaneous nerve, and the ulnar nerve. (See following figure for additional nerves that are given off by the brachial plexus.)

Note that there are 8 cervical nerves but only 7 cervical vertebrae. Cervical nerves 1-7 exit the vertebral column **above** the corresponding vertebra (cervical nerve C7 exits **above** cervical vertebra C7), whereas cervical nerve C8 exits **below** vertebra C7. All subsequent (lower) spinal nerves (thoracic and lumbar) exit below their corresponding vertebrae.

UL-15 Brachial plexus and its nerves

(opposite page)

Color and label

1 Phrenic nerve. The motor nerve to the diaphragm. It arises from branches of cervical nerves C3, C4, and C5. It passes inferiorly in front of the root of the lung, pierces the diaphragm and innervates it on its inferior surface.
2 Dorsal scapular nerve. A branch of the fifth cervical nerve. After piercing the scalenus medius muscle to reach the deep surface of the rhomboids, it supplies these two muscles and sometimes the levator scapulae as well.
3 Suprascapular nerve. A branch (with fibers from C5 and C6) of the superior trunk. It supplies the supraspinatus and infraspinatus muscles after passing backwards under the ligament that bridges the suprascapular notch.
4 Nerve to the subclavius muscle. A branch (C5,C6) of the superior trunk.
5 Upper trunk of brachial plexus
6 Lateral pectoral nerve. A branch (C5-C7) of the lateral cord supplying the clavicular and upper sternal portion of the pectoralis major muscle. Some of its fibers reach the pectoralis minor muscle through a communicating link (7) with the medial pectoral nerve.
7 Communicating link between the lateral and medial pectoral nerves
8 Lateral cord of brachial plexus
9 Musculocutaneous nerve. A major terminal branch (C5-C7) of the brachial plexus that innervates the flexor muscles of the upper arm, coracobrachialis (which it penetrates), the biceps brachii, and the brachialis. It emerges in the forearm as the lateral cutaneous nerve which supplies the skin of the lateral (radial) forearm as far as the thenar eminence. Hence its name, the "muscle-skin" nerve.
10 Lateral root of median nerve
11 Median nerve. A major nerve (C5-T1) to the flexor muscles of the forearm and hand. It supplies sensation to the radial 3 1/2 digits (including the thumb) plus motor fibers to the critically important thumb muscles, the abductor pollicis brevis, the flexor pollicis brevis, and the opponens pollicis. In the forearm it gives rise to the anterior interosseous nerve.
12 Medial root of the median nerve
13 Ulnar nerve. A major terminal nerve arising from the medial cord of the brachial plexus. As it passes superficially over the medial epicondyle of the humerus, it is vulnerable to an external tap, which is usually felt as the instantaneous painful " funny bone" sensation. It suppies the skin of the front and back of the medial hand, most of the small muscles in the hand, plus some flexor muscles in the forearm.
14 Radial nerve. The largest terminal nerve (C5-T1) of the brachial plexus. It supplies all the extensor muscles of the upper limb. Its cutaneous branches supply sensibility to the dorsal surface of the upper limb from the insertion of the deltoid to the dorsum of the wrist. It supplies the long forearm extensor and abductor muscles to the digits, but it supplies no intrinsic hand muscles.
15 Axillary nerve. A major terminal branch of the brachial plexus. It carries axons from cervical nerves C5 and C6. It leaves the posterior cord and pass backwards through the quadrangular space to innervate the deltoid and teres minor muscles.
16 Medial cord of brachial plexus
17 Medial antebrachial cutaneous nerve (C8,T1). Supplies sensibility to the skin of the medial forearm.
18 Medial brachial cutaneous nerve (C8,T1). Supplies the skin of the medial (upper) arm.
19 Medial pectoral nerve. Innervates the pectoralis major and minor muscles.
20 Posterior cord of brachial plexus
21 Inferior subscapular nerve. Innervates caudal portion of subscapularis muscle and teres major muscle.
22 Thoracodorsal nerve (also middle subscapular nerve). Arises from the posterior cord. It suppies the latissimus dorsi muscle.
23 Superior subscapular nerve. Innervates cranial portion of subscapularis muscle.
24 Anterior and posterior divisions of the 3 trunks of the brachial plexus (6 in all)
25 Middle trunk of the brachial plexus
26 Lower trunk of the brachial plexus
27 Long thoracic nerve to the serratus anterior muscle
28 Nerves to prevertebral muscles and scalene muscles

UL-15 Brachial plexus and its nerves

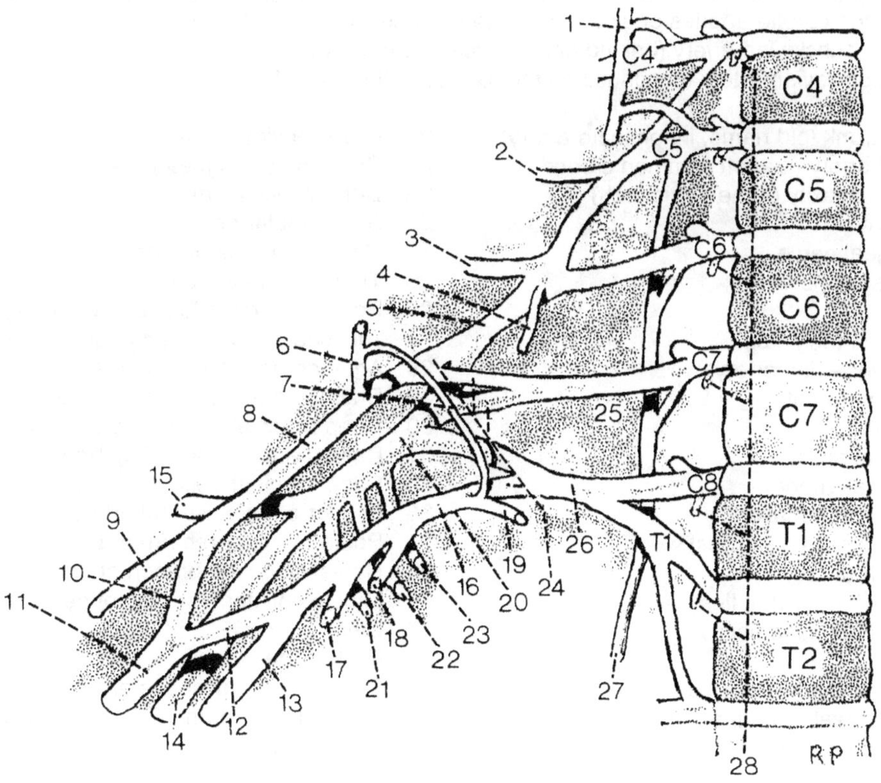

UL-16 Arteries of the posterior shoulder and arm

(opposite page)

Color and label

SC-1 First part of subclavian artery; the major artery to the upper extremity; the right subclavian artery begins at the bifurcation of the brachiocephalic trunk into the right subclavian and right common carotid arteries. The left subclavian and common carotid arteries originate from the convexity of the aortic arch.
SC-2 Second part of subclavian artery (behind anterior scalene muscle)
SC-3 Third part of subclavian artery (continues as the axillary in the shoulder)

1 Brachiocephalic trunk (old name, innominate artery)
2 Common carotid artery (the left common carotid arises from the convexity of the aortic arch)
3 Right vagus nerve
4 Recurrent laryngeal nerve (branch of the vagus nerve)
5 Vertebral artery
6 Thyrocervical trunk (origin on ventral side of subclavian artery) (see insert on upper right)
7 Inferior thyroid artery
8 Ascending cervical artery
9 Transverse cervical artery
10 Superficial branch of transverse cervical artery (supplies trapezius)
11 Ascending branch of (10)
12 Descending branch of (10); it lies deep to trapezius but superficial to rhomboids.
13 Deep branch of transverse cervical artery (it accompanies dorsal scapular nerve)
14 Dorsal scapular nerve (a small section)
15 Suprascapular artery (passes over the transverse scapular ligament)
16 Suprascapular nerve (passes under transverse scapular ligament)
17 Arterial plexus within supraspinatus muscle (not shown)
18 Arterial plexus within infraspinatus muscle (muscle not shown)
19 Axillary artery (continuation of subclavian artery)
20 Internal thoracic artery (old name, internal mammary artery)
21 Costocervical trunk
22 Supreme (or highest) intercostal artery
23 Deep cervical artery
24 Subscapular artery
25 Circumflex scapular artery
26 Thoracodorsal artery
27 Posterior circumflex humeral artery (passes through quadrangular space)
28 Anterior circumflex humeral artery
29 Brachial artery (continuation of axillary artery)
30 Deep brachial artery (profunda brachii artery)
31 Deltoid artery (ascending branch)
32 Superior ulnar collateral artery
33 Inferior ulnar collateral artery
34 Posterior ulnar recurrent artery
35 Radial collateral branch of deep brachial artery
36 Middle collateral branch of deep brachial artery
37 Ulnar artery
38 Radial artery
39 Common interosseous artery (a short thick branch of ulnar artery; divides into anterior and posterior interosseous arteries)
40 Posterior interosseous artery
41 Anterior interosseous artery
42 Recurrent interosseous artery (it may arise from the common interosseous artery)
43 Axillary nerve (cut)
44 Radial nerve (cut)
45 Ulnar nerve (a small section)

UL-16 Arteries of the posterior shoulder and arm

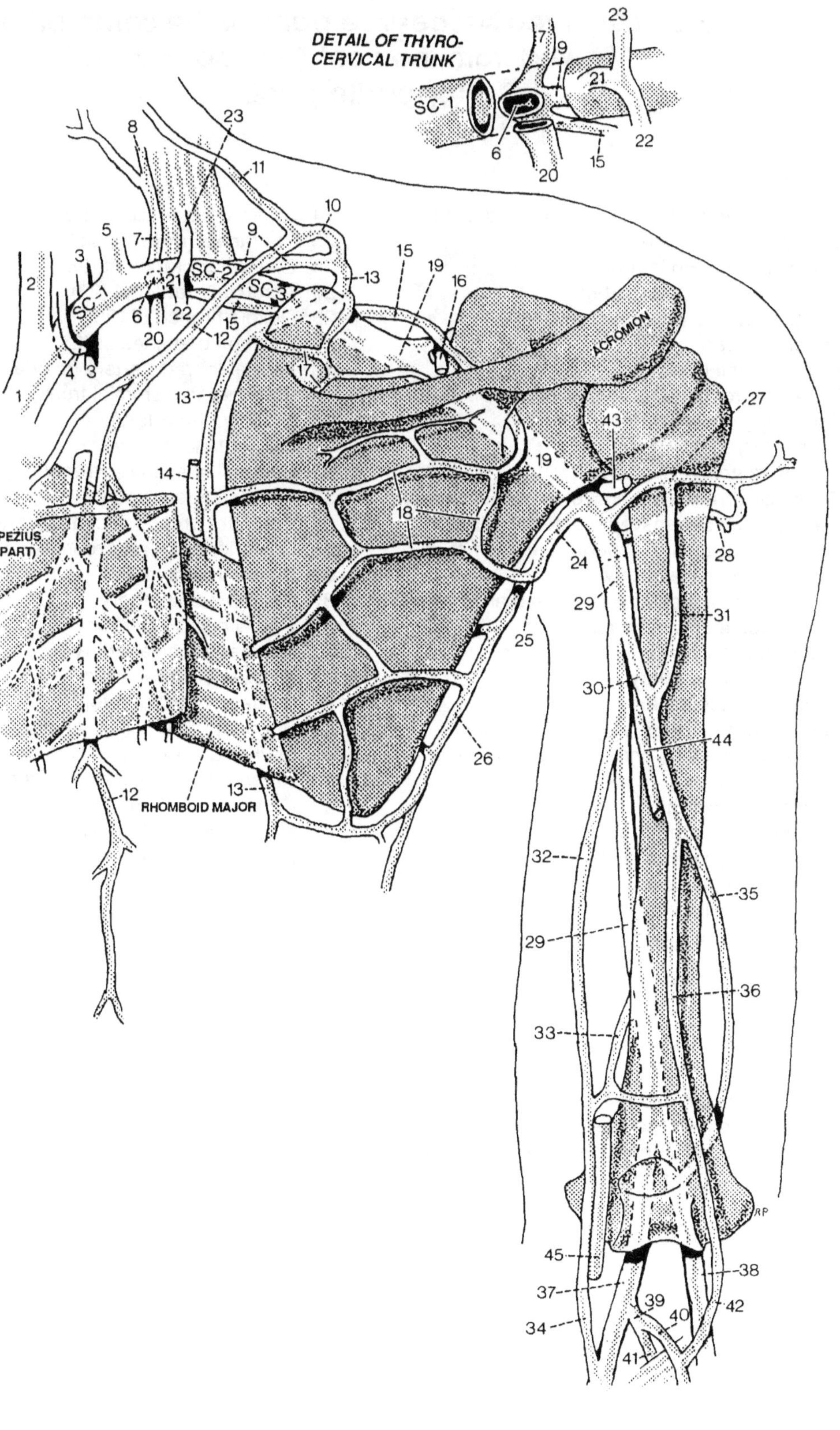

UL-17 Subclavian, axillary and brachial arteries

Actually three successive parts of the same artery
Viewed from the front (anterior aspect)
(opposite page)

Color and label

1 Ascending aorta (behind sternum and manubrium)
2 Brachiocephalic trunk
3 Left common carotid artery
4 Right common carotid artery
5 Subclavian artery
6 Vertebral artery
7 Thyrocervical trunk
8 Inferior thyroid artery
9 Ascending cervical artery
10 Inferior laryngeal artery
11 Transverse cervical artery
12 Superficial branch of transverse cervical artery
13 Deep branch of transverse cervical artery
14 Ascending branch of superficial branch of transverse cervical artery
15 Descending branch of superficial branch of transverse cervical artery
16 Suprascapular artery
17 Internal thoracic artery
18 Anterior intercostal arteries (the intercostal arteries are accompanied by intercostal veins and intercostal nerves; not shown here)
19 Perforating branches
20 Musculophrenic artery (terminal branch of the internal thoracic artery)
21 Superior epigastric artery (terminal branch of the internal thoracic artery)
22 Deep cervical artery
23 Axillary artery
24 Supreme thoracic artery
25 Thoracoacromial trunk
26 Clavicular branch of (25)
27 Acromial branch of (25)
28 Deltoid branch of (25)
29 Pectoral branches of (25)
30 Lateral thoracic artery (may also arise from thoracoacromial trunk or from subscapular artery)
31 Subscapular artery
32 Circumflex scapular artery
33 Thoracodorsal artery
34 Anterior humeral circumflex artery
35 Posterior humeral circumflex artery
36 Brachial artery
37 Deep brachial artery
38 Radial collateral artery (of deep brachial artery)
39 Middle collateral artery (of deep brachial artery)
40 Superior ulnar collateral artery
41 Inferior ulnar collateral artery
42 Anterior ulnar recurrent artery
43 Posterior ulnar recurrent artery
44 Radial recurrent artery
45 Interosseous recurrent artery
46 Posterior interosseous artery
47 Anterior interosseous artery
48 Common interosseous artery

The dissector should understand that, with very few exceptions, veins (not shown here) accompany arteries. The veins may be single or doubled and tend to be more irregular in their course than arteries. One should expect to encounter variations in the patterns of both arteries and veins that differ from the figures depicted here. In other words, no two human bodies are exactly alike. Anatomy texts and atlases portray the most common anatomy.

UL-17 Subclavian, axillary, and brachial arteries

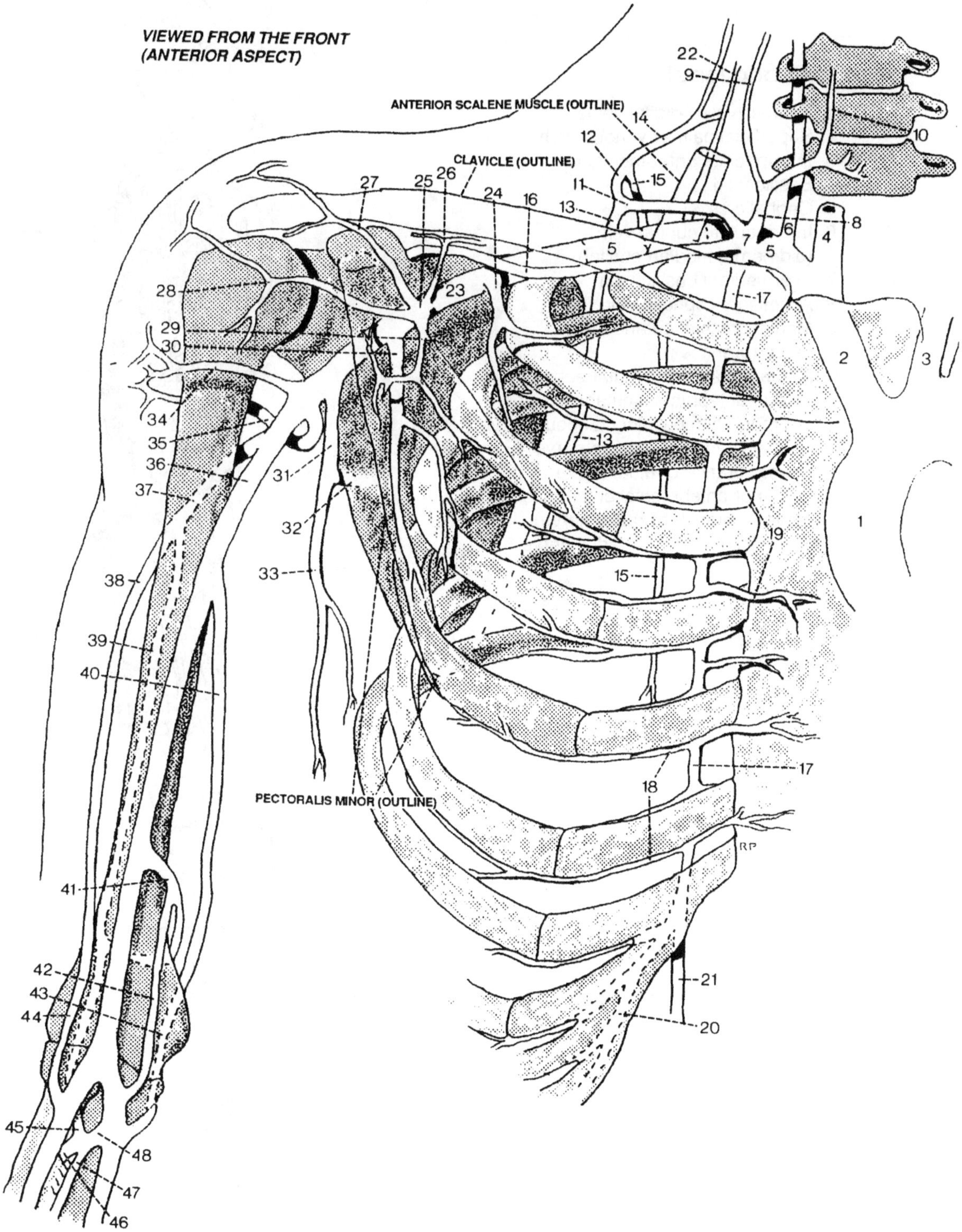

UL-18 Superficial veins and nerves of the anterior arm

Right arm - anterior surface

Color and label

1 Palmar (volar) digital veins
2 Superficial palmar venous arch
3 Intermediate antebrachial vein
4 Basilic vein
5 Cephalic vein
6 Intermediate cubital vein (old name, median cubital)
7 Intermediate basilic vein
8 Accessory cephalic vein
9 Medial brachial cutaneous nerve (branches)
10 Medial antebrachial cutaneous nerve
11 Lateral antebrachial cutaneous nerve (a branch of musculocutaneous nerve)
12 Palmar branch of median nerve
13 Palmar branch of ulnar nerve
14 Posterior antebrachial cutaneous nerve (a branch of radial nerve)
15 Superficial branch of radial nerve

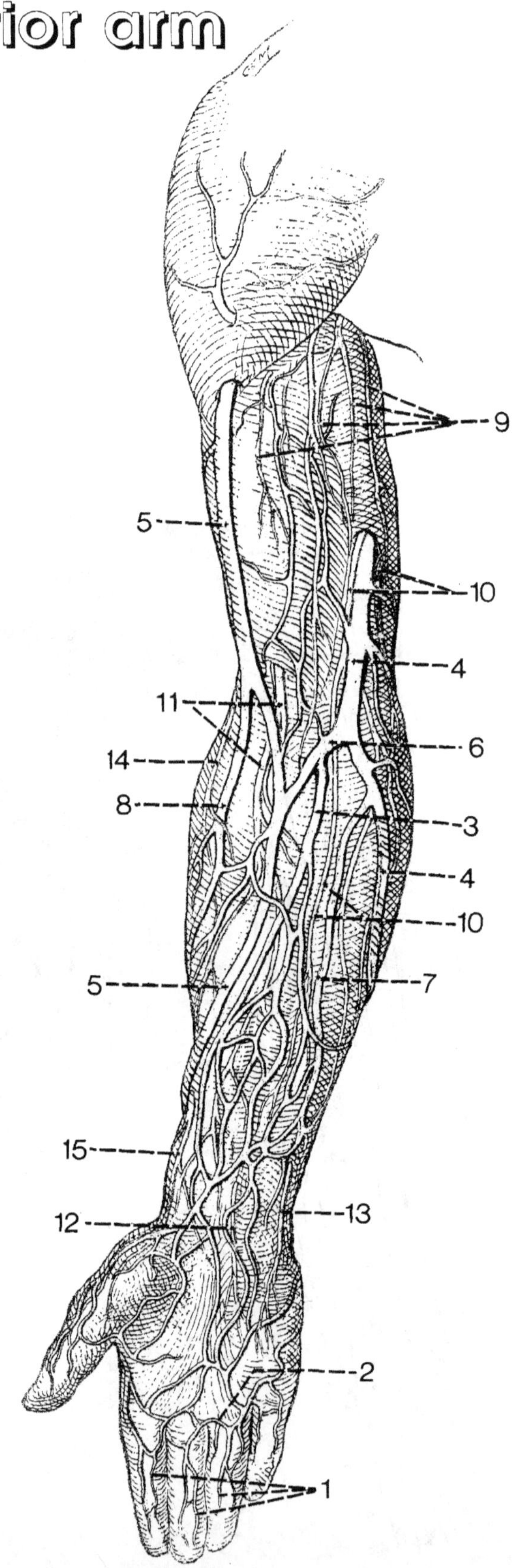

Eycleshymer and Jones

UL-19 Superficial veins and nerves of the posterior arm

Right arm - posterior surface

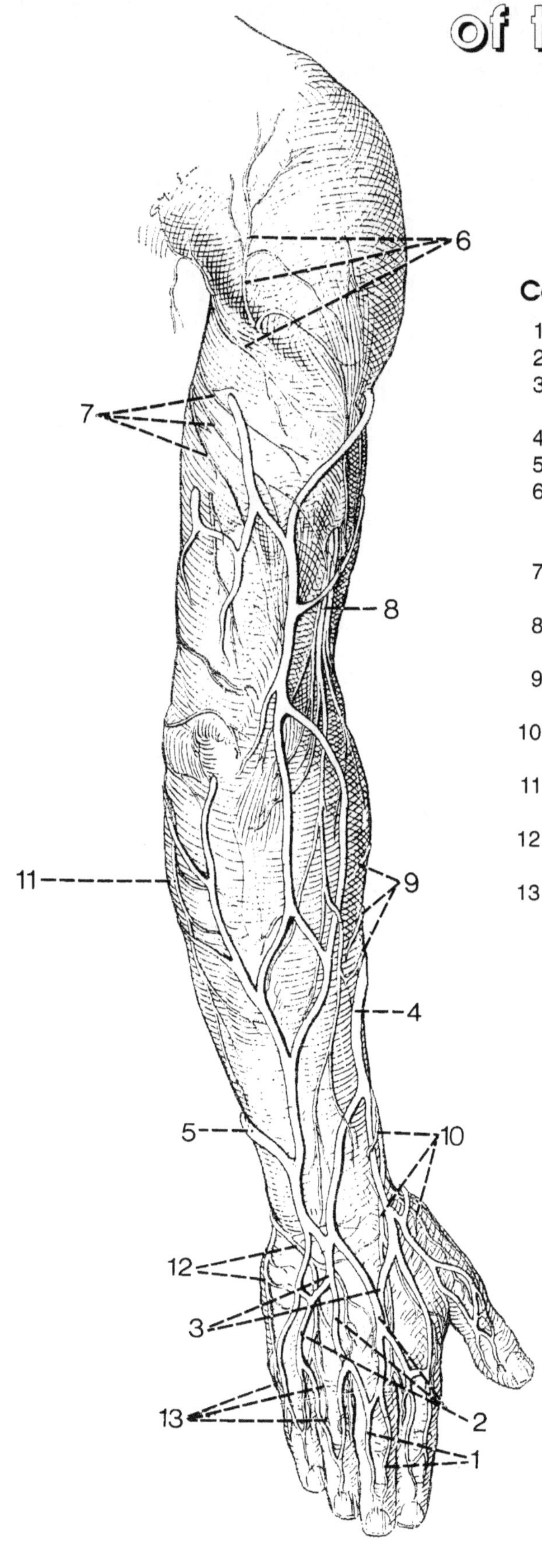

Color and label

1 Dorsal digital veins
2 Dorsal metacarpal veins
3 Dorsal venous network of the hand
4 Cephalic vein
5 Basilic vein
6 Lateral superior brachial cutaneous nerve (of axillary nerve)
7 Posterior brachial cutaneous nerve (of radial nerve)
8 Posterior antebrachial cutaneous nerve (of radial nerve)
9 Lateral antebrachial cutaneous nerve (of musculocutaneous nerve)
10 Superficial branch of radial nerve
11 Medial antebrachial cutaneous nerve
12 Branch of ulnar nerve to dorsum of the hand
13 Dorsal digital nerves

Eycleshymer and Jones

UL-20 Deep dissection of the posterior arm

Color and label

1 Scapula
2 Spine of scapula
3 Acromion of scapula
4 Infraspinatus muscle (insertion on greater tubercle of humerus; part of rotator cuff)
5 Deltoid muscle (cut)
6 Teres minor muscle (insertion; part of rotator cuff)
7 Axillary nerve emerging from quadrangular space
8 Quadrangular space
9 Posterior humeral circumflex artery (vein not shown)
10 Long head of triceps brachii muscle (the three-headed muscle)
11 Lateral head of triceps brachii
12 Medial head of triceps brachii (origin on humerus)
13 Biceps brachii
14 Radial nerve (old name, musculospiral)
15 Posterior antebrachial cutaneous nerve (branch of radial nerve)
16 Brachioradialis muscle
17 Lateral epicondyle of humerus
18 Olecranon of ulna
19 Extensor carpi radialis longus muscle
20 Anconeus muscle
21 Circumflex scapular artery (branch of subscapular artery)
22 Long head of triceps brachii
23 Teres major muscle (arm has been pulled downward)
24 Latissimus dorsi muscle
25 Brachial artery

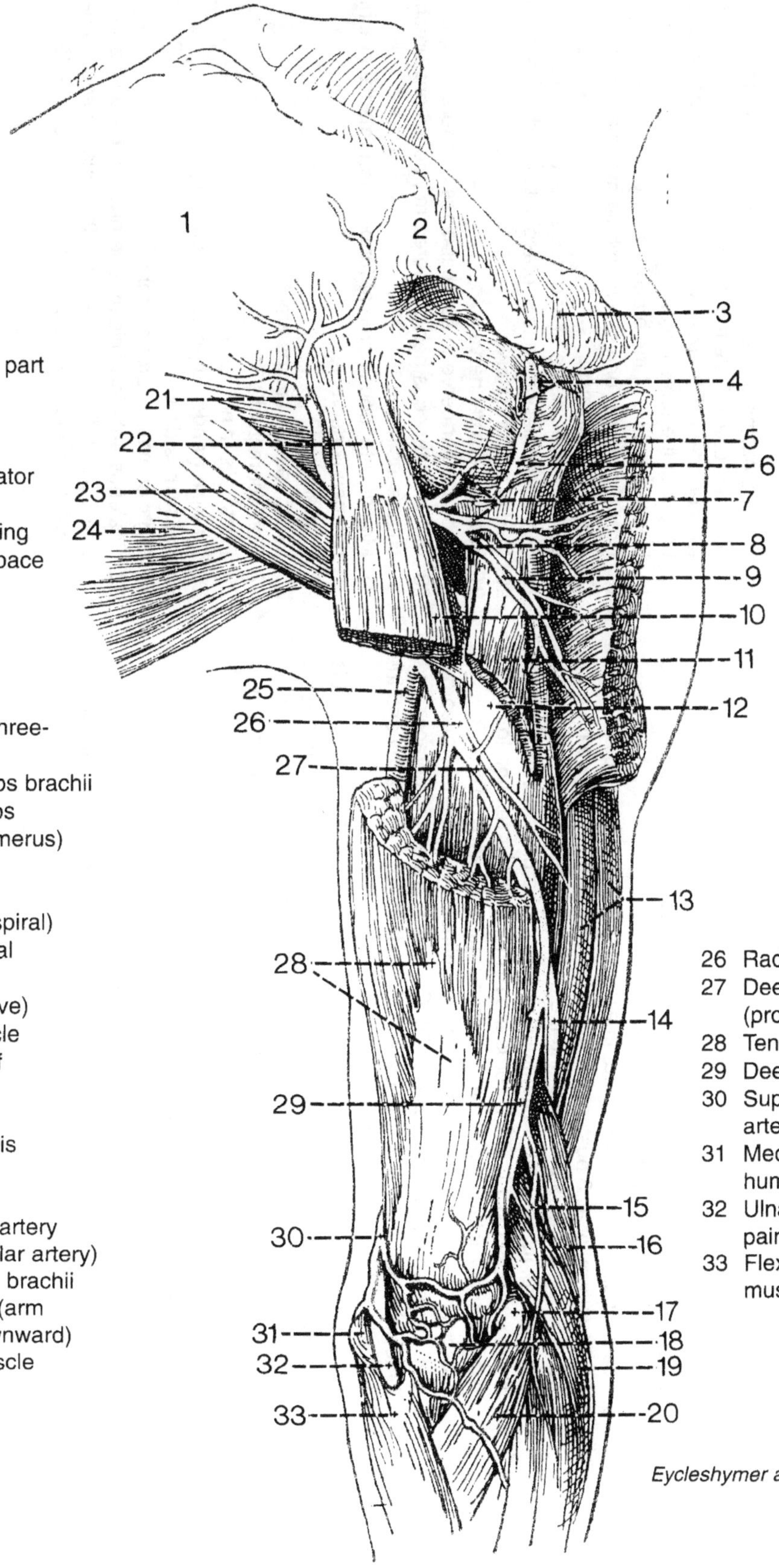

26 Radial nerve
27 Deep brachial artery (profunda brachii)
28 Tendon of triceps brachii
29 Deep brachial artery
30 Superior ulnar collateral artery
31 Medial condyle of humerus
32 Ulnar nerve ("funny bone" pain felt if tapped here)
33 Flexor carpi ulnaris muscle

Eycleshymer and Jones

UL-21 Brachial plexus III

(opposite page)

Color and label

1 Upper trunk
2 Middle trunk
3 Lower trunk
4 Lateral cord. It continues mainly as the musculocutaneous nerve. Carries fibers from spinal nerves C5, C6, C7.
5 Posterior cord; the posterior cord receives nerve fibers from spinal nerves C5-T1 by way of all 3 posterior divisions; two large nerves arise from the posterior cord: the radial nerve and the axillary nerve.
6 Medial cord; its nerve fibers continue mainly as the ulnar nerve. Carries fibers from C8 and T1. The 3 cords are named by their relation to the axillary artery, lateral, posterior, and medial (see 14 and 15).
7 Musculocutaneous nerve. It is the main continuation of the lateral cord with fibers from spinal nerves C5, C6, C7. It penetrates the coracobrachialis muscle, which it supplies along with the biceps brachii and the brachialis.
8 Median nerve. Contains fibers from spinal nerves C5,C6,C7,C8, T1. It is formed by two roots, a lateral root from the lateral cord and a medial root from the medial cord. Note how these two roots plus the musculocutaneous nerve and the ulnar nerve form an “M”. This “M” formation may occur further distally.
9 Ulnar nerve (C8,T1)
10 Radial nerve (C5,C6,C7,C8,T1)
11 Axillary nerve (C5,C6)
12 Brachial artery
13 Subclavian artery. This continues as the axillary artery at the lateral border of the first rib.
14 Dashed outline of the axillary artery (rendered transparent to show the posterior cord). Note that the posterior cord is directly posterior to the axillary artery. The axillary artery becomes the brachial artery at the lower border of the teres major.
15 Dashed outline of the brachial artery.
16 Dorsal scapular nerve to rhomboid major and minor
17 Nerve to subclavius
18 Long thoracic nerve to serratus anterior
19 Suprascapular nerve to supraspinatus and infraspinatus
20 Medial pectoral nerve
21 Lateral pectoral nerve
22 Subscapular nerve to subscapularis and teres major
23 Medial cutaneous nerve of forearm (medial antebrachial cutaneous nerve)
24 Medial cutaneous nerve of (upper) arm (medial brachial cutaneous nerve)
25 Humerus
26 Short head of biceps brachii
27 Coracobrachialis
28 Pectoralis minor (cut)
29 Clavicle (rendered partly transparent)
30 Latissimus dorsi
31 Right common carotid artery
32 Scalenus anterior. This muscle divides the subclavian artery into 3 parts: first part medial to the muscle; second part behind the muscle; third part lateral to the muscle

UL-21 Brachial plexus III

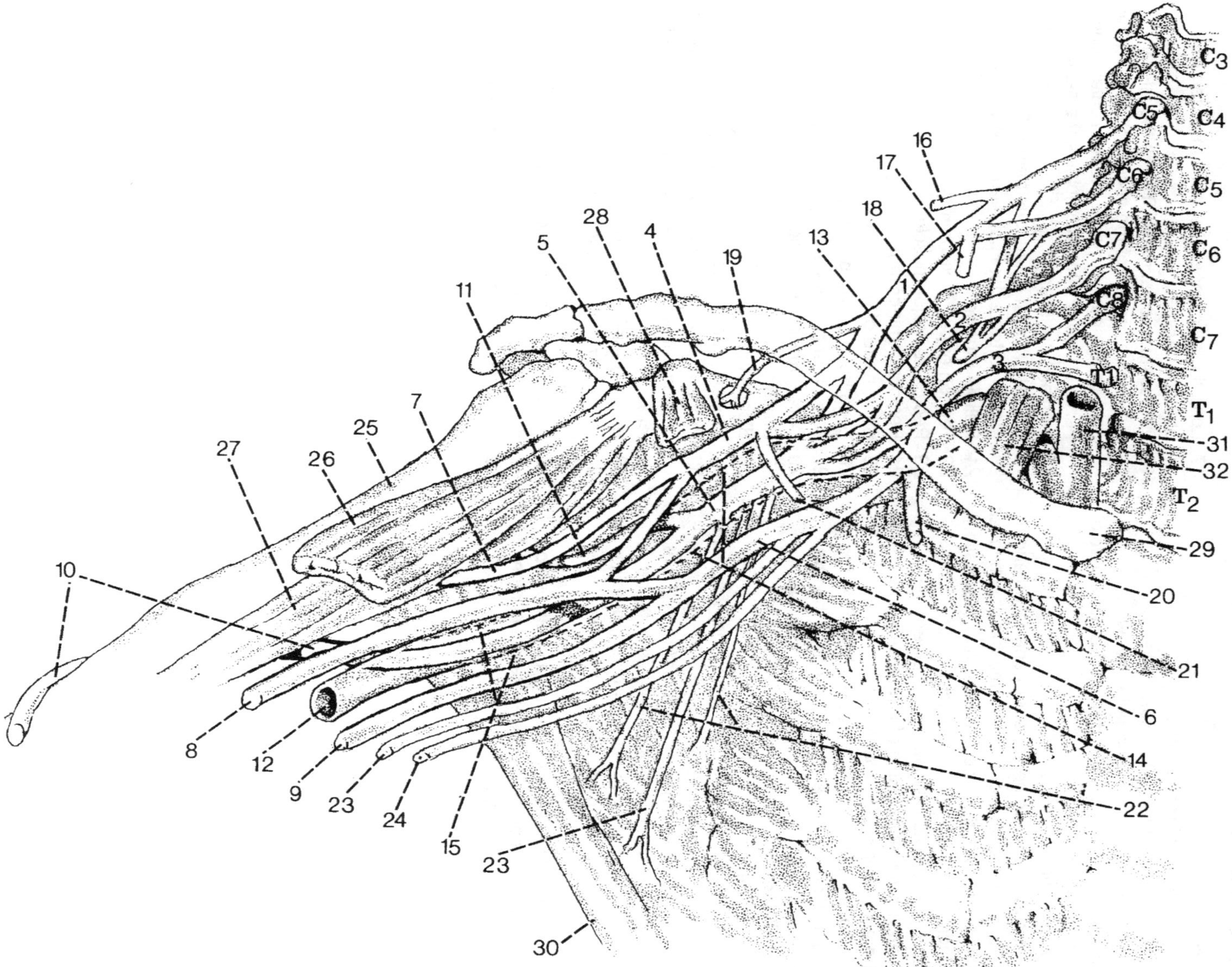

Redrawn from Gray's Anatomy, 38th ed. P.L. Williams. Edinburgh, Churchill Livingstone, 1995

UL-22 Nerves of the upper right limb

Anterior aspect (opposite page)

Color and label

1 Axillary artery
2 Lateral cord of brachial plexus
3 Medial cord of brachial plexus
4 Median nerve; note its formation by two roots, one from the lateral cord and one from the medial cord.
5 Ulnar nerve
6 Musculocutaneous nerve; after penetrating and supplying the coracobrachialis muscle, it continues on to innervate the biceps brachii and brachialis.
7 Radial nerve (superficial branch)
8 Lateral antebrachial cutaneous nerve (lateral cutaneous nerve of forearm)
9 Anterior interosseous nerve
10 Brachial artery; the axillary artery becomes the brachial artery at the inferior border of the teres major.
11 Ulnar artery
12 Radial artery
13 Median nerve entering palm after emerging from under the flexor retinaculum
14 Branch of median nerve to thenar (thumb) muscles
15 Lateral pectoral nerve; it innervates both the pectoralis major and pectoralis minor; note its connection to the medial pectoral nerve.
16 Medial pectoral nerve; after entering and innervating the pectoralis minor, it continues on to supply the costal and lower sternal portions of the pectoralis major.
17 Long thoracic nerve; it supplies the serratus anterior muscle.
18 Intercostobrachial nerve. This is the lateral cutaneous branch of the second thoracic nerve; note its joining the medial brachial cutaneous nerve (19) with which it supplies the skin of the medial (upper) arm.
19 Medial brachial cutaneous nerve
20 Medial antebrachial cutaneous nerve
21 Deltoid muscle
22 Tendon of pectoralis minor (cut)
23 Pectoralis major muscle
24 Pectoralis minor muscle
25 Short head of biceps brachii
26 Long head of biceps brachii
27 Tendon of pectoralis major muscle (cut)
28 Coracobrachialis muscle
29 Brachialis muscle
30 Biceps brachii muscle
31 Pronator teres (superficial head)(cut)
32 Pronator teres (deep head); note the median nerve passes between the two heads of the pronator teres.
33 Brachioradialis muscle
34 Flexor carpi ulnaris muscle
35 Flexor pollicis longus tendon
36 Tendon of palmaris longus (cut)
37 Flexor retinaculum
38 Digitations of the serratus anterior muscle

UL-22 Nerves of the upper right limb

Anterior aspect

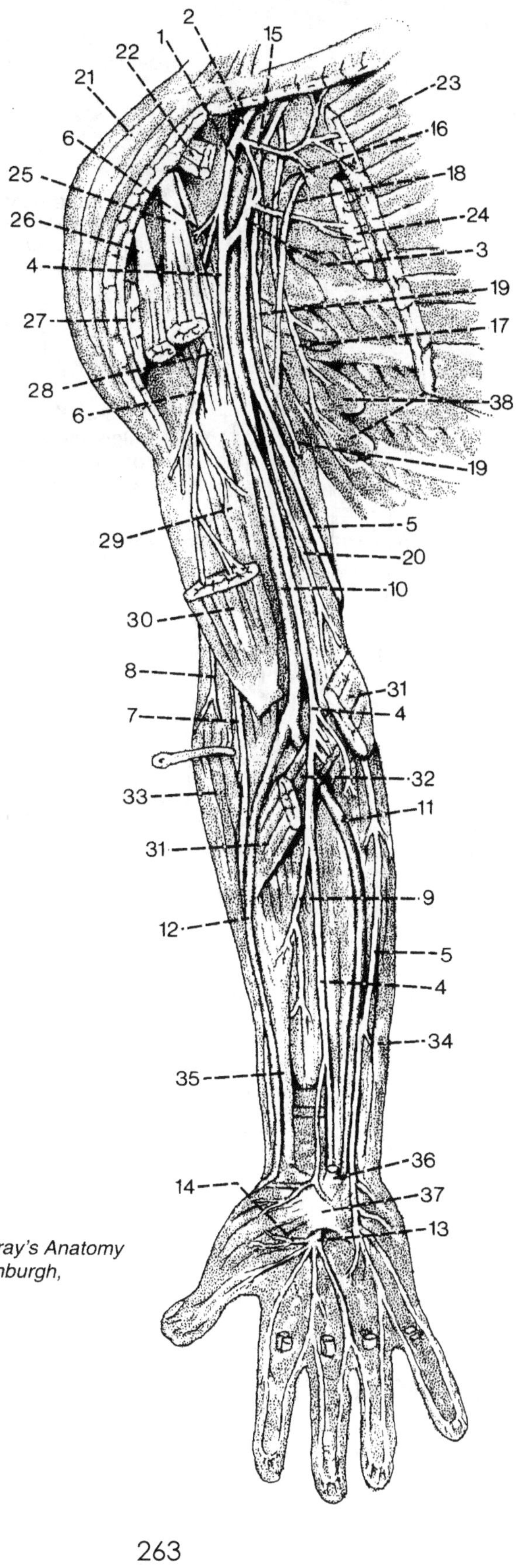

Redrawn and modified from Gray's Anatomy 38th ed. P.L. Williams ed., Edinburgh, Churchill Livingstone, 1995

UL-23 Biceps brachii: A flexor and supinator

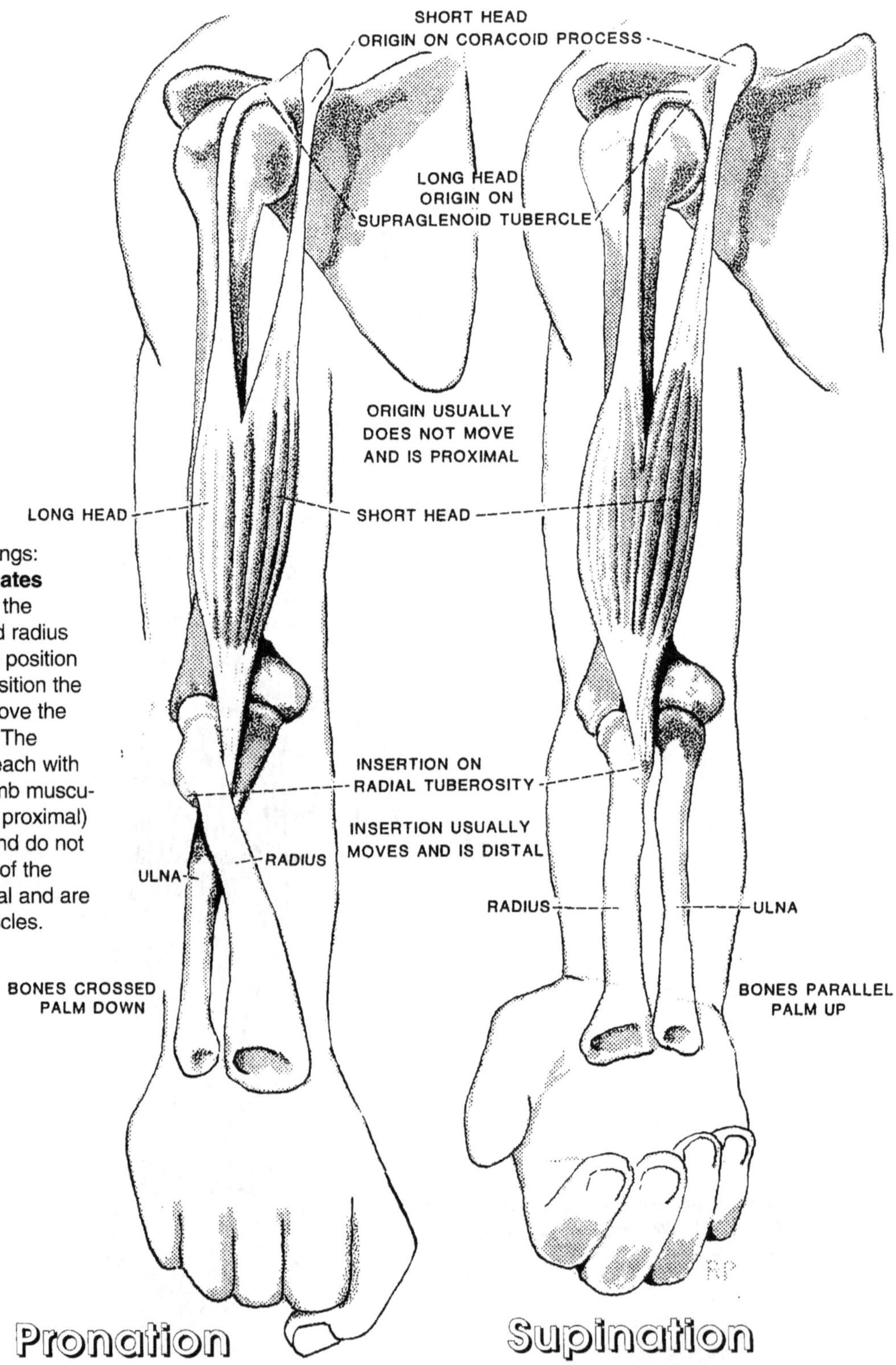

The biceps brachii does two things: it **flexes** the elbow and it **supinates** the forearm so that the palm of the hand faces up and the ulna and radius are **parallel**. This is the **supine** position of the forearm. In the **prone** position the radius is **crossed** in front or above the ulna and the palm faces down. The biceps brachii has two heads, each with its own origin. **Origins** of the limb musculature are usually nearer (more proximal) to the trunk, are more stable, and do not move, whereas the **insertions** of the limb musculature are more distal and are the action ends of the limb muscles.

UL-24 Dissection of upper arm

Anterior aspect

Color and label

1 Median nerve
2 Axillary artery (it becomes brachial artery (7) at lower border of teres major)
3 Pectoralis major muscle (arm is abducted approximately 45% from the thorax)
4 Subscapularis muscle
5 Teres major muscle
6 Subscapular nerve (above) and subscapular artery (below)
7 Brachial artery
8 Ulnar nerve
9 Superior ulnar collateral artery
10 Medial intermuscular septum. This membranous partition separates the anterior flexor muscles from the posterior extensor triceps brachii, as does the lateral intermuscular septum (not shown). The ulnar nerve penetrates the medial intermuscular septum, which has been partially removed.
11 Inferior ulnar collateral artery
12 Bicepital aponeurosis
13 Medial epicondyle of humerus
14 Pronator teres (humeral or superficial head)
15 Ulnar artery. After passing under the bicepital aponeurosis, the brachial artery divides into the radial and ulnar arteries.
16 Flexor carpi ulnaris (humeral head)
17 Median nerve in forearm. Entering the forearm the median nerve passes under the bicepital aponeurosis and between the two heads of the pronator teres.
18 Cephalic vein
19 Deltoid muscle
20 Brachialis muscle
21 Biceps brachii muscle
22 Lower portion of brachialis muscle.This strong flexor of the forearm inserts on the ulnar tuberosity.
23 Tendon of biceps inserting on the radial tuberosity
24 Brachial artery emerging from under bicepital aponeurosis
25 Recurrent radial artery
26 Brachioradialis muscle
27 Superficial radial nerve
28 Radial artery

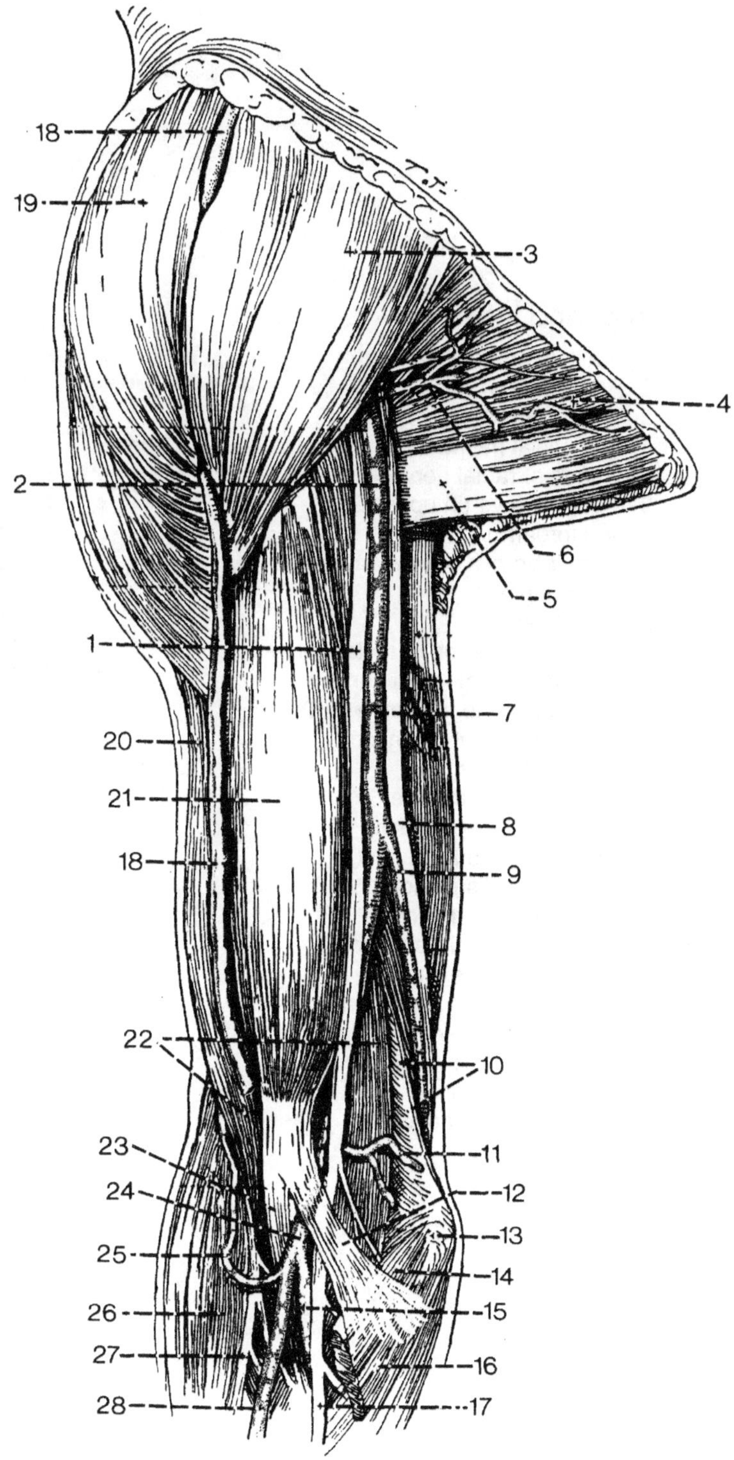

Eycleshymer and Jones with modification

UL-25 Anterior forearm dissection

Color and label

1 Brachial artery
2 Radial artery
3 Ulnar artery
4 Superficial palmar branch of radial nerve
5 Median nerve (in upper arm and forearm)
6 Palmar branch of median nerve
7 Ulnar nerve
8 Radial nerve
9 Superficial branch of radial nerve
10 Deep branch of radial nerve
11 Musculocutaneous nerve (cut); becomes lateral cutaneous nerve of forearm
12 Biceps brachii muscle
13 Tendon of biceps brachii
14 Bicipital aponeurosis (cut)
15 Brachioradialis muscle
16 Pronator teres muscle
17 Flexor carpi radialis muscle
18 Palmaris longus muscle
19 Flexor digitorum superficialis
20 Flexor carpi ulnaris muscle
21 Abductor pollicis longus muscle
22 Supinator muscle
23 Extensor carpi radialis longus muscle

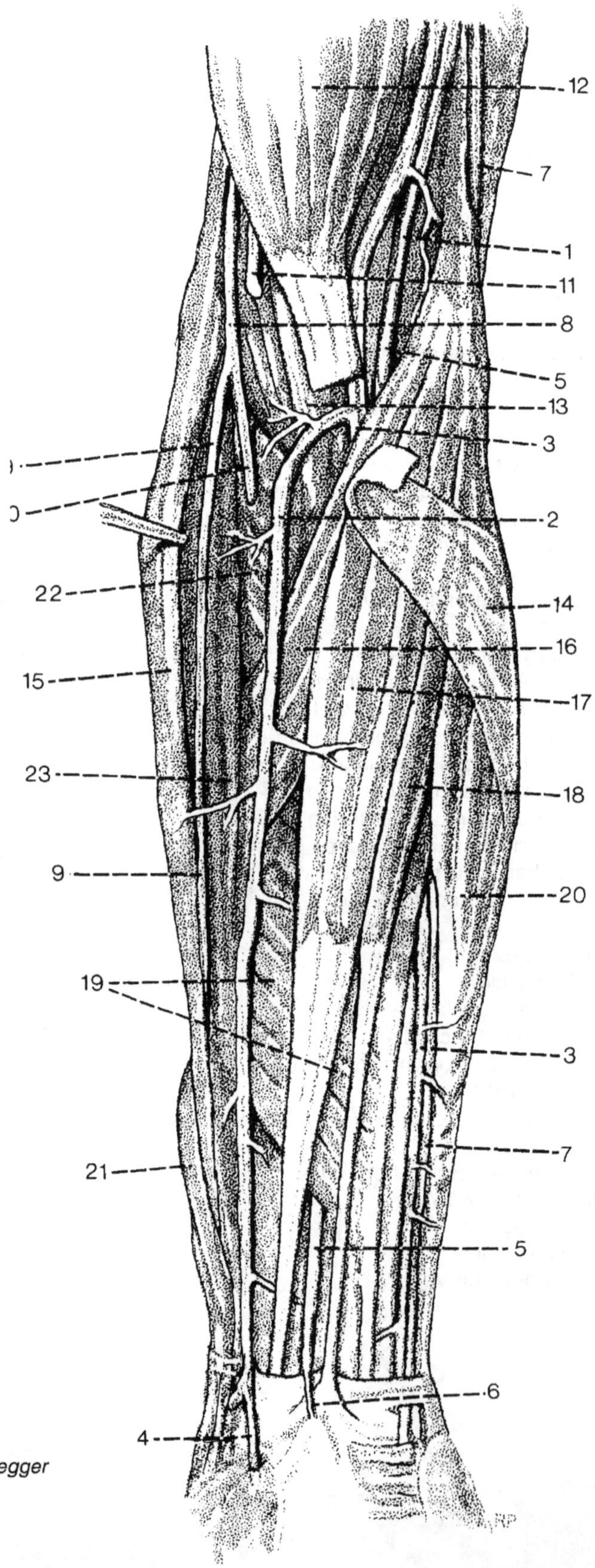

Redrawn from Wolf-Heidegger

UL-26 Arteries and nerves of the anterior forearm

Color and label

1 Brachial artery
2 Ulnar artery
3 Radial artery
4 Ulnar recurrent artery
5 Common interosseous artery
6 Anterior interosseous artery
7 Posterior interosseous artery
8 Recurrent radial artery
9 Radial collateral artery
10 Inferior ulnar collateral artery
11 Superior ulnar collateral artery
12 Superficial palmar branch of ulnar artery
13 Deep palmar branch of ulnar artery
14 Superficial palmar branch of radial artery
15 Radial nerve
16 Median nerve
17 Anterior interosseous nerve; supplies deep flexor muscles of the forearm
18 Palmar branch of median nerve
19 Ulnar nerve
20 Superficial branch of median nerve
21 Deep branch of ulnar nerve
22 Lateral antebrachial cutaneous nerve (continuation of musculocutaneous nerve) (cut)
23 Deep branch of radial nerve
24 Superficial branch of radial nerve
25 Biceps brachii muscle
26 Tendon of biceps brachii
27 Bicipital aponeurosis (cut)
28 Common head of forearm flexors (cut)
29 Brachioradialis muscle (cut)
30 Flexor carpi ulnaris (cut)
31 Abductor pollicis longus muscle
32 Flexor pollicis longus muscle
33 Pronator quadratus muscle
34 Flexor digitorum profundus muscle; note that its four tendons remain flat as they pass into the hand
35 Four tendons of flexor digitorum superficialis (cut); note that tendons 3 and 4 to the middle and ring finger are anterior to tendons 2 and 5, which go to the index and little finger. Remember, when demonstrating with your own fingers and palm facing up: "34 is higher than 25".

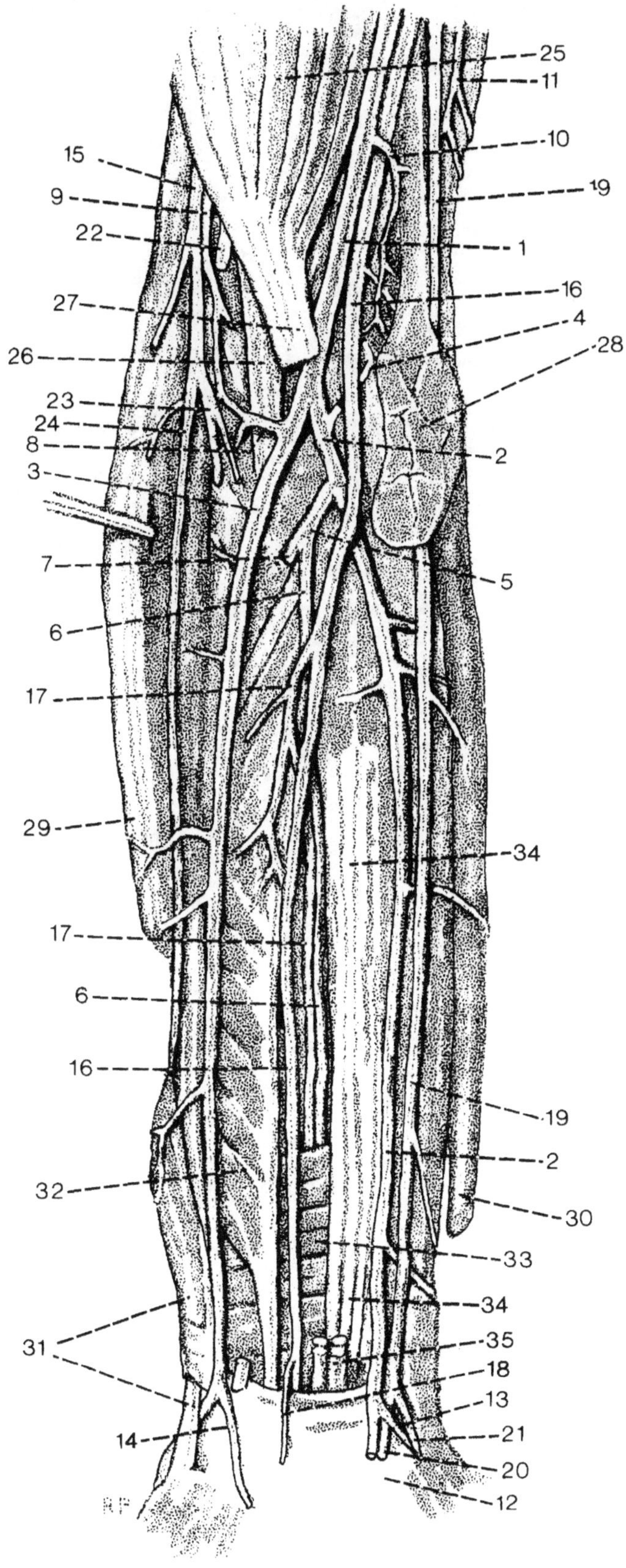

Redrawn from Wolf-Heidegger

UL-27 Brachial plexus and major nerves of the arm

(highly schematic)

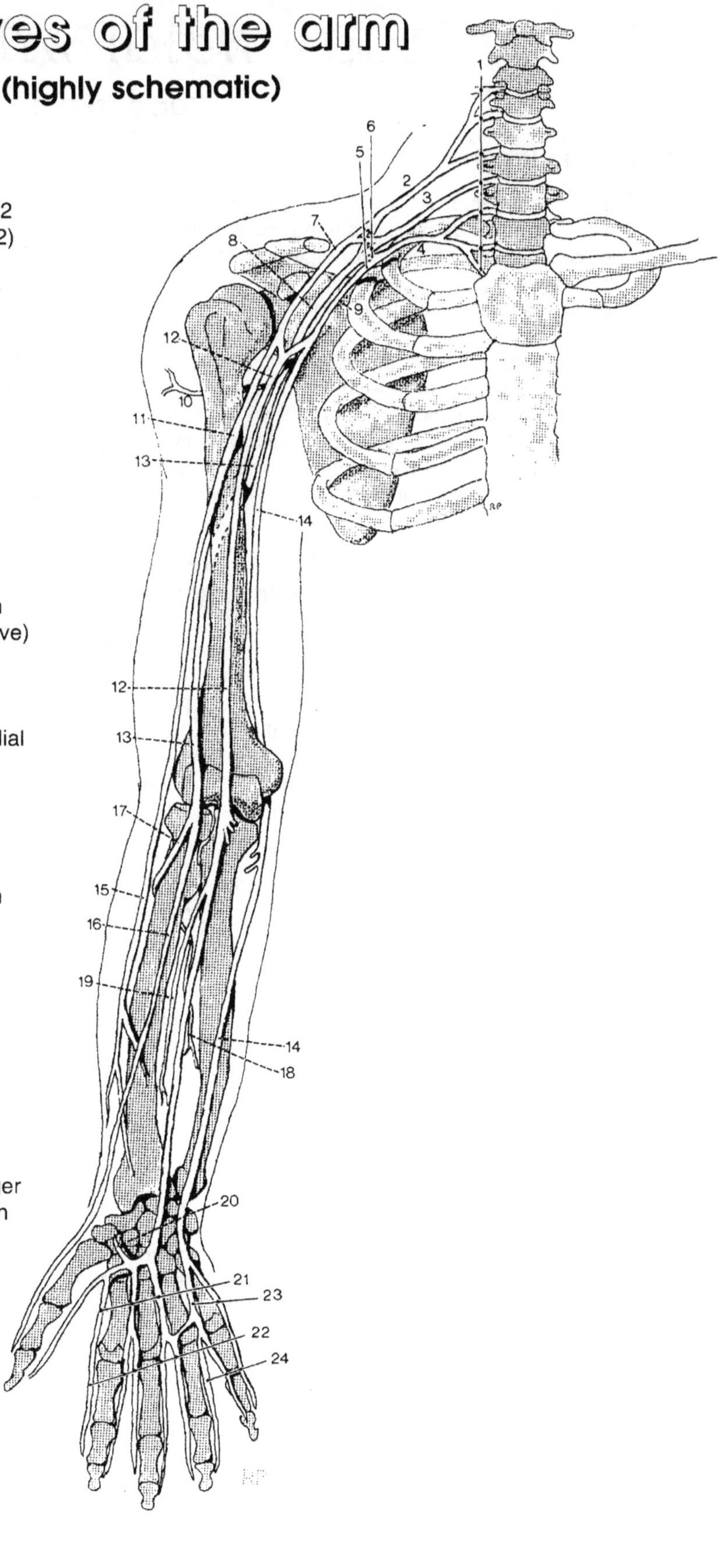

Color and label

1 Anterior rami of spinal nerves C4-T2 (small contributions from C4 and T2)
2 Superior trunk of brachial plexus
3 Middle trunk of brachial plexus
4 Inferior trunk of brachial plexus
5 Anterior divisions of three trunks
6 Posterior divisions of three trunks
7 Lateral cord
8 Posterior cord
9 Medial cord
10 Axillary nerve
11 Musculocutaneous nerve
12 Median nerve
13 Radial nerve
14 Ulnar nerve
15 Lateral cutaneous nerve of forearm (lateral antebrachial cutaneous nerve)
16 Superficial branch of radial nerve
17 Deep branch of radial nerve
18 Posterior interosseous nerve (continuation of deep branch of radial nerve; passes in back of interosseous membrane)
19 Anterior interosseous nerve of median nerve (passes in front of interosseous membrane)
20 Thenar muscular branch of median nerve
21 Common palmar digital nerves (branches of median nerve)
22 Proper palmar digital nerves (of median nerve)
23 Common palmar digital nerves (branches of ulnar nerve)
24 Proper palmar digital nerves (of ulnar nerve)

Usually the skin of the fourth (ring) finger (or digit) is supplied by both the median nerve (laterally) and the ulnar nerve (medially).

UL-28 Pronator teres and superficial wrist flexors

(opposite page)

Color and label

1 Median nerve; supplies all the forearm wrist flexors except the flexor carpi ulnaris (ulnar nerve) and the two medial heads of the flexor digitorum profundus (ulnar nerve).
2 Pronator teres muscle(humeral or superficial head)
3 Pronator teres muscle (ulnar or deep head); both heads supplied by median nerve.
4 Flexor carpi radialis muscle (median nerve)
5 Palmaris longus muscle (median nerve)
6 Palmar aponeurosis; a strong triangular portion of deep fascia in the palm of the hand. It receives the tendon of the palmaris longus.
7 Flexor carpi ulnaris muscle (ulnar nerve)
8 Pisiform (pea-shaped) bone. One of the carpal bones. The flexor carpi ulnaris inserts on it.
9 Flexor retinaculum. It forms the roof of the carpal tunnel through which run the flexor tendons of the fingers and the median nerve,
10 Brachioradialis (radial nerve)
11 Extensor carpi radialis longus (radial nerve)

Muscles are described in terms of their
Origin, Insertion, Action, Innervation

Muscle	Origin	Insertion	Action	Innervation
Flexor carpi radialis	medial epicondyle of humerus by common flexor tendon, and the antebrachial fascia and the intermuscular fascia	base of second metacarpal plus a slip to the third metacarpal	flexes and abducts the hand	median nerve
Palmaris longus	common flexor tendon (medial humeral epicondyle) and antebrachial fascia	flexor retinaculum and palmar aponeurosis	flexes the hand and tenses the palmar aponeurosis	median nerve
Brachioradialis	upper two thirds of the supracondylar ridge of the humerus and the front of the lateral intermuscular septum	base of styloid process of radius	flexes forearm especially in the semiprone position and helps in pronation when the arm is supine and flexed	branch of radial nerve with fibers from nerves C5 and C6
Flexor carpi ulnaris humeral head	common flexor tendon (medial humeral epicondyle)	pisiform bone and by the pisohamate and pisometacarpal ligaments to the hamate bone and the base of the fifth metacarpal bone.	helps flex and adduct the hand	ulnar nerve
Flexor carpi ulnaris ulnar head	medial side of the olecranon and upper two thirds of the posterior margin of the ulna			

UL-28 Pronator teres and superficial wrist flexors

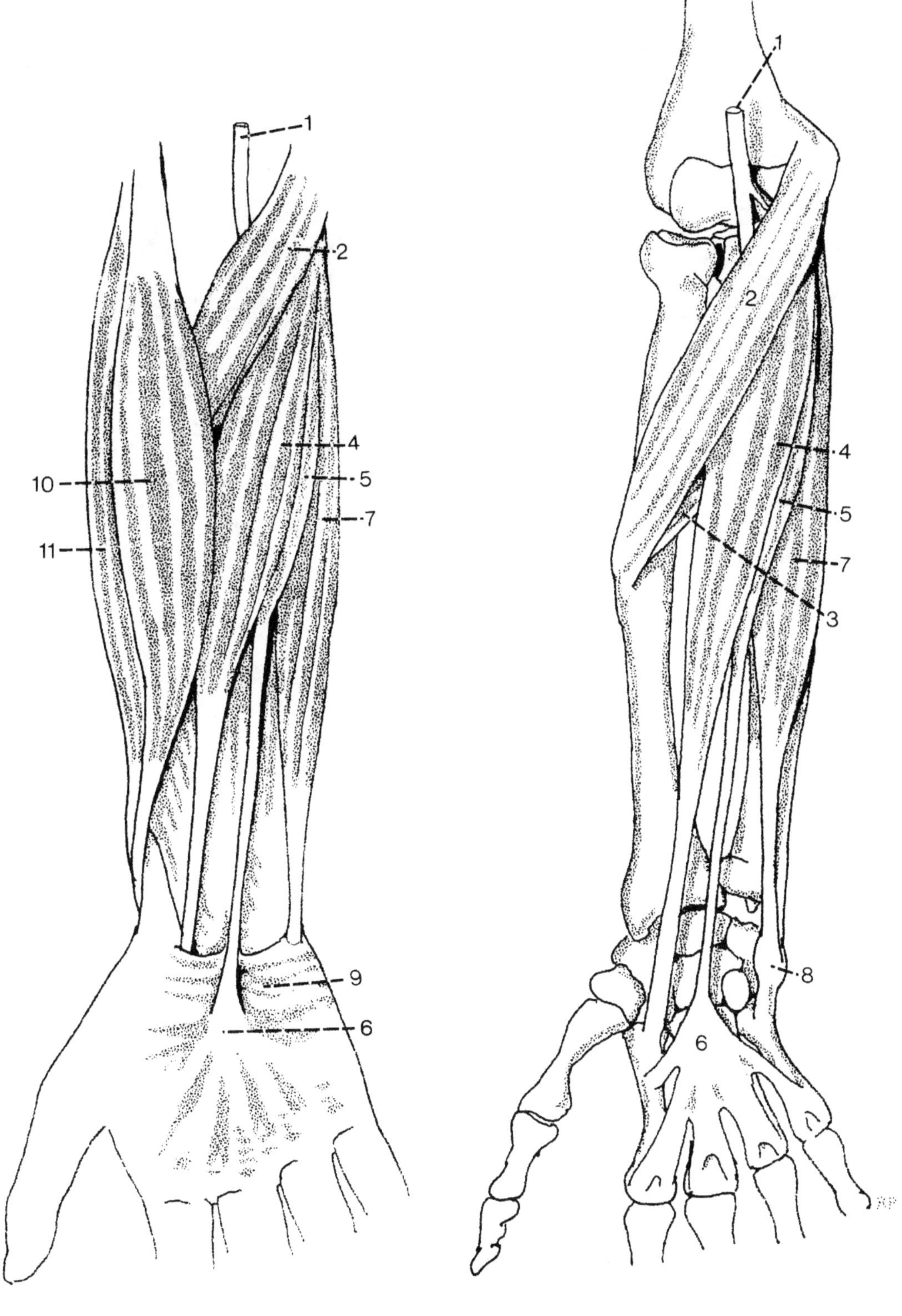

UL-29 Musculocutaneous nerve and the muscles it supplies

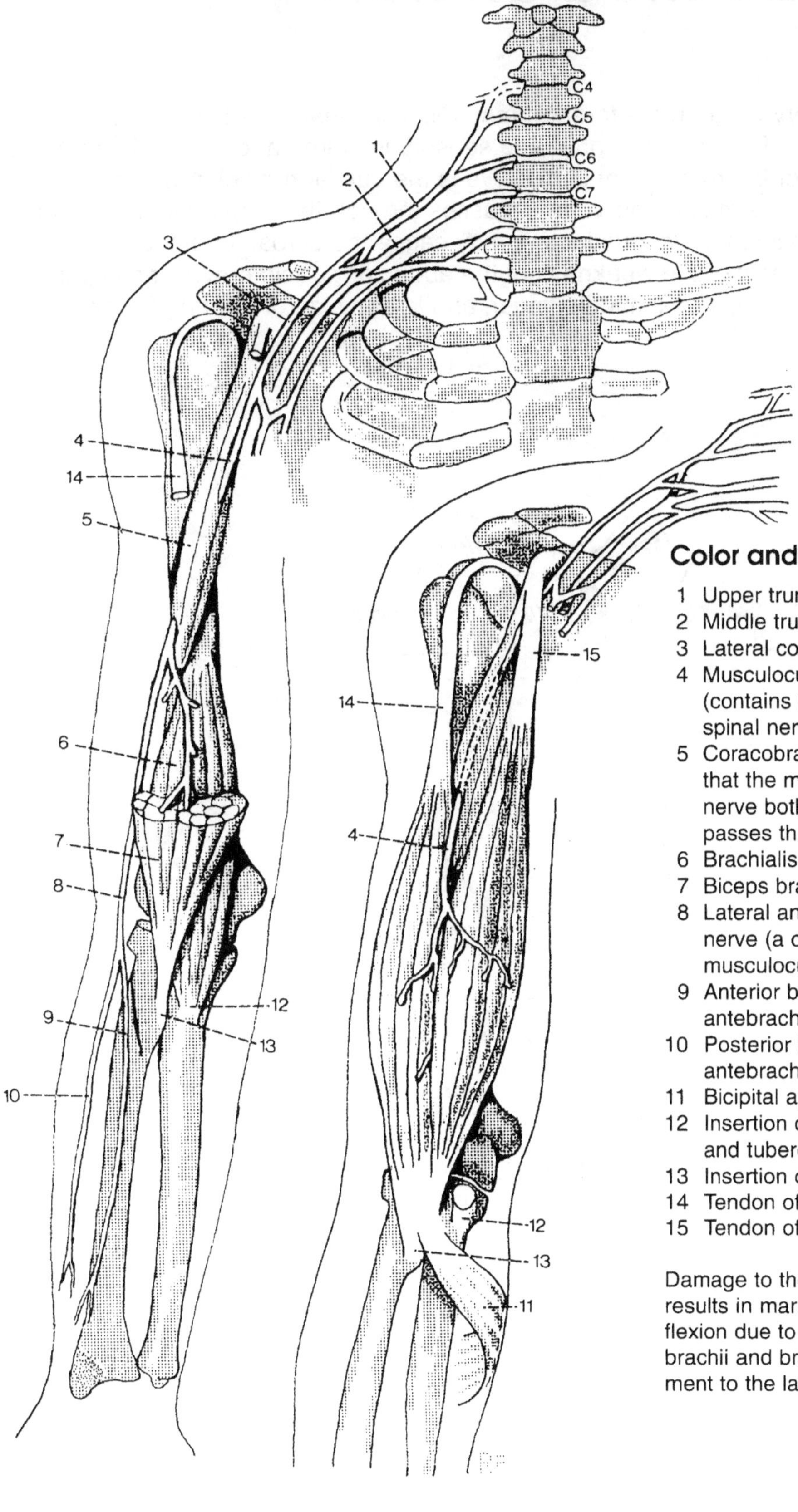

Color and label

1 Upper trunk of brachial plexus
2 Middle trunk of brachial plexus
3 Lateral cord of brachial plexus
4 Musculocutaneous nerve (contains nerve fibers from spinal nerves C5-C7)
5 Coracobrachialis muscle (notice that the musculocutaneous nerve both supplies and passes through this muscle)
6 Brachialis muscle
7 Biceps brachii
8 Lateral antebrachial cutaneous nerve (a continuation of the musculocutaneous nerve)
9 Anterior branch of lateral antebrachial cutaneous nerve
10 Posterior branch of lateral antebrachial cutaneous nerve
11 Bicipital aponeurosis
12 Insertion of brachialis on coronoid process and tuberosity of ulna
13 Insertion of biceps on radial tuberosity
14 Tendon of long head of biceps
15 Tendon of short head of biceps

Damage to the musculocutaneous nerve results in marked weakness of elbow flexion due to paralysis of the biceps brachii and brachialis and a sensory impairment to the lateral aspect of the forearm.

UL-30 Muscular distribution of the median nerve

Damage to the median nerve high in the forearm may result in weakness in pronation and weakness in the long finger flexors (weak grip) and sensory impairment on the palm of the hand. The most common entrapment of median nerve is the **carpal tunnel syndrome** caused by compression of the median nerve as it passes through the carpal tunnel into the hand under the flexor retinaculum. Various factors may cause the carpal tunnel to become narrowed. This results in wasting and weakness of the abductor pollicis brevis and impairment of sensation in the thumb, index, middle finger, and lateral side of the ring finger.

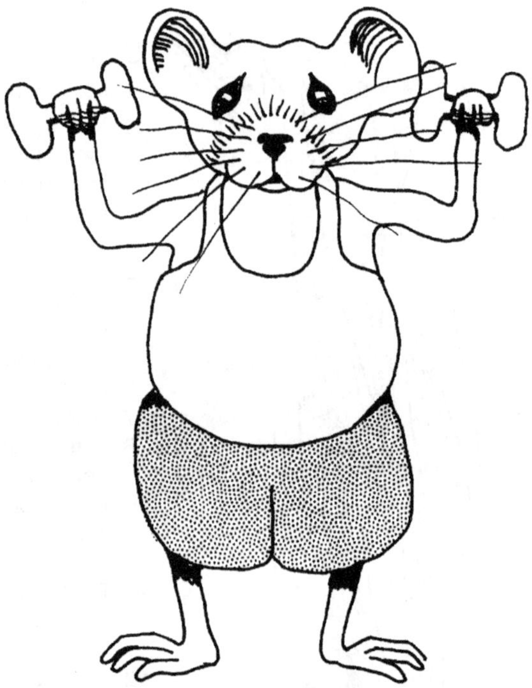

Muscle means "little mouse."

UL-30 Muscular distribution of the median nerve

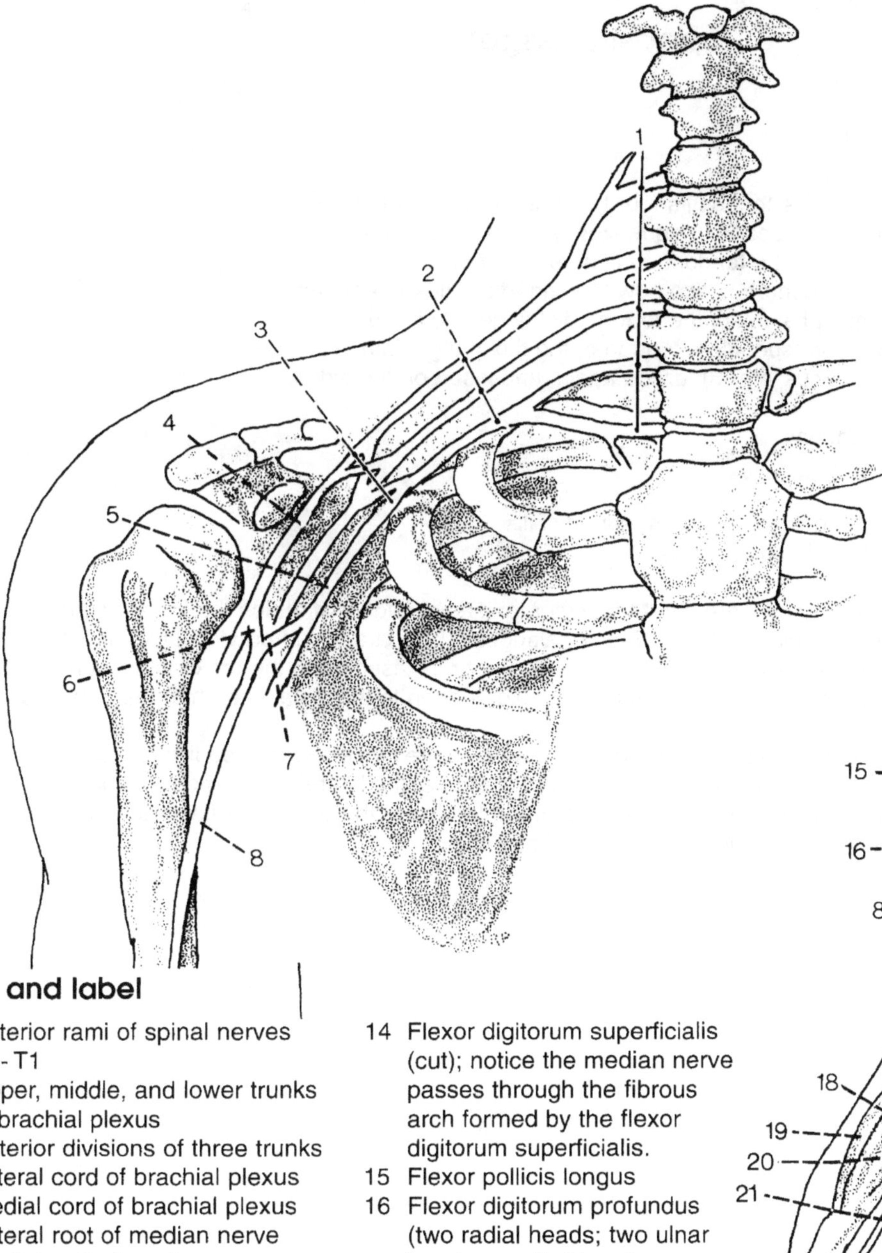

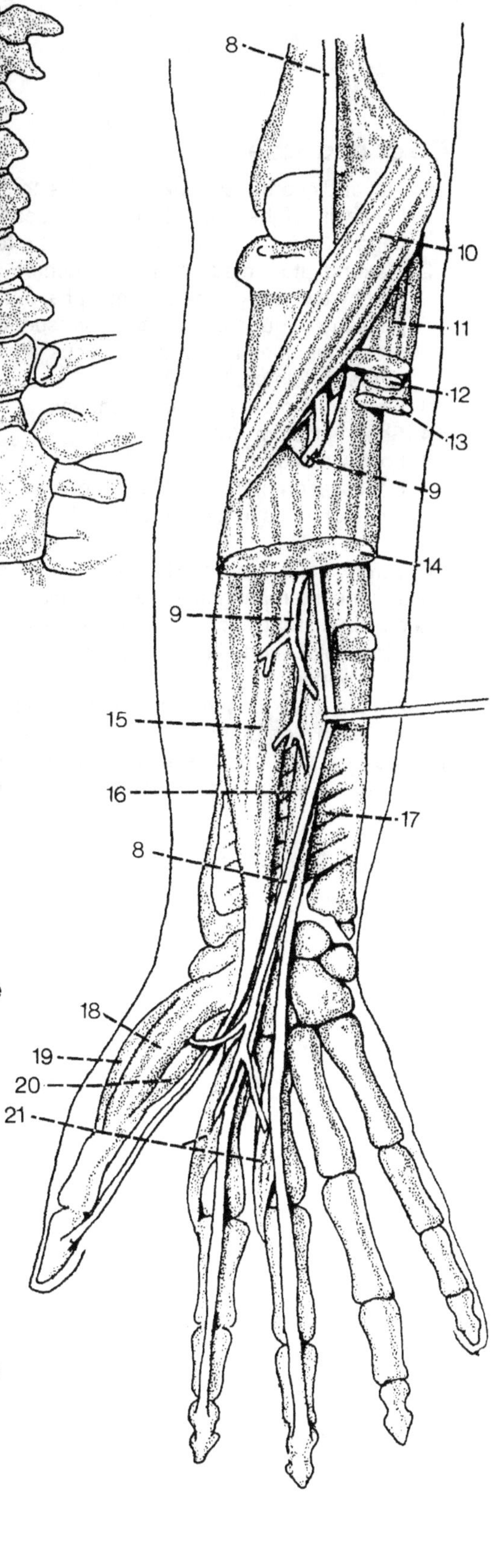

Color and label

1 Anterior rami of spinal nerves C5- T1
2 Upper, middle, and lower trunks of brachial plexus
3 Anterior divisions of three trunks
4 Lateral cord of brachial plexus
5 Medial cord of brachial plexus
6 Lateral root of median nerve
7 Medial root of median nerve
8 Median nerve
9 Anterior interosseous nerve (branch of median nerve)
10 Pronator teres
11 Flexor carpi radialis (cut)
12 Palmaris longus (cut)
13 Flexor carpi ulnaris (cut; ulnar nerve innervation)
14 Flexor digitorum superficialis (cut); notice the median nerve passes through the fibrous arch formed by the flexor digitorum superficialis.
15 Flexor pollicis longus
16 Flexor digitorum profundus (two radial heads; two ulnar heads supplied by ulnar nerve)
17 Pronator quadratus
18 Abductor pollicis brevis
19 Opponens pollicis
20 Flexor pollicis brevis
21 Lumbrical muscles (two lateral or radial muscles)

UL-31 Flexor digitorum superficialis muscle

(opposite page)

Color and label

1 Flexor digitorum superficialis; notice that as its four tendons pass through the concavity of the carpal tunnel, they become "squeezed" so that the tendons to fingers 3 and 4 become anterior to the tendons to fingers 2 and 5.
2 Flexor digitorum superficialis tendon(s); notice how the superficial flexor tendons end by dividing on the proximal phalanx of the four medial fingers to allow passage through them of the corresponding tendon of the flexor digitorum profundus; they then reunite, decussate (6), divide again, and insert on the sides of the middle phalanx (7).
3 Flexor digitorum profundus tendons
4 Short vinculum* (pl. vincula)
5 Long vinculum†
6 Decussation of the tendon of the flexor digitorum superficialis
7 Insertion of its tendon on sides of middle phalanx

**Vinculum*, Latin, a band. The short vincula are short triangular tendinous folds that attach the finger flexor tendons to the interphangeal joints and adjacent parts of the phalanges. There are two short vincula in each finger; the proximal short vinculum attaches the superficial flexor tendon near its insertion to the proximal interphangeal joint; the distal short vinculum attaches the deep (profundus) flexor tendon to the distal interphangeal joint and adjacent bones.
†There are three long vincula in each finger. The proximal long vincula are two slender threadlike bands connecting each side of the superficial flexor tendon to the synovial sheath at the lateral border near the base of the proximal phalanx. The single distal long vinculum connects the tendon of the profundus flexor to the posterior part of the synovial sheath at the distal end of the proximal phalanx.

UL-31 Flexor digitorum superficialis muscle

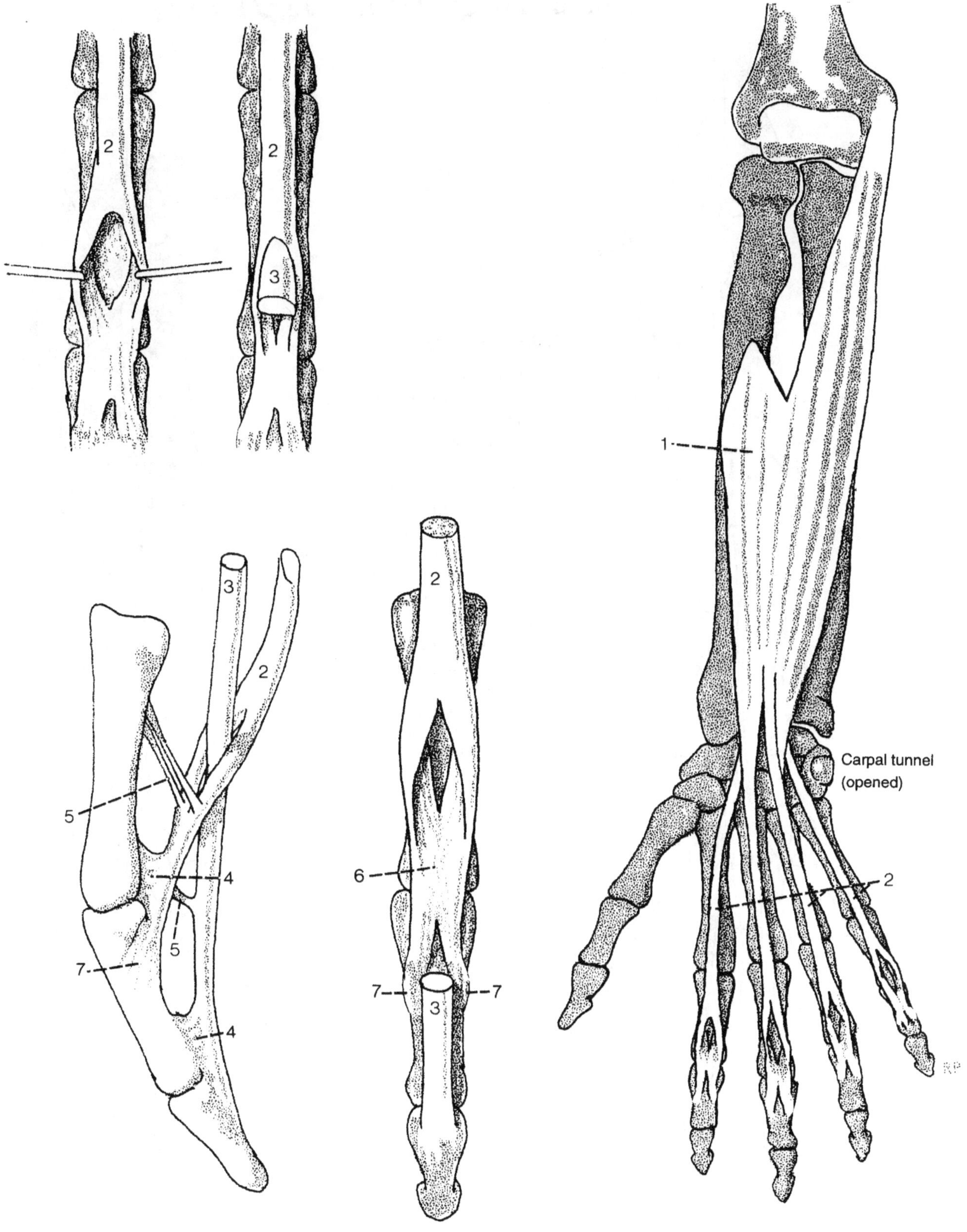

UL-32 Flexor pollicis longus, flexor digitorum profundus, and median nerve

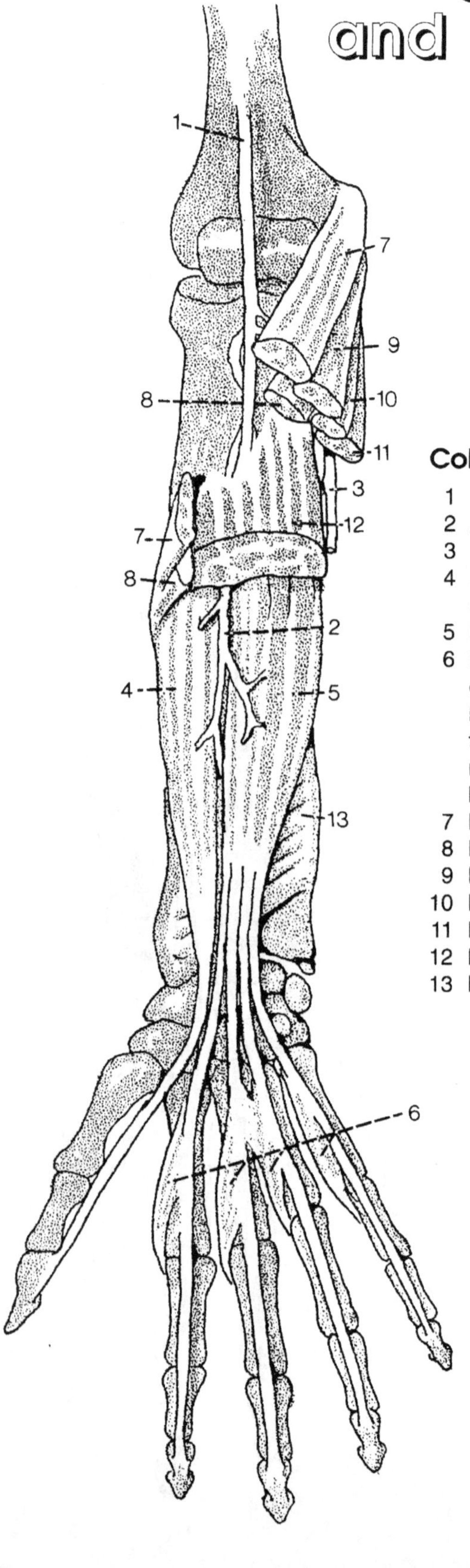

Color and label

1 Median nerve
2 Anterior interosseous nerve
3 Ulnar nerve (cut)
4 Flexor pollicis longus (long flexor of the thumb)
5 Flexor digitorum profundus
6 Lumbrical muscles of the hand. The two lateral lumbricals are innervated by the median nerve. The two medial lumbricals are supplied by the ulnar nerve.
7 Pronator teres (humeral head)
8 Pronator teres(ulnar head)
9 Flexor carpi radialis
10 Palmaris longus
11 Flexor carpi ulnaris
12 Flexor digitorum superficialis
13 Pronator quadratus

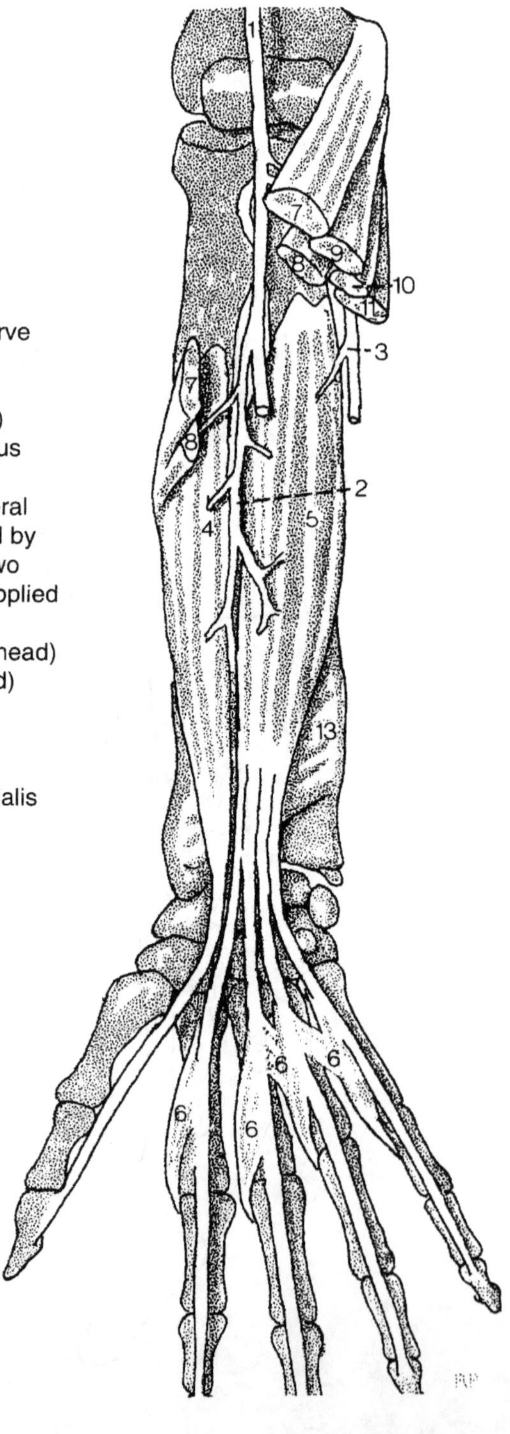

UL-33 Median nerve and deep dissection of the forearm

Color and label

1 Median nerve
2 Anterior antebrachial interosseous nerve (also anterior interosseous nerve of the forearm). It supplies the flexor pollicis longus, flexor digitorum profundus (two lateral heads), and the pronator quadratus, plus sensory receptors on the interosseous membrane and distally the radioulnar, radiocarpal, and carpal joints.
3 Ulnar nerve
4 Flexor pollicis longus muscle
5 Flexor digitorum profundus muscle
6 Lumbrical muscles of the fingers. Notice how the four lumbrical muscles arise from the four tendons of the deep finger flexor; only the two lateral (radial) lumbricals are supplied by the median nerve (figure on right). The two medial lumbricals (ulnar nerve innervation) arise from two adjacent profundus tendons rather than from a single profundus tendon.
7 Pronator teres (humeral head)
8 Pronator teres (ulnar head)
9 Flexor carpi radialis muscle
10 Palmaris longus muscle
11 Flexor carpi ulnaris muscle
12 Flexor digitorum superficialis muscle
13 Pronator quadratus muscle
14 Opponens pollicis muscle
15 Abductor pollicis brevis muscle
16 Flexor pollicis brevis muscle
17 Motor branch of median nerve to thenar muscles
18 Common digital nerves
19 Proper digital nerves

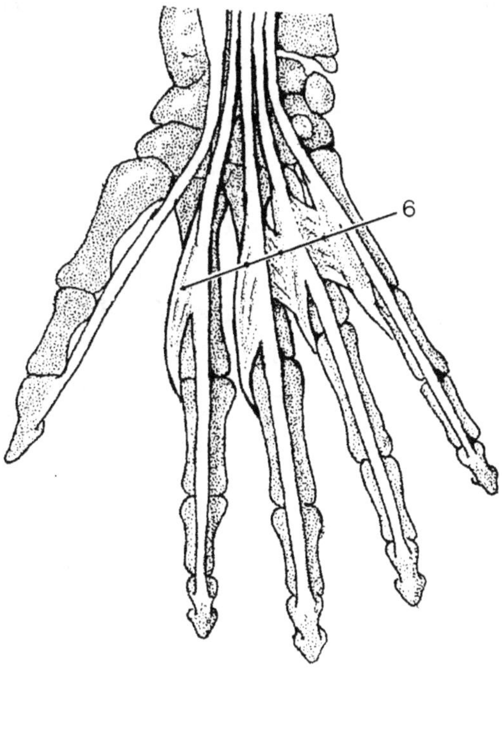

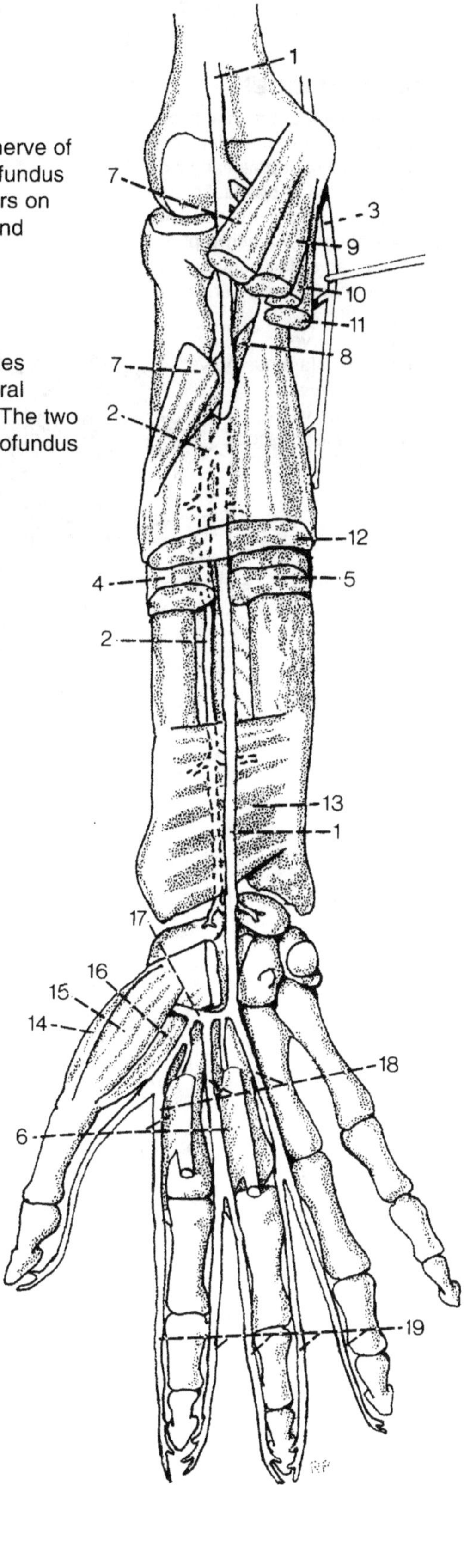

UL-34 Motor distribution of the ulnar nerve

Color and label

1 Upper trunk of brachial plexus
2 Middle trunk of brachial plexus
3 Lower trunk of brachial plexus
4 Medial cord of brachial plexus
5 Posterior cord of brachial plexus
6 Lateral cord of brachial plexus
7 Ulnar nerve (the continuation of the medial cord with fibers mainly from C8 and T1)
8 Median nerve
9 Musculocutaneous nerve
10 Radial nerve
11 Axillary nerve
12 Medial intermuscular septum

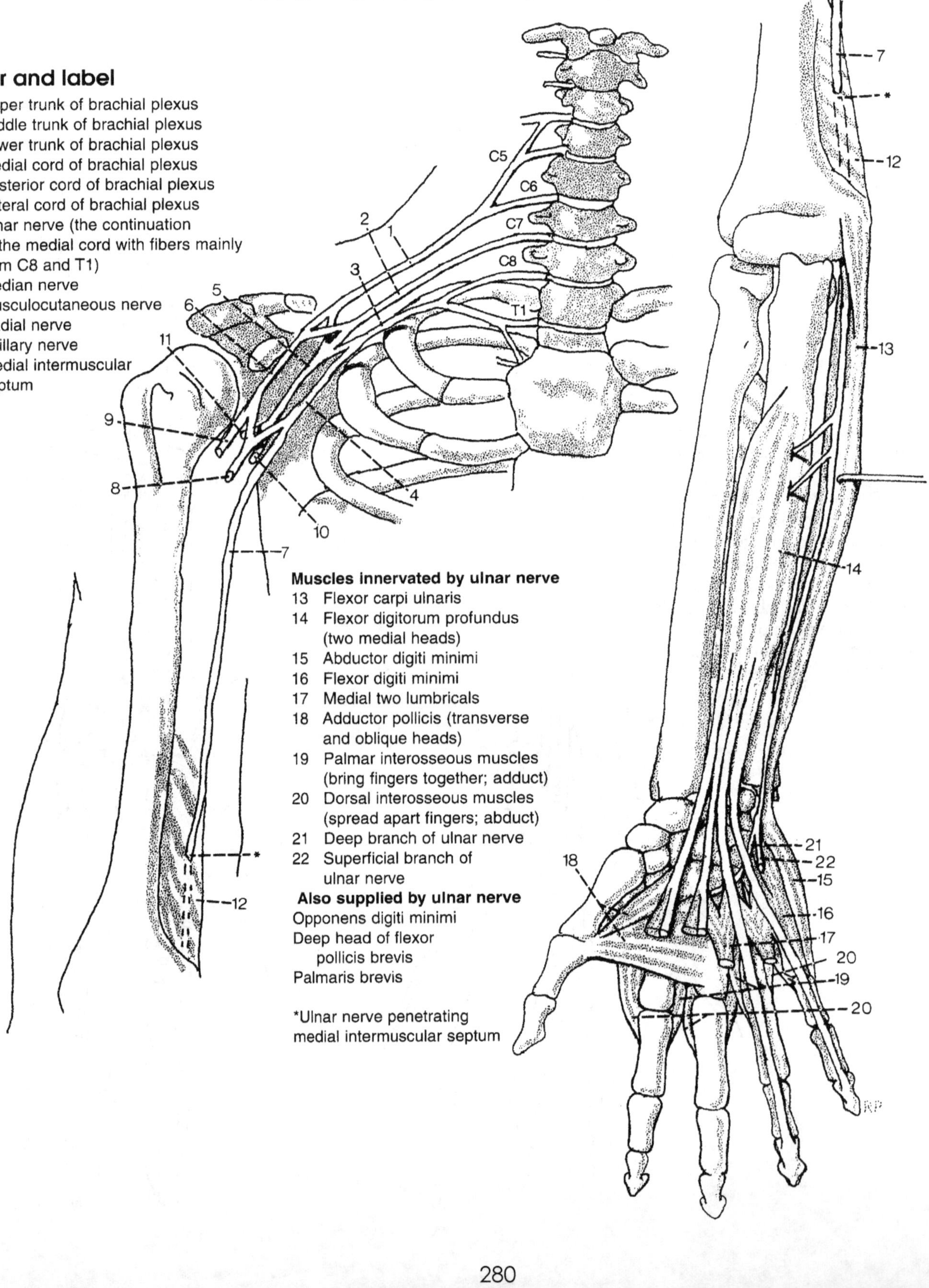

Muscles innervated by ulnar nerve

13 Flexor carpi ulnaris
14 Flexor digitorum profundus (two medial heads)
15 Abductor digiti minimi
16 Flexor digiti minimi
17 Medial two lumbricals
18 Adductor pollicis (transverse and oblique heads)
19 Palmar interosseous muscles (bring fingers together; adduct)
20 Dorsal interosseous muscles (spread apart fingers; abduct)
21 Deep branch of ulnar nerve
22 Superficial branch of ulnar nerve

Also supplied by ulnar nerve

Opponens digiti minimi
Deep head of flexor pollicis brevis
Palmaris brevis

*Ulnar nerve penetrating medial intermuscular septum

UL-35 Motor distribution of the radial nerve I

Superficial muscles

The radial nerve is the largest nerve in the arm. The radial nerve and the axillary nerve both arise from the posterior cord of the brachial plexus. Because it spirals downward directly on the humerus, the radial nerve may be injured in fractures of the humerus. The radial nerve innervates all the extensors of the elbow, wrist, and fingers. It does not, however, supply any intrinsic hand musculature.

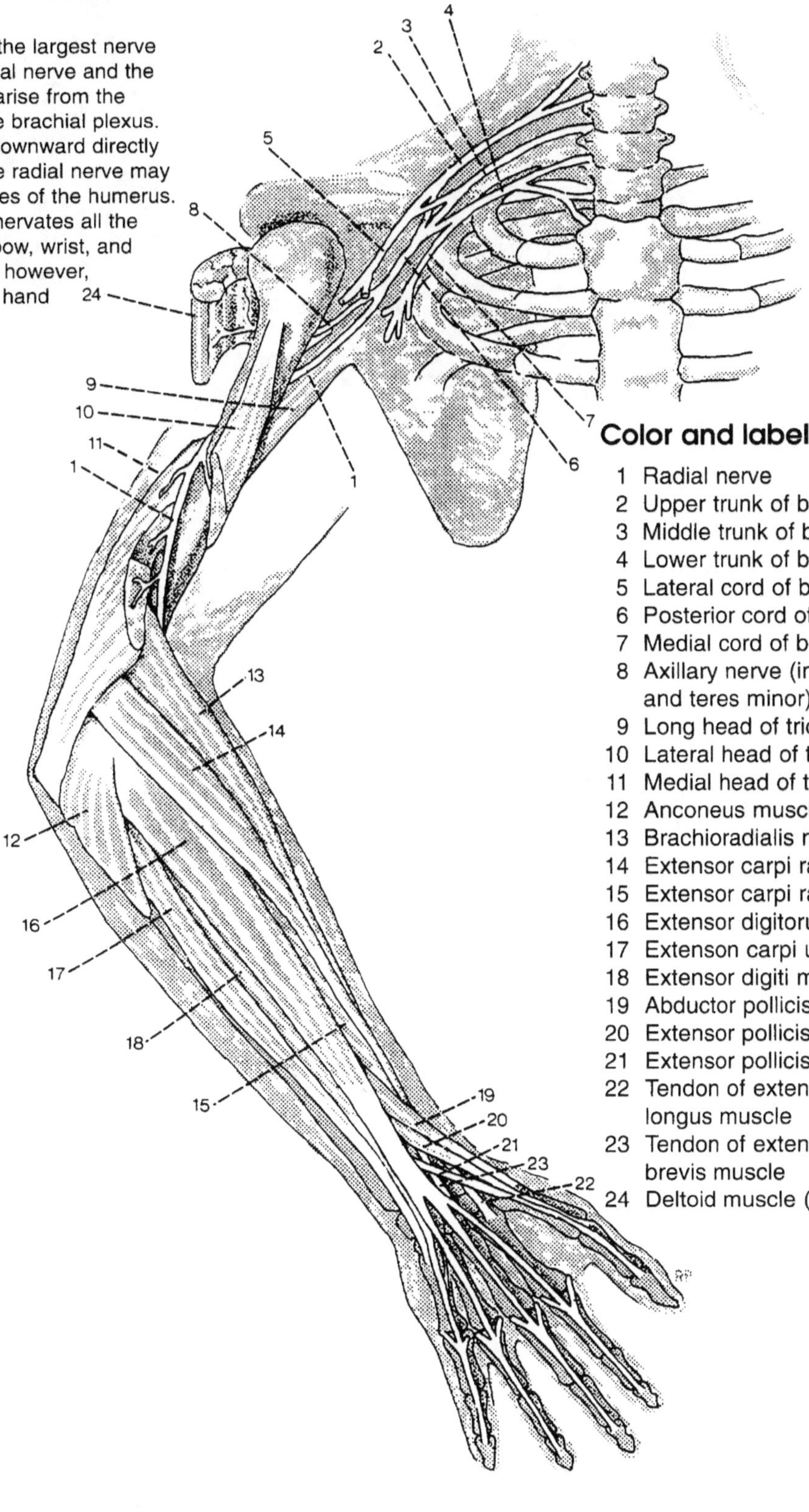

Color and label

1 Radial nerve
2 Upper trunk of brachial plexus
3 Middle trunk of brachial plexus
4 Lower trunk of brachial plexus
5 Lateral cord of brachial plexus
6 Posterior cord of brachial plexus
7 Medial cord of brachial plexus
8 Axillary nerve (innervates deltoid and teres minor)
9 Long head of triceps brachii muscle
10 Lateral head of triceps brachii (cut)
11 Medial head of triceps brachii
12 Anconeus muscle
13 Brachioradialis muscle
14 Extensor carpi radialis longus muscle
15 Extensor carpi radialis brevis muscle
16 Extensor digitorum muscle
17 Extenson carpi ulnaris muscle
18 Extensor digiti minimi
19 Abductor pollicis longus muscle
20 Extensor pollicis brevis muscle
21 Extensor pollicis longus muscle
22 Tendon of extensor carpi radialis longus muscle
23 Tendon of extensor carpi radialis brevis muscle
24 Deltoid muscle (a small portion)

UL-36 Motor distribution of radial nerve II

Deep muscles

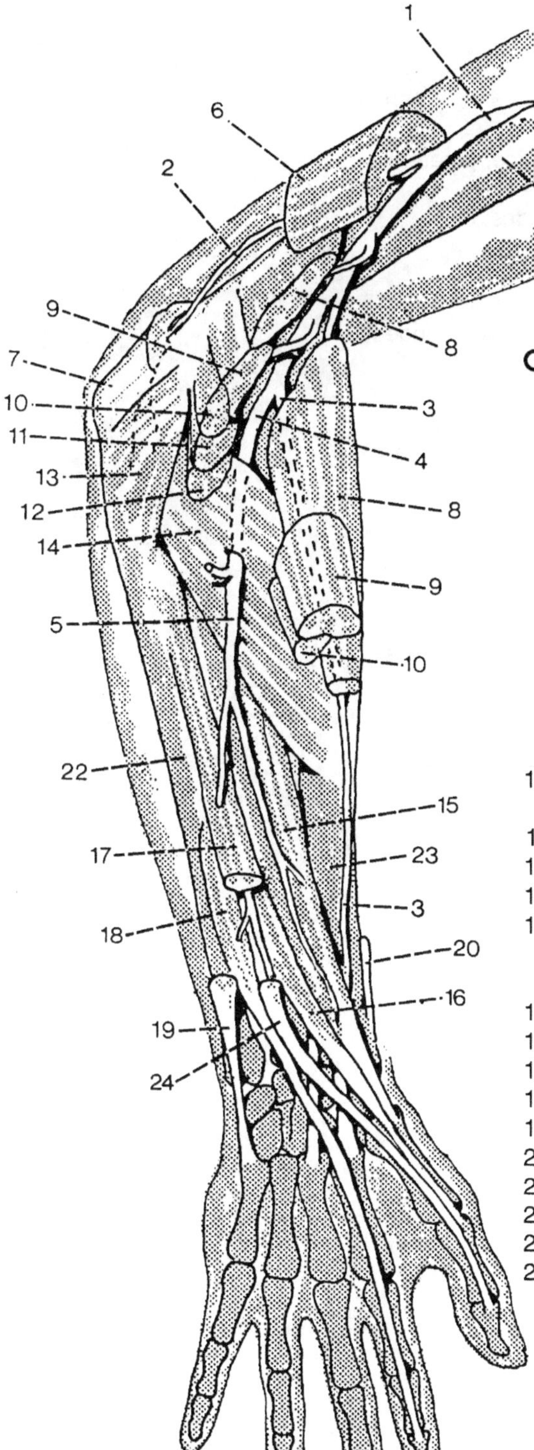

Color and label

1 Radial nerve in radial groove
2 Nerve to anconeus
3 Superficial branch of radial nerve
4 Deep branch of radial nerve
5 Posterior interosseous nerve (continuation of deep branch of radial nerve)
6 Triceps brachii (a small section)
7 Insertion of triceps on olecranon of ulna
8 Brachioradialis muscle (cut)
9 Extensor carpi radialis longus muscle (cut)
10 Extensor carpi radialis brevis muscle (cut)
11 Extensor digitorum muscle (cut)
12 Extensor carpi ulnaris muscle (cut)
13 Anconeus muscle
14 Supinator muscle (deep branch of radial nerve both supplies and penetrates it)
15 Abductor pollicis longus
16 Extensor pollicis brevis muscle
17 Extensor pollicis longus muscle (cut)
18 Extensor indicis muscle
19 Tendon of extensor carpi ulnaris
20 Tendon of brachioradialis
21 Humerus
22 Ulna
23 Radius
24 Tendon of extensor pollicis longus (cut)

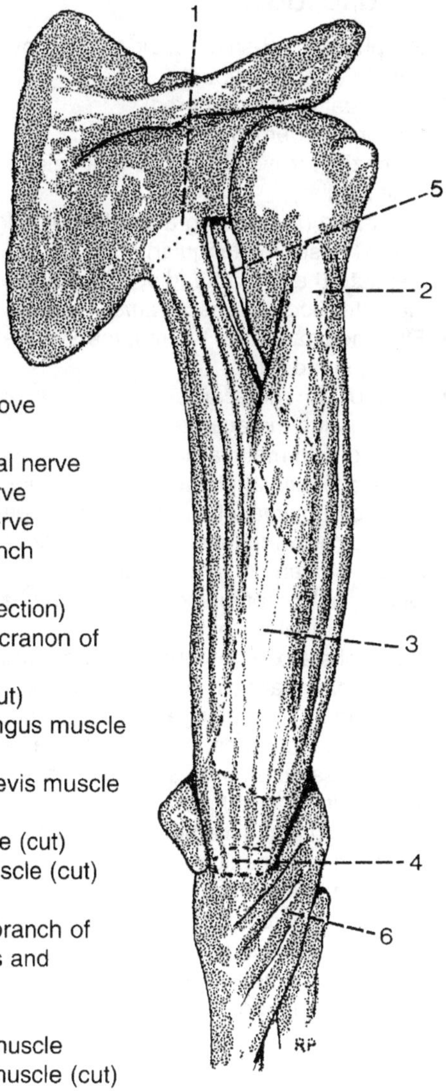

Triceps brachii

Color and label

1 Triceps brachii long head origin (on scapula)
2 Triceps lateral head origin (on back of upper humerus)
3 Triceps medial head origin (on back of lower humerus)
4 Insertion of triceps brachii on olecranon of ulna
5 Radial nerve
6 Anconeus muscle

UL-37 Bones of the hand

Palmar (ventral) aspect of right hand
(opposite page)

Color and label

1 Scaphoid (boat-shaped; old name, navicular)
2 Lunate (moon-shaped)
3 Triquetral (three-cornered)
4 Pisiform (resembling a pea)
5 Trapezium (resembling a Greek small table called a *trapezion*; old name, greater multangular)
6 Trapezoid (resembling a quadrilateral figure which has two parallel sides; old name, lesser multangular)
7 Capitate (having a head or a headlike enlargement)
8 Hamate (hook-shaped; *hamus*, Latin, a hook)
9 First metacarpal (of thumb); the five metacarpal bones are the largest and strongest bones in the hand.
10 Base of fifth metacarpal
11 Body of fifth metacarpal
12 Head of fifth metacarpal (each metacarpal bone has a base, body, and head)
13 Base of proximal phalanx of index finger
14 Body of proximal phalanx of index finger
15 Head of proximal phalanx of index finger
16 Middle phalanx of index finger
17 Distal phalanx of index finger (each phalanx has a base, body, and head)
18 Proximal phalanx of thumb
19 Distal phalanx of thumb; the thumb, which is the most mobile and useful finger, has only two phalanges, whereas each of the other four digits has three phalanges, resulting in 14 phalanges in each hand.
20 Radial sesamoid bone (resembling a sesame seed)
21 Ulnar sesamoid bone (sesamoid bones develop within tendons and remain in them)
22 Tuberosity of distal phalanx
23 Hamulus (Latin, little hook) of hamate bone
24 Tubercle of trapezium
25 Tubercle of scaphoid
26 Carpometacarpal joint; the thumb carpometacarpal joint is a saddle joint
27 Metacarpophalangeal joint (abbreviated MP joint or MCP joint)
28 Proximal interphalangeal joint (PIP joint)
29 Distal interphalangeal joint (DIP)

UL-37 Bones of the hand

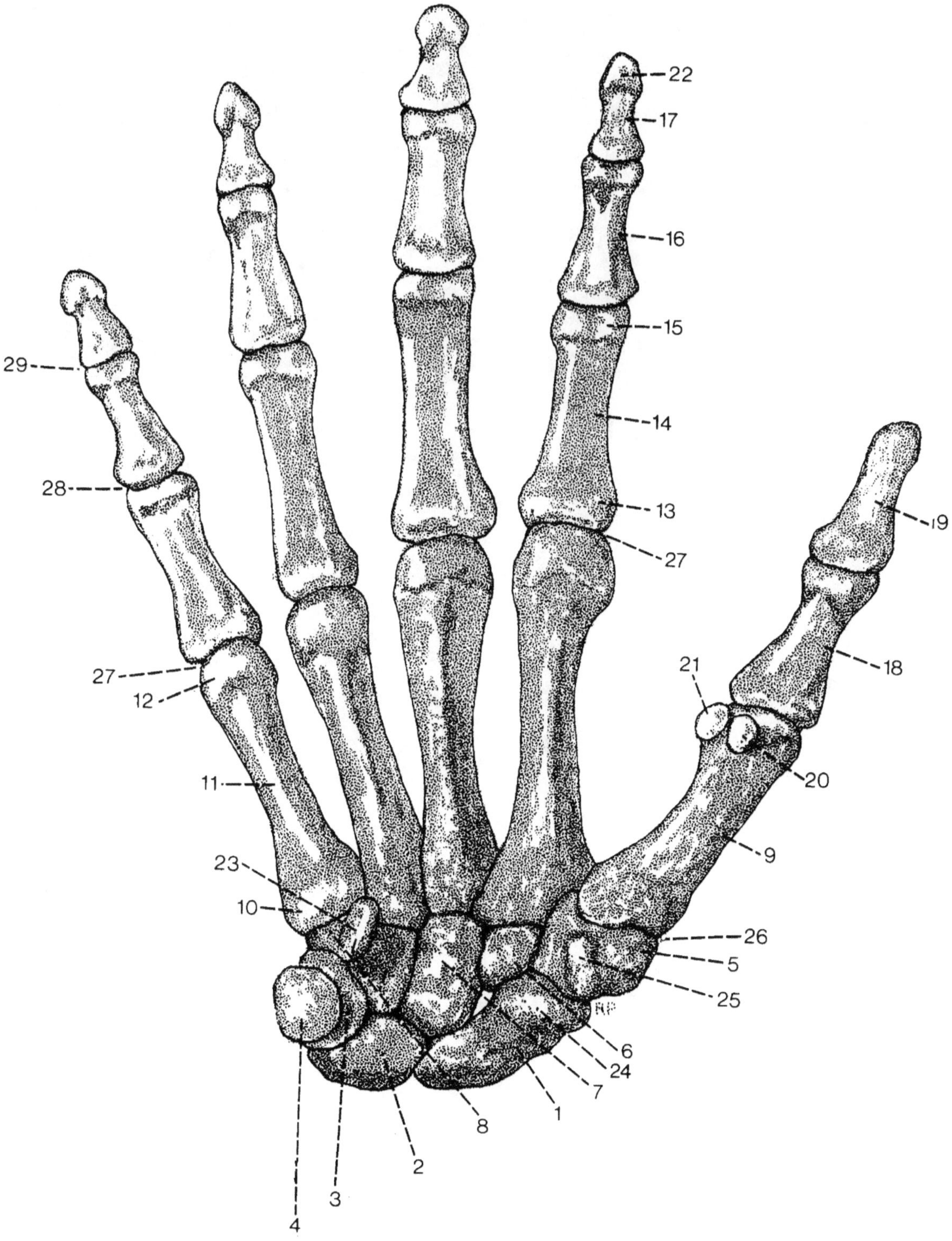

UL-38 Palmar aponeurosis and anchoring connective tissue

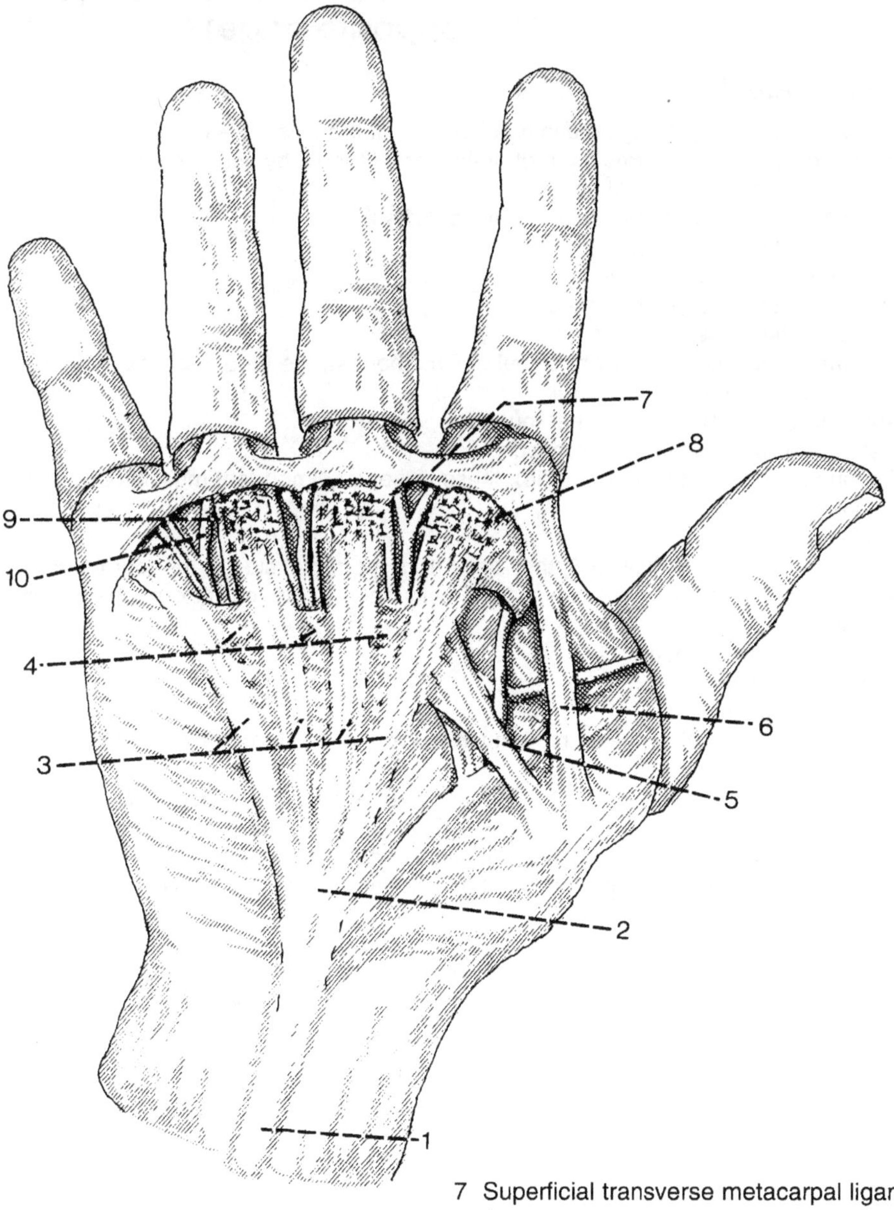

Color and label

1 Tendon of palmaris longus muscle. When present, this muscle, by way of its long tendon, inserts into the apex of the palmar aponeurosis.
2 Palmar aponeurosis. The thick triangular sheet of deep fascia in the palm of the hand. It is firmly bound to the overlying skin by its superficial fibers. Its deeper fibers join the fibrous flexor sheaths of the fingers.
3 Longitudinal fibers of palmar aponeurosis
4 Transverse fibers of palmar aponeurosis
5 Proximal commissural ligament
6 Distal commissural ligament
7 Superficial transverse metacarpal ligament (or natatory ligament)
8 Longitudinal fibers of the palmar aponeurosis inserting into the skin of the palm (cut when skin is removed). These superficial longitudinal fibers insert into the dermis of the distal palm, thus anchoring the skin of the palm and resisting centrifugal pulling or degloving forces that occur in, e.g., swinging a baseball bat.
9 Digital nerve (proper digital nerve)
10 Digital artery (proper digital artery)

Redrawn from Gray's Anatomy, 38 edition. P L Williams ed. Edinburgh, Churchill Livingstone, 1995.

UL-39 Flexor retinaculum and superficial hand muscles

After removal of palmar aponeurosis (opposite page)

Color and label

1 Flexor retinaculum; strong fibrous band in front of the wrist. It is continuous with the antebrachial fascia. It forms the roof of the carpal tunnel by spanning the hollowed space formed by the carpal bones.
2 Tendons of flexor digitorum superficialis to digits 2-5
3 Tendon of flexor carpi radialis
4 Tendon of flexor pollicis longus
5 Tendon of abductor pollicis longus
6 Tendon of flexor carpi ulnaris
7 Pisiform bone (one of the eight carpal or wrist bones); the tendon of flexor carpi ulnaris inserts on it.
8 Abductor pollicis brevis (a thenar muscle)
9 Flexor pollicis brevis (a thenar muscle)
10 Opponens pollicis (a thenar muscle); these three very important muscles form the thenar eminence.
11 Adductor pollicis
12 Lumbrical muscles to digits 2-5; they arise from the radial side of the four tendons of flexor digitorum profundus, which lie directly deep to the four flexor superficialis tendons.
13 First dorsal interosseous
14 Flexor digiti minimi
15 Abductor digiti minimi
16 Opponens digiti minimi; these three muscles (14, 15, 16) form the hypothenar eminence.
17 Cruciate (or crossing) fibers of fibrous tendon sheath; cruciate fibers occur at the interphalangeal joints and allow the sheaths to fold at the joints as the fingers flex.
18 Fibrous and synovial tendon sheaths of middle finger (opened)
19 Tendon of flexor digitorum profundus of middle finger; note its insertion on the distal phalanx.
20 Arrow in carpal tunnel
21 Annular fibers of fibrous tendon sheath. These are stronger and thicker than the cruciate fibers and hold the flexor tendons firmly against the phalanges, thus preventing them from bowing.

UL-39 Flexor retinaculum and superficial hand muscles

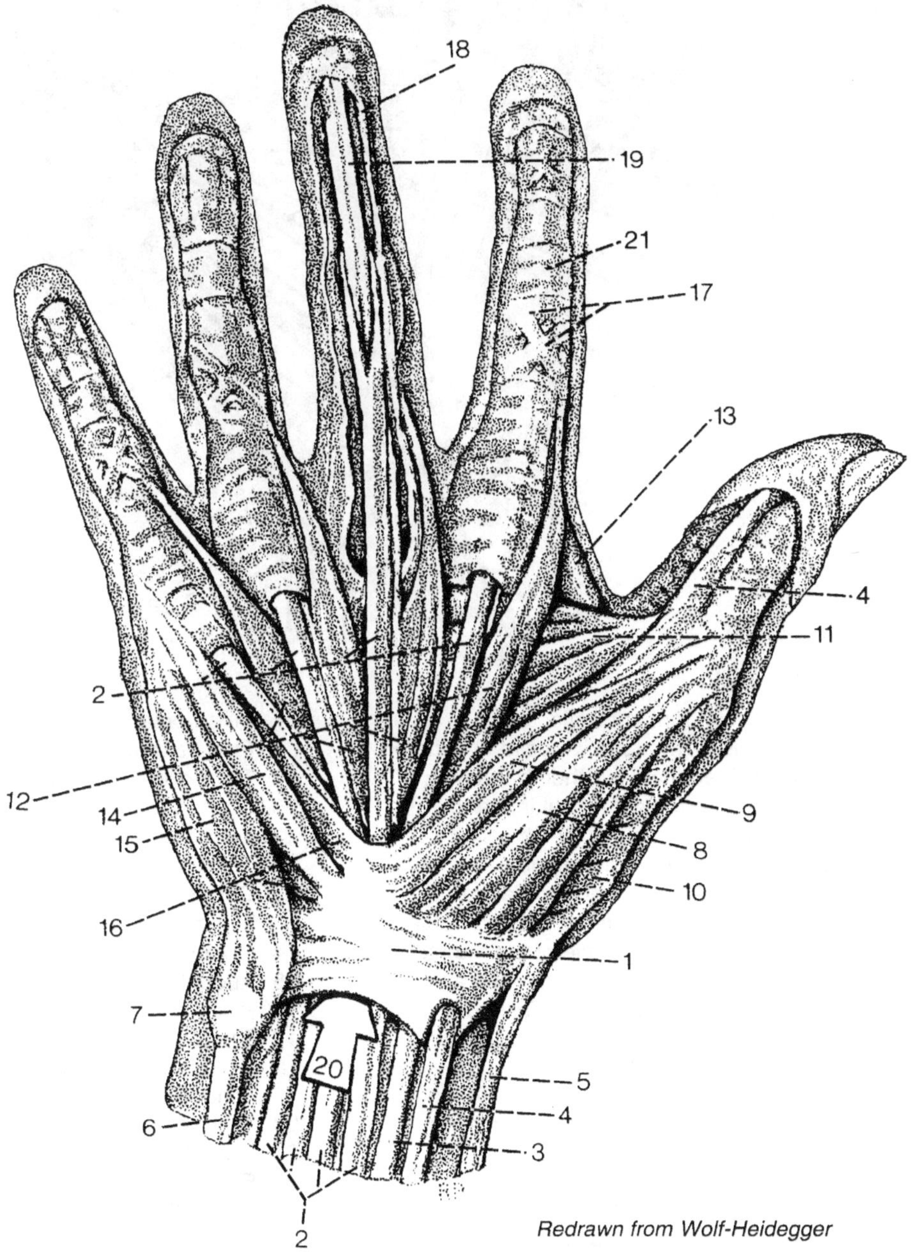

Redrawn from Wolf-Heidegger

UL-40 Deep thenar, hypothenar, and interosseous muscles

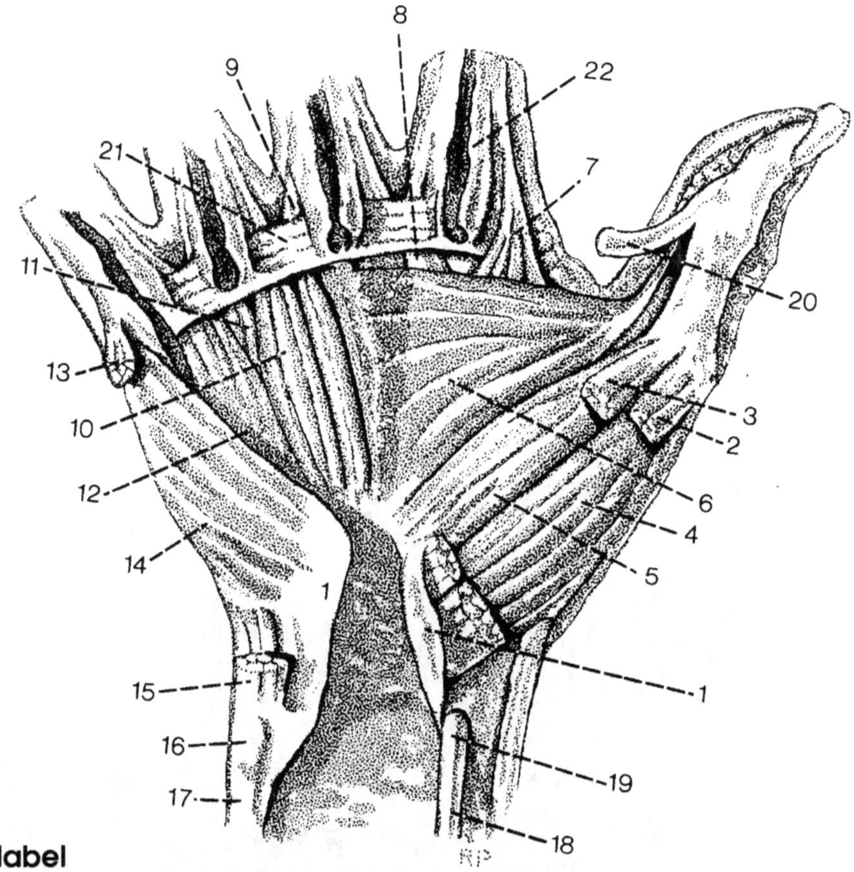

Color and label

1 Flexor retinaculum (cut and reflected)
2 Abductor pollicis brevis (cut). Supplied by the median nerve, it abducts the thumb, rotating it medially, flexes the proximal phalanx, and extends the terminal phalanx. (Also called short abductor muscle of the thumb)
3 Flexor pollicis brevis (cut); (superficial head). Supplied by recurrent branch of median nerve. (Also called short flexor muscle of the thumb)
4 Opponens pollicis. Supplied by the median nerve, it flexes, abducts, and medially rotates the first metacarpal in opposition. (Also called opposing muscle of the thumb)
5 Flexor pollicis brevis (deep head). The deep head is usually supplied by the deep branch of the ulnar nerve.
6 Adductor pollicis. It arises by two heads: an oblique head (caput obliquum) and a transverse head (caput transversum). It is supplied by the deep branch of the ulnar nerve. It adducts and flexes the first metacarpal bone of the thumb, and flexes the proximal metacarpal of the thumb, especially in gripping movements.
7 First dorsal interosseous
8 First palmar interosseous
9 Third dorsal interosseous
10 Second palmar interosseous
11 Fourth dorsal interosseous
12 Third palmar interosseous
13 Common insertion of abductor digiti minimi and flexor digiti minimi (cut)
14 Opponens digiti minimi
15 Abductor digiti minimi (origin)
16 Pisiform bone
17 Tendon of flexor carpi ulnaris
18 Tendon of flexor carpi radialis
19 Tendon of abductor pollicis longus
20 Tendon of flexor pollicis longus
21 Deep transverse carpal ligament
22 Fibrous tendon sheath (cut open and both superficial and deep tendons removed)

Redrawn from Wolf-Heidegger

UL-41 Interosseous and related muscles

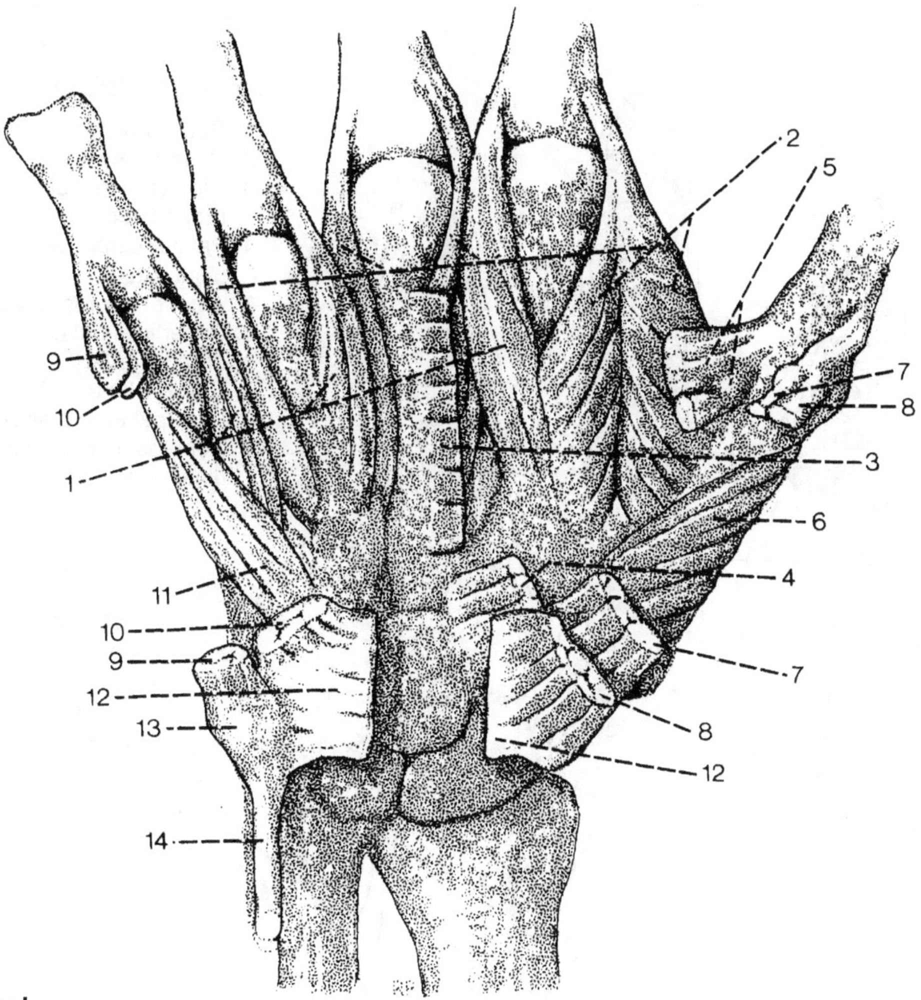

Color and label

1 Palmar interosseous muscles. The traditional view is that there are three of these muscles (as depicted here). However, some authors find that there are actually four, and that the first has been mistakenly overlooked as part of either the flexor pollicis brevis or the adductor pollicis. The palmar interossei adduct (bring together) digits 2,4, and 5 toward the middle finger. They also flex the MP joint (metacarpophalangeal) and extend the PIP joint (proximal interphalangeal) and the DIP (distal interphalangeal) joint. They are supplied by the deep branch of the ulnar nerve.

2 Dorsal interosseous muscles. Four bipennate* muscles. They are supplied by the ulnar nerve. They abduct the second and fourth finger from the middle finger, which itself remains stationary. Like the palmar interossei, they flex the first phalanges and extend the middle and distal phalanges.

3 Adductor pollicis (transverse head, cut)
4 Adductor pollicis (oblique head, cut)
5 Adductor pollicis insertion with ulnar sesamoid bone
6 Opponens pollicis
7 Flexor pollicis brevis with radial sesamoid bone (cut)
8 Abductor pollicis brevis (cut)
9 Abductor digiti minimi (cut)
10 Flexor digiti minimi (cut)
11 Opponens digiti minimi
12 Flexor retinaculum (cut)
13 Pisiform bone
14 Tendon of flexor carpi ulnaris

*Shaped like a feather with a central shaft between its two vanes.

Redrawn from Wolf- Heidegger

UL-42 Arteries of the hand

Simplified; smaller branches are not shown

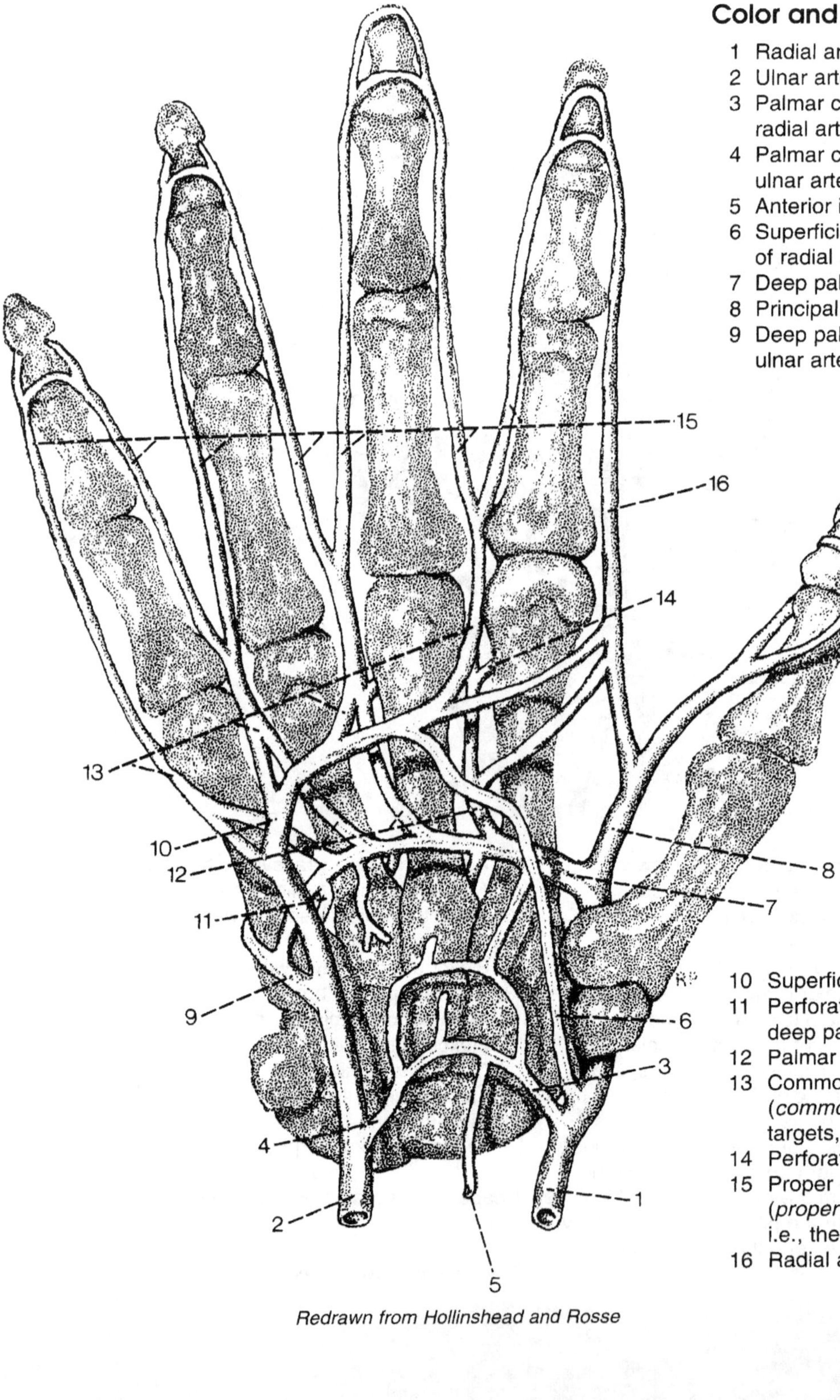

Redrawn from Hollinshead and Rosse

Color and label

1 Radial artery
2 Ulnar artery
3 Palmar carpal branch of radial artery
4 Palmar carpal branch of ulnar artery
5 Anterior interosseous artery
6 Superficial palmar branch of radial artery
7 Deep palmar arch
8 Principal thumb artery
9 Deep palmar branch of ulnar artery
10 Superficial palmar arch
11 Perforating branch of deep palmar arch
12 Palmar metacarpal arteries
13 Common digital arteries (*common* denotes several targets, not just a single digit)
14 Perforating branch
15 Proper digital arteries (*proper* denotes its sole destination, i.e., the digit)
16 Radial artery of index finger

UL-43 Deep palmar arch and deep branch of ulnar nerve

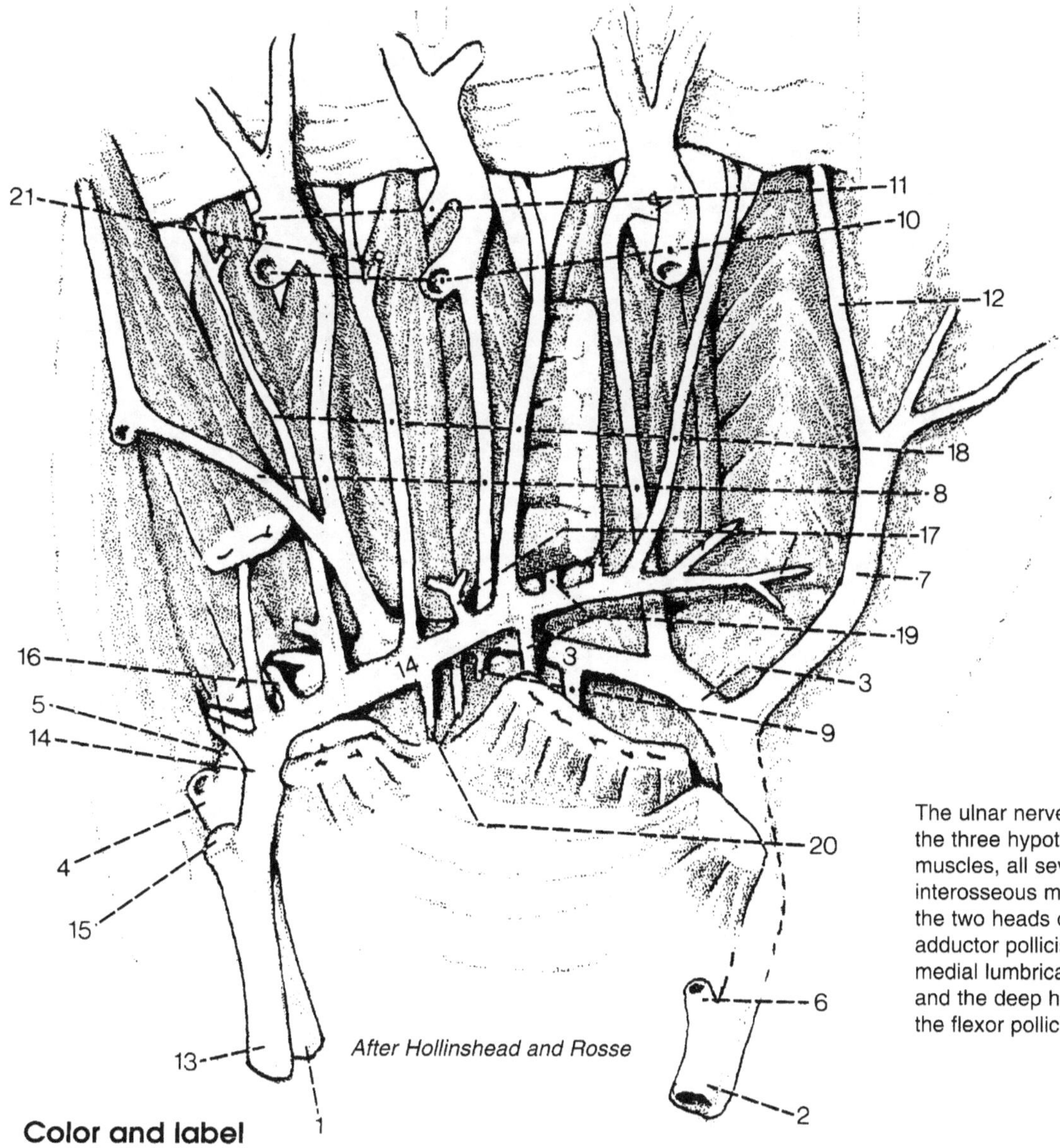

After Hollinshead and Rosse

The ulnar nerve supplies the three hypothenar muscles, all seven interosseous muscles, the two heads of the adductor pollicis, the two medial lumbricals, and the deep head of the flexor pollicis brevis.

Color and label

1 Ulnar artery
2 Radial artery
3 Deep palmar arch
4 Superficial palmar arch (cut)
5 Deep palmar branch of ulnar artery
6 Superficial palmar branch of radial artery (cut)
7 Princeps pollicis artery (main artery of the thumb)
8 Palmar metacarpal arteries
9 Perforating branches from deep palmar arch
10 Common digital arteries (cut)
11 Perforating branches of metacarpal arteries
12 Radialis indicis artery (radial artery of the index finger)
13 Ulnar nerve
14 Deep branch of ulnar nerve
15 Superficial branch of ulnar nerve (cut)
16 Ulnar nerve branches to hypothenar muscles
17 Branches to interosseous muscles
18 Articular branches to metacarpophalangeal joints
19 Branches to two heads of adductor pollicis
20 Carpal twigs to carpal bones and joints
21 Nerves to two medial lumbricals

UL-44 Nerves and arteries of the palm

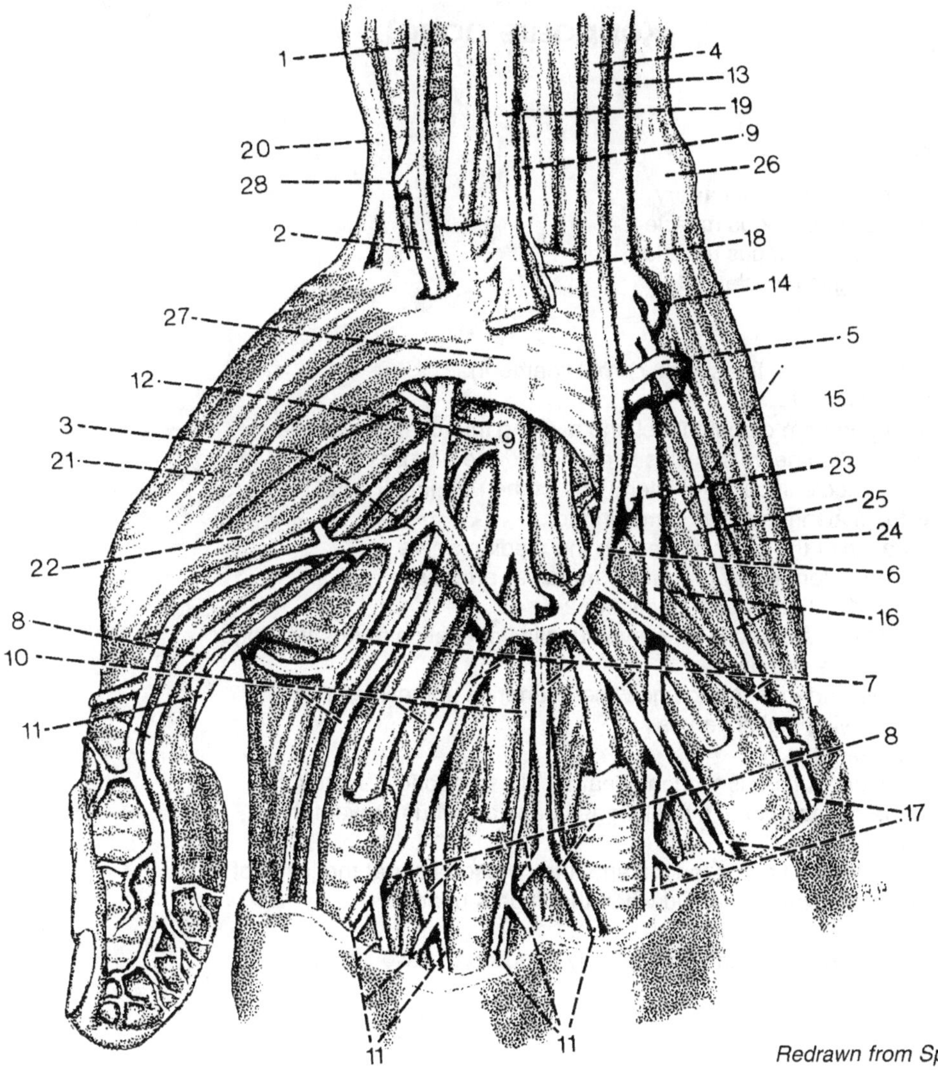

Redrawn from Spalteholz and Spanner

Color and label

1 Radial artery
2 Superficial palmar branch of radial artery
3 Principal thumb artery (princeps pollicis)
4 Ulnar artery
5 Deep branch of ulnar artery
6 Superficial palmar arch
7 Common palmar digital arteries
8 Proper palmar digital arteries
9 Median nerve
10 Common palmar digital nerves (from median nerve)
11 Proper palmar digital nerves (from median nerve)
12 Thenar muscular branch of median nerve (recurrent branch)
13 Ulnar nerve
14 Deep branch of ulnar nerve
15 Superficial branch of ulnar nerve
16 Common palmar digital nerves (from ulnar nerve)
17 Proper palmar digital nerves (from ulnar nerve)
18 Palmar branch of median nerve
19 Tendon of palmaris longus
20 Tendon of abductor pollicis longus
21 Abductor pollicis brevis
22 Flexor pollicis brevis
23 Communicating branch between median and ulnar nerves
24 Abductor digiti minimi
25 Flexor digiti minimi
26 Pisiform bone
27 Flexor retinaculum
28 Deep palmar branch of radial artery

UL-45 Superficial palmar arch
Median and ulnar nerves

(opposite page)

Color and label

1 Superficial palmar branch of radial artery
2 Tendon of extensor pollicis longus muscle
3 Tendon of abductor pollicis longus muscle
4 Tendon of palmaris longus muscle (cut)
5 Ulnar artery
6 Ulnar nerve
7 Flexor retinaculum (old name, transverse carpal ligament)
8 Abductor digiti minimi muscle
9 Median nerve emerging from carpal tunnel and dividing into common palmar digital nerves. The median nerve supplies sensation to the palmar surface of the thumb, index finger, middle finger, and lateral half of the ring finger, plus the dorsal surface of the distal phalanges of the same fingers.
10 Communicating branch of the ulnar nerve with the median nerve.
11 Superficial palmar arch (formed by the radial and ulnar arteries)
12 Flexor tendons (superficial and deep) to fingers 2-5
13 Proper palmar digital nerves. The ulnar nerve supplies sensation to the fifth finger and the medial half of the ring finger.
14 Common palmar digital arteries. Notice how these arteries sometimes pass through the accompanying digital nerves.
15 Proper palmar digital arteries
16 Annular (ring-like) fibers of fibrous tendon sheaths. These strongly anchor the flexor tendons to the metacarpal and phalanges bones and thus prevent the tendons from bowing.
17 Cruciate (crossing) fibers of fibrous tendon sheaths. These occur at the joints of the fingers and allow the sheaths to fold when the fingers bend.
18 Adductor pollicis muscle
19 First lumbrical muscle. The median nerve usually supplies the two lateral lumbricals.
20 Flexor pollicis brevis muscle
21 Branch of the median nerve to the thenar muscles
22 Abductor pollicis brevis muscle

UL-45 Superficial palmar arch Median and ulnar nerves

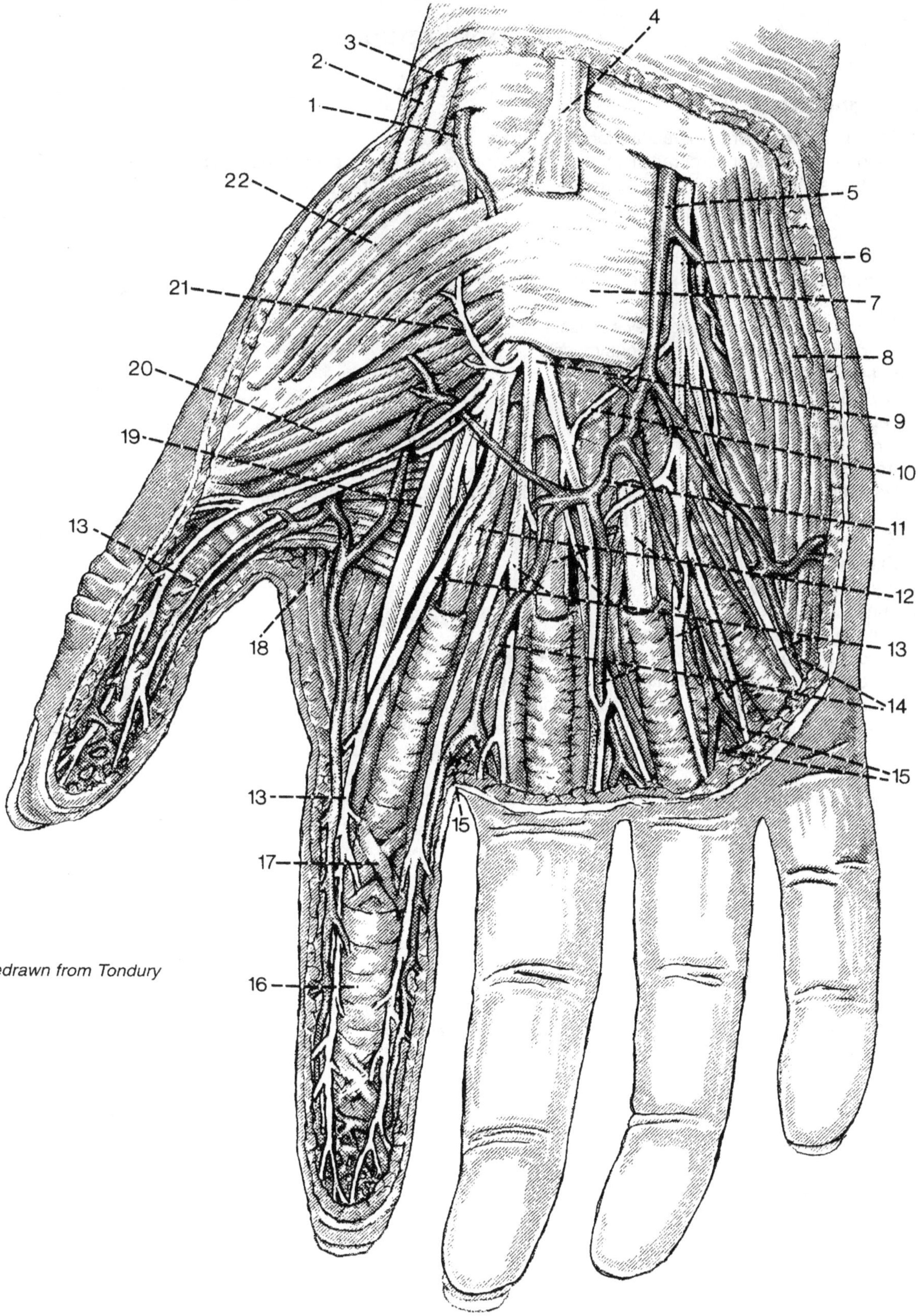

Redrawn from Tondury

UL-46 Extensor tendons on dorsum of hand

(opposite page)

Color and label

1 Tendon of extensor carpi radialis longus muscle
2 Tendon of extensor carpi radialis brevis muscle; these two extensors of the wrist insert on the two strongest bones in the hand, the 2nd and 3rd metacarpals; they also stabilize the wrist by working with the finger flexors.
3 Abductor pollicis longus muscle
4 Extensor pollicis brevis muscle
5 Tendon of extensor pollicis longus muscle
6 Radius
7 Tendon of extensor pollicis brevis muscle
8 Tendon of abductor pollicis longus muscle
9 Extensor retinaculum
10 Styloid process of radius
11 Tendon of flexor carpi radialis muscle
12 First dorsal interosseous muscle
13 Adductor pollicis muscle
14 Dorsal digital expansion of the extensor digitorum tendon to the index finger
15 Four tendons of the extensor digitorum muscle
16 Extensor carpi ulnaris muscle
17 Extensor digiti minimi muscle
18 Styloid process of ulna
19 Lunate wrist bone
20 Tendon of extensor carpi ulnaris
21 Tendons of extensor digitorum muscle to fingers 2-5
22 Tendon of extensor indicis muscle to index finger
23 Tendon of extensor digiti minimi muscle; fingers 2 and 5 each have an additional extensor muscle, giving them the ability to extend separately from the other fingers.
24 Dorsal interosseous muscles

Tr Trapezium wrist bone
Td Trapezoid wrist bone
C Capitate wrist bone
H Hamate wrist bone
S Scaphoid wrist bone
Tq Triquetral wrist bone (triquetrum)

All the extensor arm muscles are innervated by the radial nerve or its posterior interosseous branch.

UL-46 Extensor tendons on dorsum of hand

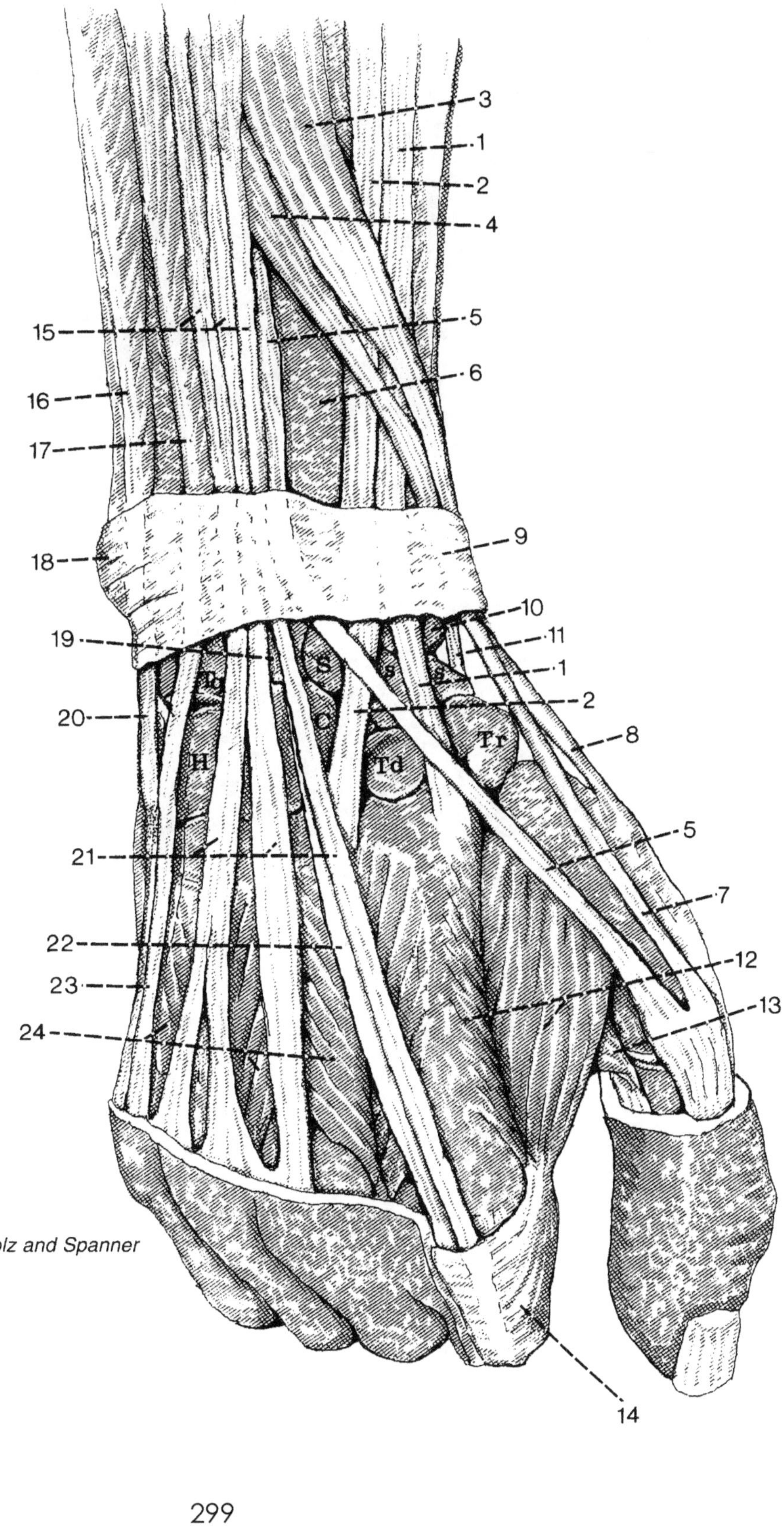

Redrawn from Spalteholz and Spanner

UL-47 Radial artery and superficial branch of radial nerve

Color and label

1 Cutaneous branch of radial nerve
2 Brachioradialis muscle
3 Tendon of flexor carpi radialis
4 Tendon of palmaris longus muscle
5 Radial artery
6 Palmar branch of median nerve
7 Median nerve
8 Tendon of abductor pollicis longus muscle
9 Superficial palmar branch of radial artery
10 Opponens pollicis muscle
11 Abductor pollicis muscle
12 Extensor pollicis brevis tendon
13 Extensor pollicis longus tendon. Notice that these two extensor tendons of the thumb define the anatomical "snuff box," through which traverses the radial artery.
14 First dorsal interosseous muscle
15 First metacarpal bone
16 Thumb (digit 1)
17 Index finger (digit 2)
18 Second metacarpal bone
19 Cutaneous branch of radial nerve
20 Superficial branch of radial nerve
21 Extensor pollicis brevis muscle
22 Extensor retinaculum
23 Extensor carpi radialis brevis tendon (inserts on 3rd metacarpal)
24 Extensor carpi radialis longus tendon (inserts on 2nd metacarpal)
25 First dorsal metacarpal artery

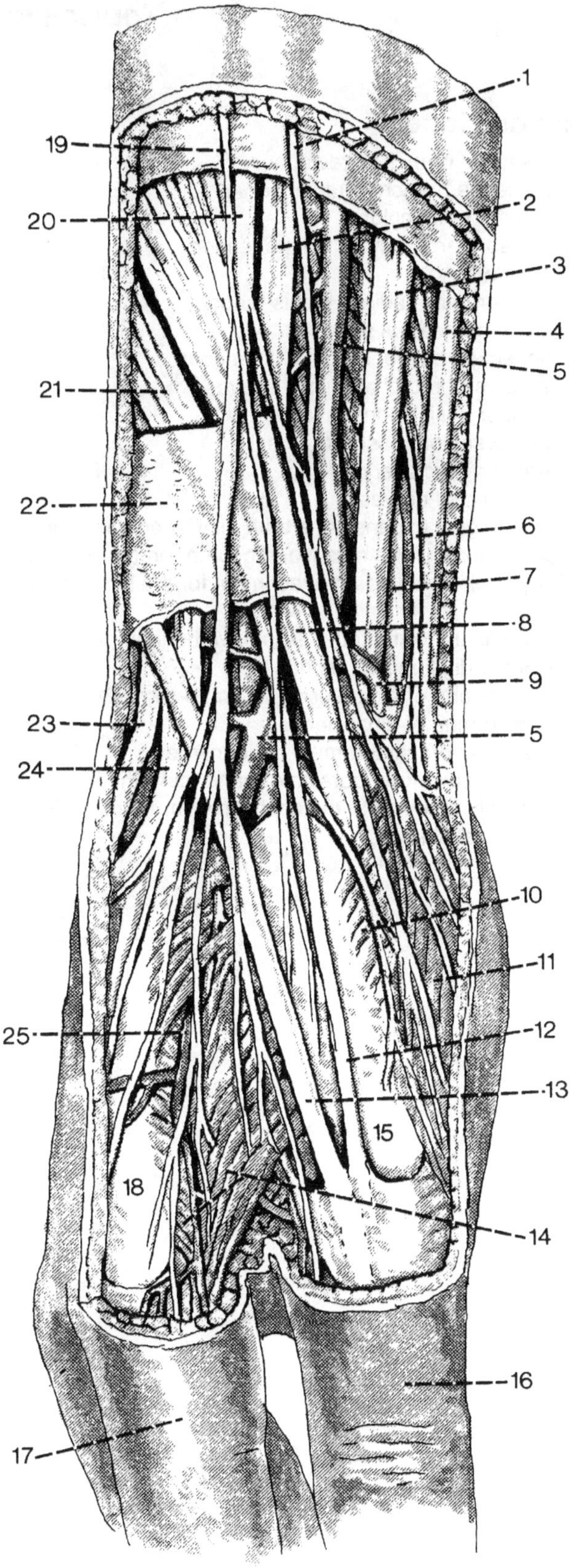

Redrawn from Tondury

UL-48 Dorsum of hand

After removal of fascia and dorsal venous plexus (opposite page)

Color and label

1 Superficial branch of radial nerve
2 Cutaneous branch of radial nerve
3 Extensor retinaculum
4 Extensor carpi radialis longus tendon
5 Radial artery
6 Extensor carpi radialis brevis tendon
7 Dorsal metacarpal artery
8 Connection between dorsal cutaneous branches of radial and ulnar nerves
9 Extensor pollicis longus tendon
10 First dorsal interosseous muscle
11 Extensor indicis tendon
12 Dorsal digital nerves
13 Dorsal digital expansion; a triangular aponeurotic extension of each of the four tendons of the extensor digitorum on the proximal phalanges of digits 2-5. They each serve as an attachment for the lumbricals and the interosseous muscles.
14 Dorsal digital veins (cut; veins have been largely removed)
15 Extensor digiti minimi tendon
16 Four tendons of extensor digitorum to digits 2-5
17 Dorsal ramus of ulnar nerve
18 Dorsal antebrachial rami of radial nerve
19 Venous network on dorsum of hand (cut); these coalesce and drain proximally mainly into the cephalic vein (thumb side) and basilic vein (little finger side).

UL-48 Dorsum of hand

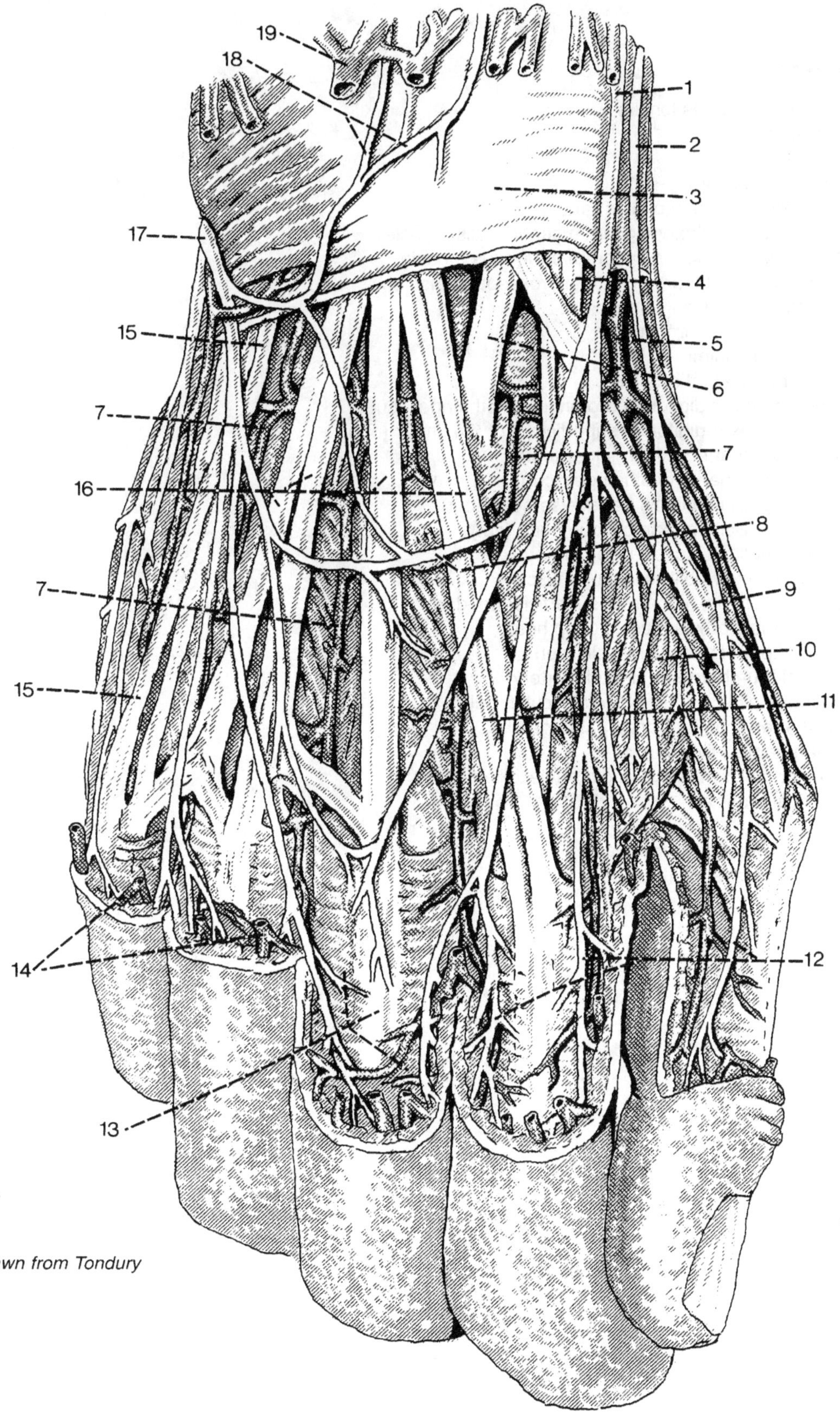

Redrawn from Tondury

UL-49 Palmar hand. Deep dissection

(opposite page)

Color and label

1 Tendon of palmaris longus
2 Ulnar artery
3 Ulnar nerve
4 Flexor retinaculum
5 Deep palmar branch of ulnar artery
6 Four tendons of flexor digitorum superficialis muscle
7 Four tendons of flexor digitorum profundus muscle
8 Deep branch of ulnar nerve to interosseous muscles
9 Opponens digiti minimi muscle
10 Abductor digiti minimi muscle
11 Flexor digiti minimi
12 Palmar metacarpal arteries
13 Tendon of flexor digitorum profundus of 5th finger (cut)
14 Tendon of flexor digitorum superficialis of 5th finger (cut)
15 Proper digital artery of 5th finger (cut)
16 Proper digital nerve of 5th finger (cut)
17 Adductor pollicis muscle transverse head (cut)
18 Adductor pollicis muscle oblique head (cut)
19 Adductor pollicis muscle insertion (cut)
20 Tendon of flexor pollicis longus muscle
21 Flexor pollicis brevis muscle superficial head (cut)
22 Flexor pollicis brevis muscle deep head
23 Abductor pollicis brevis muscle (cut)
24 Principal thumb artery (off radial artery)
25 Opponens pollicis artery (partially cut in half)
26 Radial artery origin of deep palmar arch
27 Median nerve (divisions cut)
28 Abductor pollicis muscle origin on flexor retinaculum
29 Lumbrical muscles

P Palmar interosseous muscles
D Dorsal interosseous muscles

UL-49 Palmar hand. Deep dissection

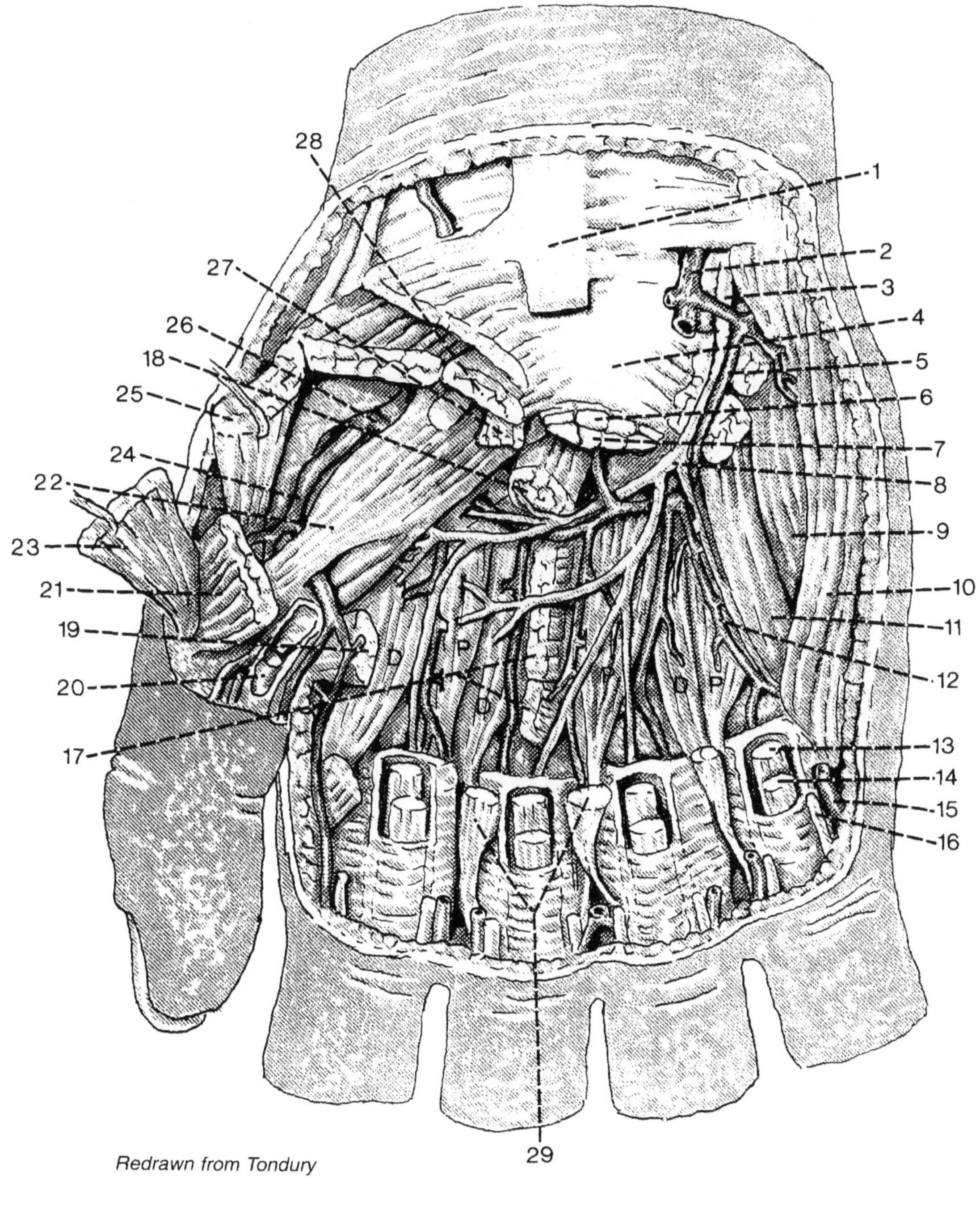

Redrawn from Tondury

UL-50 Extensor tendons on dorsum of hand

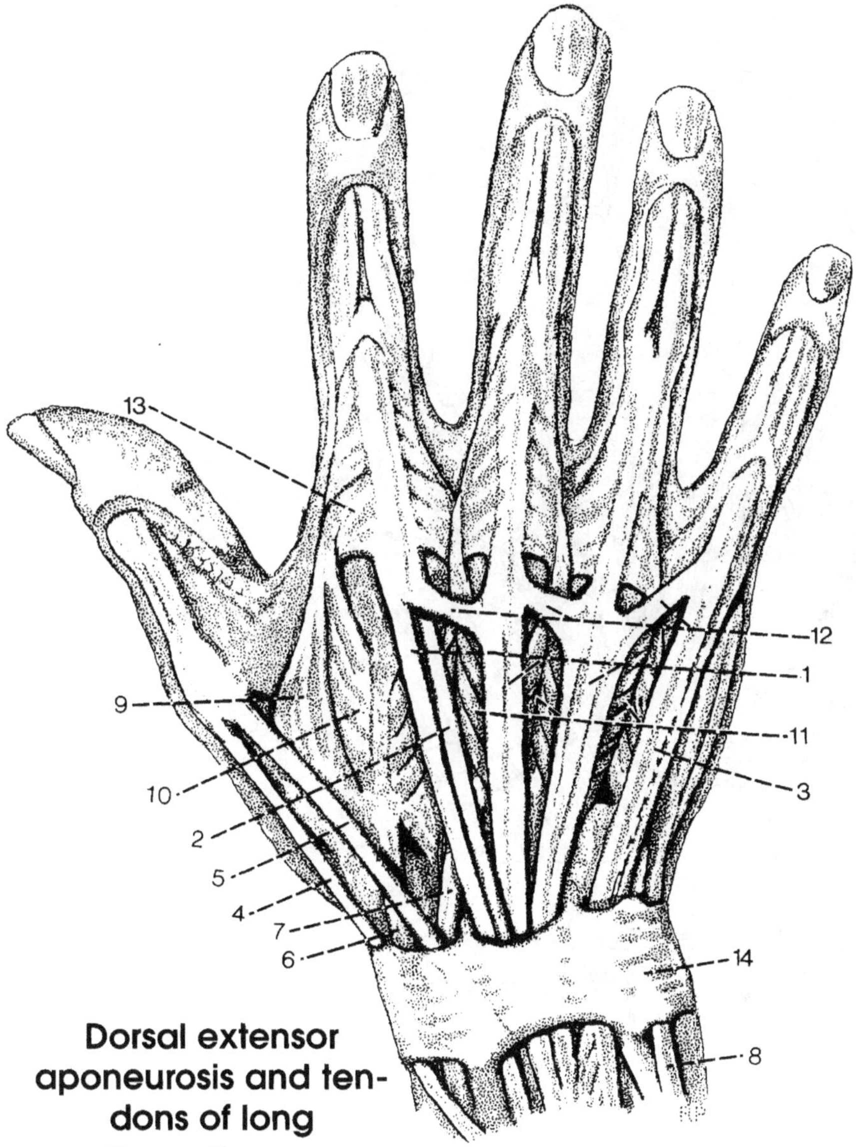

Color and label

1 Tendons of extensor digitorum fingers 2-5
2 Tendon of extensor indicis
3 Tendon of extensor digiti minimi
4 Tendon of extensor pollicis brevis
5 Tendon of extensor pollicis longus
6 Tendon of extensor carpi radialis longus
7 Tendon of extensor carpi radialis brevis
8 Tendon of extensor of carpi ulnaris
9 First dorsal interosseous (lateral head)
10 First dorsal interosseous (medial head)
11 Dorsal interosseous muscles 2,3,4 *
12 Intertendinous connections
13 Dorsal extensor aponeurosis (also called dorsal digital expansion and extensor hood)
14 Extensor retinaculum

* The interossei attach to both the dorsal extensor aponeurosis as well as to the proximal phalanx.

Dorsal extensor aponeurosis and tendons of long finger flexors

(right middle finger; radial or thumb aspect)

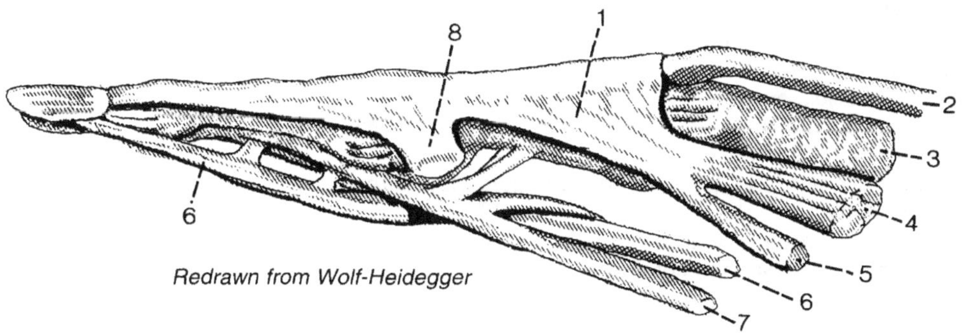

Redrawn from Wolf-Heidegger

Color and label

1 Dorsal extensor aponeurosis
2 Tendon of extensor digitorum
3 Metacarpal bone of middle finger
4 Dorsal interosseous muscle II
5 Lumbrical muscle II
6 Tendon of flexor digitorum profundus muscle
7 Tendon of flexor digitorum superficialis muscle
8 Cruciform (crossing) fibers of the fibrous digital sheath (cut and reflected, allowing long flexor tendons to be pulled away from phalanges)

UL-51 Synovial flexor tendon sheaths

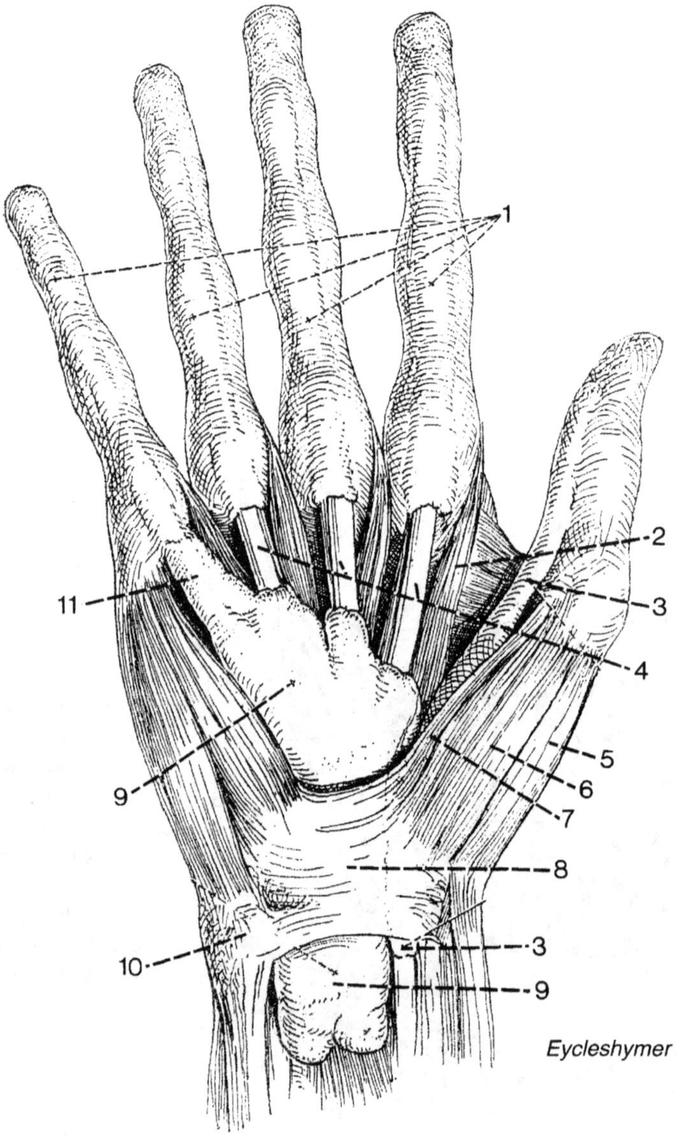

Eycleshymer and Jones

Color and label

1 Digital synovial tendon sheaths
2 First lumbrical muscle
3 Synovial tendon sheath for flexor pollicis longus
4 Flexor tendons (deep and superficial) to fingers 2,3,4
5 Opponens pollicis
6 Abductor pollicis brevis
7 Flexor pollicis brevis
8 Flexor retinaculum
9 Common synovial sheath for flexors to fingers 2,3,4,5
10 Pisiform bone
11 Abductor digiti minimi synovial sheath; note its continuity with the common synovial sheath.

UL-52 Synovial extensor tendon sheaths

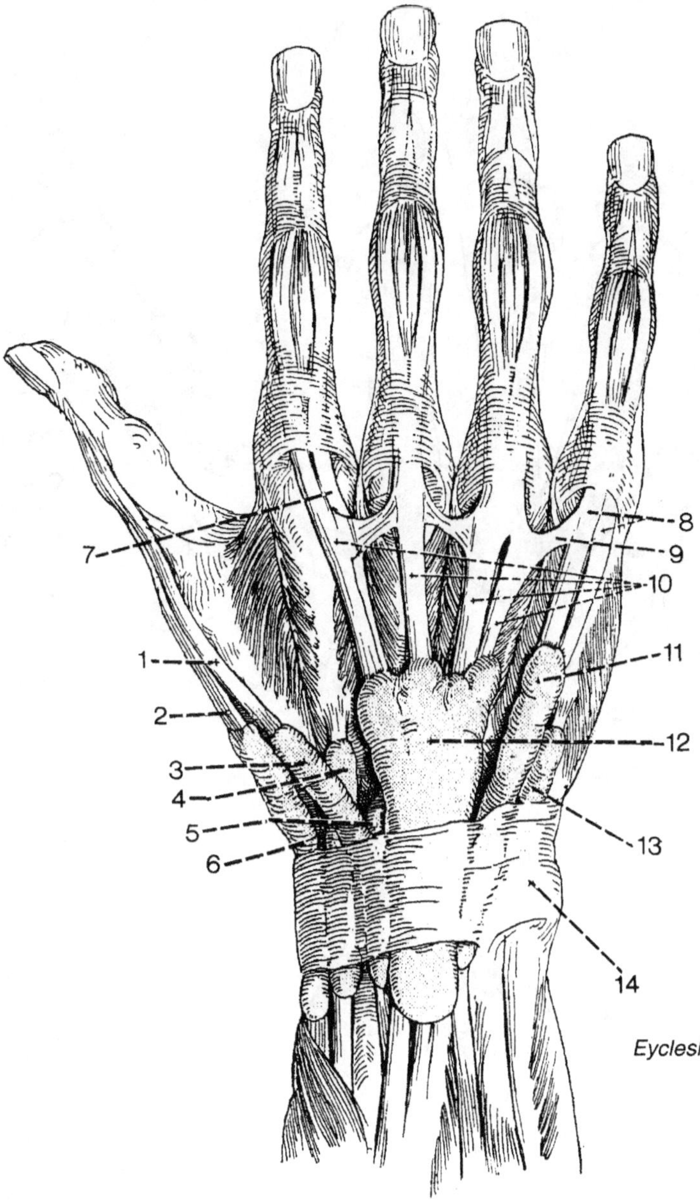

Eycleshymer and Jones

Color and label

1 Tendon of extensor pollicis longus
2 Tendon of extensor pollicis brevis
3 Extensor pollicis longus synovial tendon sheath
4 Extensor carpi radialis longus synovial tendon sheath
5 Extensor carpi radialis brevis synovial tendon sheath
6 Extensor pollicis brevis synovial tendon sheath
7 Tendon of extensor indicis
8 Tendon of extensor digiti minimi; notice these two "extra" extensor tendons to fingers 2 and 5 lie on the ulnar (or medial) sides of the two corresponding extensor digitorum tendons and impart an additional extensor independence to these two digits.
9 Intertendinous connection
10 Extensor digitorum tendons to fingers 2-5. Its action on finger 5 is usually conveyed via an intertendinous link to extensor digiti minimi tendon.
11 Synovial tendon sheath of extensor digiti minimi
12 Synovial tendon sheath for extensor digitorum and extensor indicis
13 Synovial tendon sheath for extensor carpi ulnaris
14 Extensor retinaculum

UL-53 Thumb muscles I

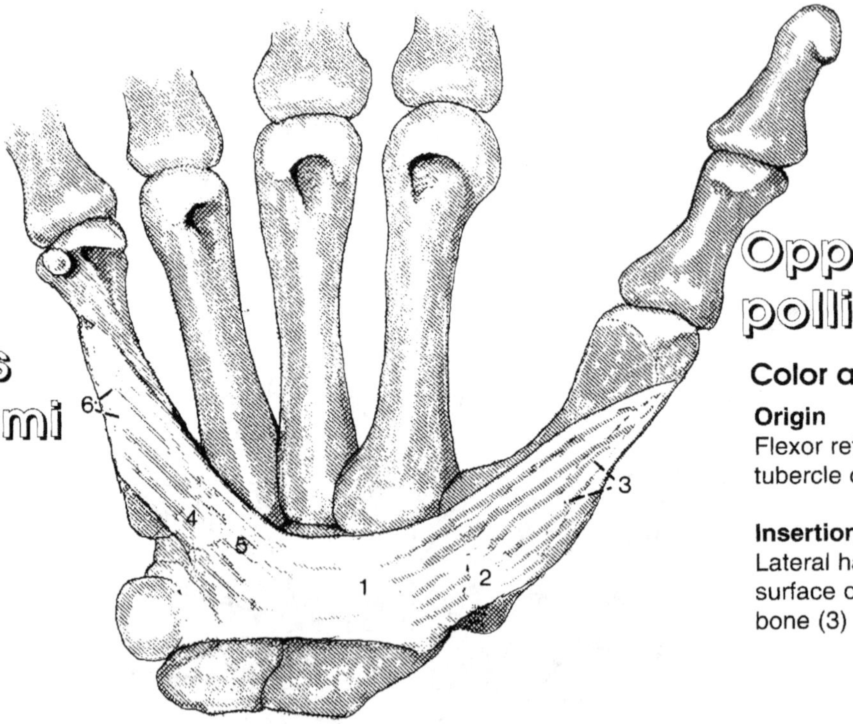

Opponens digiti minimi

Color and label

Origin
Distal margin of hook of the hamate (4) and its adjacent flexor retinaculum (5)

Insertion
Medial margin of 5th metacarpal bone (6)

Opponens pollicis

Color and label

Origin
Flexor retinaculum (1) and tubercle of trapezium (2)

Insertion
Lateral half of anterior surface of first metacarpal bone (3)

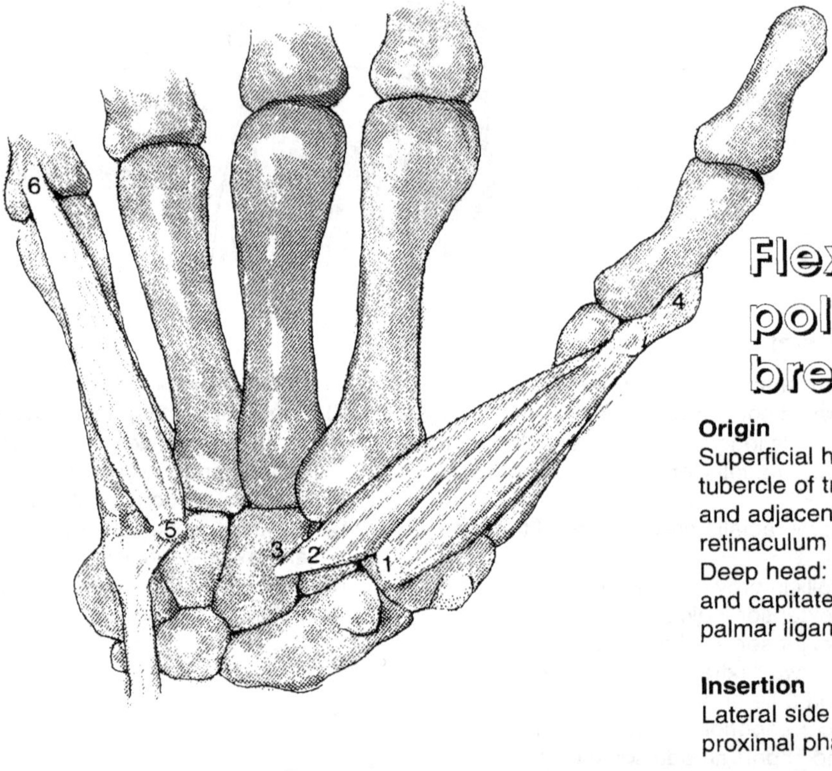

Flexor digiti minimi

Origin
Hook of hamate (5)

Insertion
Medial side of base of proximal phalanx (6) of little finger

Flexor pollicis brevis

Origin
Superficial head: tubercle of trapezium (1) and adjacent part of flexor retinaculum (not shown)
Deep head: trapezoid (2) and capitate bones (3) and palmar ligaments (not shown)

Insertion
Lateral side of base of proximal phalanx of thumb (4)

UL-54 Thumb muscles II

Adductor digiti minimi muscle

Adductor pollicis brevis muscle

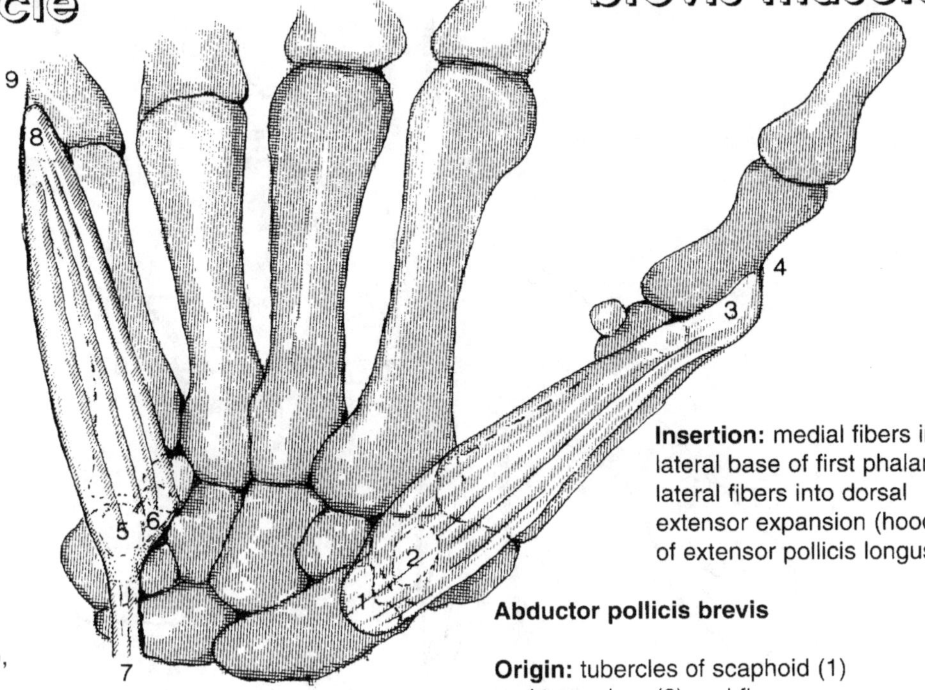

Abductor digiti minimi

Insertion: medial side of proximal phalanx of little finger (8) and medial border of dorsal expansion of extensor digiti minimi muscle (9)

Abductor digiti minimi

Origin: pisiform bone (5), pisohamate ligament (6), and tendon of flexor carpi ulnaris muscle (7)

Insertion: medial fibers into lateral base of first phalanx (3); lateral fibers into dorsal extensor expansion (hood) (4) of extensor pollicis longus muscle

Abductor pollicis brevis

Origin: tubercles of scaphoid (1) and trapezium (2) and flexor retinaculum (removed)

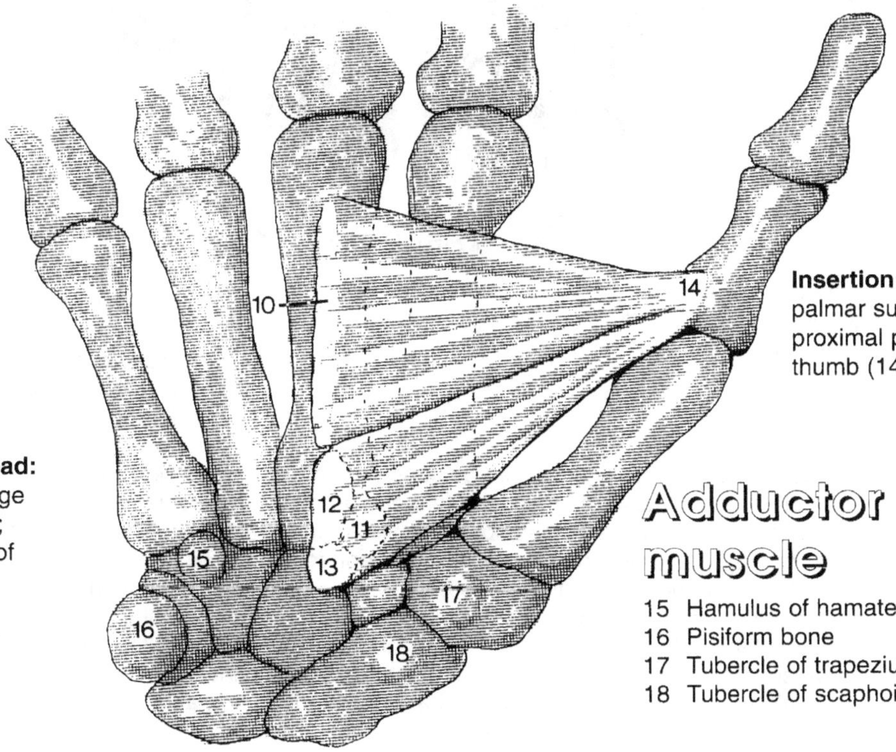

Insertion: ulnar side of palmar surface of base of proximal phalanx of thumb (14)

Origin: transverse head: distal 2/3 of palmar ridge of 3rd metacarpal (10); **oblique head:** bases of 2nd (11) and 3rd (12) metacarpals, capitate bone (13), and palmar ligament (not shown)

Adductor pollicis muscle

15 Hamulus of hamate bone
16 Pisiform bone
17 Tubercle of trapezium bone
18 Tubercle of scaphoid bone

UL-55 Palmar interosseous muscles

Palmar aspect of right hand

Redrawn from Spalteholz and Spanner

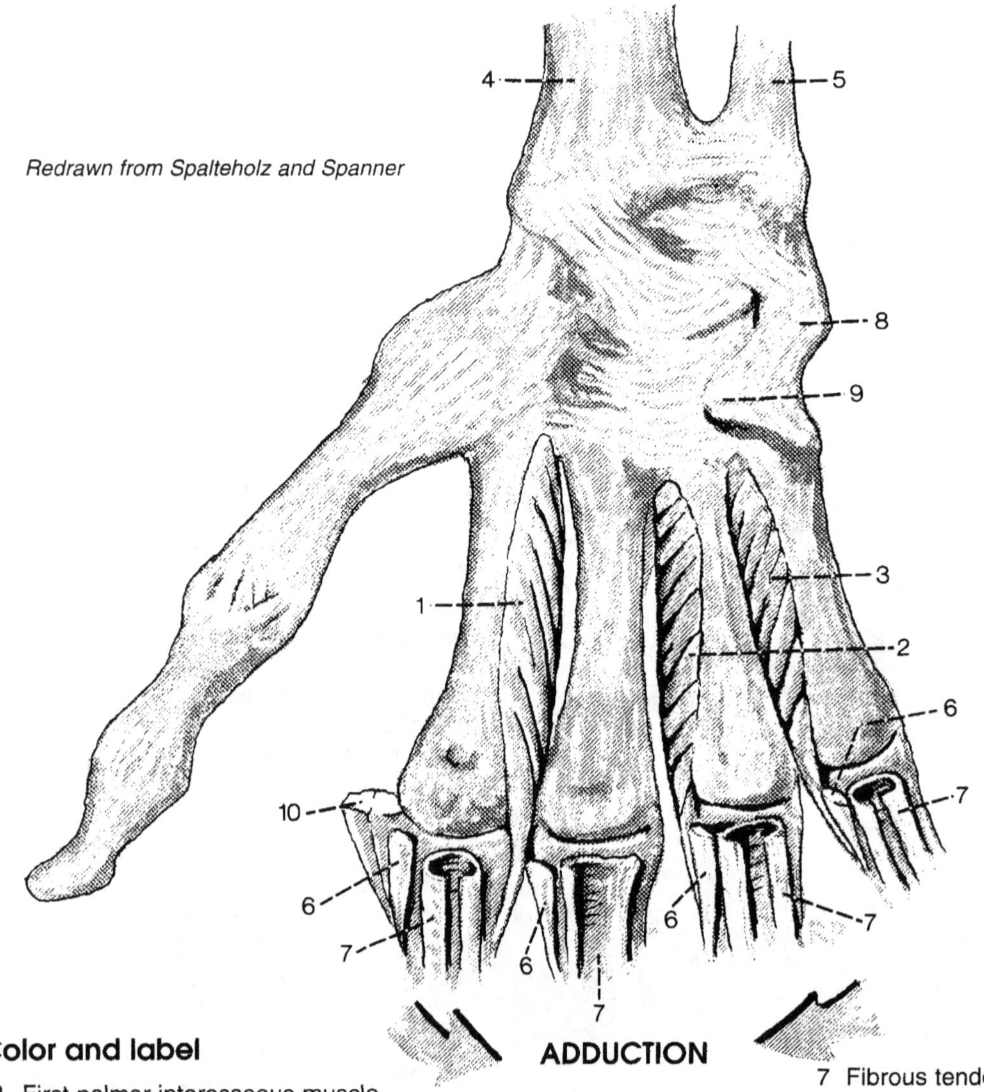

Color and label

1 First palmar interosseous muscle
2 Second palmar interosseous muscle
3 Third palmar interosseous muscle
4 Radius
5 Ulna
6 Lumbrical muscles (cut)
7 Fibrous tendon sheaths for superficial and deep flexor tendons (cut open and tendons removed)
8 Pisiform bone
9 Hook of hamate bone
10 First dorsal interosseous muscle (cut)

The palmar interosseous muscles, usually described as consisting of three muscles, as depicted here, are described by some authors as consisting of four muscles. According to these authors,* the first palmar interosseous, which is usually considered part of either the flexor pollicis or the adductor pollicis, arises from the medial side of the palmar surface of first metacarpal bone near its base (not shown here). The present account depicts three palmar interosseous muscles rather than four. The first arises from the medial surface of the second metacarpal and inserts into the medial side of the base of the proximal phalange and the medial side of the dorsal digital expansion of the index finger. The second arises from the lateral surface of the fourth metacarpal and inserts onto the lateral side of the dorsal digital expansion of the ring finger. The third arises from the lateral side of the fifth metacarpal and inserts into the lateral side of the dorsal digital expansion of the fifth finger. The palmar interossei **adduct** the 2nd, 4th, and 5th fingers toward the middle finger. They also flex the proximal phalanx and extend the middle phalanx and distal phalanx of the four medial fingers.

* Gray's Anatomy 38 Ed, 1995, Churchill Livingstone

UL-56 Dorsal interosseous muscles of the hand

Dorsal aspect right hand

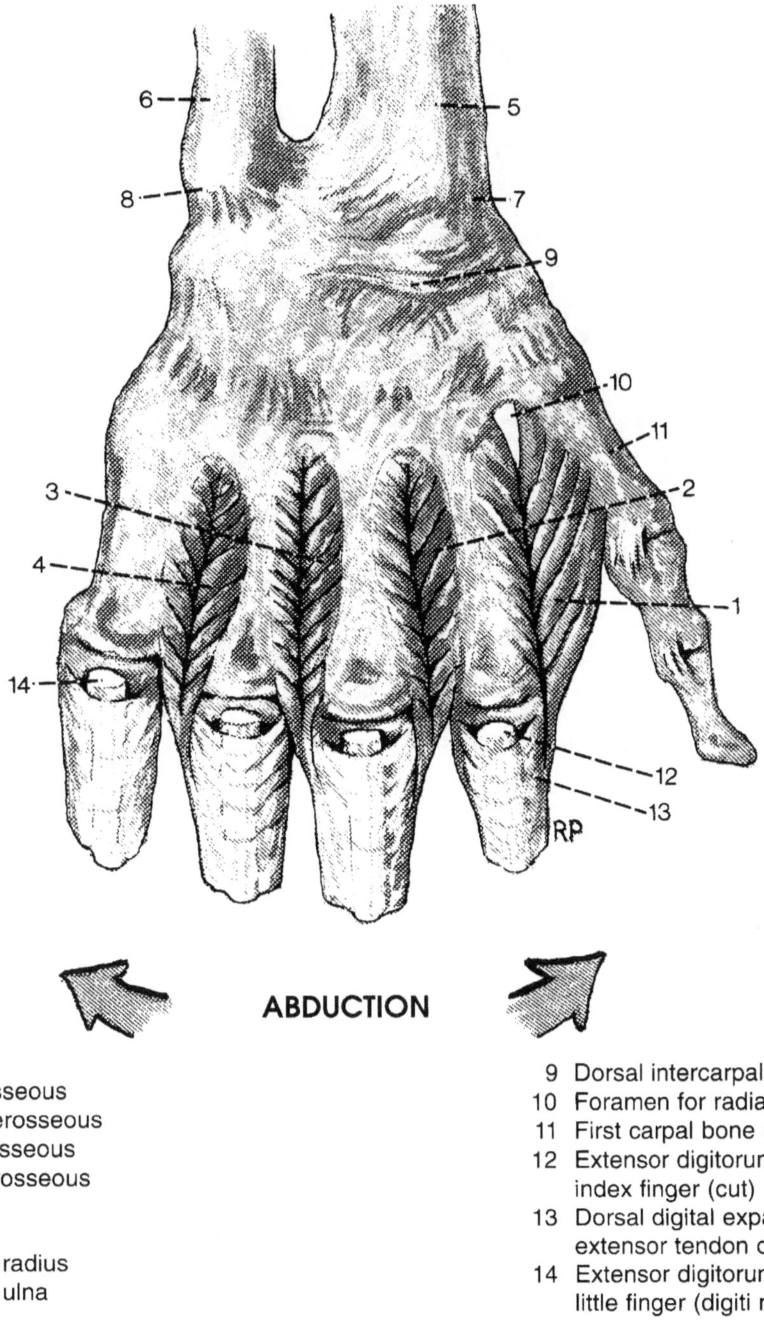

Color and label

1 First dorsal interosseous
2 Second dorsal interosseous
3 Third dorsal interosseous
4 Fourth dorsal interosseous
5 Radius
6 Ulna
7 Styloid process of radius
8 Styloid process of ulna
9 Dorsal intercarpal ligaments
10 Foramen for radial artery
11 First carpal bone (of thumb)
12 Extensor digitorum tendon of index finger (cut)
13 Dorsal digital expansion of extensor tendon of index finger
14 Extensor digitorum tendon of little finger (digiti minimi) (cut)

The dorsal interosseous muscles are four bipennate muscles in each hand. They each arise from adjacent sides of two metacarpal bones and insert onto the bases of proximal phalanges and dorsal digital (extensor tendon) expansions. The first inserts on the radial side of the index finger; the second and third on the radial and ulnar sides, respectively, of the middle finger. The fourth inserts onto the ulnar side of the ring finger (4th). They are innervated by the deep branch of the ulnar nerve. They **abduct** the second and fourth fingers from the middle finger. They flex the proximal phalanges (MP joint) and extend the middle (PIP joint) and distal phalanges (DIP joint).

UL-57 Some finger movements

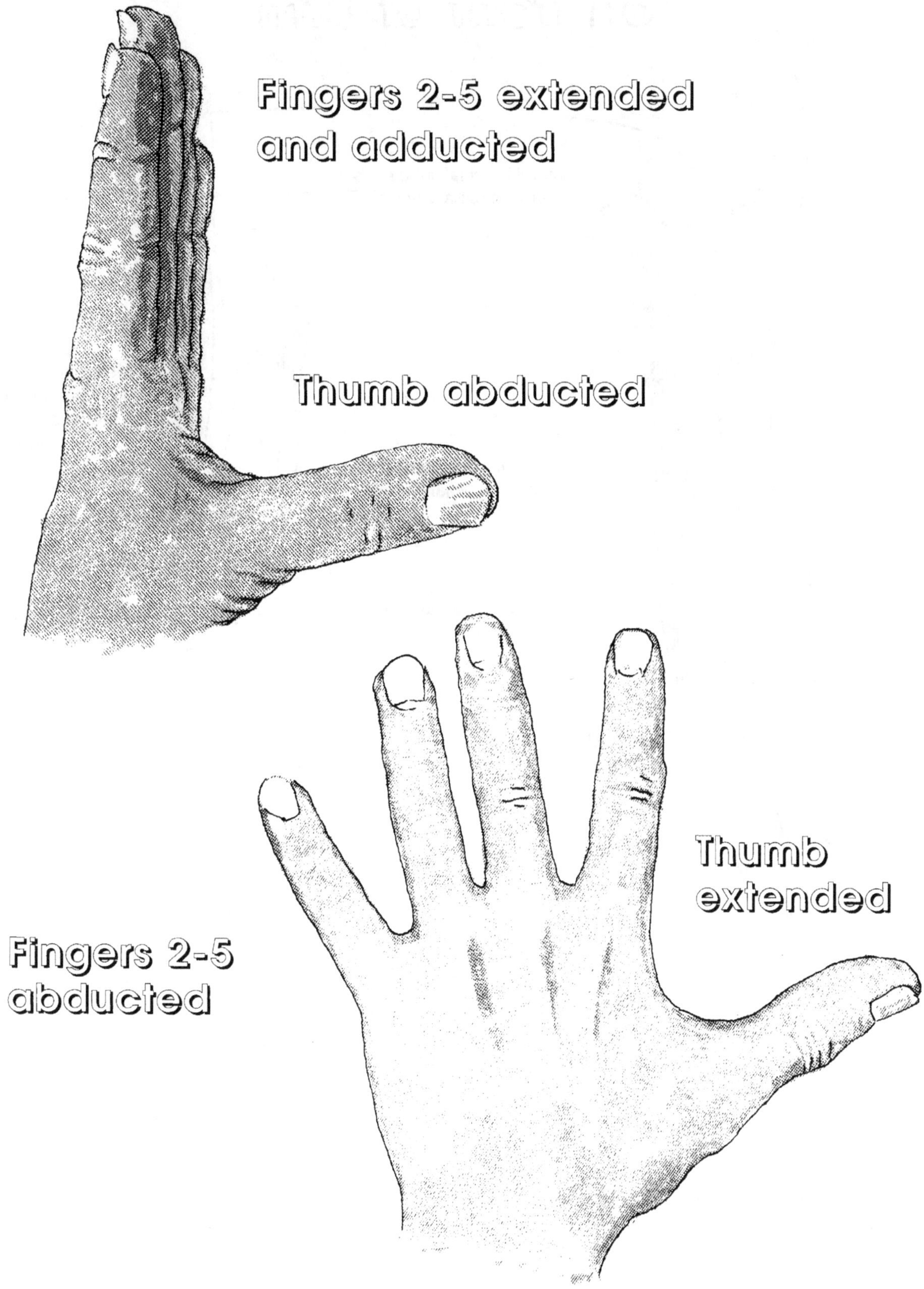

UL-58 Cutaneous nerve distribution on front of arm

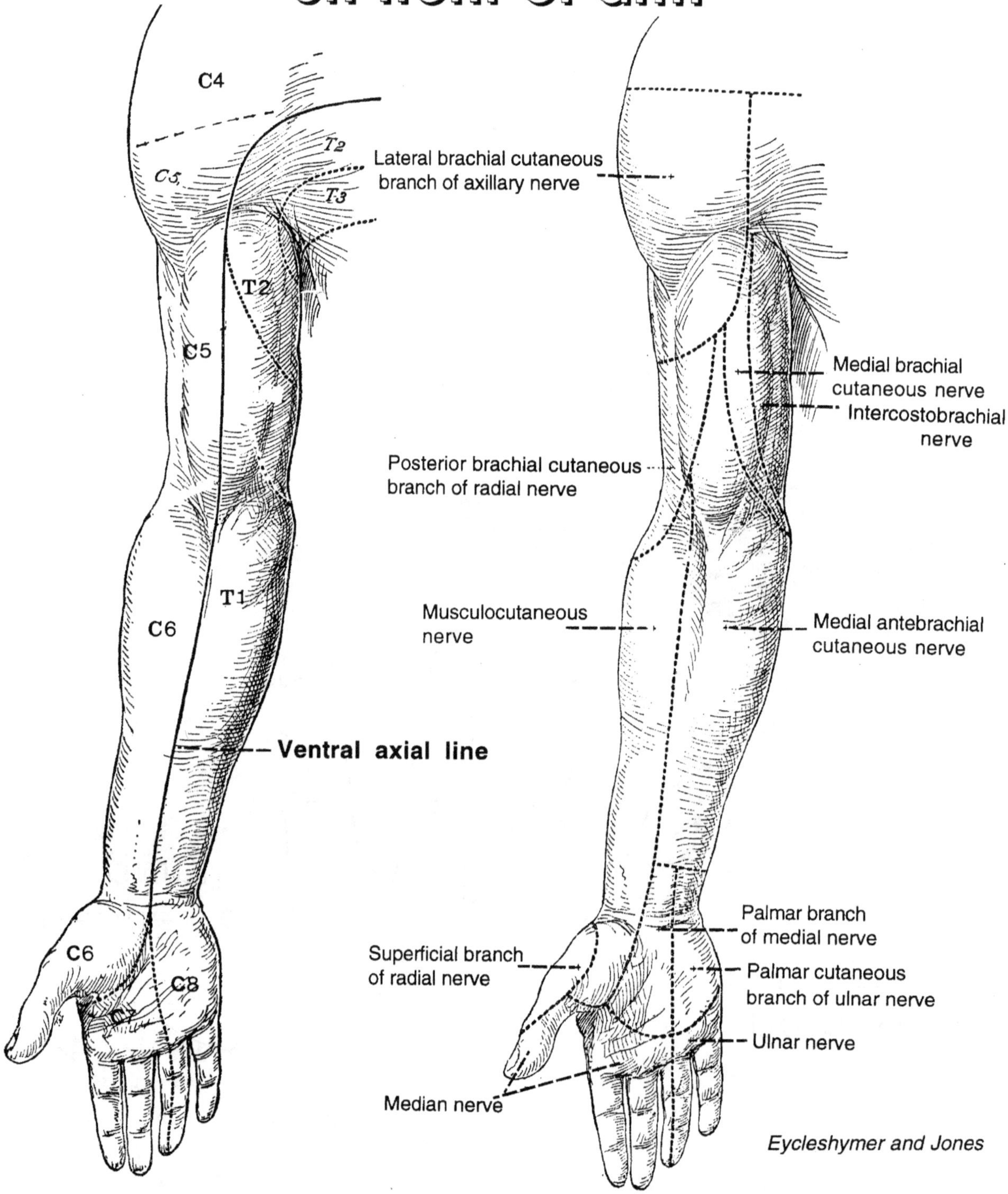

The figure on the left shows the segmental cutaneous distribution of the **principal** cervical (C) and thoracic (T) spinal nerves to the skin of the anterior arm. There is considerable overlap from adjacent spinal nerves both above and below the indicated nerve level. However, there is very little overlap of the ventral axial line. The figure on the right shows the areas of distribution of the cutaneous nerves.

UL-59 Distribution of cutaneous nerves on back of upper limb

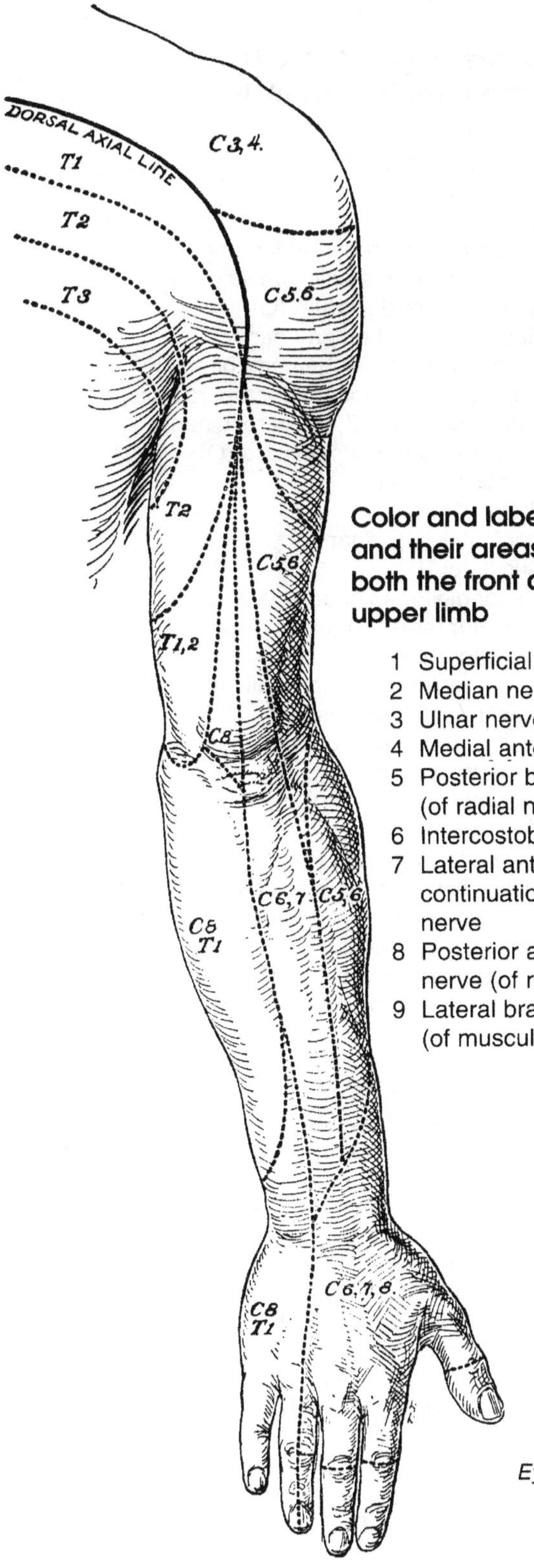

Color and label the nerves and their areas of distribution on both the front and back of the upper limb

1. Superficial branch of radial nerve
2. Median nerve
3. Ulnar nerve
4. Medial antebrachial cutaneous nerve
5. Posterior brachial cutaneous nerve (of radial nerve)
6. Intercostobrachial nerve
7. Lateral antebrachial cutaneous nerve; continuation of musculocutaneous nerve
8. Posterior antebrachial cutaneous nerve (of radial nerve)
9. Lateral brachial cutaneous nerve (of musculocutaneous nerve)

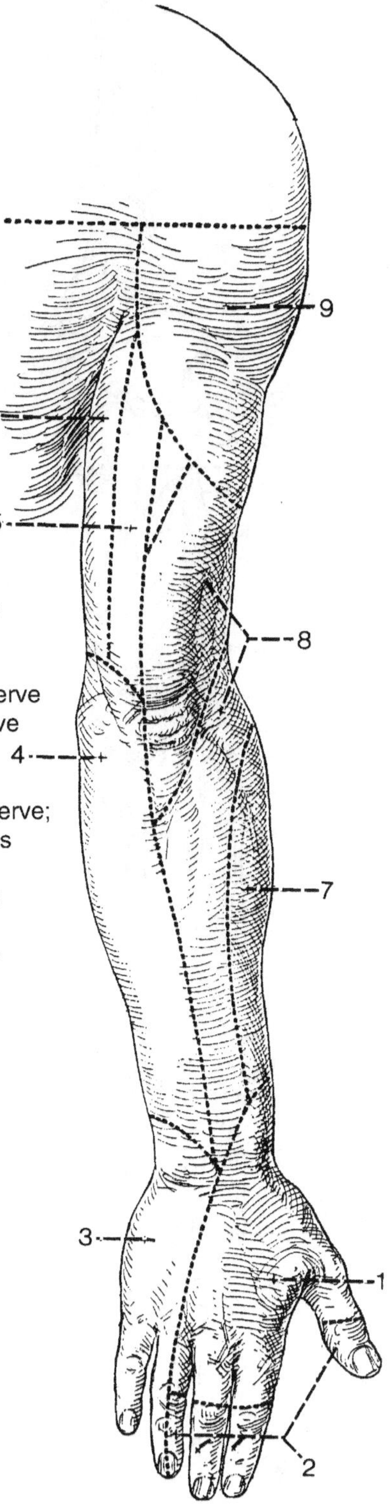

Eycleshymer and Jones

UL-60 Muscle attachments of the anterior arm

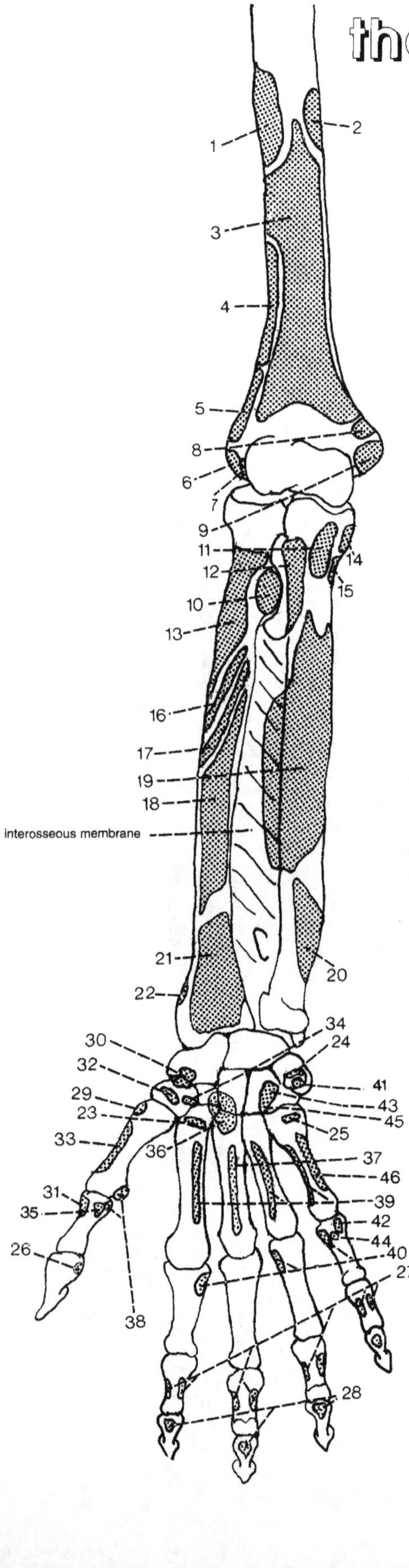

Color the origins (O) RED and the insertions (I) BLUE

1 Deltoid (I)
2 Coracobrachialis (I)
3 Brachialis (O)
4 Brachioradialis (O)
5 Extensor carpi radialis longus (O)
6 Extensor carpi radialis brevis (O) and extensor digitorum (O)
7 Supinator (O), humeral part
8 Pronator teres (O), humeral head
9 Common origin for flexor carpi radialis, palmaris longus, flexor carpi ulnaris, flexor digitorum superficialis (O)
10 Biceps brachii (I)
11 Brachialis (I)
12 Supinator (O), ulnar part
13 Supinator (I)
14 Flexor digitorum superficialis (O), ulnar origin
15 Pronator teres (O), ulnar head
16 Pronator teres (I)
17 Flexor digitorum superficialis (O), radial origin
18 Flexor pollicis longus (O)
19 Flexor digitorum profundus (O)
20 Pronator quadratus (O)
21 Pronator quadratus (I)
22 Brachioradialis (I)
23 Flexor carpi radialis (I)
24 Flexor carpi ulnaris insertion on pisiform bone (I)
25 Flexor carpi ulnaris insertion on 5th metacarpal (I)
26 Flexor pollicis longus (I)
27 Flexor digitorum superficialis (I)
28 Flexor digitorum profundus (I)
29 Abductor pollicis longus (I)
30 Abductor pollicis brevis (O)
31 Abductor pollicis brevis (I)
32 Opponens pollicis (O)
33 Opponens pollicis (I)
34 Flexor pollicis brevis (O)
35 Flexor pollicis brevis (I)
36 Adductor pollicis (O), oblique head
37 Adductor pollicis (O), transverse head
38 Adductor pollicis (I)
39 Palmar interosseous (O)
40 Palmar interosseous (I)
41 Abductor digiti minimi (O)
42 Abductor digiti minimi (I)
43 Flexor digiti minimi brevis (O)
44 Flexor digiti minimi brevis (I)
45 Opponens digiti minimi (O)
46 Opponens digiti minimi (I)

UL-61 Muscle attachments of the posterior arm

Color the origins (O) RED and the insertions (I) BLUE

1 Sternocleidomastoid (O)
2 Pectoralis major (O)
3 Deltoid (O)
4 Trapezius (I)
5 Omohyoid (O)
6 Supraspinatus (O)
7 Levator scapulae (I)
8 Rhomboid minor (I)
9 Rhomboid major (I)
10 Infraspinatus (O)
11 Teres major (O)
12 Teres minor (O)
13 Deltoid (I)
14 Infraspinatus (I)
15 Teres minor (I)
16 Triceps brachii lateral head (O)
17 Triceps brachii long head (O)
18 Triceps brachii medial head (O)
19 Anconeus (O)
20 Flexor carpi ulnaris (O)
21 Triceps brachii (I); all three heads
22 Anconeus (I)
23 Flexor digitorum superficialis (O)
24 Flexor digitorum profundus (O)
25 Supinator (O)
26 Abductor pollicis longus (O)
27 Extensor pollicis longus (O)
28 Extensor indicis (O)
29 Supinator (I)
30 Pronator teres (I)
31 Extensor pollicis brevis (I)
32 Common aponeurosis for origin of extensor carpi ulnaris, flexor carpi ulnaris, flexor digitorum profundus
33 Extensor carpi ulnaris (I)
34 Extensor carpi radialis longus (I)
35 Extensor carpi radialis brevis (I)
36 First dorsal interosseous (O)
37 Second dorsal interosseous (O)
38 Third dorsal interosseous (O)
39 Fourth dorsal interosseous (O)
40 Extensor pollicis brevis (I)
41 Extensor pollicis longus (I)
42 First dorsal interosseous (I)
43 Second dorsal interosseous (I)
44 Third dorsal interosseous (I)
45 Fourth dorsal interosseous (I)
46 Extensor digitorum (I)
47 Extensor indicis (I) *(common insertion)*
48 Extensor digiti minimi *(common insertion)*

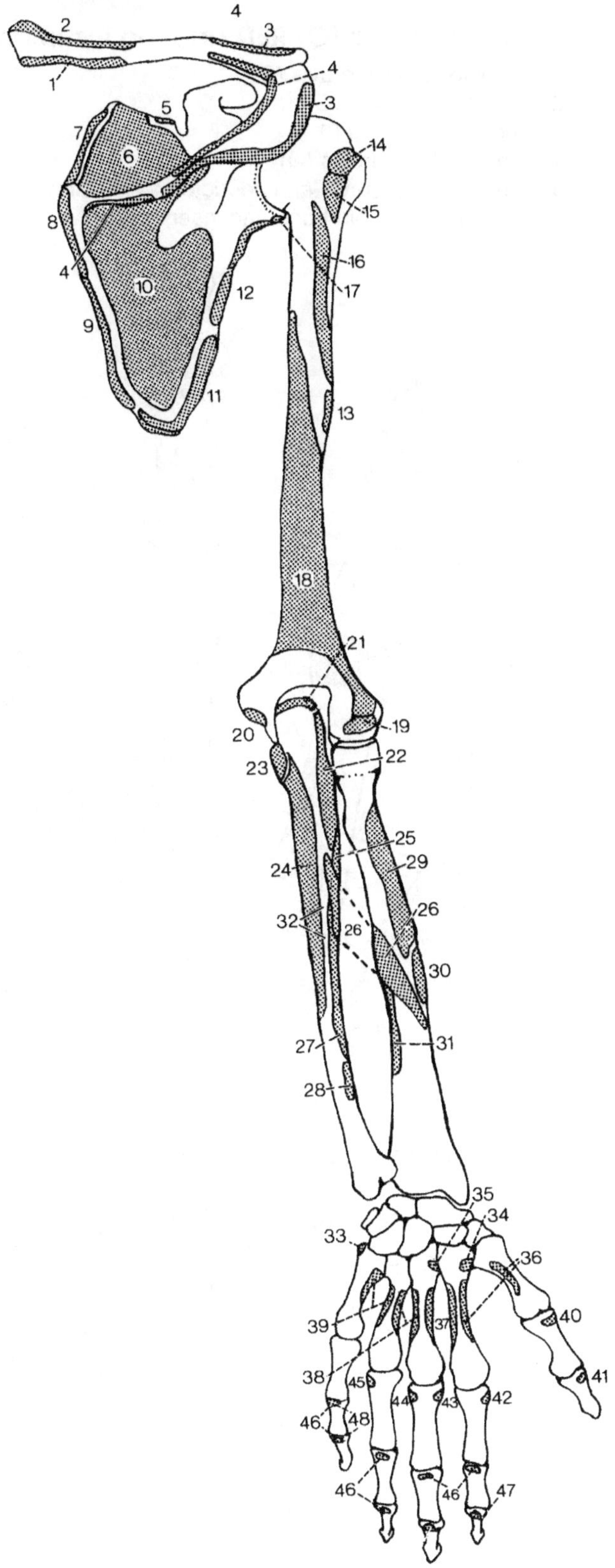

UL-62 Muscle attachments on the anterior hand

Color the origins (O) RED and the insertions (I) BLUE

1 Adductor pollicis brevis (O)
2 Opponens pollicis (O)
3 Opponens pollicis (I)
4 Flexor pollicis brevis (O)
5 Flexor pollicis brevis and adductor pollicis brevis common sesamoid bone and insertion (I)

6 Adductor pollicis *(oblique head)* (O)
7 Adductor pollicis *(transverse head)* (O)
8 Adductor pollicis sesamoid bone and insertion (I)
9 Dorsal interosseous (1,2,3,4) (O)
10 Dorsal interosseous (1,2,3,4) inserts on "hood" of extensor tendons (I)
11 Palmar (ventral) interosseous (1,2,3) (O)
12 Palmar (ventral) interosseous (1,2,3) (I)
13 Flexor digiti minimi (O) and pisohamate ligament
14 Abductor digiti minimi (O)
15 Opponens digiti minimi (O)
16 Opponens digiti minimi (I)
17 Abductor digiti minimi (I)
18 Flexor digiti minimi (I)

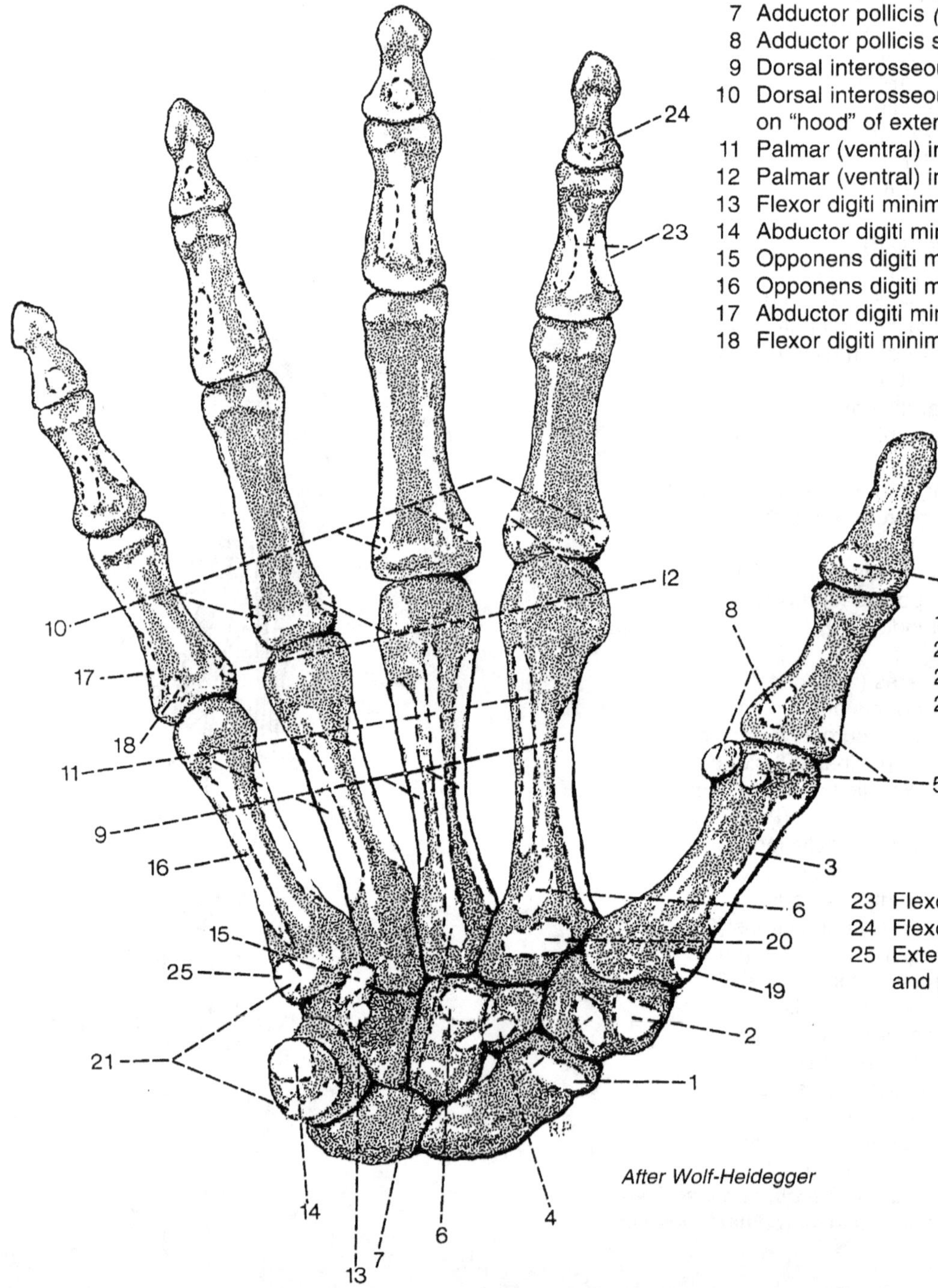

19 Abductor pollicis longus (I)
20 Flexor carpi radialis (I)
21 Flexor carpi ulnaris (I)
22 Flexor pollicis longus (I)

23 Flexor digitorum superficialis (I)
24 Flexor digitorum profundus (I)
25 Extensor carpi ulnaris (I) and pisometacarpal ligament

After Wolf-Heidegger

UL-63 Frontal (coronal) section of the right wrist and hand

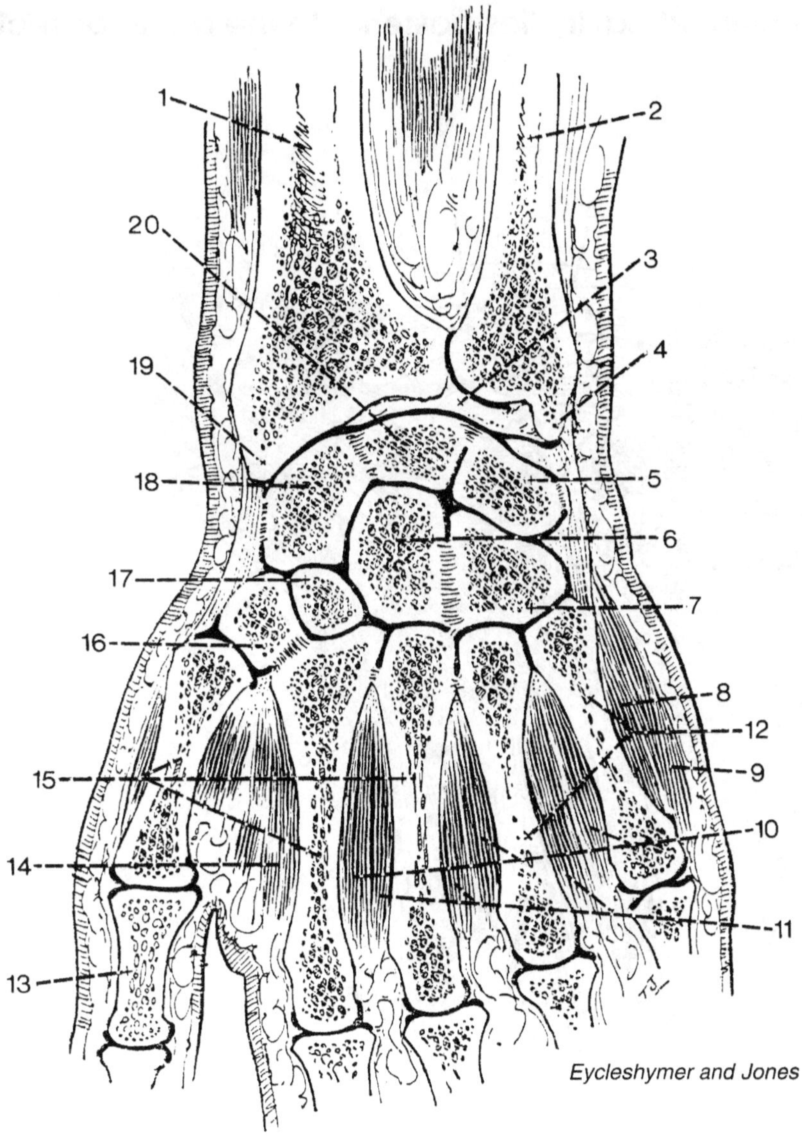

Eycleshymer and Jones

Color and label

1 Radius
2 Ulna
3 Articular disk
4 Styloid process of ulna
5 Triquetral bone (plane of section does not pass through pisiform)
6 Capitate bone
7 Hamate bone
8 Opponens digiti muscle
9 Abductor digiti minimi muscle
10 Palmar interosseous muscles
11 Dorsal interosseous muscles
12 Fourth and fifth metacarpal bones
13 Proximal phalanx of thumb
14 First dorsal interosseous muscle
15 First, second, and third metacarpal bones
16 Trapezium bone (old name, greater multangular)
17 Trapezoid bone (old name, lesser multangular)
18 Scaphoid bone (old name, navicular)
19 Styloid process of radius
20 Lunate bone

UL-64 Coronal section of the right shoulder

(The glenoid cavity lies posterior to the plane of section)

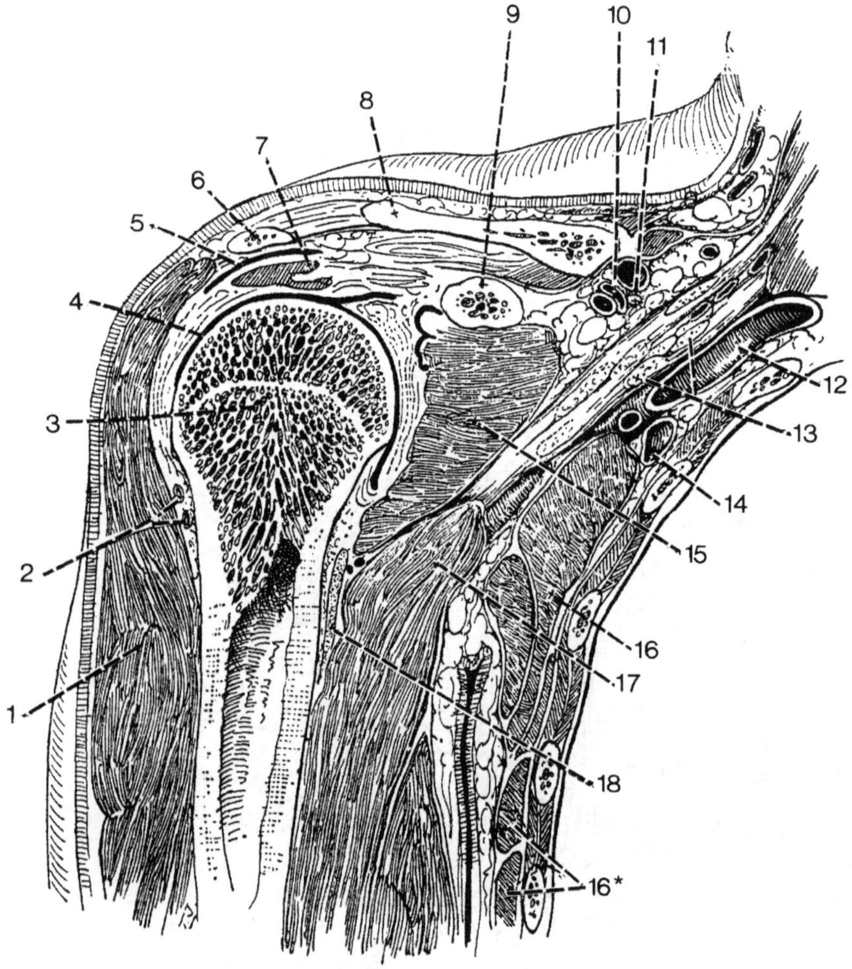

Color and label

1 Deltoid muscle
2 Posterior circumflex humeral artery and vein
3 Head of humerus
4 Articular cavity
5 Bursa
6 Acromion
7 Supraspinatus muscle
8 Clavicle
9 Coracoid process
10 Transverse scapular artery
11 Suprascapular nerve
12 Subclavian artery
13 Brachial plexus
14 Subclavian vein
15 Subscapular muscle
16 Serratus anterior muscle (*digitations; part of origin)
17 Triceps brachii muscle (long head)
18 Tendon of latissimus dorsi

UL-65 Ligaments of right shoulder joint

Anterior view

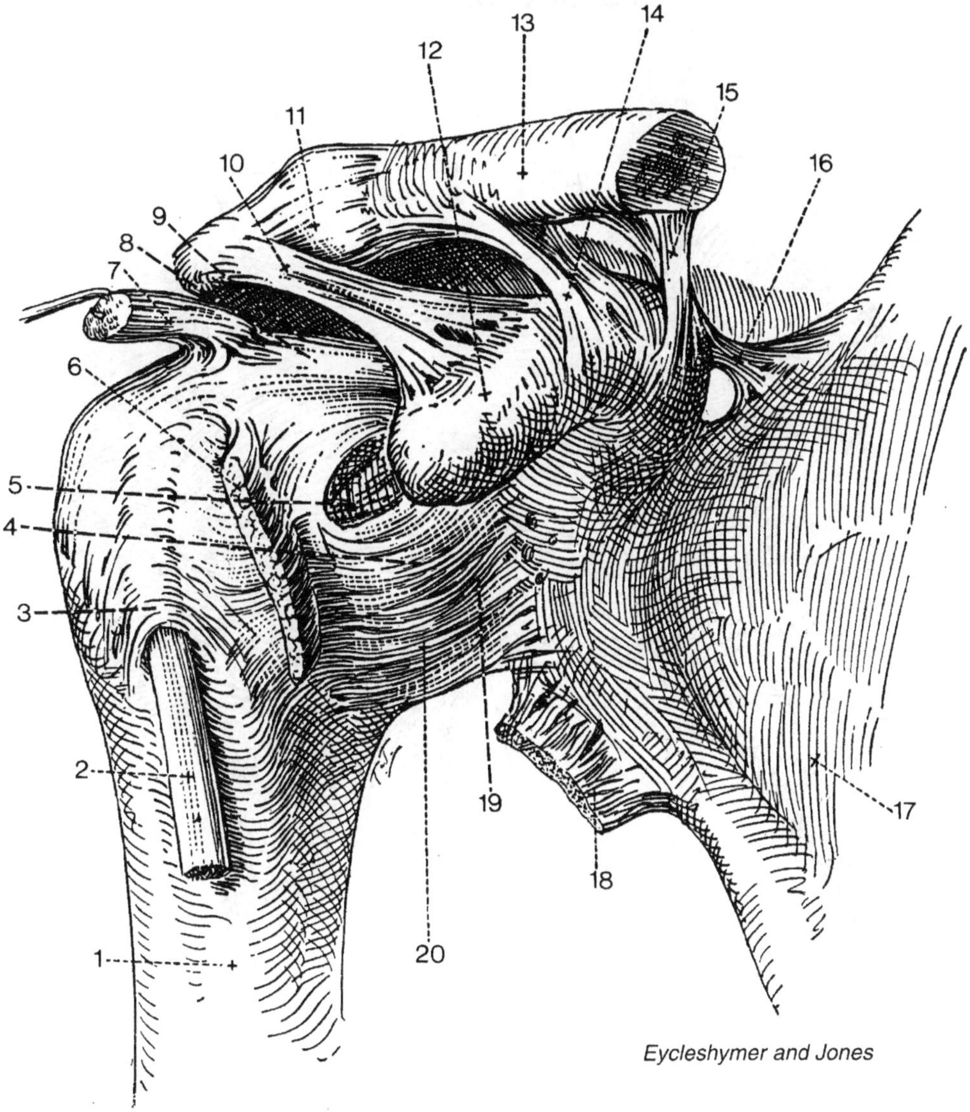

Color and label

1 Humerus
2 Biceps brachii (long head, tendon)
3 Transverse humeral ligament
4 Middle glenohumeral ligament
5 Opening of subscapular bursa
6 Subscapularis muscle
7 Supraspinatus muscle (tendon, cut and pulled laterally)
8 Superior glenohumeral ligament
9 Coracohumeral ligament
10 Coracoacromial ligament
11 Acromioclavicular ligament
12 Coracoid process
13 Clavicle
14 Trapezoid ligament
15 Conoid ligament
16 Superior transverse scapular ligament
17 Scapula
18 Triceps brachii (long head)
19 Inferior glenohumeral ligament
20 Fibrous capsule of shoulder joint

UL-66 Ligaments of the right shoulder joint

Posterior view

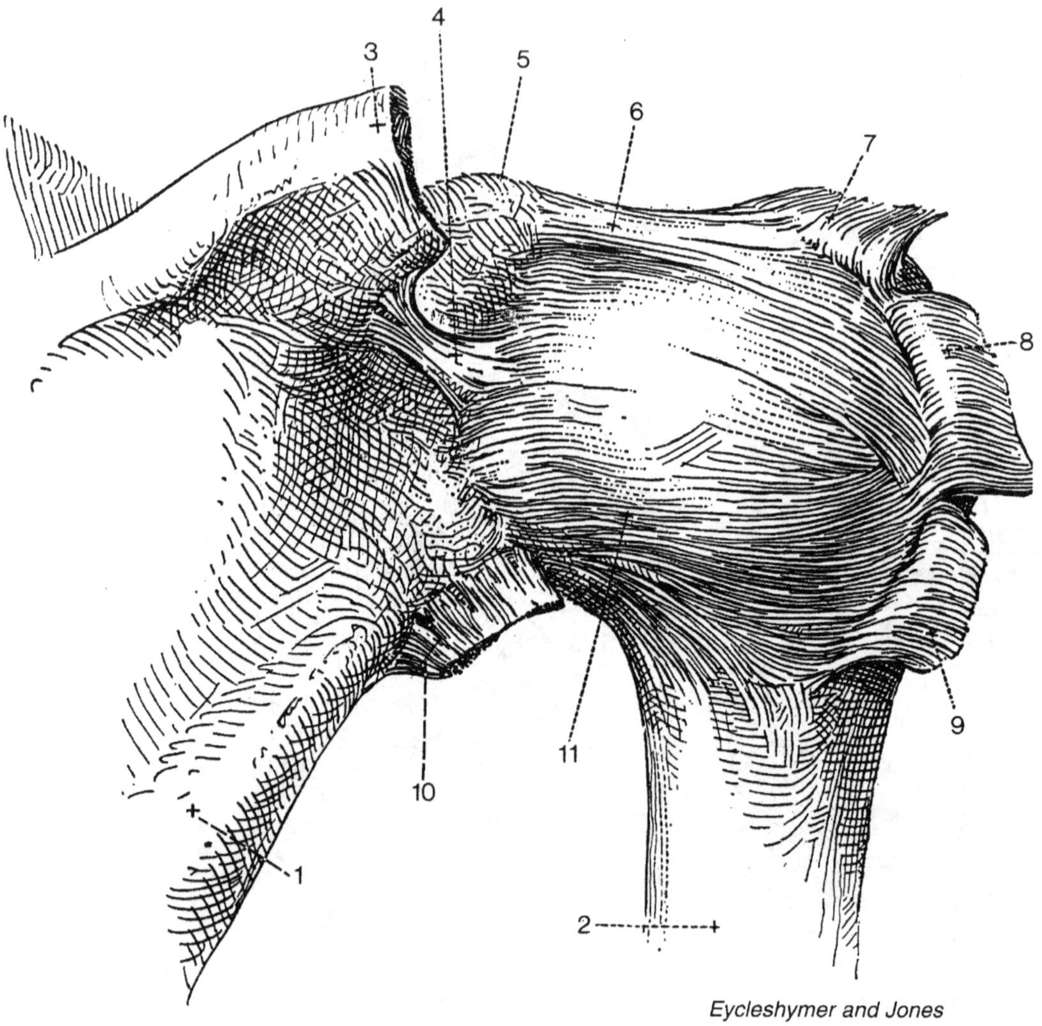

Eycleshymer and Jones

Color and label

1 Scapula (lateral part)
2 Humerus
3 Spine of scapula (acromion has been cut off)
4 Inferior transverse scapular ligament
5 Coracoid process
6 Coracohumeral ligament
7 Supraspinatus muscle (cut and reflected)*
8 Infraspinatus muscle (cut and reflected)*
9 Teres minor muscle (cut and reflected)*
10 Long head of triceps brachii (cut)
11 Articular capsule

*These three muscles plus the **subscapularis** make up the **rotator cuff.**

UL-67 Ligaments of the right elbow

Viewed from the ulnar side

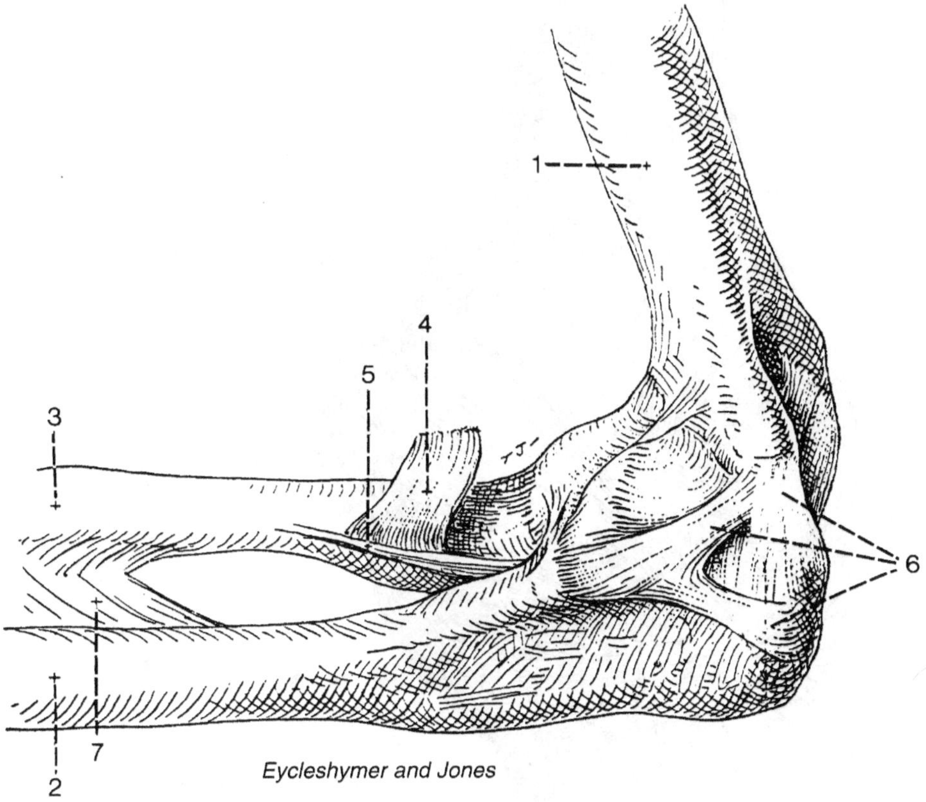

Eycleshymer and Jones

Color and label

1 Humerus
2 Ulna
3 Radius (forearm is supinated)
4 Tendon of biceps brachii inserting on radial tuberosity
5 Oblique cord
6 Ulnar collateral ligament
7 Interosseous membrane

UL-68 Ligaments of the right elbow

Anterior aspect

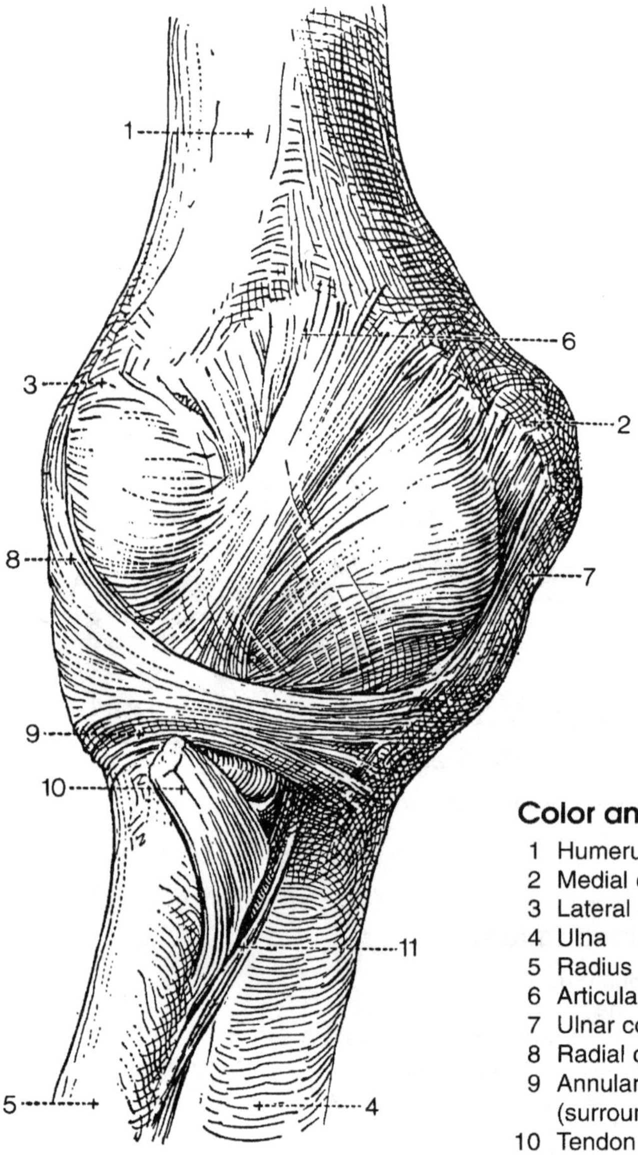

Eycleshymer and Jones

Color and label

1 Humerus
2 Medial epicondyle
3 Lateral epicondyle
4 Ulna
5 Radius
6 Articular capsule
7 Ulnar collateral ligament
8 Radial collateral ligament
9 Annular ligament of radius (surrounds head of radius)
10 Tendon of biceps brachii (cut)
11 Oblique cord

UL-69 Sagittal section of right elbow

Viewed from the radial side

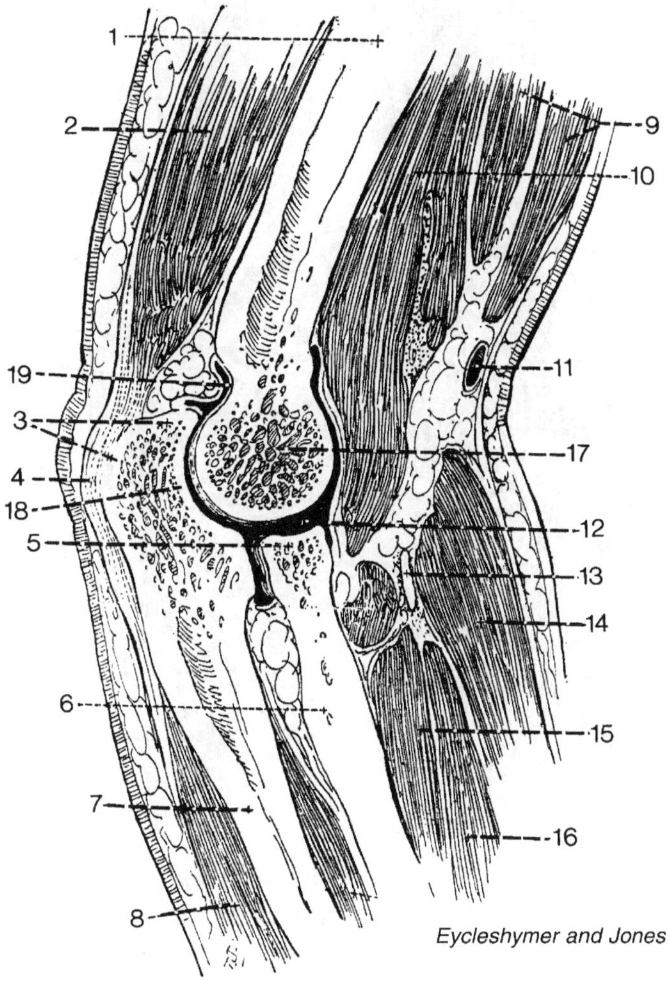

Eycleshymer and Jones

Color and label

1 Humerus
2 Triceps brachii muscle
3 Olecranon of ulna
4 Tendon of triceps brachii insertion on olecranon
5 Head of radius
6 Radius
7 Ulna
8 Flexor digitorum profundus muscle
9 Biceps brachii muscle
10 Brachilais muscle
11 Cephalic vein
12 Joint cavity
13 Radial nerve
14 Brachioradialis muscle
15 Supinator muscle
16 Extensor carpi radialis brevis muscle
17 Trochlea of humerus
18 Trochlear notch of ulna
19 Olecranon fossa of humerus

UL-70 Frontal section of right elbow

Viewed from the front

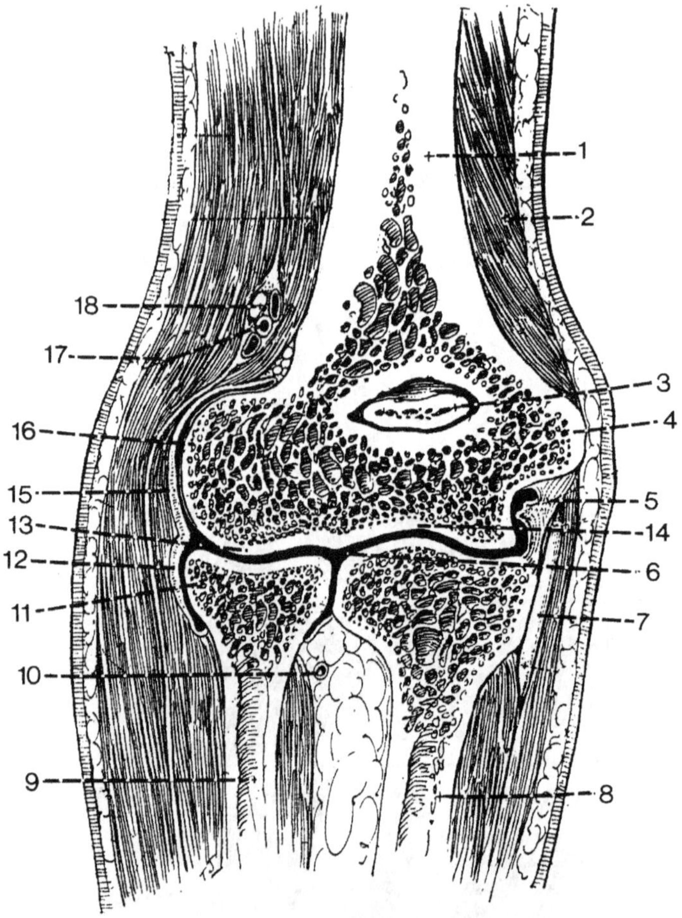

Elbow is extended so that olecranon lies in olecranon fossa of humerus

Color and label

1 Humerus
2 Brachialis muscle
3 Olecranon of ulna (in olecranon fossa of humerus; tip of the trochlear notch; cut)
4 Medial epicondyle of humerus
5 Articular capsule (internal to ulnar collateral ligament)
6 Articular cavity (joint cavity)
7 Ulnar nerve
8 Ulna
9 Radius
10 Common interosseous artery (branch of ulnar artery)
11 Head of radius
12 Anular ligament of radius
13 Capitulum of humerus
14 Trochlea of humerus
15 Radial collateral ligament
16 Lateral epicondyle of humerus
17 Radial collateral artery (branch of deep brachial artery) and accompanying veins
18 Radial nerve

Eycleshymer and Jones with modification

UL-71 Ligaments of the right wrist

Palmar aspect

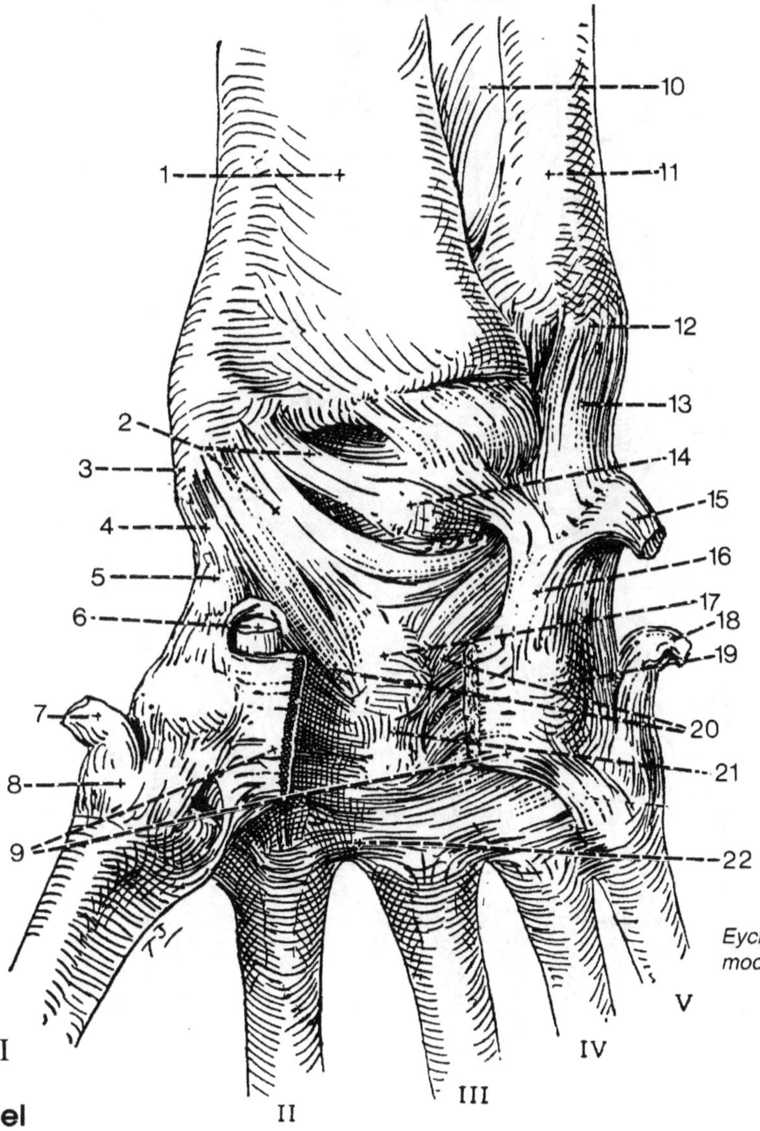

Eycleshymer and Jones with modification

Color and label

1 Radius
2 Palmar radiocarpal ligament
3 Styloid process of radius
4 Radial collateral carpal ligament
5 Tubercle of trapezoid bone
6 Tendon of flexor carpi radialis insertion onto base of second metacarpal
7 Tendon of abductor pollicis longus insertion onto lateral side of base of first metacarpal and trapezium
8 Carpometacarpal joint of thumb
9 Flexor retinaculum (cut) (old name, transverse carpal ligament)
10 Interosseous membrane
11 Ulna
12 Styloid process of ulna
13 Ulnar carpal collateral ligament
14 Lunate bone
15 Tendon of flexor carpi ulnaris (cut) insertion onto the pisiform and by the pisohamate ligament and pisometacarpal ligament to the hamate bone and the base of the fifth metacarpal, respectively
16 Pisohamate ligament
17 Capitate bone
18 Tendon of extensor carpi ulnaris insertion on medial side of base of fifth metacarpal
19 Hamulus of hamate bone
20 Carpal radiating ligament
21 Palmar carpometacarpal ligament
22 Palmar (inter) metacarpal ligaments

UL-72 Ligaments of the right wrist

Posterior aspect

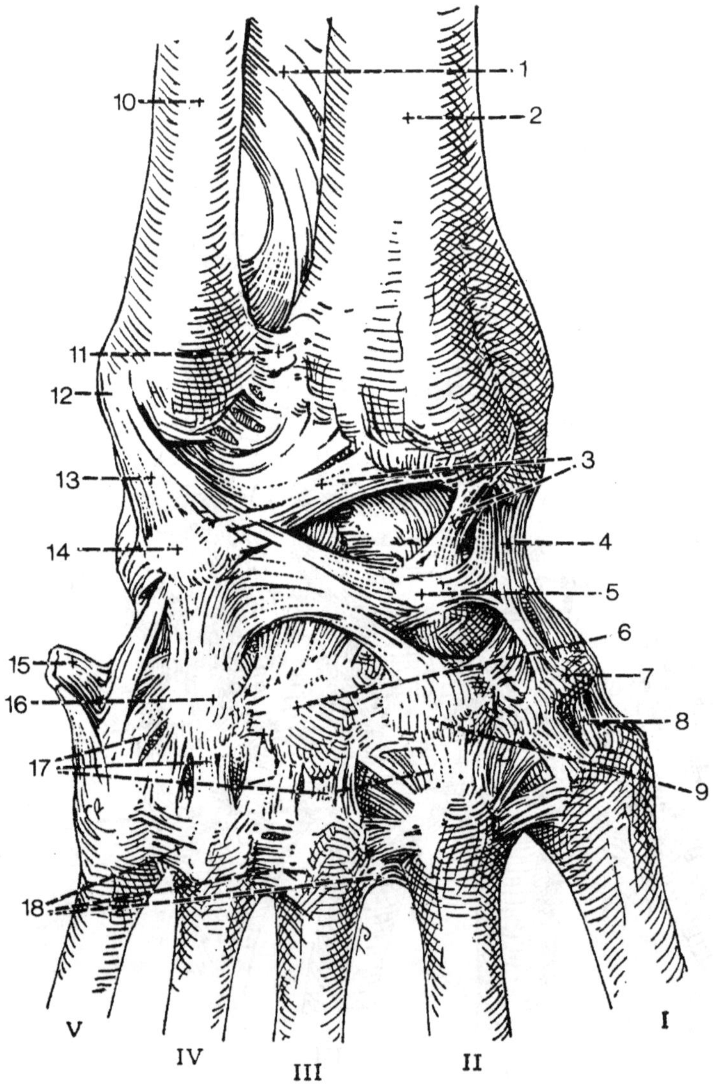

Metacarpal bones

Color and label

1 Antebrachial (forearm) interosseous membrane
2 Radius
3 Dorsal radiocarpal ligament
4 Radial carpal collateral ligament
5 Scaphoid bone (old name, navicular)
6 Capitate bone
7 Trapezium bone (old name, greater multangular)
8 Carpometacarpal joint of thumb (pollicis)
9 Trapezoid bone (old name, lesser multangular)
10 Ulna
11 Distal radial-ulnar joint (articulation)
12 Styloid process of ulna
13 Ulnar carpal collateral ligament
14 Triquetral bone
15 Tendon (cut) of extensor carpi ulnaris (insertion on base of fifth metacarpal)
16 Hamate bone
17 Dorsal carpometacarpal ligaments
18 Dorsal (inter) metacarpal (bases) ligaments

Eycleshymer and Jones

UL-73 Hand dissection

Oblique view; palmar aspect
Skin and palmar aponeurosis removed

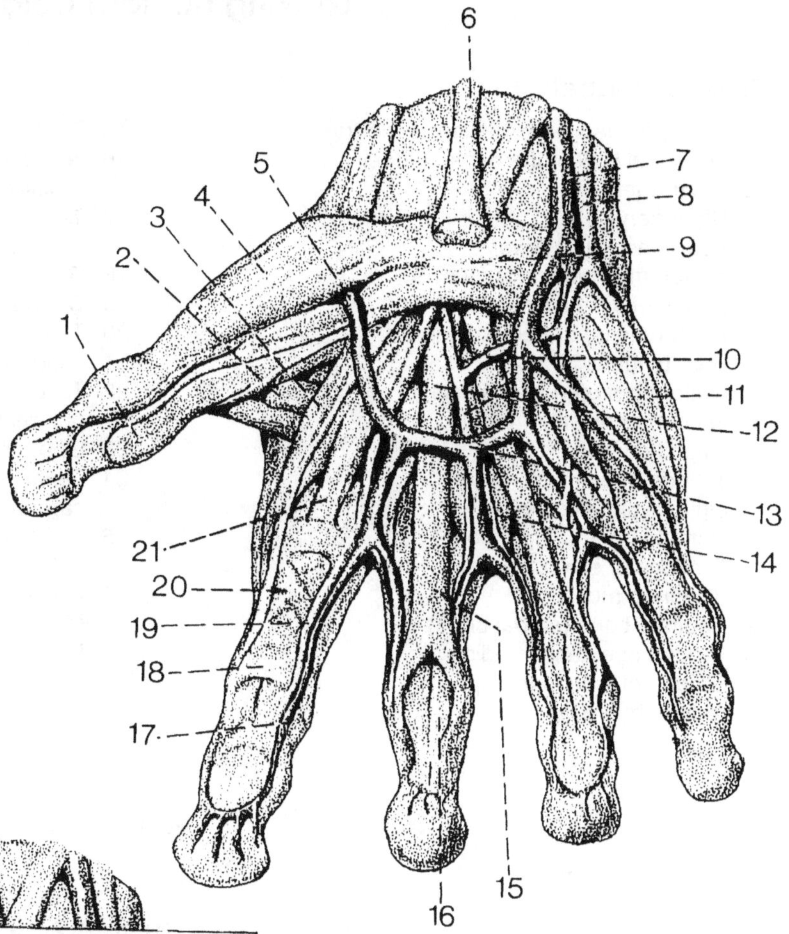

Color and label

1 Tendon of flexor pollicis longus muscle
2 Adductor pollicis muscle
3 First lumbrical muscle
4 Abductor pollicis muscle
5 Radial artery
6 Cut end of tendon of palmaris longus
7 Ulnar artery
8 Ulnar nerve
9 Flexor retinaculum
10 Communicating branch of ulnar nerve with median nerve
11 Hypothenar muscles
12 Common palmar digital branches of median nerve
13 Superficial palmar (arterial) arch
14 Common palmar digital nerve and artery
15 Tendon of flexor digitorum superficialis muscle to 3rd finger
16 Tendon of flexor digitorum profundus
17 Proper palmar digital artery
18 Anular fibers of fibrous tendon sheath
19 Proper palmar digital nerve
20 Cruciate fibers of fibrous tendon sheath
21 Tendon of flexor digitorum superficialis muscle

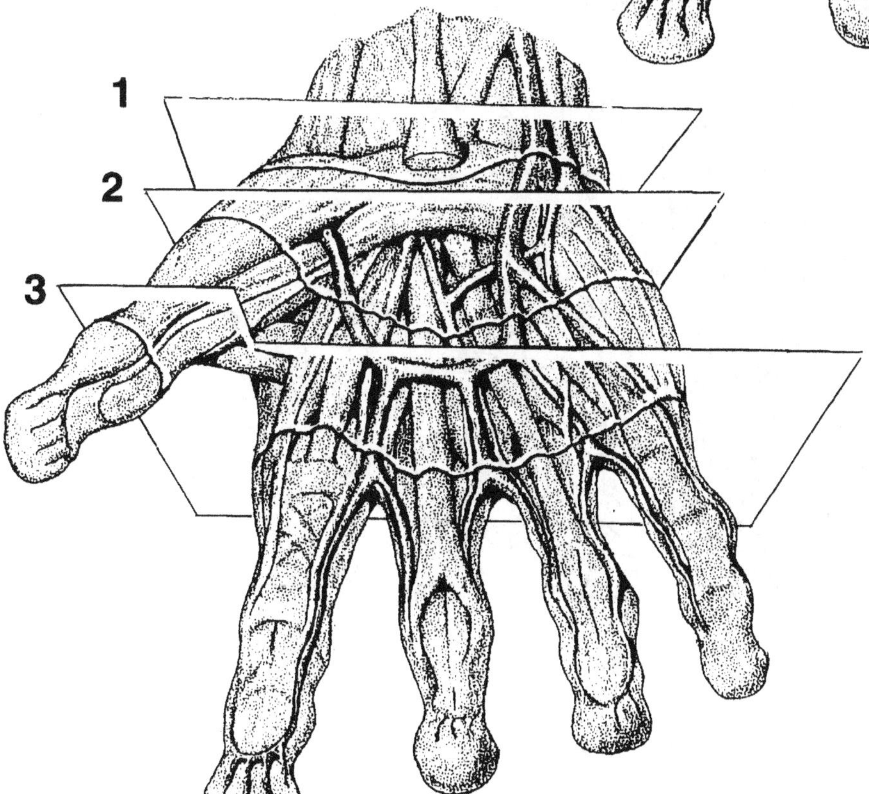

UL-74 Wrist cross section

Looking up from below

Color and label

1 Flexor retinaculum; this forms the "roof" or ventral wall of the carpal tunnel
2 Ulnar artery
3 Ulnar nerve
4 Four tendons of flexor digitorum superficialis muscle
5 Hypothenar muscles
6 Hook (uncus) of hamate bone
7 Four tendons of flexor digitorum profundus muscle
8 Tendon of extensor carpi ulnaris muscle
9 Tendon of extensor digiti minimi muscle
10 Hamate bone (carpal bone)
11 Tendons of extensor digitorum muscle
12 Capitate bone (carpal bone)
13 Tendon of extensor indicis
14 Tendon of extensor carpi radialis brevis
15 Trapezoid bone (carpal bone)
16 Tendon of extensor carpi radialis longus muscle
17 Tendon of extensor pollicis longus muscle
18 Radial artery (in "snuff box")
19 Cephalic vein
20 Trapezium (carpal bone)
21 Tendon of extensor
22 Tendon of abductor pollicis longus muscle
23 Opponens pollicis muscle
24 Tendon of flexor carpi radialis muscle
25 Tendon of flexor pollicis longus muscle
26 Abductor pollicis brevis muscle
27 Median nerve
28 Flexor pollicis brevis muscle
29 "Snuff box"

Ventral

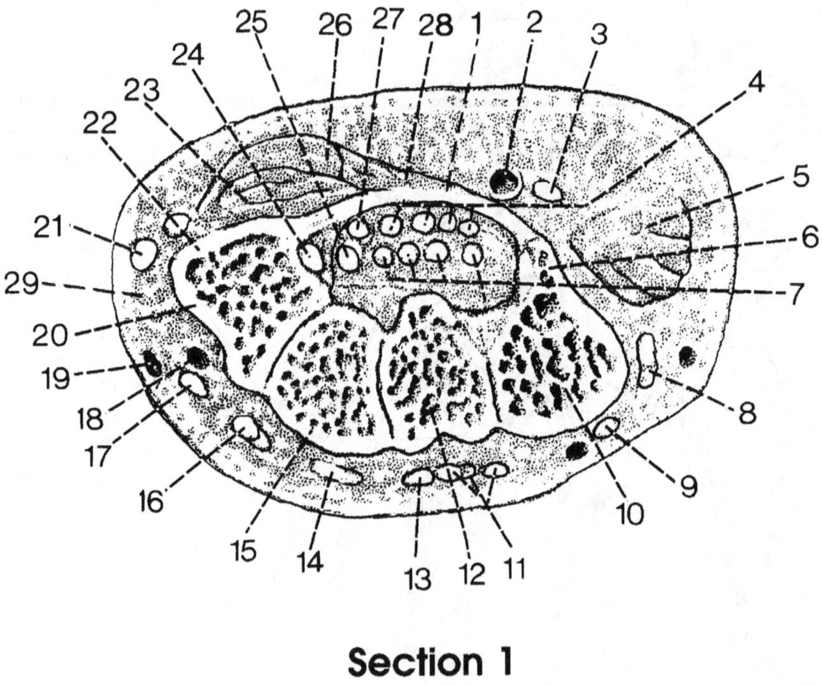

Section 1

UL-75 Hand cross section I

Looking up from below

Color and label

1 First metacarpal bone
2 Opponens pollicis muscle
3 Abductor pollicis brevis muscle
4 Tendon of flexor pollicis longus muscle
5 Flexor pollicis brevis muscle
6 Median nerve and first lumbrical muscle
7 Tendons of flexor digitorum superficialis and flexor digitorum profundus to index finger
8 Palmar aponeurosis
9 Ulnar nerve and arterial branch off superficial palmar arch
10 Superficial and deep flexor tendons to fifth finger
11 Flexor digiti minimi muscle
12 Abductor digiti minimi muscle
13 Opponens digiti minimi muscle
14 Ventral (palmer or volar) interosseous muscle
15 Fifth metacarpal bone
16 Fourth dorsal interosseous muscle
17 Tendons of superficial flexor muscle and deep (profundus) flexor muscle to fourth finger (deep tendon is surrounded by third lumbrical muscle)
18 Fourth metacarpal bone
19 Third dorsal interosseous muscle
20 Tendons of superficial and deep flexor muscles to third finger (deep tendon is surrounded by second lumbrical muscle)
21 Third metacarpal bone
22 Second dorsal interosseous muscle
23 First ventral (palmar or volar) interosseous muscle
24 Second metacarpal bone
25 First dorsal interosseous muscle
26 Adductor pollicis muscle
27 Cephalic vein
28 Radial artery
29 Tendon of extensor pollicic brevis
30 Tendon of extensor pollicis longus
31 Tendon of extensor digitorum to 4th digit

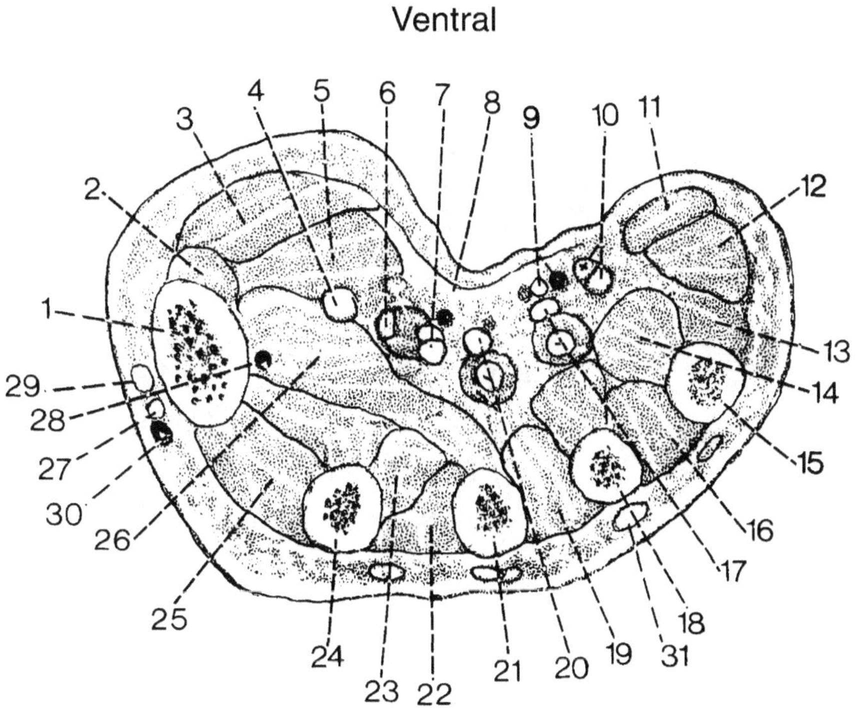

Section 2

UL-76 Hand cross section II

Looking up from below

Color and label

1 Tendon of extensor pollicis longus muscle
2 Distal phalanx of thumb
3 Tendon of flexor pollicis longus muscle
4 Superficial flexor tendons to digits 2-5
5 Deep flexor tendons to digits 2-5
6 Tendon of extensor digiti minimi
7 Extensor digitorum tendon to fifth finger
8 Fifth metacarpal
9 Extensor digitorum tendon to fourth finger
10 Fourth metacarpal bone
11 Extensor digitorum tendon to third finger
12 Extensor indicis tendon to second finger
13 Third metacarpal
14 Extensor digitorum tendon to second (index) finger
15 Second metacarpal
16 First lumbrical muscle
17 First dorsal interosseous muscle
18 Compartments for interosseous muscles
19 Neurovascular bundles to each finger

Ventral

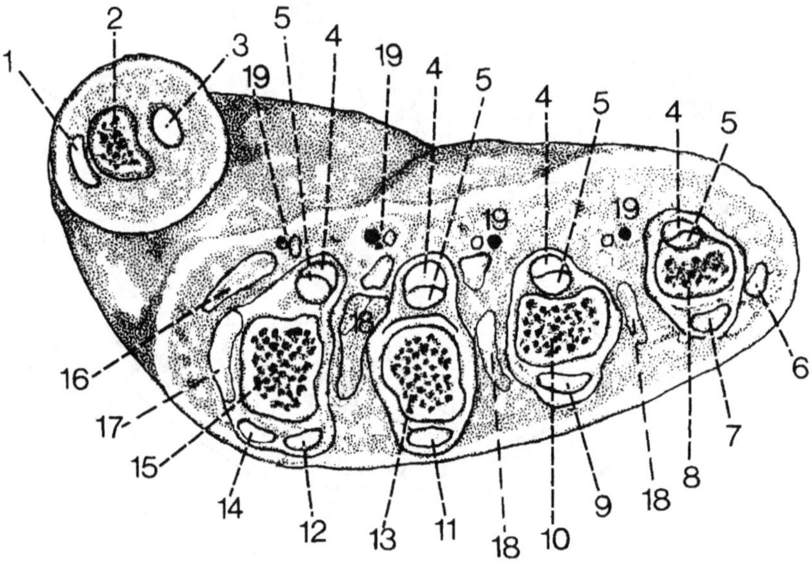

Section 3

Part V: Back

Bk-1 Superficial back muscles

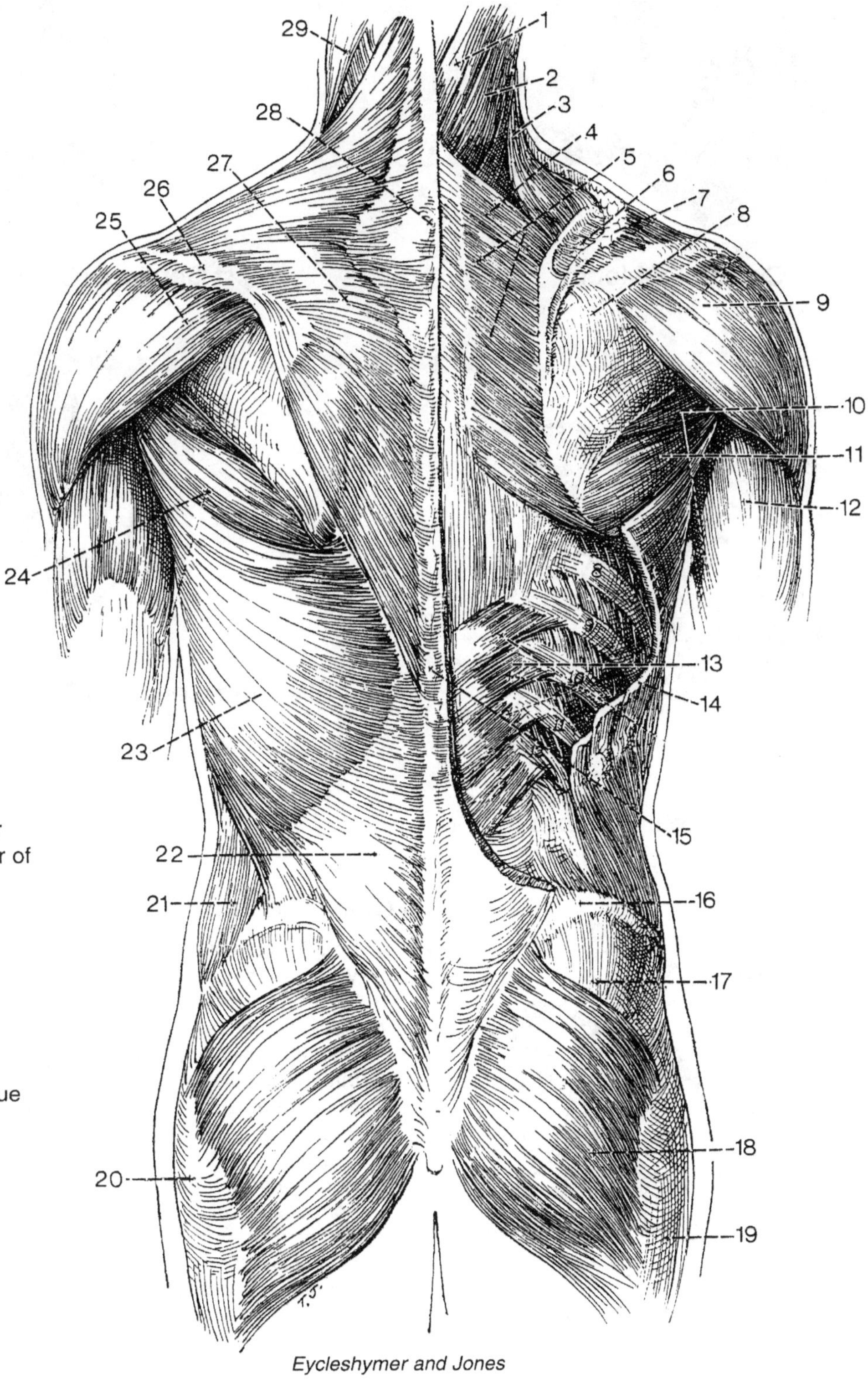

Eycleshymer and Jones

Color and label

1 Splenius capitus
2 Splenius cervicus
3 Levator scapulae
4 Rhomboid minor
5 Rhomboid major
6 Supraspinatus
7 Trapezius (cut)
8 Infraspinatus fascia
9 Deltoid
10 Teres minor
11 Teres major
12 Triceps brachii
13 Serratus posterior inferior (part of intermediate layer of back muscles)
14 Latissimus dorsi (cut)
15 12th thoracic vertebrae
16 Iliac crest
17 Lumbar trigone
18 Gluteus maximus
19 Iliotibial tract
20 Major trochanter
21 External abdominal oblique
22 Lumbodorsal fascia
23 Latissimus dorsi
24 Teres major
25 Deltoid
26 Spine of scapula
27 Trapezius
28 Spinous process of cervical vertebra C 7
29 Sternocleidomastoid

Bk-2 Typical vertebrae

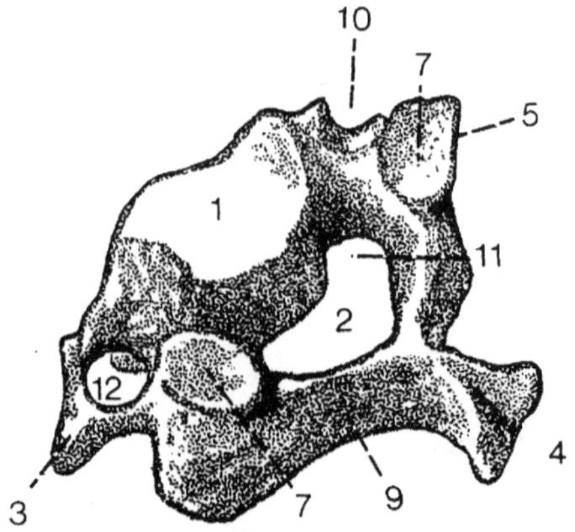

Cervical Vertebra

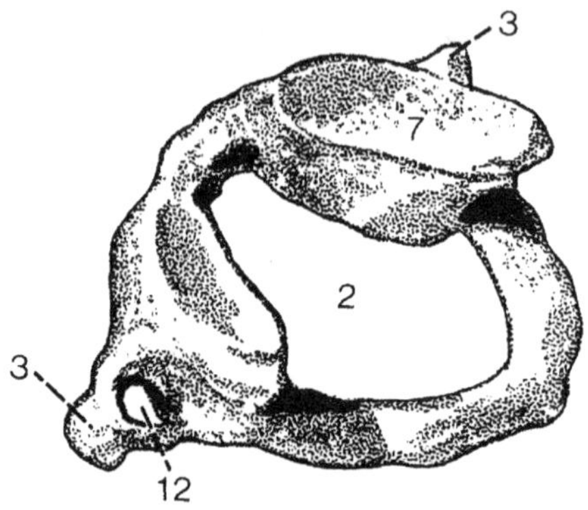

First Cervical (C1) Vertebra (Atlas)

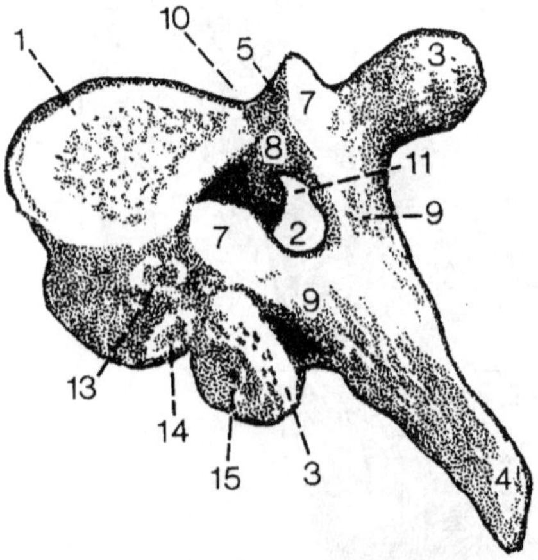

Thoracic Vertebra

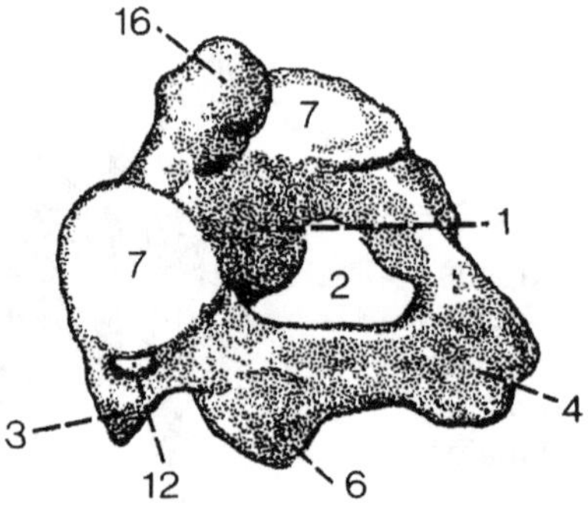

Second Cervical (C2) Vertebra (Axis)

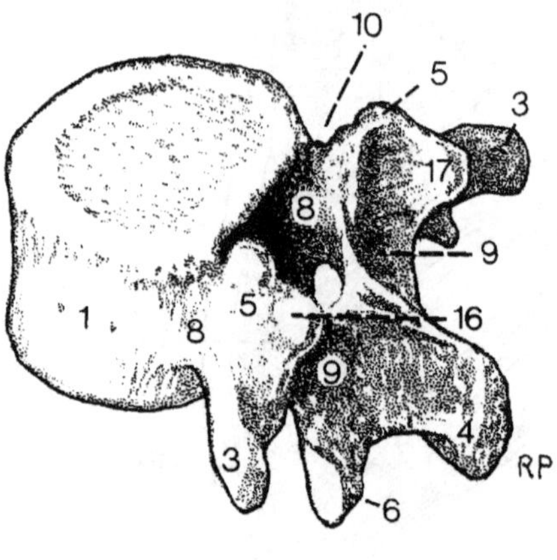

Lumbar Vertebra

Color and label

1 Body of vertebra
2 Vertebral foramen
3 Transverse process
4 Spinous process
5 Superior articular process
6 Inferior articular process
7 Superior articular facet
8 Pedicle
9 Lamina
10 Superior vertebral notch (for passage of spinal nerve)
11 Inferior vertebral notch (for passage of spinal nerve)
12 Transverse foramen (for vertebral artery) (only in cervical vertebrae)
13 Superior demifacet (for head of rib) (only in thoracic vertebrae)
14 Inferior demifacet (for head of rib) (only in thoracic vertebrae)
15 Facet on transverse process (for tubercle of rib) (only in thoracic vertebrae)
16 Mamillary process (only in lumbar vertebrae)

Bk-3 Rib-vertebra articulation

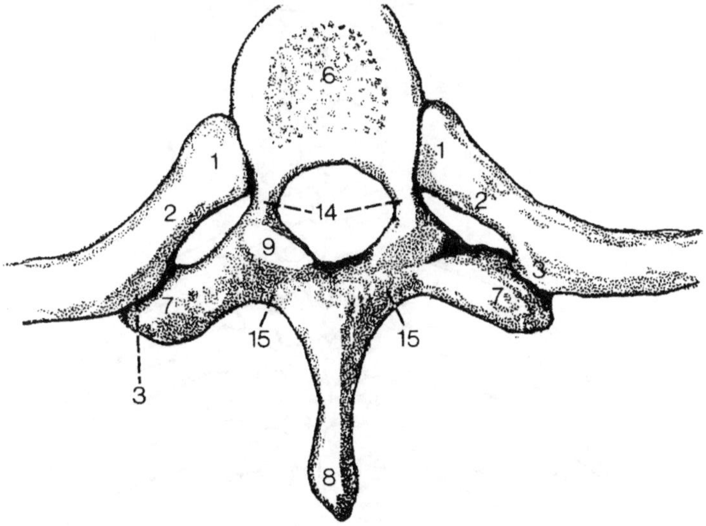

Outline of left rib superimposed on two thoracic vertebrae

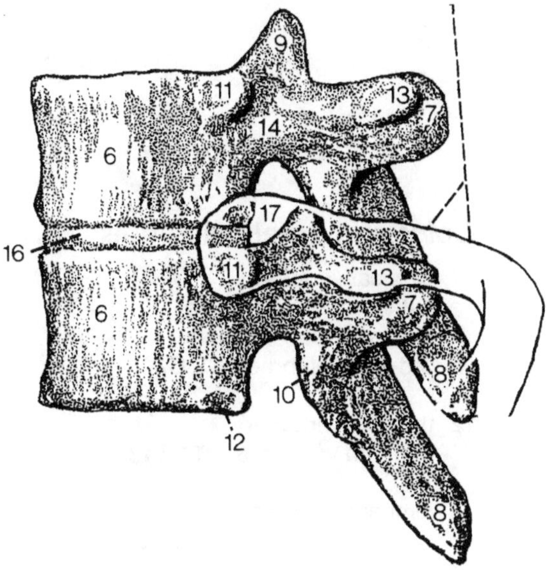

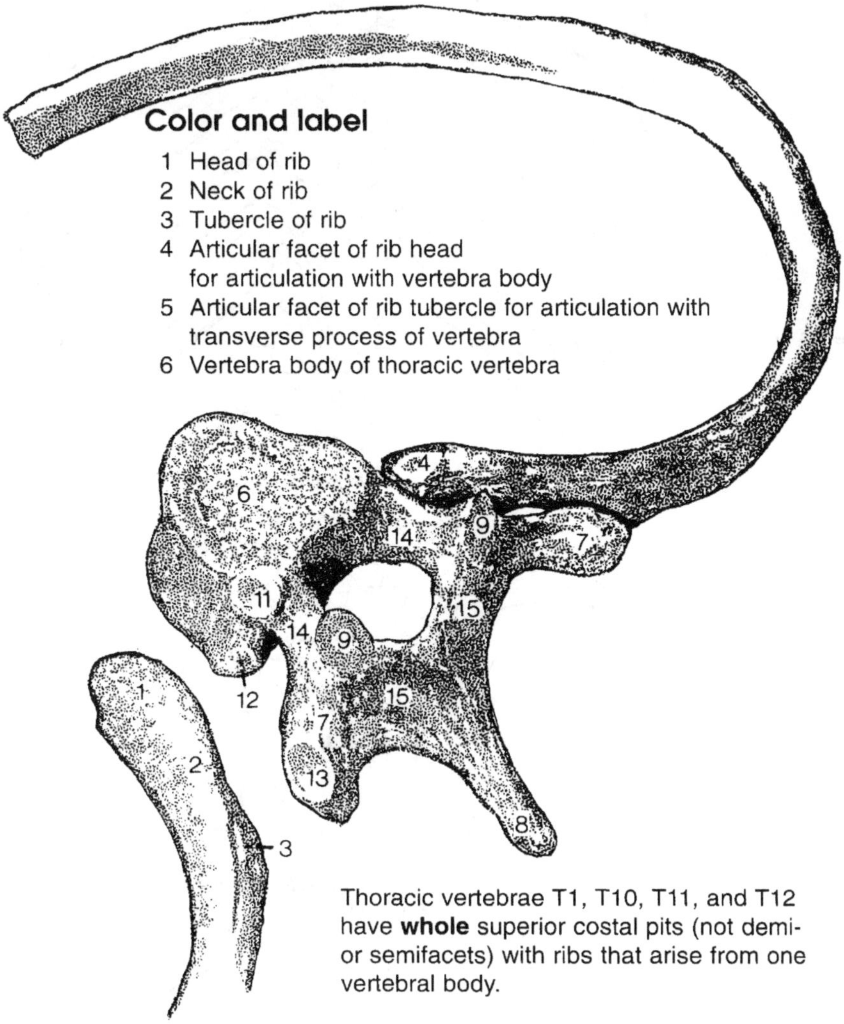

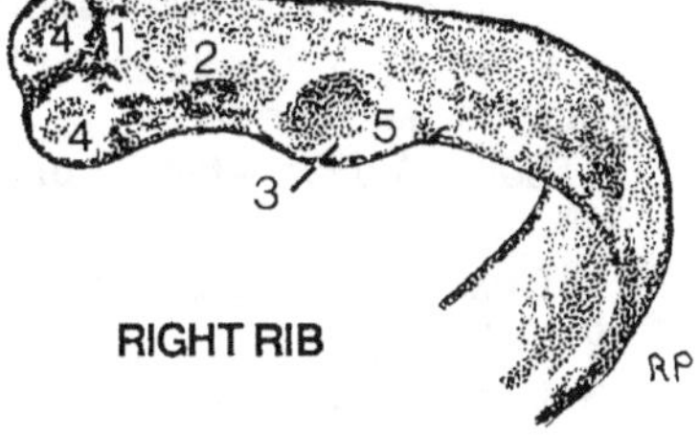

RIGHT RIB

Color and label

1 Head of rib
2 Neck of rib
3 Tubercle of rib
4 Articular facet of rib head for articulation with vertebra body
5 Articular facet of rib tubercle for articulation with transverse process of vertebra
6 Vertebra body of thoracic vertebra
7 Transverse process of vertebra
8 Spinous process
9 Superior articular process and articular surface
10 Inferior articular process and articular surface
11 Superior costal pit (or fovea) for head of rib (demifacet in vertebrae T2-T9)
12 Inferior costal pit for head of rib (demifacet in vertebrae T1-T8)
13 Transverse costal pit or articular facet for articulation with tubercle of rib
14 Pedicle of vertebral arch
15 Lamina
16 Intervertebral disk between two vertebrae bodies
17 Intervertebral foramen
18 Vertebral foramen (contains spinal cord)

Thoracic vertebrae T1, T10, T11, and T12 have **whole** superior costal pits (not demi- or semifacets) with ribs that arise from one vertebral body.

Bk-4 Vertebral column

Dorsal aspect

Color and label bold items

7 cervical vertebae
  1st vertebra - **C1, atlas**
  2nd vertebra - **C2, axis**
  3rd-7th vertebrae - **C3-C7**

12 thoracic vertebrae
  8th-19th vertebrae - **T1-T12**

5 lumbar vertebrae
  20th-24th vertebrae - **L1-L5**

5 fused sacral vertebrae
  25th-29th vertebrae - **sacrum**

3-5 coccygeal vertebrae
  30th-33rd (variable) - **coccyx**

1 Coxal bone (hip bone)
2 Ischial spine
3 Ischial tuberosity
4 Iliac crest
Sacrum + two coxal bones=bony pelvis

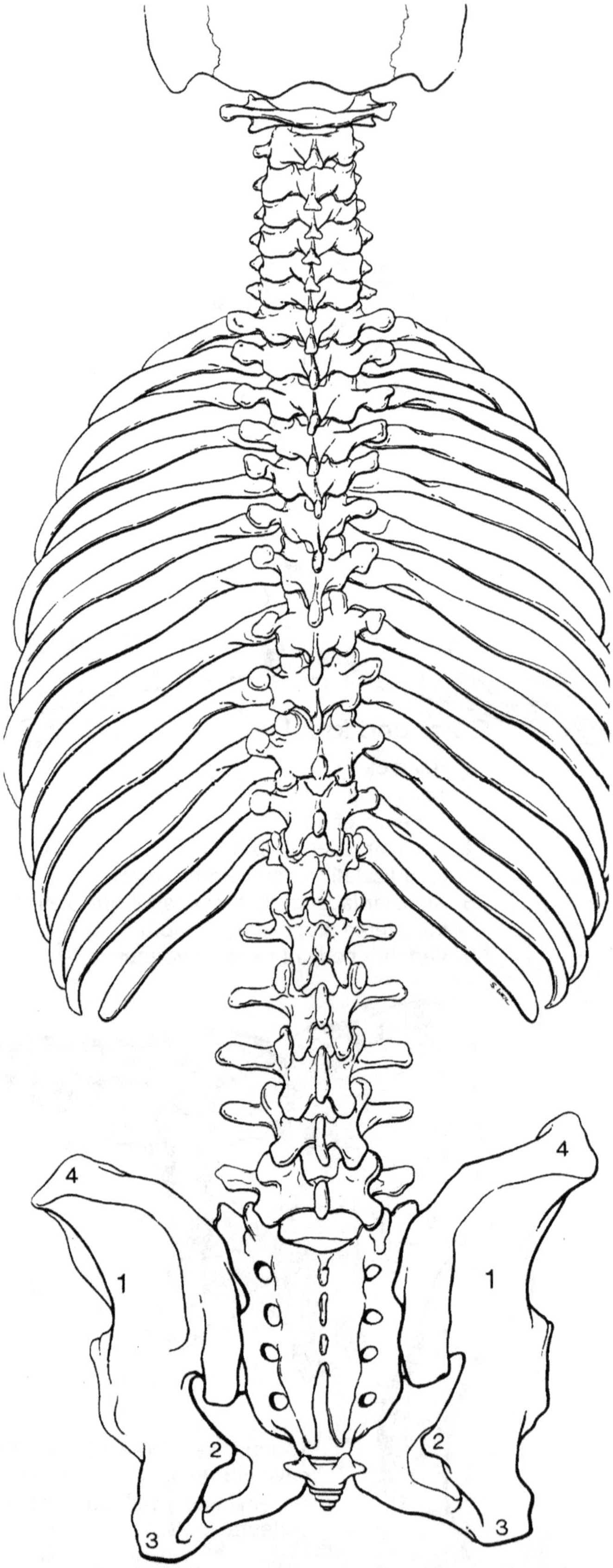

Bk-5 Back muscles I

Superficial layer

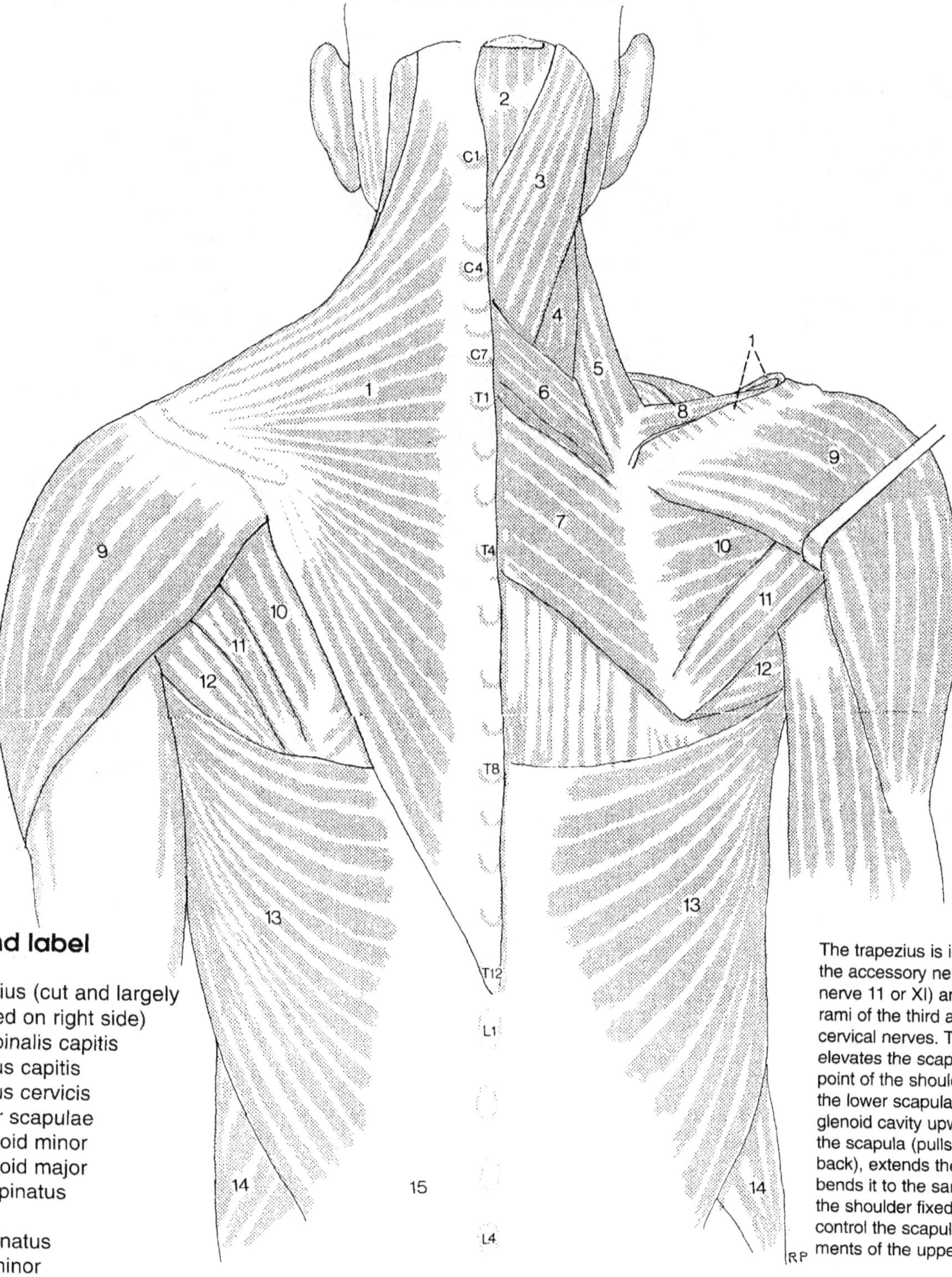

Color and label

1 Trapezius (cut and largely removed on right side)
2 Semispinalis capitis
3 Splenius capitis
4 Splenius cervicis
5 Levator scapulae
6 Rhomboid minor
7 Rhomboid major
8 Supraspinatus
9 Deltoid
10 Infraspinatus
11 Teres minor
12 Teres major
13 Latissimus dorsi
14 External abdominal oblique
15 Thoracolumbar fascia

The trapezius is innervated by the accessory nerve (cranial nerve 11 or XI) and the ventral rami of the third and fourth cervical nerves. The trapezius elevates the scapula and the point of the shoulder, helps rotate the lower scapula laterad and the glenoid cavity upward, retracts the scapula (pulls shoulder back), extends the head and bends it to the same side with the shoulder fixed, and helps to control the scapula in movements of the upper limb.

Bk-6 Back muscles II

Intermediate layers

Color and label

1 Splenius capitus
2 Semispinalis capitis
3 Splenius cervicis
4 Levator scapulae (cut on right side)
5 Serratus posterior superior
6 Rhomboid minor
7 Rhomboid major
8 Trapezius (largely removed)
9 Deltoid (largely removed on right)
10 Supraspinatus
11 Infraspinatus
12 Teres minor
13 Teres major
14 Triceps brachii, long head
15 Triceps brachii, lateral head

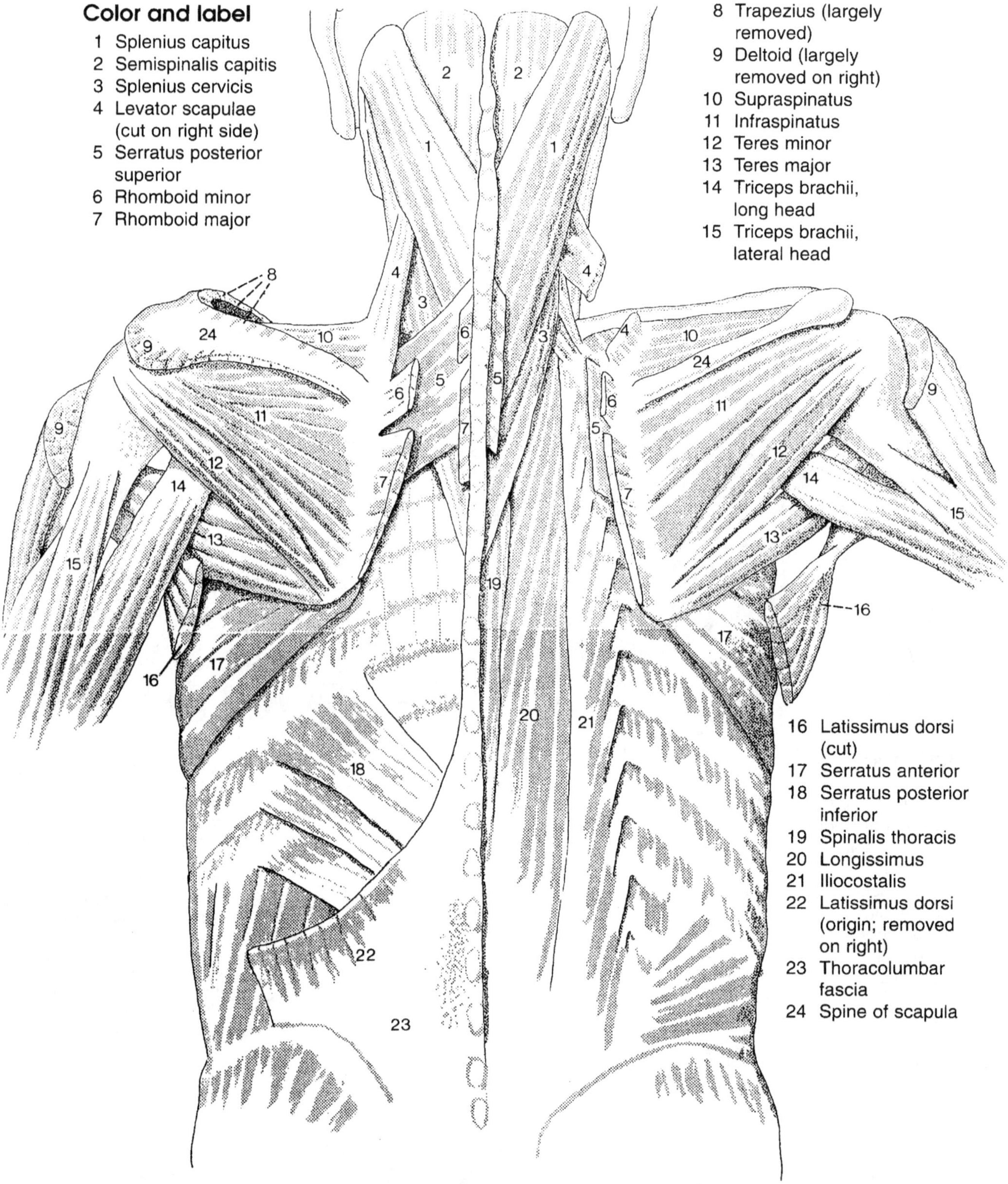

16 Latissimus dorsi (cut)
17 Serratus anterior
18 Serratus posterior inferior
19 Spinalis thoracis
20 Longissimus
21 Iliocostalis
22 Latissimus dorsi (origin; removed on right)
23 Thoracolumbar fascia
24 Spine of scapula

Bk-7 Back muscles III

Erector spinae

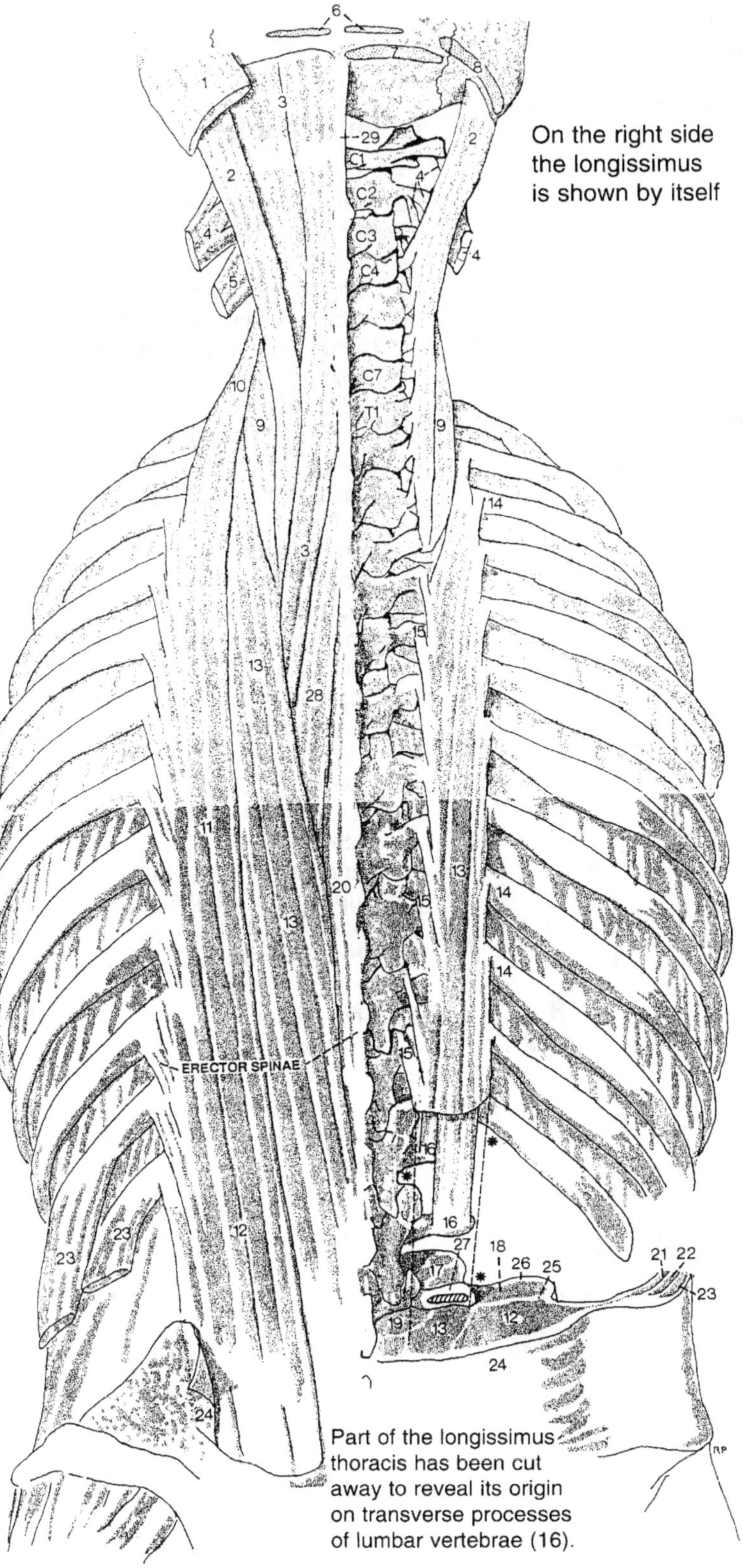

Color and label

1 Splenius capitis
2 Longissimus capitis
3 Semispinalis capitis
4 Splenius cervicis
5 Levator scapulae
6 Insertion of trapezius (on occipital bone)
7 Insertion of semispinalis
8 Insertion of splenius capitis
9 Longissimus cervicis
10 Iliocostalis cervicis
11 Iliocostalis thoracis
12 Iliocostalis lumborum (cut)
13 Longissimus thoracis (cut)
14 Insertion of longissimus thoracis onto ribs 3-12
15 Insertion of longissimus thoracis onto transverse processes of thoracic vertebrae
16 Attachments of longissimus thoracis on lumbar vertebrae L1 ans L2
17 Psoas major (cut)
18 Quadratus lumborum (cut)
19 Multifidus and rotatores (cut)
20 Spinalis thoracis
21 Transversus abdominis (cut)
22 Internal abdominal oblique
23 External abdominal oblique
24 Posterior layer of thoracolumbar fascia
25 Anterior layer of thoracolumbar fascia
26 Transversalis fascia
27 Transverse process of lumbar vertebra L3 with attachment of longissimus
28 Semispinalis cervicis and thoracis
29 Ligamentum nuchae (nuchal ligament)

*The erector spinae (old name, sacrospinalis) lies between the anterior and posterior layers of the thoracolumbar fascia.

Bk-8 Back muscles IV–deepest muscles

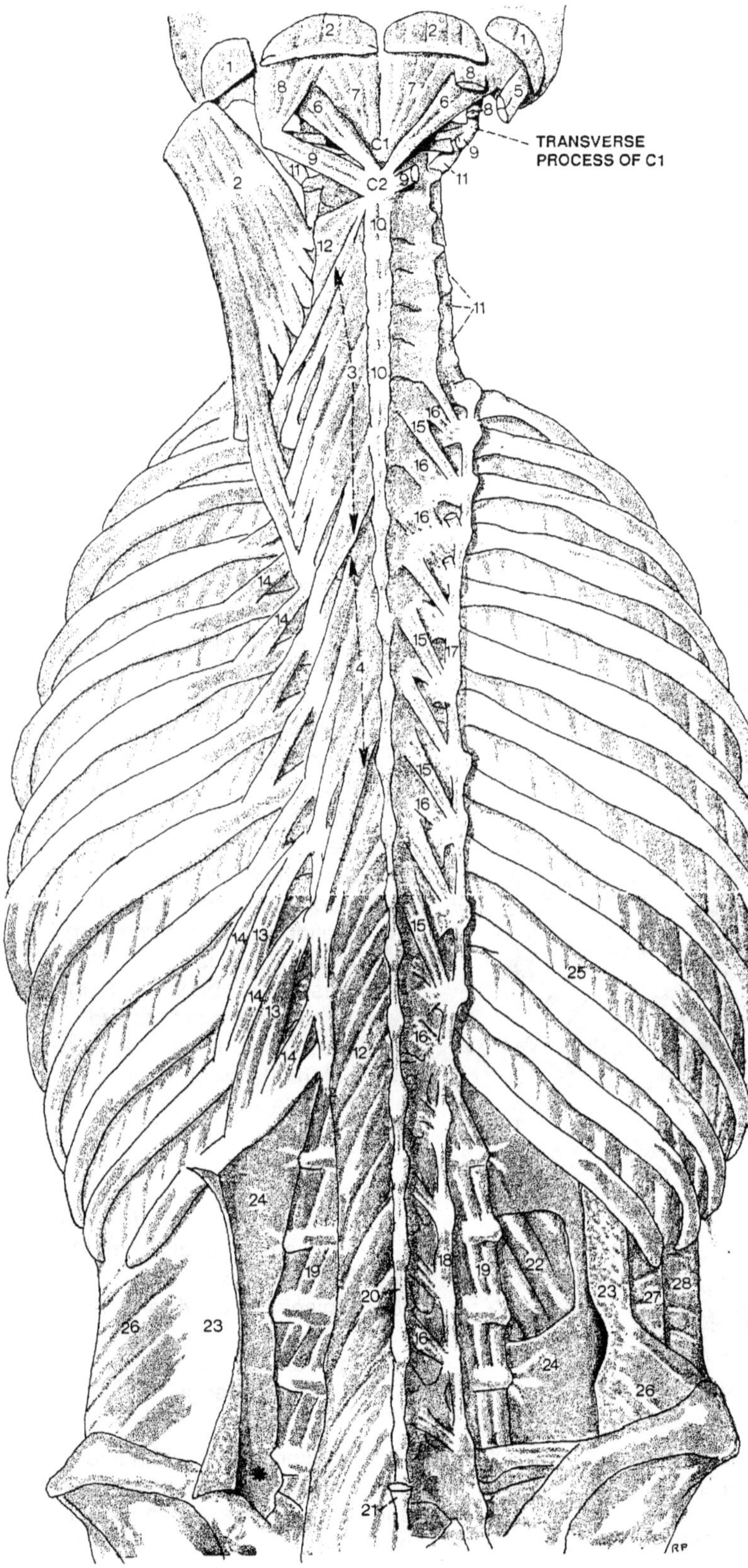

Color and label

1 Splenius capitis (cut)
2 Semispinalis capitis (cut)
3 Semispinalis cervicis
4 Semispinalis thoracis
5 Longissimus capitis
6 Rectus capitis posterior major
7 Rectus capitis posterior minor
8 Obliquus capitis superior
9 Obliquus capitis inferior
10 Interspinalis cervicis
11 Intertransversarii cervicis (posterior)
12 Multifidis
13 Long levator costorum (long costal levators)
14 Short levator costorum (short costal levators)
15 Long rotatores
16 Short rotatores
17 Intertranversarii thoracis
18 Intertranversarii lumborum (medial)
19 Intertranversarii lumborum (lateral)
20 Interspinalis lumborum
21 Supraspinous ligament (cut)
22 Quadratus lumborum
23 Thoracolumbar fascia (posterior layer, cut)
24 Thoracolumbar fascia (anterior layer)
25 External intercostal
26 External abdominal oblique
27 Internal abdominal oblique
28 Transversus abdominis

Bk-9 Back muscles V: the multifidus

The multifidus muscles extend from the posterior sacrum to the spinous process of the second cervical vertebra (C2, axis). The general arrangement of muscle bundles is shown on the left. Here four muscle bundles arise from a single origin, the mamillary process of the 5th lumbar vertebra. The longest bundle (1) reaches up to and inserts on the spinous process of vertebra T12. The next longest bundle (2) inserts on the spinous process of L1. Bundle 3 inserts on vertebra L2, and bundle 4 inserts on vertebra L3. The origins of the multifidi are the back of the sacrum (indicated by shaded area on posterior sacrum), the mamillary processes of the five lumbar vertebrae, the transverse process of the twelve thoracic vertebrae, and the articular processes of the lower four cervical vertebrae. The multifidi are innervated by the dorsal (primary) rami of spinal nerves.

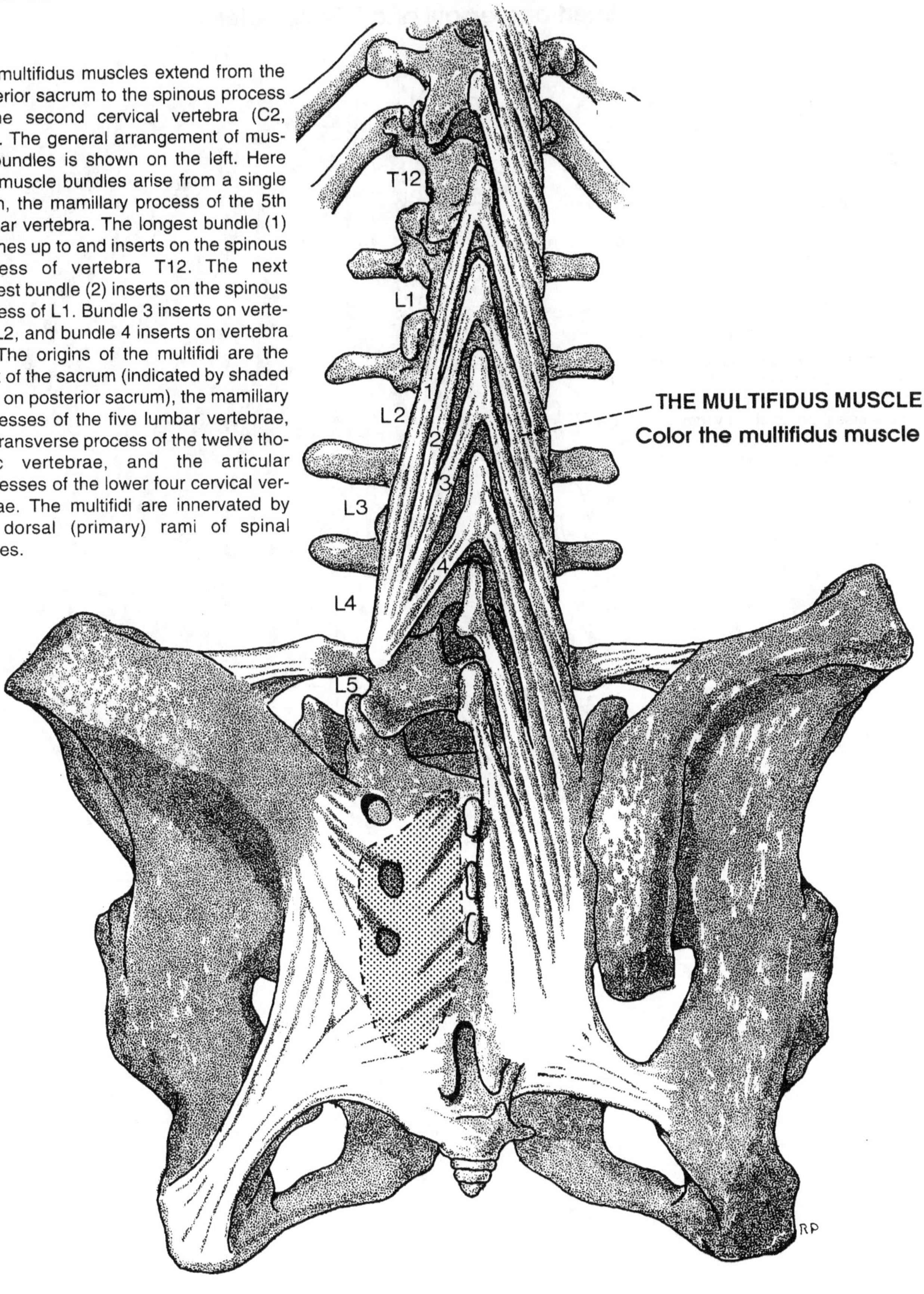

Bk-10 Back muscles VI

intertransversarii and interspinales

Color and label

1 Lateral intertransversarii
2 Medial intertransversarii
3 Interspinales doubled on the lumbar spine)
4 External intercostals
5 Quadratus lumborum
6 External abdominal oblique
7 Gluteus maximus
8 Gluteus medius
9 Multifidus (cut, origin on back of sacrum)

The intertransversarii (intertransverse muscles) are short muscles that extend from the transverse process of one vertebra to the transverse process of the vertebra immediately above (1). The lumbar vertebrae are also connected by additional *medial* intertransversarii, which extend from the mamillary process and accessory process of one lumbar vertebra to the same two processes of the vertebra immediately above (2).

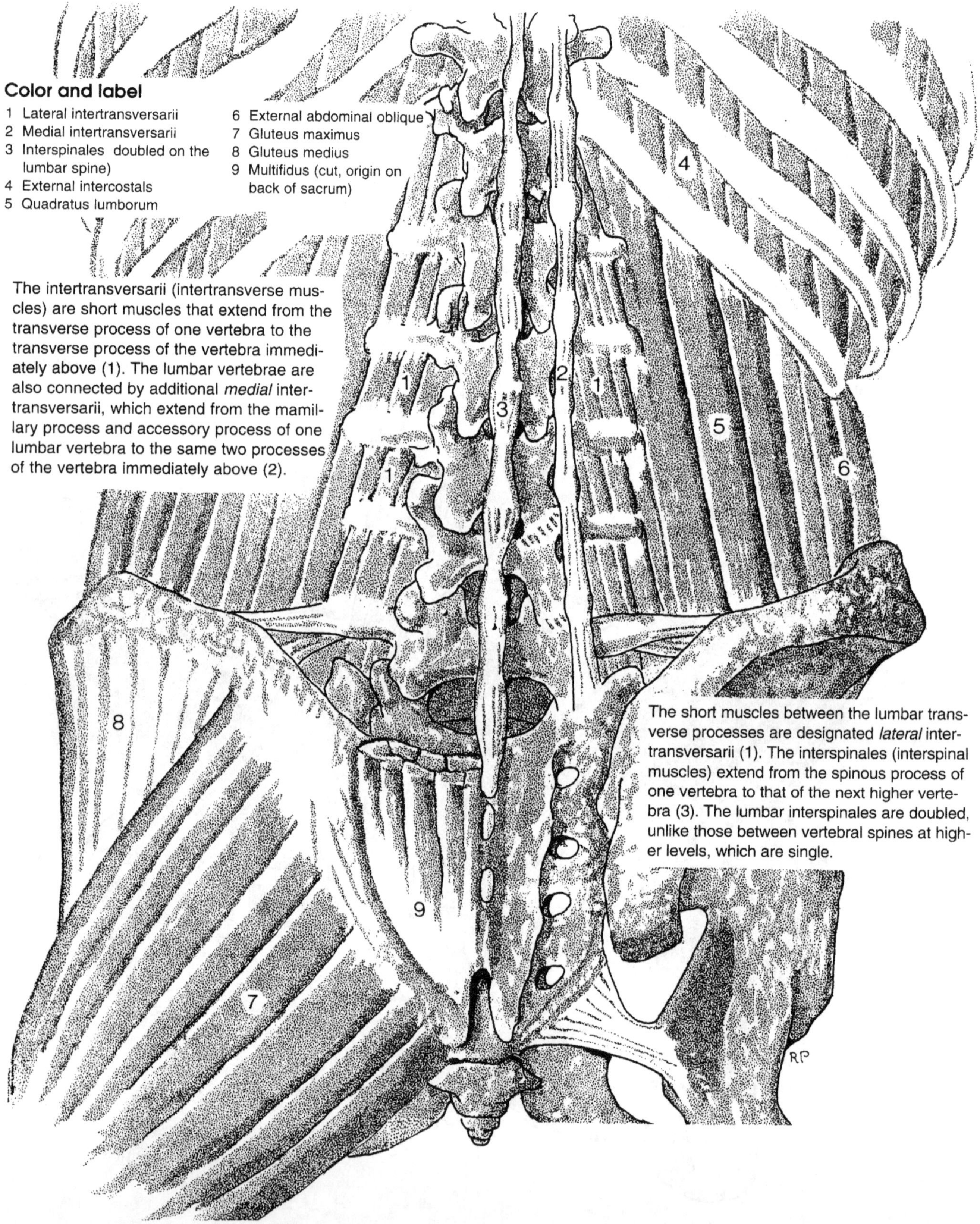

The short muscles between the lumbar transverse processes are designated *lateral* intertransversarii (1). The interspinales (interspinal muscles) extend from the spinous process of one vertebra to that of the next higher vertebra (3). The lumbar interspinales are doubled, unlike those between vertebral spines at higher levels, which are single.

Bk-11 Ligaments of the posterior sacrum

Color and label

1 Sacrotuberous ligament
2 Sacrospinous ligament
3 Iliolumbar ligament
4 Posterior sacroiliac ligament
5 Supraspinous ligament (runs from posterior tip of one vertebral spinous process to that of adjacent vertebrae for entire length of vertebral column)
6 Joint capsule surrounding gliding synovial joints between articular processes of vertebrae (only two are shown here)
7 Spine of ischium
8 Ischial tuberosity

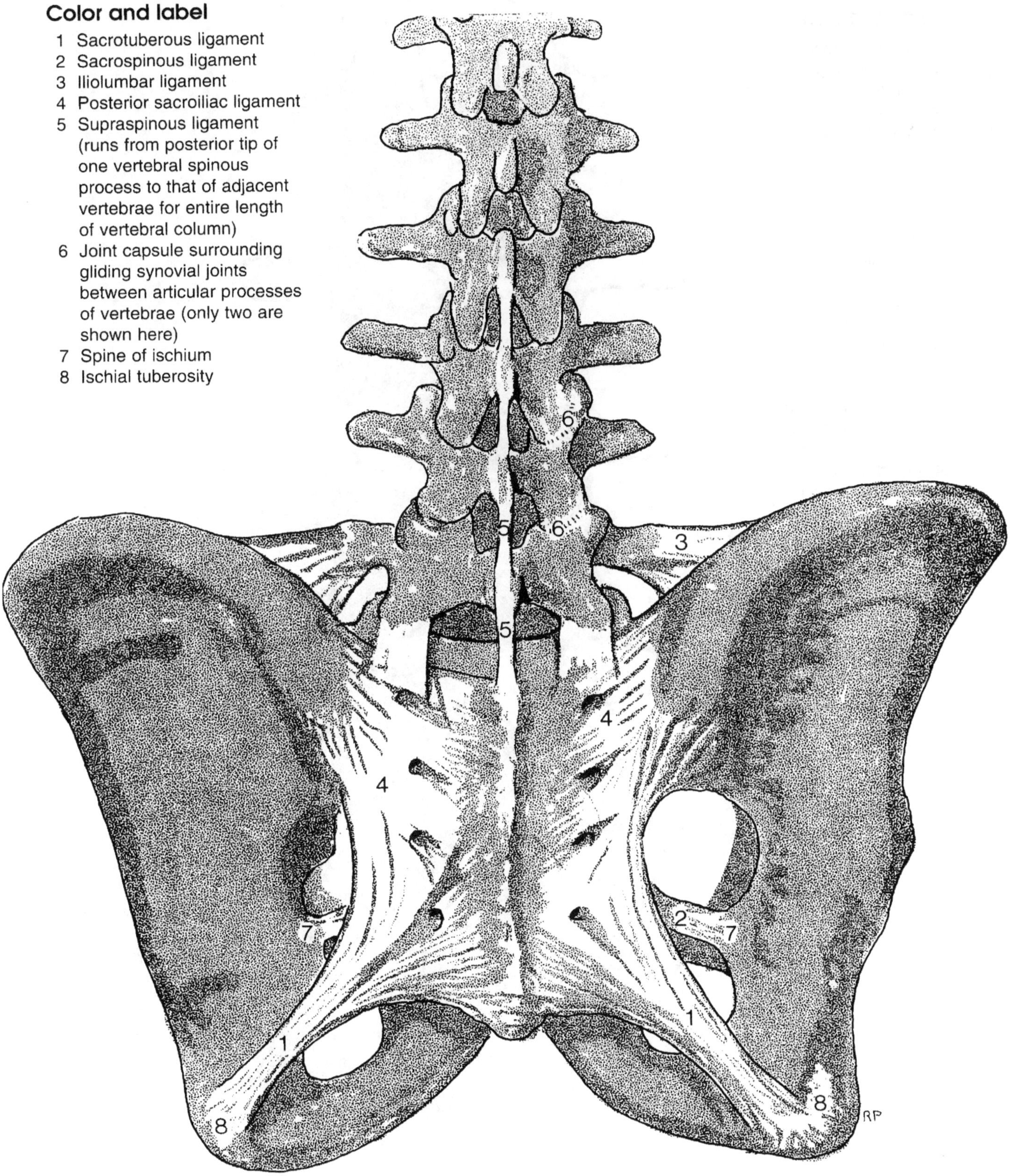

Bk-12 Lumbar vertebrae

Dorsal aspect

Color and label

1 Spinous process
2 Transverse process
3 Superior articular process
4 Inferior articular process
5 Superior articular facet (covered with hyaline cartilage; this forms a gliding synovial joint with the facet of the inferior articular process of the next higher vertebra)
6 Lamina
7 Mamillary process
8 Accessory process
9 Body
10 Posterior superior iliac spine
LI First lumbar vertebra
L2 Second lumbar vertebra
L3 Third lumbar vertebra
L4 Fourth lumbar vertebra
L5 Fifth lumbar vertebra

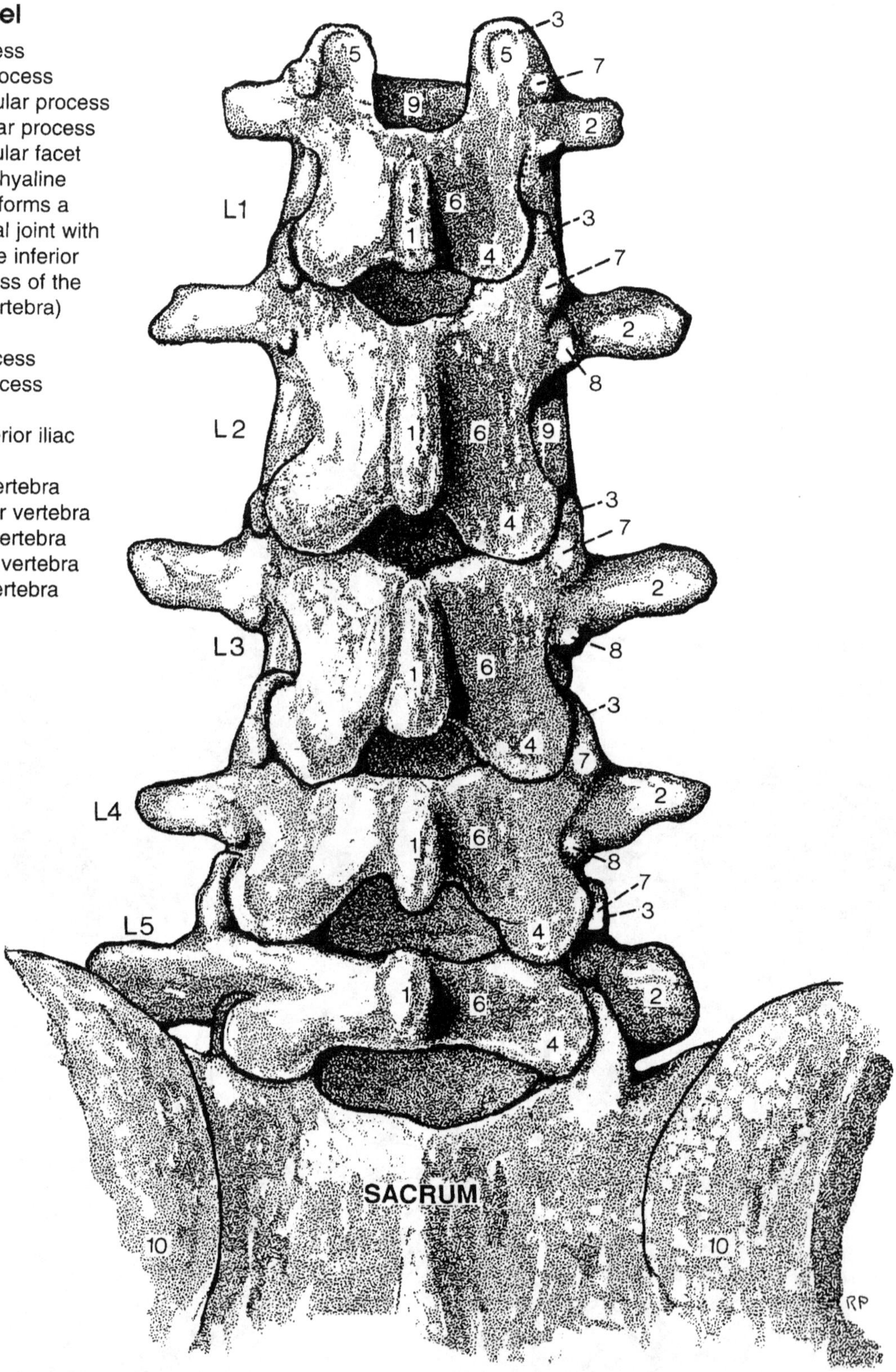

Bk-13 Sacrum

Fifth Lumbar Vertebra

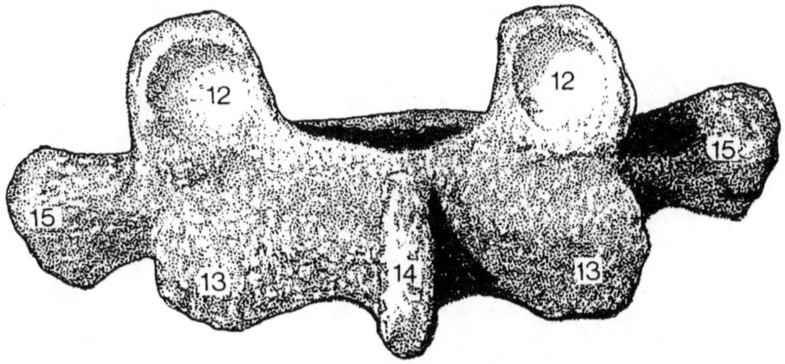

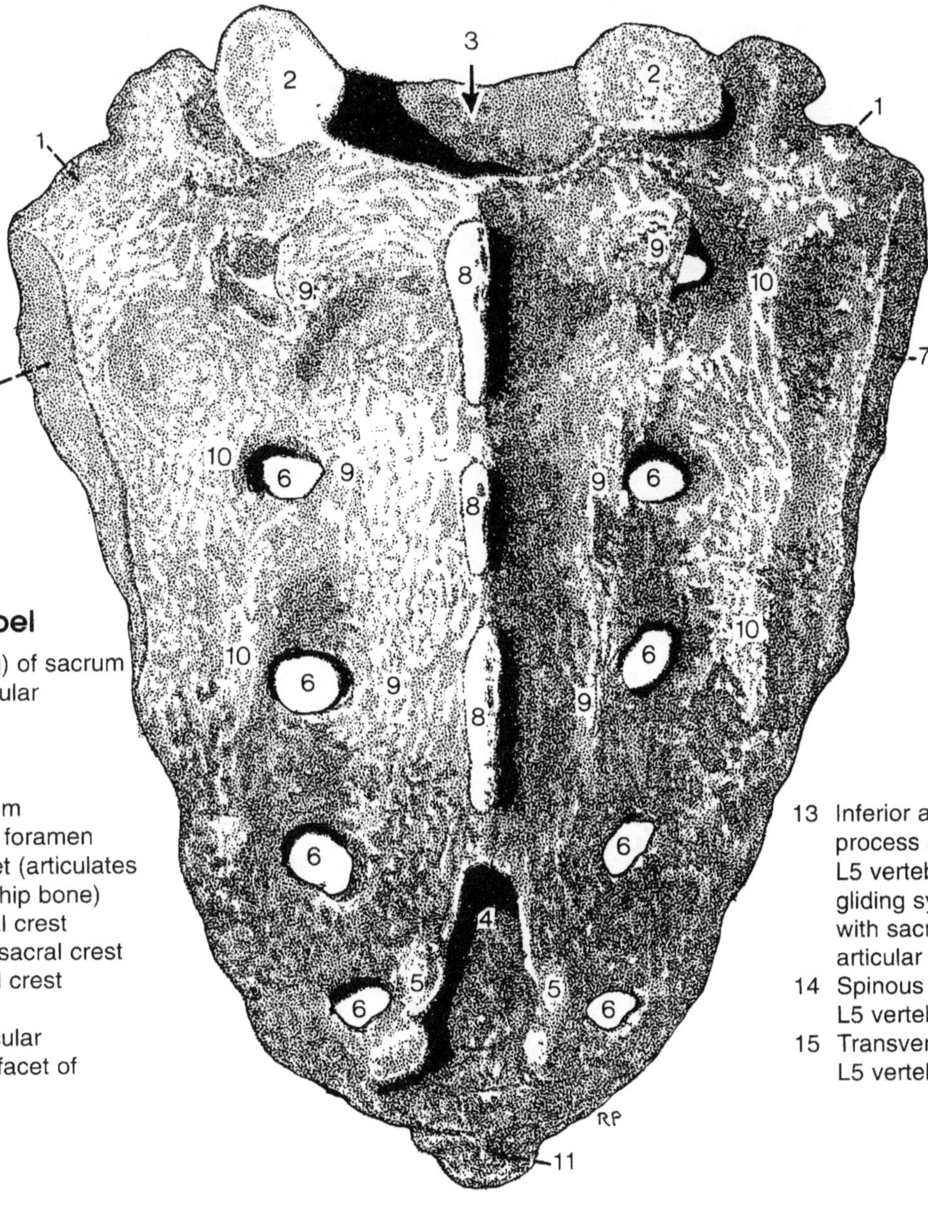

Color and label

1 Ala (Lat. wing) of sacrum
2 Superior articular process
3 Sacral canal
4 Sacral hiatus
5 Horn of sacrum
6 Dorsal sacral foramen
7 Auricular facet (articulates with coxal or hip bone)
8 Median sacral crest
9 Intermediate sacral crest
10 Lateral sacral crest
11 Coccyx
12 Superior articular process and facet of
L5 vertebra
13 Inferior articular process and facet of L5 vertebra (forms a gliding synovial joint with sacral superior articular process)
14 Spinous process of L5 vertebra
15 Transverse process of L5 vertebra

Bk-14 Cross section of cervical spinal cord

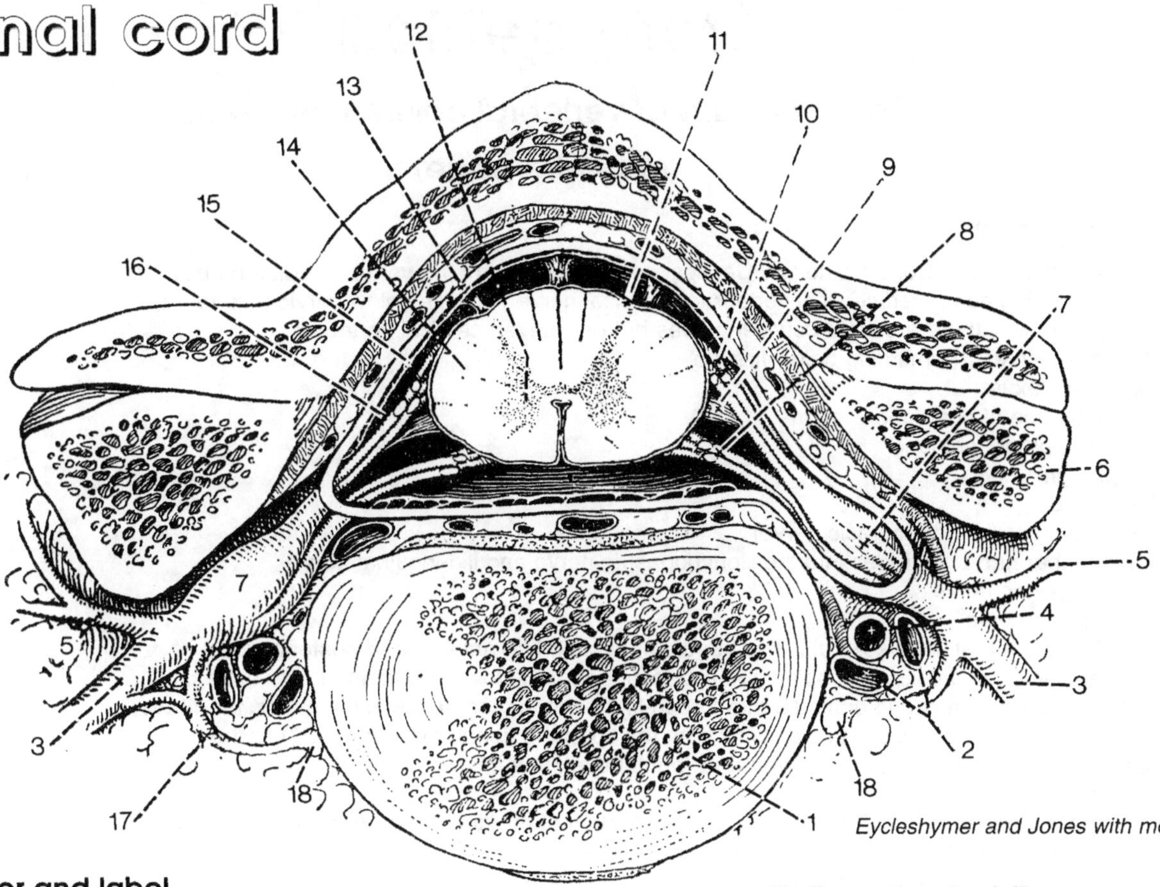

Eycleshymer and Jones with modification

Color and label

1 Body of fourth cervical vertebra
2 Vertebral veins
3 Ventral ramus of cervical nerve C4
4 Vertebral artery
5 Dorsal ramus of cervical nerve C4
6 Superior articular process of cervical vertebra C5
7 Spinal ganglion (also dorsal root ganglion); this contains the neuron cell bodies of the sensory nerve fibers in nerves.
8 Ventral root of spinal nerve; this consists of the outgoing nerve fibers (axons) to muscles and glands
9 Dentate ligament; a notched sheet of pia mater attaching the lateral border of the spinal cord to the inner wall of the vertebral canal.
10 Dorsal root of spinal nerve; this consists of incoming (afferent) sensory nerve fibers. Each spinal nerve is formed by two roots, a dorsal sensory root, and a ventral motor root.
11 Pia mater; a delicate fibrous membrane firmly attached to the circumference of the spinal cord and brain.
12 Gray matter of spinal cord; largely consists of neuron cell bodies.
13 Dura mater; a tough fibrous sheath that surrounds the spinal cord and brain.
14 White matter; largely consists of longitudinal myelinated axons.
15 Arachnoid mater (also arachnoidea, or simply arachnoid); the web-like middle membrane closely applied to the inner surface of the dura mater.
16 Subarachnoid space; space between the pia mater and the arachnoid filled with cerebrospinal fluid; traversed by thin arachnoid trabeculae.
17 Ramus communicans; contains postganglionic sympathetic nerve fibers and some cardiac pain fibers.
18 Sympathetic trunk

Definitions

Neuron: a nerve cell
Ganglion: a collection of nerve cell bodies outside the central nervous system (brain and spinal cord)
Axon: nerve fiber that carries the nerve impulse
Nerve: a bundle of nerve fibers connecting the central nervous system to other parts of the body

Bk-15 Spinal cord displayed from behind

Posterior parts of vertebral column removed

(opposite page)

Color and label

1 Cervical nerves C5, C6, C7, and C8. Cervical nerves C1-C7 exit the vertebral column above the corresponding numbered cervical vertebrae. Cervical nerve C8 exits below cervical vertebra C7. This is why there are eight cervical nerves but only seven cervical vertebrae.
2 Thoracic nerve T1; emerging below first rib
3 Brachial plexus
4 Superior lobe of right lung
5 Inferior lobe of right lung
6 Diaphragm
7 Twelth rib
8 Subcostal nerve (12th thoracic nerve)
9 First lumbar nerve; it divides into the iliohypogastric nerve and ilio-inguinal nerve.
10 Iliohypogastric nerve
11 Ilio-inguinal nerve
12 Cauda equina (Latin, horse's tail). The bundle of descending anterior and posterior roots of lumbar, sacral, and coccygeal spinal nerves destined for the lower trunk and lower extremity. In the middle of the cauda equina a thin thread-like prolongation of spinal pia mater, the **filum terminale internum**, extends downward from the tip of the conus medullaris (27) to the lower border of the second sacral vertebra (not labeled; see following figure).
13 First sacral vertebra
14 Filum terminale externum. The downward prolongation of the dura mater from the second sacral vertebra to the first coccygeal vertebral segment.
15 First coccygeal vertebra (segment).
16 Ischial tuberosity
17 Internal pudendal artery and vein and pudendal nerve
18 Sciatic nerve (also nervus ischiadicus): the largest nerve in the body formed by nerves L4-S3. It divides usually in the lower third of the thigh into the tibial nerve and common peroneal nerves.
19 Levator ani muscle
20 Cervical vertebrae C4 and C5
21 First rib (costa I)
22 Head of humerus (caput humeri)
23 Pedicle of third thoracic vertebra. The pedicles of all the vertebrae have been cut, thus removing their laminae and transverse and spinous processes.
24 Fourth rib
25 Spinal cord (medulla spinalis). The spinal cord extends from the foramen magnum to the upper lumbar vertebrae, usually to the intervertebral disc L1-L2.
26 Twelth thoracic vertebrae
27 Conus medullaris; the cone-shaped lower end of the spinal cord at the level of the upper lumbar vertebrae.
28 Third lumbar vertebra
29 Dura mater; the outermost, toughest, and most fibrous of the three membranes that cover the brain and spinal cord.
30 Lumbosacral trunk; carries fibers from lumbar nerves L4 and L5 that join sacral nerves S1,S2, and S3 to form the sciatic nerve.
31 First sacral nerve
32 Superior gluteal nerve (artery and vein not shown)
33 Sciatic nerve
34 Anus

Bk-15 Spinal cord displayed from behind

Posterior parts of vertebral column removed

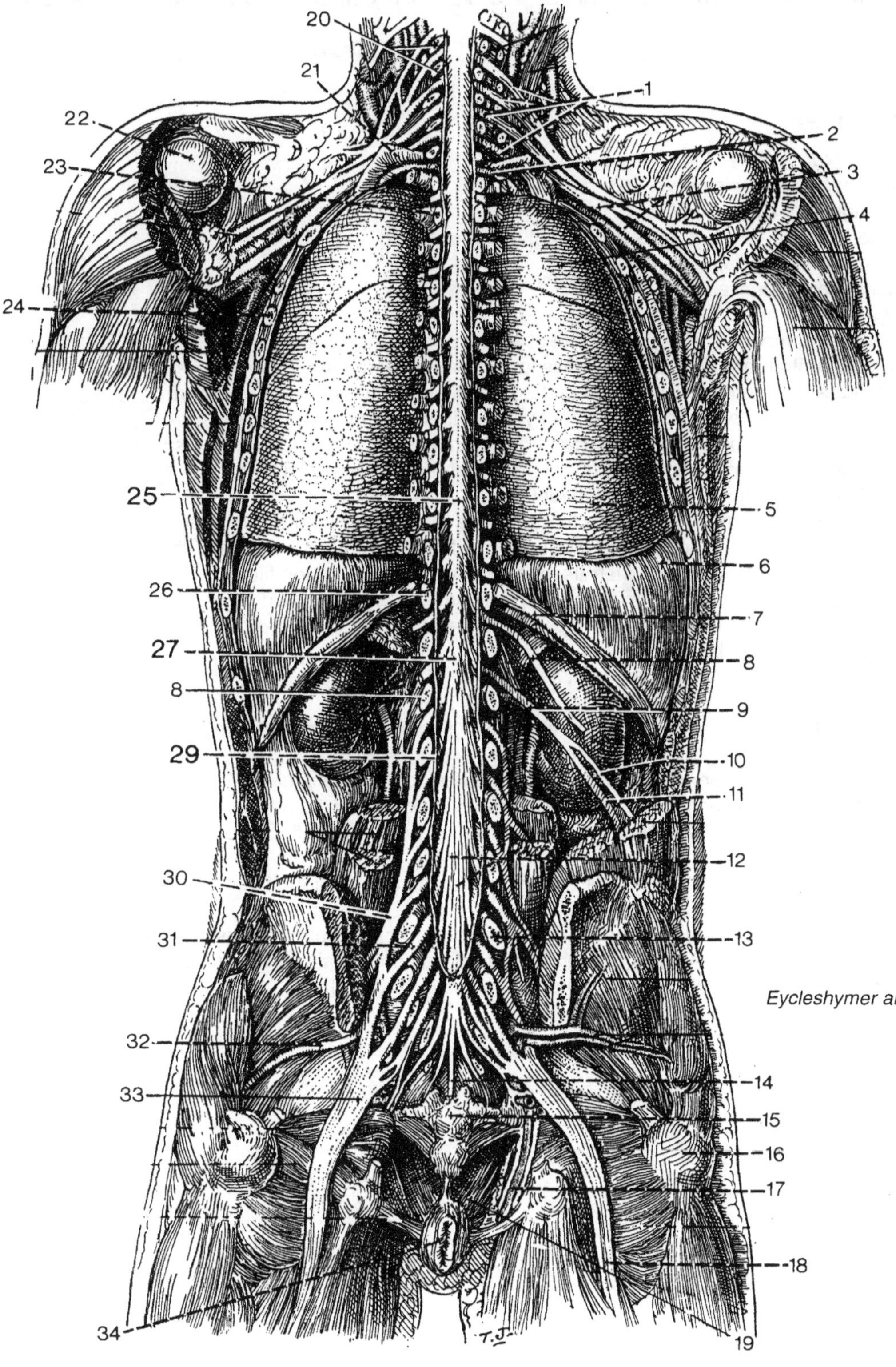

Eycleshymer and Jones

Bk-16 The cauda equina of the spinal cord

The posterior parts of the lumbar vertebrae have been removed, the dura mater cut open, and the posterior portion of the sacrum cut away to reveal the sacral canal.

(opposite page)

Color and label

1 Dura mater (cut)
2 Subcostal nerve (thoracic nerve T12)
3 Spinal ganglion of lumbar nerve L1
4 Conus medullaris; the tapering caudal end of the spinal cord
5 Iliohypogastric nerve; derived from L1
6 Ilio-inguinal nerve; derived from L1
7 Spinal ganglion of nerve L3
8 Dorsal ramus of nerve L3. The dorsal rami of spinal nerves tend to be much smaller than ventral rami. The dorsal *rami* supply motor fibers to the extensor muscles of the back and sensory fibers to the medial skin of the back. Each spinal nerve is formed by a *dorsal* and *ventral* root whose fibers are almost exclusively sensory and motor respectively. Each spinal nerve (nerve trunk) then gives off a small *dorsal ramus* and continues as a much larger *ventral ramus.* Nerves such as the intercostal, femoral, and sciatic are continuations of ventral rami.
9 Filum terminale internum. Long slender thread of pia mater extending downward from the tip of the conus medullaris to the fundus of the dural sac at the level of the second sacral vertebra where it penetrates the dura and fuses with the filum externum of the dura mater to form the coccygeal ligament, which in turn fuses with the periosteum of the posterior surface of the the coccyx.
10 Spinal gangion of nerve L5
11 Femoral nerve (derived from nerves L2, L3, and L4)
12 Dural sac
13 Sacral nerve S1 (anterior ramus; sensory and motor fibers) contributing to the sciatic nerve
14 Sacral nerve S2 (same components as S1) contributing to the sciatic nerve
15 Sacral nerve S3 (same components as S1) contributing to the sciatic nerve
16 Sciatic nerve (formed by fibers from the anterior rami of nerves L4, L5, S1, S2, S3)
17 Sacral nerve S5
18 Filum terminale externum (filum terninale internum has fused inside the filum terminale externum)
19 Sacral nerve S4
20 Cauda equina; descending dorsal (sensory) and ventral (motor) root filaments and roots of the lower spinal nerves. As they descend, the root filaments coalesce into roots.
21 Lumbosacral trunk; fibers from nerves L4 and L5 joining sacral nerves S1, S2, and S3, forming the sciatic nerve.

Bk-16 The cauda equina

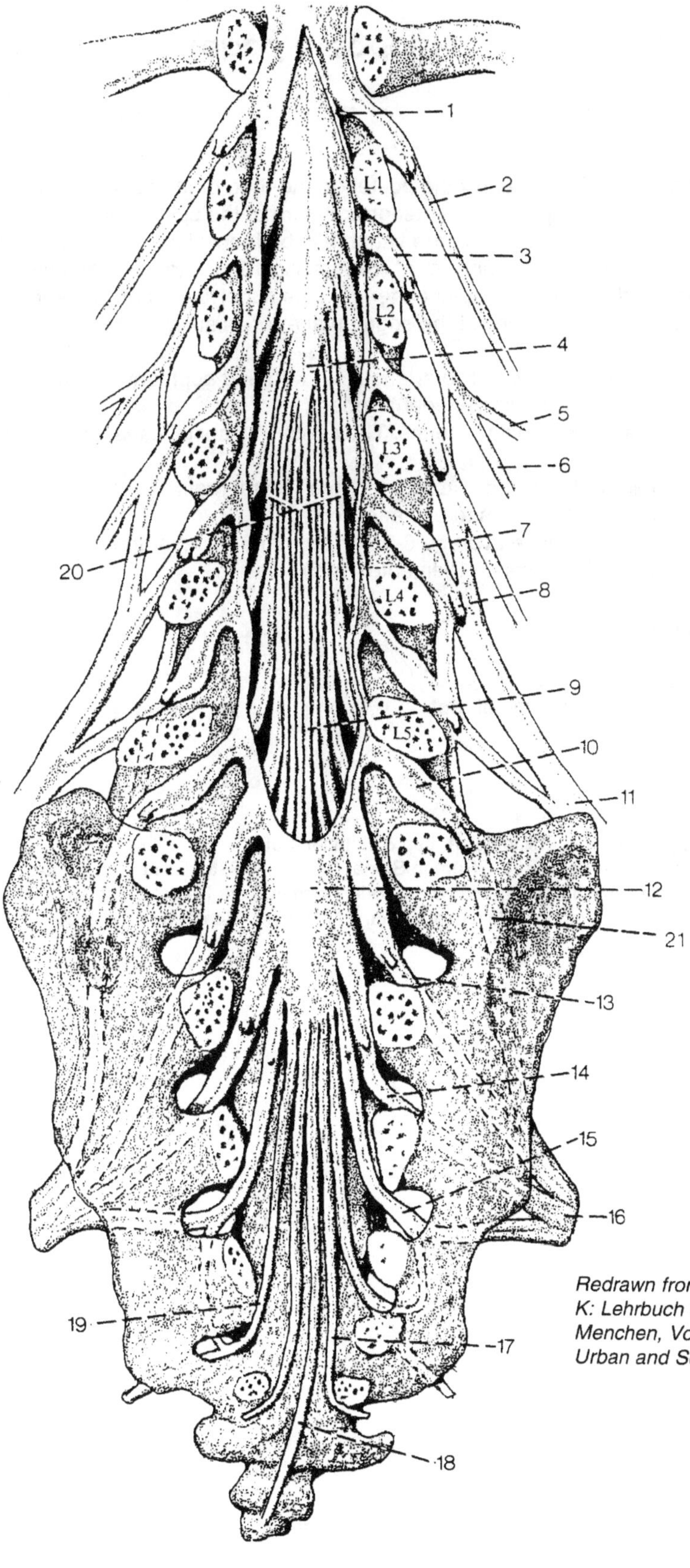

Redrawn from Benninghoff A, Goerttler K: Lehrbuch der Anatomie des Menchen, Vol. 3, 9th ed. Munich, Urban and Schwarzenberg, 1975.

Bk-17 Arterial supply and vascular pattern to a portion of the spinal cord

(opposite page)

Color and label

1 Posterior spinal arteries. These supply the posterior one-third of the spinal cord.
2 Anterior spinal artery. This supplies the anterior one-third of the spinal cord.
3 Anterior medullary feeder artery. These are variable in both position (level) and in number (they average a total of 8 for the whole spinal cord (Dommisse 1975, cited in Clemente 1985). These feeder arteries join with the anterior spinal arteries, thus supplying them with additional blood. They arise from the spinal branches of the segmental arteries such as the posterior intercostal arteries.
4 Posterior medullary feeder artery. These arteries join with and augment the posterior spinal arteries. They arise like the anterior medullary feeder arteries.
5 Spinal rami (branches) of segmental arteries. They enter the spinal canal bilaterally at every intervertebral level.
6 Anterior (ventral) radicular branches. They supply the ventral roots.
7 Dorsal (posterior) radicular branches to posterior roots.
8 Sulcal (or central) arteries. These average 5-9 per segment and average 210 for all 31 spinal cord segments (Tvetan 1976, cited in Clemente 1985).
9 Coronal arteries
10 Superficial pial plexus
11 Penetrating vessels
12 Spinal ganglion (dorsal root ganglion)
13 Dorsal filaments (rootlets) and dorsal root
14 Ventral filaments (rootlets)

References

Clemente CD (ed): Gray's Anatomy, Philadelphia, Lea & Febiger, 1985
Dommisse GF: The Arteries and Veins of the Human Spinal Cord from Birth. Edinburgh, Churchill Livingstone, 1975.
Tvetan L: Spinal cord vascularity. III. The spinal cord arteries in man. Acta Radiol Diagn (Stockh) 17:257-273, 1976.
Windle WF (ed): The Spinal Cord and Its Reaction to Injury. New York, Marcel Dekker, 1980.

Bk-17 Arterial supply and vascular pattern to a portion of the spinal cord

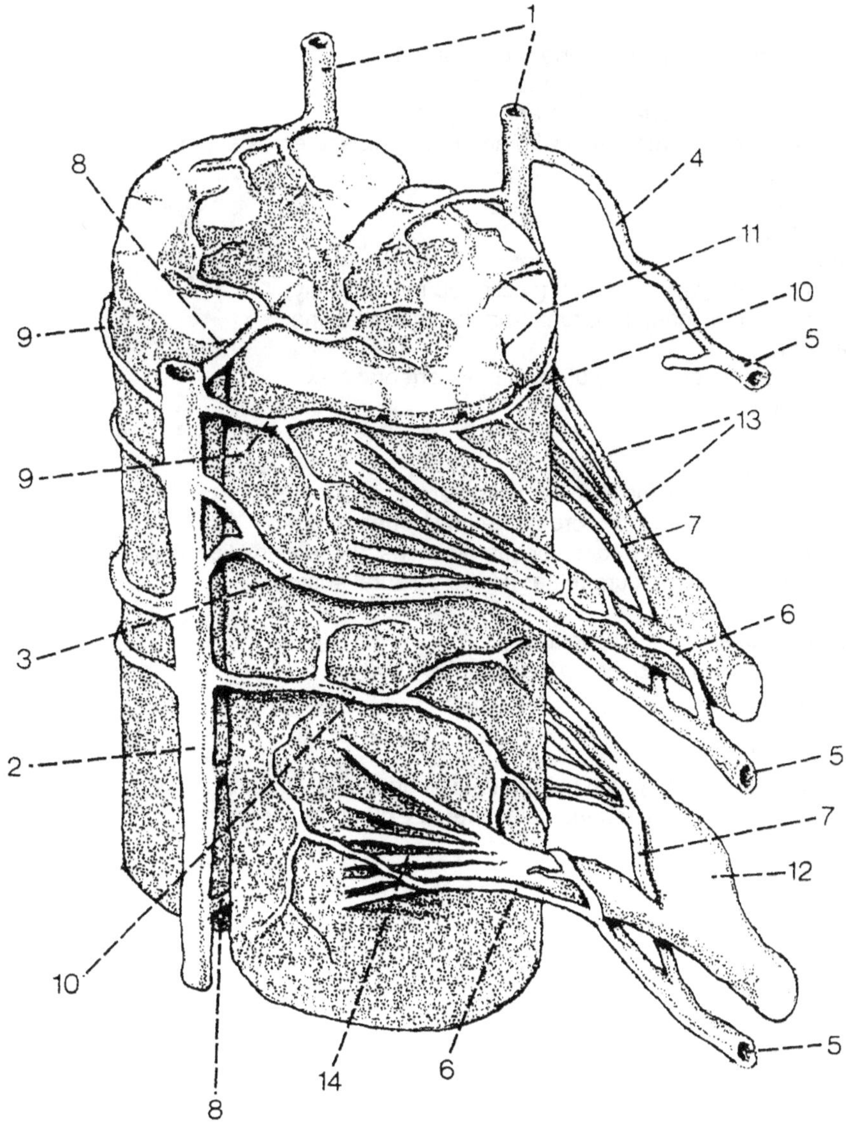

After Windle

Bk-18 The intervertebral disks and internal vertebral venous plexus

Vertebral cana cut open; cauda equina and dura mater removed (opposite page)

Color and label

1 Superior articular processes of lumbar vertebrae L1 and L2
2 Lumbar artery (dorsal ramus penetrating transverse process)
3 Transverse process of lumbar vertebrae L1 and L2 (cut)
4 Inferior articular process of L1 articulating with and largely obscured by superior articular process of L2
5 Spinous process of L2
6 Inferior articular process (cut)
7 Supraspinal ligament
8 Spinous processes of vertebrae L3 and L5 (sectioned midsagittally)
9 Ligamentum flavum ("yellow ligament"); runs from lamina to lamina.
10 Interspinous ligament
11 Annulus fibrosus; the outer fibrous ring of each intervertebral disk
12 Anterior longitudinal ligament
13 Lumbar artery
14 Posterior longitudinal ligament
15 Intervertebral foramen; nerve L1 (not shown) exits here.
16 Nucleus pulposus; the inner, semifluid core of the intervertebral disks.
17 The anterior and posterior inner vertebral venous plexuses; these veins lie within the vertebral canal, exterior to the dura mater (in the epidural space).
18 Lumbar artery (cut)
19 Anterior longitudinal ligament (cut midsagittally)
20 Herniation of nucleus pulposus into the spongiosa of L4 body
21 Body of lumbar vertebra L4
22 Pedicle of L4
23 Anulus fibrosus (cut midsagittally)
24 Herniation of nucleus pulposus beneath the posterior longitudinal ligament. This type of herniation often impinges upon the spinal nerve exiting the foramen (here: nerve L4).
25 Spinal ramus of lumbar artery

Bk-18 The intervertebral disks and internal vertebral venous plexus

Vertebral cana cut open; cauda equina and dura mater removed

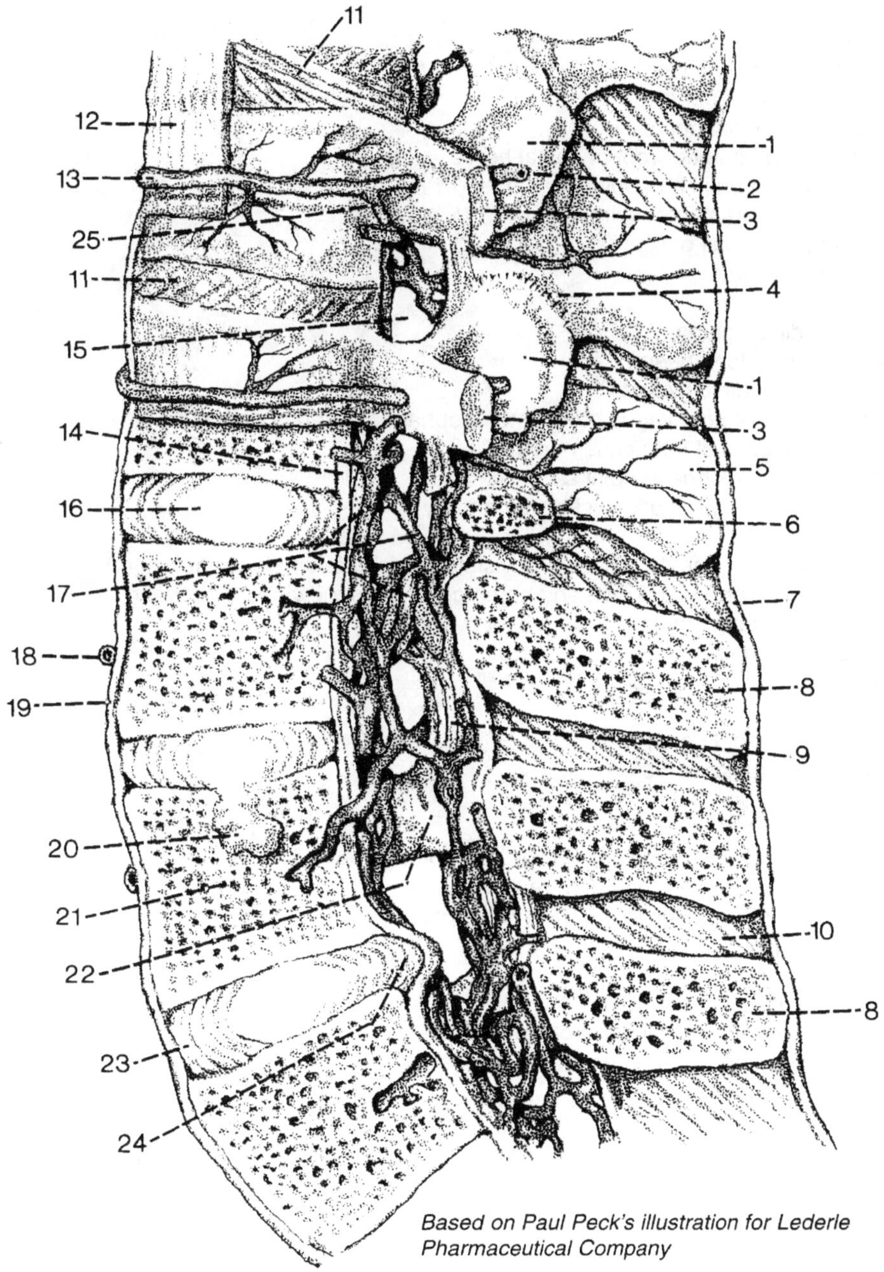

Based on Paul Peck's illustration for Lederle Pharmaceutical Company

Bk-19 Spinal cord, meninges, and internal vertebral venous plexus

(opposite page)

Color and label

1 Dura mater
2 Arachnoid membrane
3 Anterior spinal artery and vein
4 Dorsal ramus of spinal nerve
5 Anterior ramus of spinal nerve
6 Spinal ganglion and anterior root of spinal nerve
7 Posterior meningeal branch of spinal nerve
8 Anterior meningeal bramch of spinal nerve
9 Internal vertebral venous plexus
10 Epidural adipose tissue
11 Vertebral body
12 Anterior longitudinal ligament
13 Hemiazygos vein (often absent)
14 Thoracic aorta and aortic plexus
15 Esophageal plexus of right vagus nerve and esophageal arteries and veins
16 Esophagus and plexus of left vagus nerve
17 Diaphragmatic portion of pericardial sac
18 Thoracic duct (largest lymphatic vessel in the body)
19 Azygos vein
20 Inferior vena cava and hepatic veins (liver visible immediately below diaphragm)
21 Pericardiacophrenic artery and vein and phrenic nerve ('sandwiched" between parietal pleura and pericardium)
22 Greater splanchnic nerve
23 Sympathetic trunk
24 Spinal cord
25 Dorsal rootlets of spinal nerve
26 Ventral rootlets of spinal nerve
27 Superior articular process
28 Denticulate ligament
29 Spinal ganglion (contains nerve cell bodies of incoming nerve fibers)
30 Pedicle of vertebra (cut; vertebral arch removed)
31 Facet for tubercle of rib on vertebral transverse process
32 Sympathetic ganglion
33 Facet for head of rib
34 Intercostal vein, artery, and nerve
35 Central tendon (centrum tendineum) of diaphragm
36 Spinal branches of intercostal artery

Bk-19 Spinal cord, meninges, and internal vertebral venous plexus

Vertebral canal opened in thoracic region; meniniges cut to reveal spinal cord and spinal nerve origin

Redrawn from Sobotta/Figge. Atlas of Human Anatomy, 9th ed. Munich, Urban & Schwarzenberg, 1977.

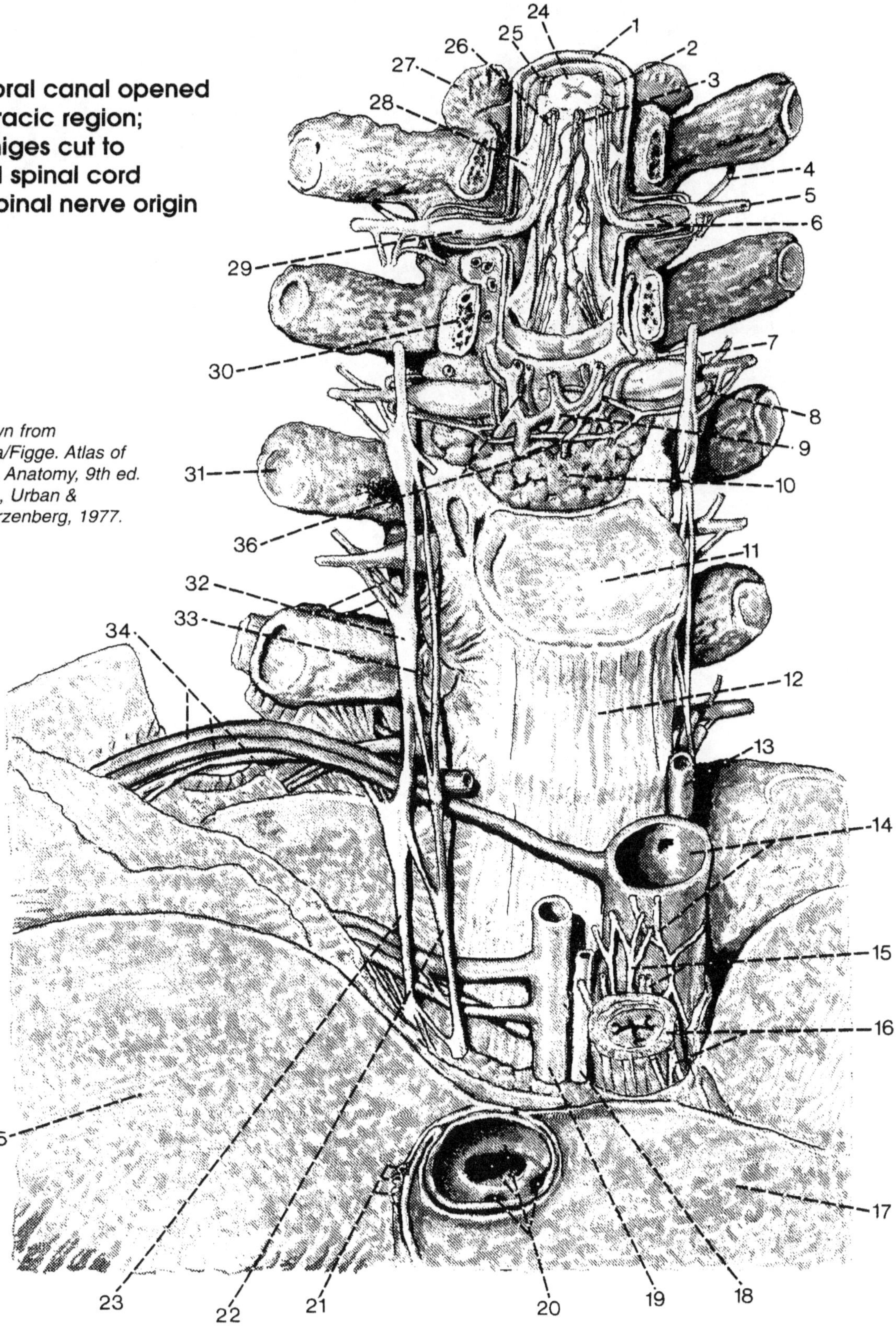

Bk-20 Typical lumbar vertebra

Color and label

1 Body
2 Pedicle
3 Lamina
4 Spinous process
5 Superior articular process
6 Inferior articular process
7 Mammillary process
8 Transverse process
9 Accessory process
10 Articular surface of superior articular process
11 Articular surface of inferior articular process
12 Vertebral foramen
13 Superior vertebral notch
14 Inferior vertebral notch

Superior view

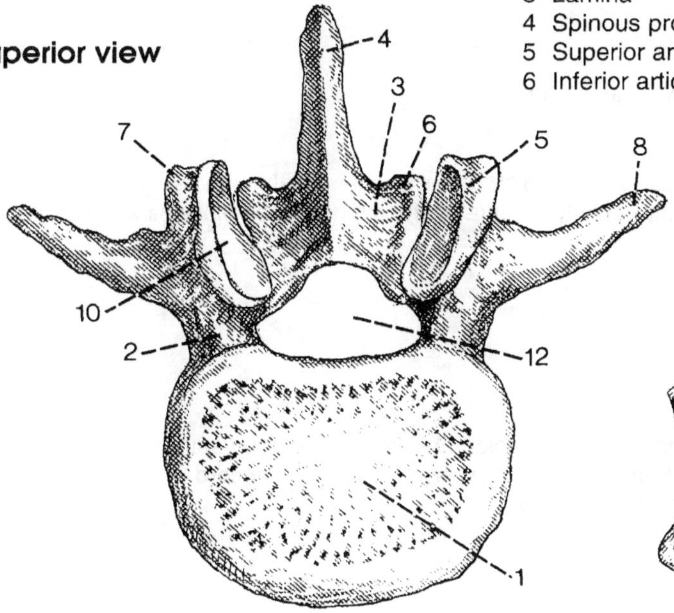

Lateral view

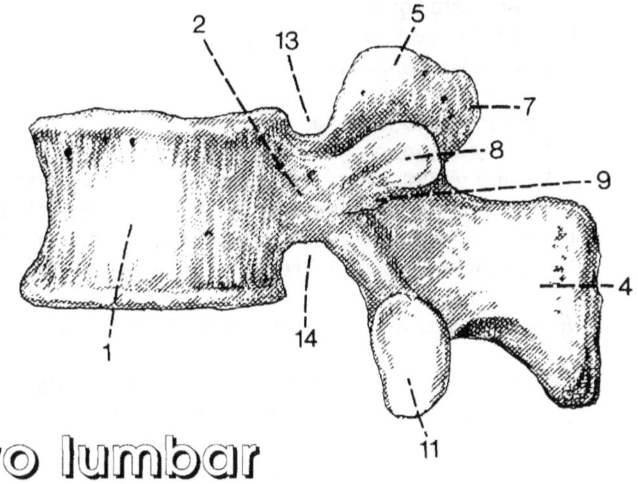

Median section of two lumbar vertebrae and their ligaments

Color and label

1 Pedicle
2 Superior articular process
3 Spinous process
4 Ligamentum flavum (yellow ligament)
5 Interspinous ligament
6 Supraspinous ligament
7 Capsular ligament (around joint between superior and inferior articular processes)
8 Lamina
9 Intervertebral foramen; formed by the inferior vertebral notch of the vertebra above and the superior vertebral notch of the vertebra below. Site of the spinal ganglion and outlet for spinal nerve.
10 Posterior longitudinal ligament
11 Anterior longitudinal ligament
12 Anulus fibrosus of the intervertebral disk; the outer laminae of fibrous tissue and cartilage
13 Nucleus pulposus; the inner core of the intervertebral disk consisting of soft, gelatinous, and highly elastic substance.
14 Body of vertebra

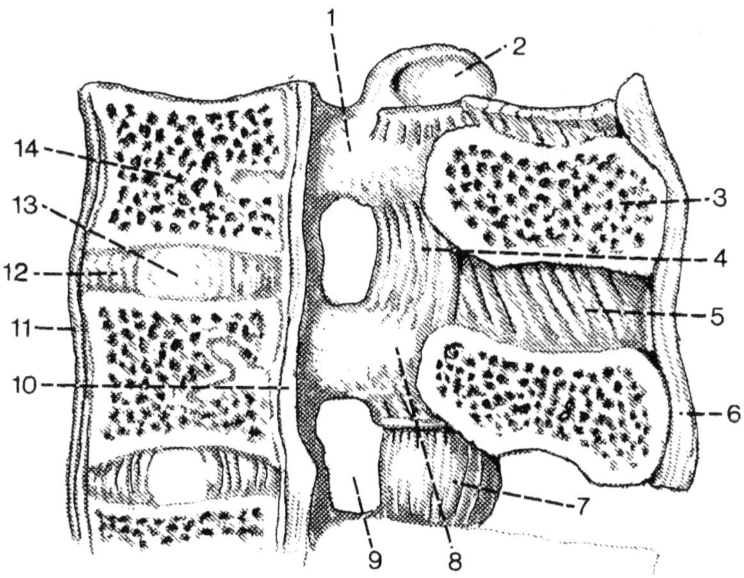

After M. Trotter and R.R. Peterson in Morris' Human Anatomy, 12th ed. B.J. Anson ed. New York, McGraw-Hill, 1966.

Bk-21 Spinal cord and spinal nerves

(opposite page)

Color and label

Figure A

1 Gray matter of spinal cord
2 Motor neuron (size exaggerated) in anterior horn of gray matter
3 Dorsal rootlets and dorsal root of spinal nerve
4 Dorsal ramus of spinal nerve
5 Ventral ramus of spinal nerve; note that the ventral ramus, which becomes the spinal nerve, is considerably larger than the dorsal ramus; the latter mainly innervates the intrinsic back muscles and medial skin of the back.
6 Denticulate ligament
7 Pedicle of vertebra (cut)
8 Arachnoid membrane
9 Dura mater
10 Epidural venous plexus
11 Body of vertebra
12 Ventral rootlets and ventral root; note that the dorsal root is considerably larger than the ventral root.
13 White matter and pia mater (thickness exaggerated) covering external surface of spinal cord
14 Spinal ganglion; contains cell bodies of incoming sensory nerve
15 Subarachnoid space; between arachnoid membrane and pia mater; filled with cerebrospinal fluid.

Figure B. Motor and sensory nerve fibers in spinal nerves (highly schematic)

1 Motor neuron and its fiber (axon) to limb muscles
2 Motor neuron and its axon to back muscles
3 Sensory neuron and its axon from skin of limb
4 Sensory neuron and its axon from skin of back; note that these neurons have a single fiber that divides into a peripheral and branch from the skin and a central branch that enters the spinal cord.
5 Interneuron
6 Second-order sensory neuron conveying information up spinal cord
7 Descending fiber carrying motor commands
8 Interneuron
9 Motor neuron
10 Dorsal root
11 Ventral root
12 Dorsal ramus
13 Ventral ramus; actually the ventral ramus is much larger than the dorsal ramus.
14 Intrinsic back muscles
15 Muscles of limbs and trunk (except back)
16 Skin of medial back
17 Skin of arm, leg, and trunk (except medial back)

Bk-21 Spinal cord and spinal nerves

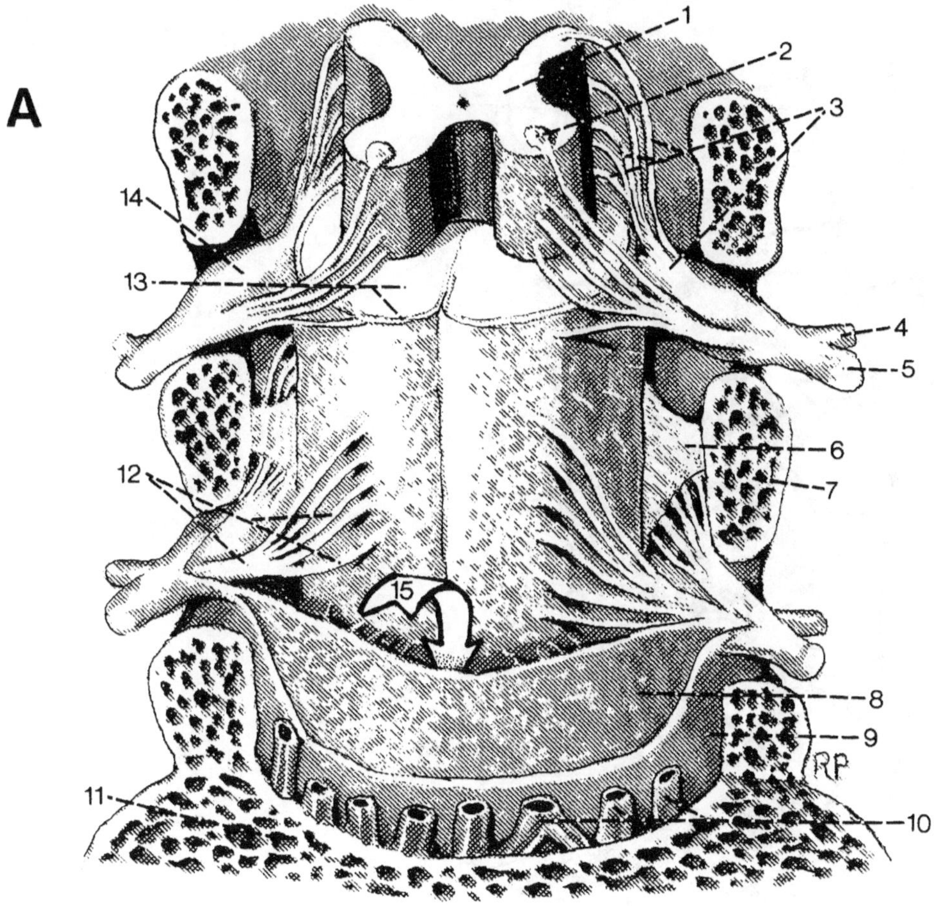

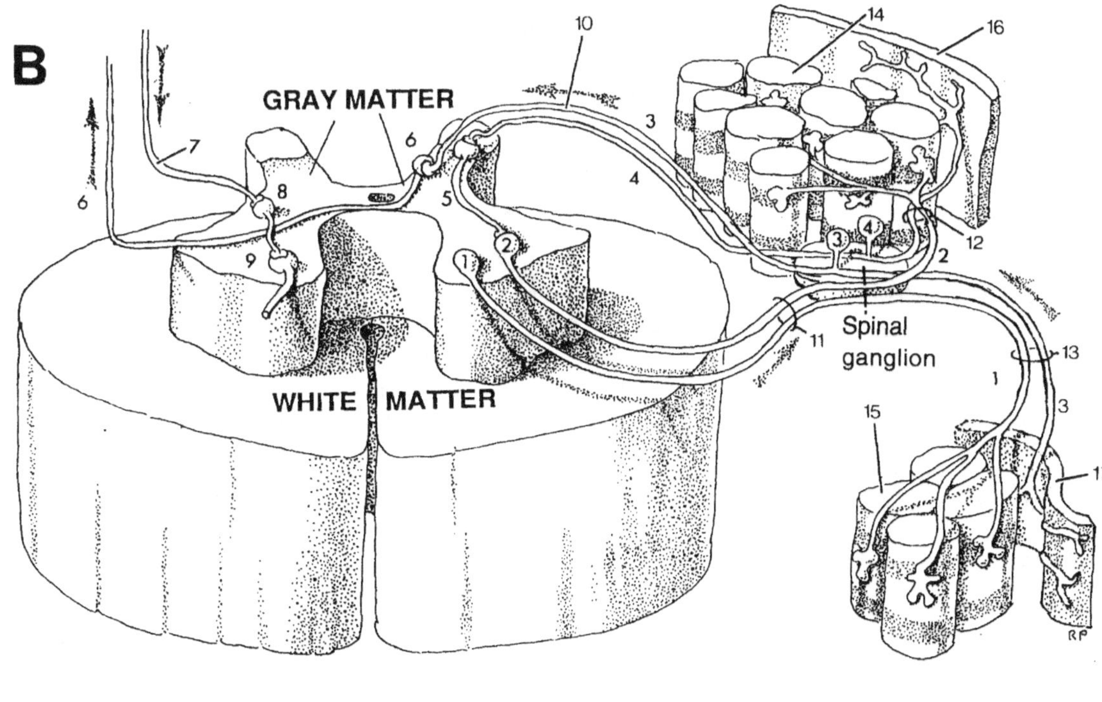

Bk-22 Lumbosacral spine I

Viewed from the left

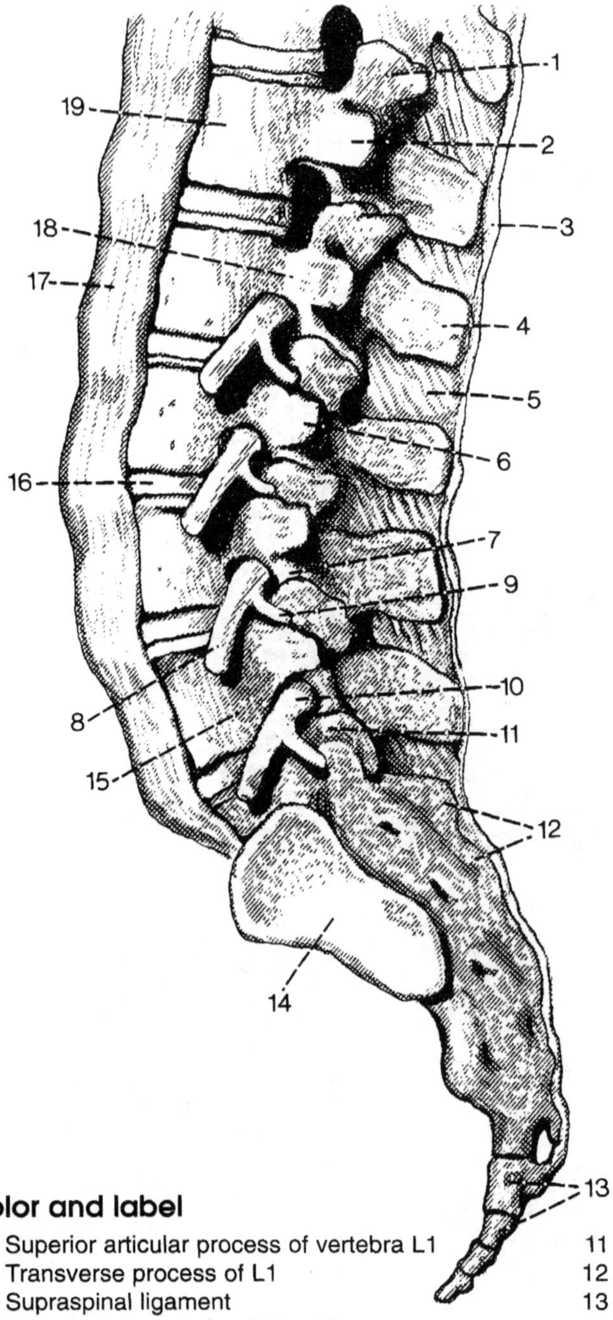

Redrawn from Netter

Color and label

1 Superior articular process of vertebra L1
2 Transverse process of L1
3 Supraspinal ligament
4 Spinous process of vertebra L2
5 Interspinal ligament
6 Superior articular process of L3
7 Inferior articular process of L4
8 Lumbar nerve (anterior ramus) L4
9 Posterior ramus of nerve L4
10 Spinal ganglion of lumbar nerve L5
11 Superior sacral articular process
12 Median sacral crest
13 Coccyx
14 Auricular facet of sacrum; forms sacroiliac joint with ilium
15 Body of vertebra L5
16 Intervertebral disc; between L3 and L4
17 Anterior longitudinal ligament
18 Pedicle of vertebra L2
19 Body of vertebra L1

Bk-23 Lumbosacral spine II

Posterior aspect

Color and label

1 Posterior longitudinal ligament
2 Intervertebral disc (between vertebrae L1 and L2)
3 Pedicle (cut)
4 Superior articular process of vertebra L3
5 Transverse process
6 Lamina
7 Inferior articular process
8 Superior articular process of L4
9 Spinous process of L4
10 Ligamentum flavum
11 Superior sacral articular process
12 Iliolumbar ligament
13 Posterior superior iliac spine

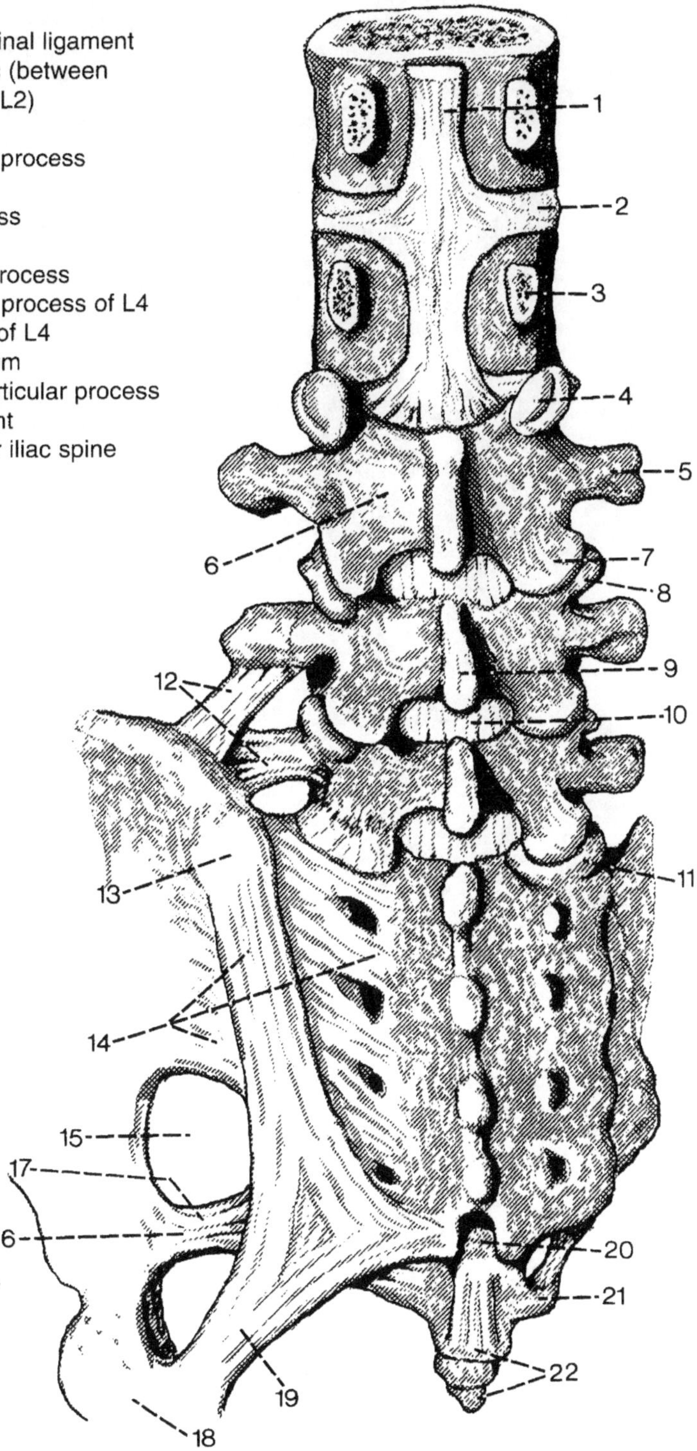

Redrawn from Netter

14 Dorsal sacroiliac ligament
15 Greater sciatic foramen
16 Ischial spine
17 Sacrospinal ligament
18 Lesser sciatic foramen
19 Sacrotuberal ligament; note how the sacrospinal ligament and the sacrotuberal ligament convert the greater and lesser sciatic *notches* into the greater and lesser sciatic *foramina.*
20 Sacral hiatus
21 Ala of the coccyx
22 Coccyx

Part VI: The Lower Limb

LL-1 Bones of the lower extremity

Including coxal bone

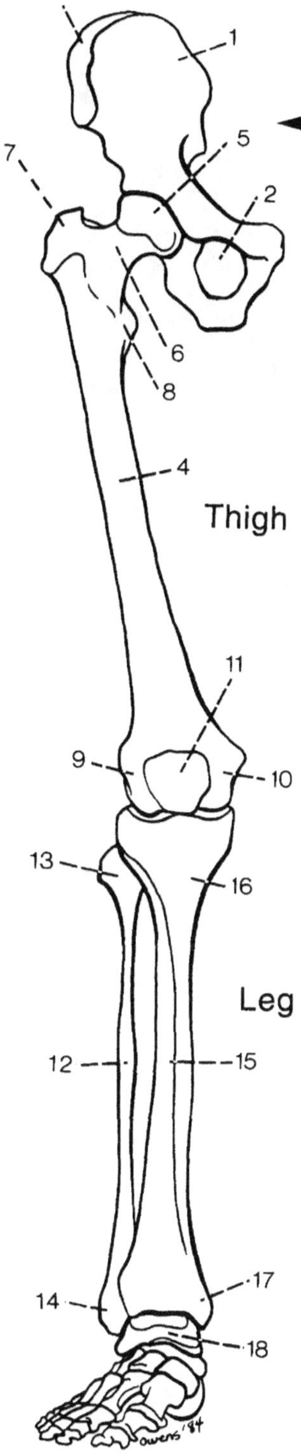

Right leg
Anterior view

Color and label

1 Coxal bone (hip bone)
2 Obturator foramen
3 Iliac crest
4 Femur
5 Head of femur
6 Neck of femur
7 Greater trochanter
8 Lesser trochanter
9 Lateral epicondyle
10 Medial epicondyle
11 Patella
12 Fibula
13 Head of fibula
14 Lateral malleolus
15 Tibia
16 Tibial tuberosity
17 Medial malleolus
18 Talus

Right leg
Posterior view

1 Ischial tuberosity
2 Greater trochanter
3 Lesser trochanter
4 Intertrochanteric crest
5 Linea aspera
6 Adductor tubercle
7 Medial condyle
8 Lateral condyle
9 Tibia
10 Fibula
11 Talus
12 Calcaneus

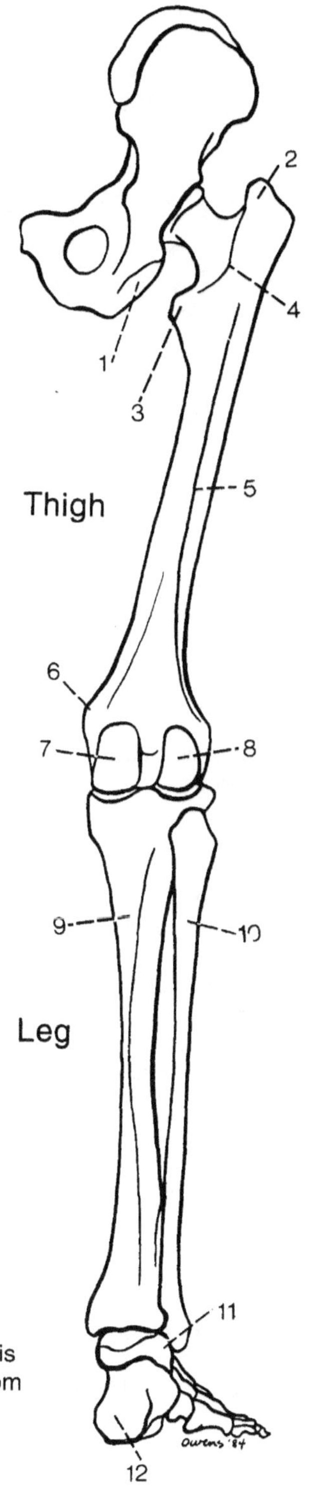

Note that in anatomy the lower extremity is divided into an upper **thigh,** extending from the hip to the knee, and lower **leg** that extends from the knee to the ankle.

LL-2 Superficial muscles of the right thigh

Anterior view

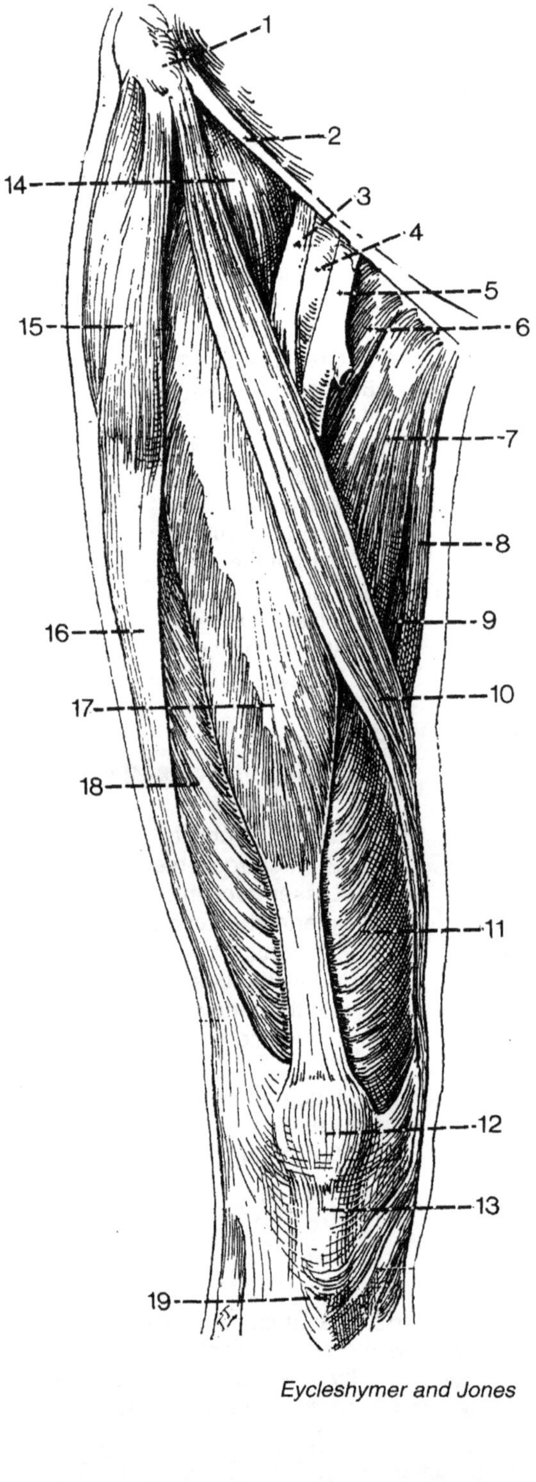

Eycleshymer and Jones

Color and label

1 Anterior superior iliac spine
2 Inguinal ligament
3 Femoral nerve
4 Femoral artery
5 Femoral vein
6 Pectineus muscle
7 Adductor magnus muscle
8 Gracilis muscle
9 Adductor magnus muscle
10 Sartorius muscle
11 Vastus medialis muscle (part of quadriceps femoris)
12 Patella (knee cap)
13 Patellar ligament
14 Iliopsoas muscle
15 Tensor fascia lata muscle
16 Iliotibial tract
17 Rectus femoris muscle (part of quadriceps femoris)
18 Vastus lateralis (part of quadriceps femoris)
19 Tibial tuberosity (insertion of quadriceps femoris)

LL-3 Superficial muscles of the right thigh

Lateral view

Color and label

1 Sartorius muscle
2 Tensor facia lata muscle
3 Greater trochanter (of femur; palpable beneath the skin)
4 Rectus femoris muscle
5 Iliotibial tract
6 Vastus lateralis muscle
7 Gluteus maximus muscle
8 Biceps femoris muscle (long head)
9 Biceps femoris muscle (short head)
10 Semimembranosus muscle
11 Tendon of biceps femoris
12 Gastrocnemius muscle (lateral head)
13 Soleus muscle
14 Patella
15 Insertion of biceps femoris on head of fibula
16 Tibial tuberosity

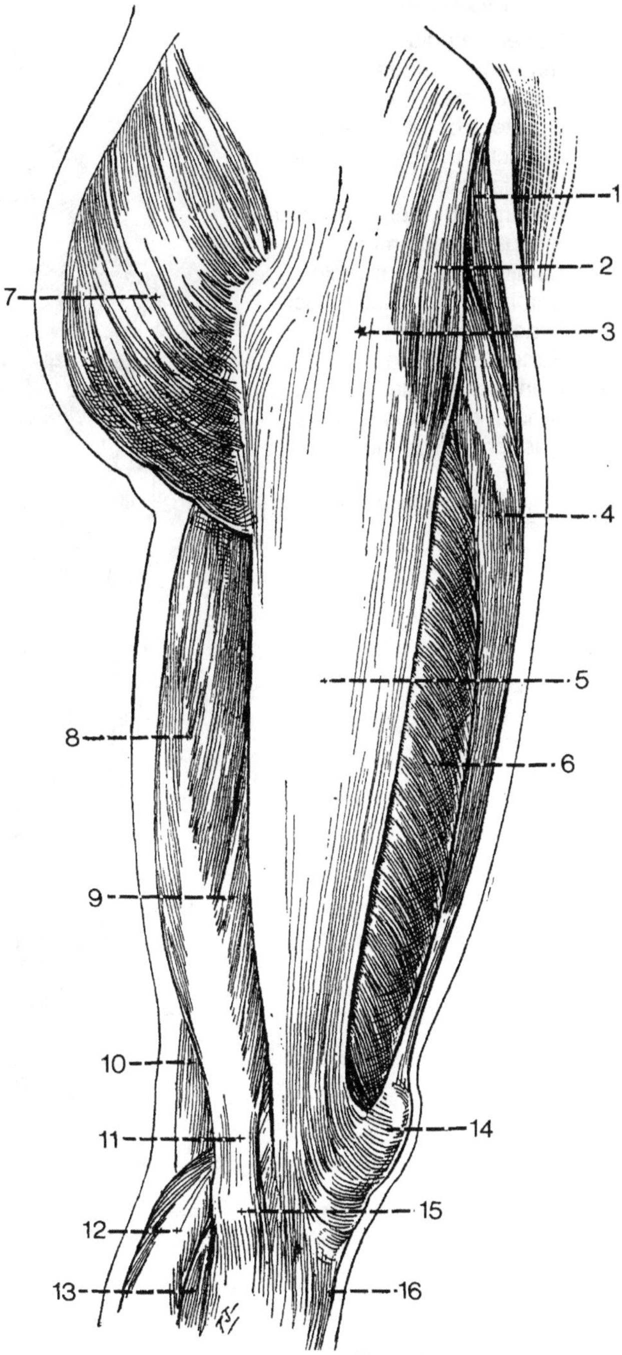

Eycleshymer and Jones

LL-4 Superficial muscles of the right thigh

Posterior view

Color and label

1 Gluteus medius muscle (under gluteal fascia)
2 Gluteus maximus muscle
3 Greater trochanter of femur
4 Adductor magnus muscle
5 Iliotibial tract
6 Semimembranosus muscle
7 Biceps femoris muscle
8 Semitendinosus muscle
9 Semimembranosus muscle
10 Gracilis muscle
11 Sartorius muscle
12 Plantaris muscle
13 Tendon of biceps femoris
14 Gastrocnemius muscle

Eycleshymer and Jones

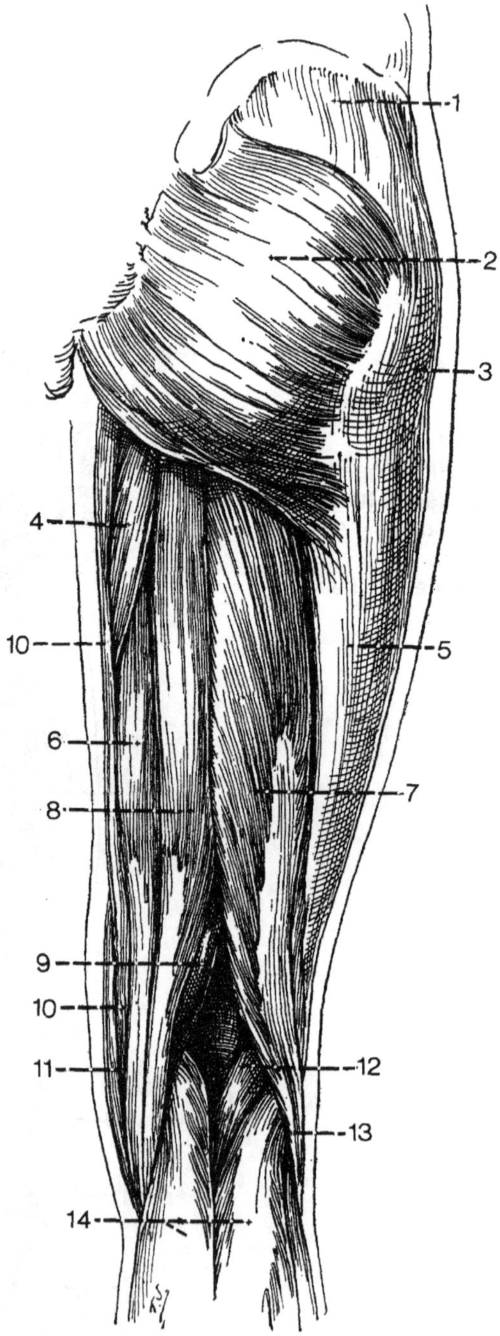

LL-5 Superficial muscles of the leg

Anterior aspect

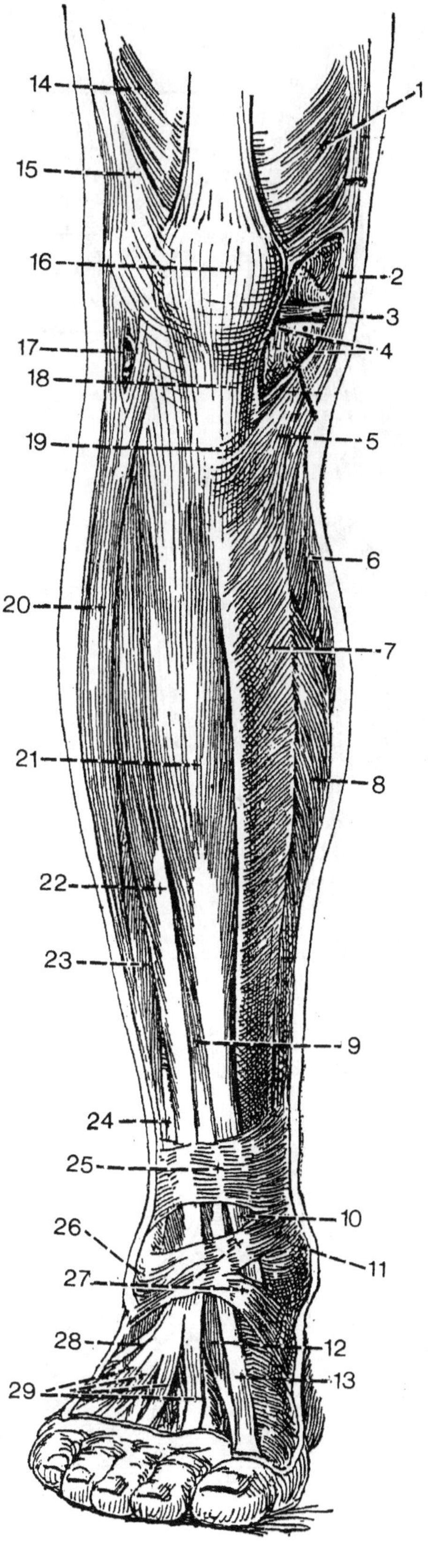

Color and label

1 Vastus medialis muscle
2 Tibial collateral ligament
3 Medial meniscus
4 Medial patellar retinaculum (cut open to expose medial meniscus)
5 Sartorius tendon (insertion on tibia)
6 Gastrocnemius muscle
7 Medial surface of tibia
8 Soleus muscle
9 Extensor hallucis longus muscle
10 Tendon of tibialis anterior
11 Medial malleolus
12 Extensor hallucis brevis muscle
13 Tendon of extensor hallucis longus
14 Vastus lateralis muscle
15 Iliotibial tract
16 Patella
17 Fibular collateral ligament
18 Patellar ligament
19 Tibial tuberosity
20 Peroneus longus muscle
21 Tibialis anterior muscle
22 Extensor digitorum longus muscle
23 Peroneus brevis muscle
24 Fibula
25 Superior extensor muscular retinaculum
26 Lateral malleolus
27 Inferior extensor muscular retinaculum
28 Tendon of peroneus tertius
29 Tendons of extensor digitorum

Eycleshymer and Jones

LL-6 Superficial muscles of the right leg

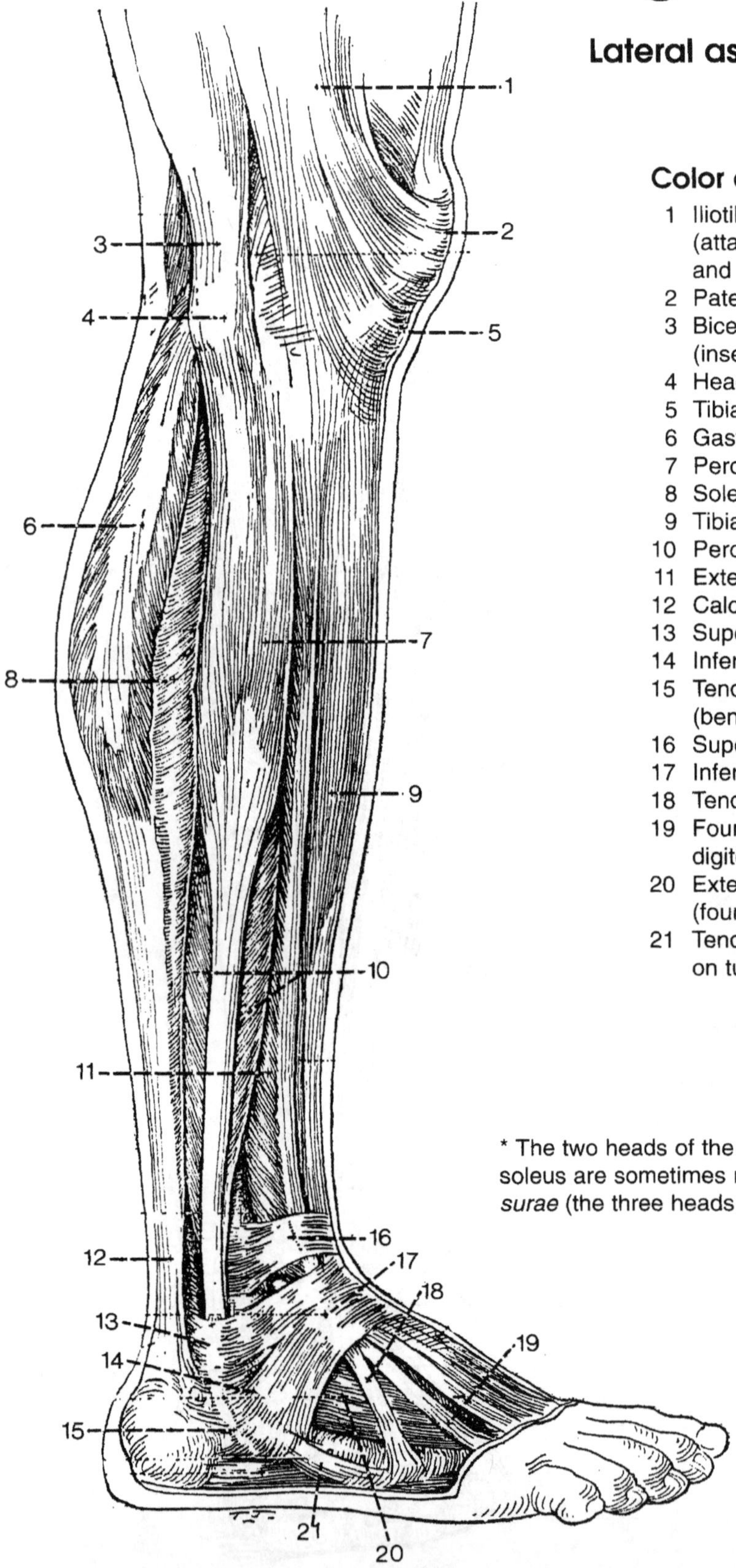

Lateral aspect

Color and label

1 Iliotibial tract (attaching to lateral condyle of tibia and fascia of vastus lateralis)
2 Patella
3 Biceps femoris muscle (inserting on head of fibula)
4 Head of fibula
5 Tibial tuberosity
6 Gastrocnemius muscle*
7 Peroneus longus muscle
8 Soleus muscle*
9 Tibialis anterior muscle
10 Peroneus brevis muscle
11 Extensor digitorum longus muscle
12 Calcaneus tendon (Achilles tendon)
13 Superior peroneal retinaculum
14 Inferior peroneal retinaculum
15 Tendon of peroneus longus (beneath retinaculum)
16 Superior extensor retinaculum
17 Inferior extensor retinaculum
18 Tendon of peroneus tertius
19 Four tendons of extensor digitorum longus
20 Extensor digitorum brevis muscles (four)
21 Tendon of peroneus brevis (inserting on tuberosity of fifth metatarsal)

* The two heads of the gastrocnemius plus the soleus are sometimes referred to as the *triceps surae* (the three heads of the calf)

Eycleshymer and Jones

LL-7 Superficial muscles of posterior leg

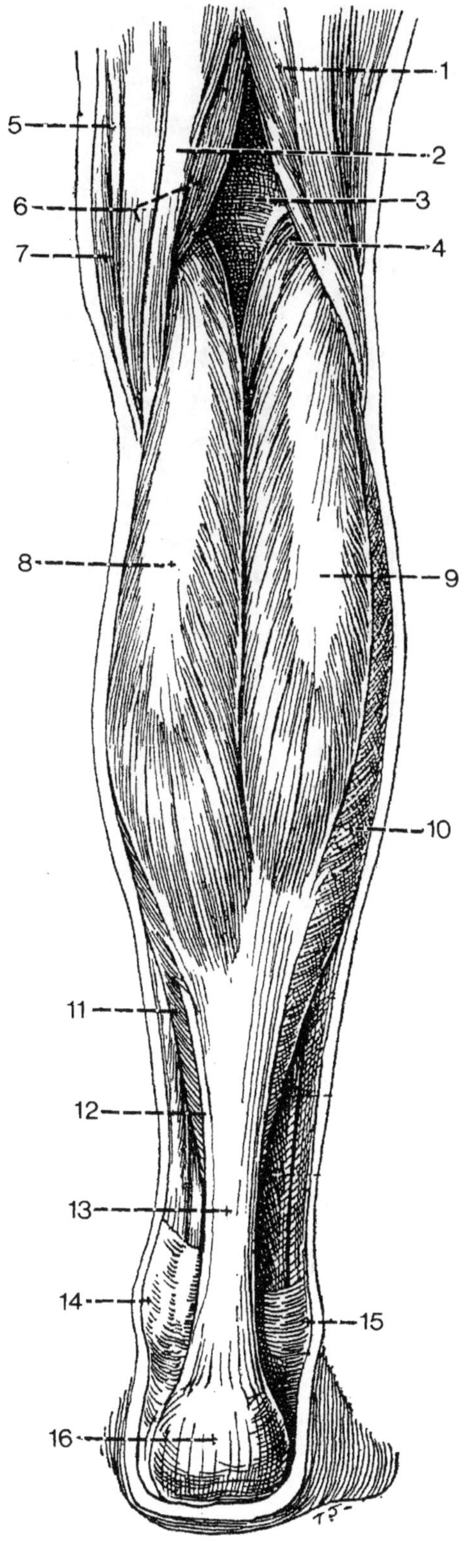

Color and label

1 Biceps femoris muscle
2 Semitendinosus muscle
3 Popliteal fossa
4 Plantaris muscle
5 Gracilis muscle
6 Semimembranosus muscle
7 Sartorius muscle
8 Gastrocnemius muscle (medial head)
9 Gastrocnemius muscle (lateral head)
10 Soleus muscle (deep to gastrocnemius)
11 Soleus muscle (deep to gastrocnemius)
12 Tendon of plantaris muscle; this small muscle has a long thin tendon that descends with the calcaneal tendon and inserts separately on the calcaneal tuberosity.
13 Calcaneal tendon (Achilles tendon)
14 Medial malleolus of tibia
15 Lateral malleolus of fibula
16 Calcaneal tuberosity

Eycleshymer and Jones

LL-8 Muscles of medial right leg

Color and label

1 Gracilis muscle
2 Semimembranosus muscle
3 Semitendinosus muscle
4 Tendon of gracilis
5 Tendon of semimembranosus
6 Semitendinosus tendon
7 Gastrocnemius muscle (medial head)
8 Soleus muscle
9 Flexor digitorum longus muscle
10 Flexor hallucis longus muscle
11 Tibialis posterior tendon (within synovial sheath)
12 Flexor digitorum longus tendon (within synovial sheath)
13 Calcaneal tendon (Achilles tendon)
14 Flexor hallucis longus tendon (within synovial sheath)
15 Flexor retinaculum
16 Abductor hallucis muscle (cut)
17 Tendon of flexor hallucis longus (within synovial sheath)
18 Tendon of tibialis anterior
19 Abductor hallucis (cut)
20 Sartorius muscle
21 Vastus medials muscle
22 Patella (knee cap)
23 Patellar ligament
24 Pes anserinus*
25 Tibialis anterior muscle
26 Tibia
27 Medial malleolus
28 Inferior extensor retinaculum
29 Tendon of tibialis anterior (within synovial sheath)
30 Synovial sheaths of extensor digitorum longus tendons
31 Synovial sheath of extensor hallucis longus
32 Extensor digitorum longus tendons (four in number)
33 Tendon of extensor hallucis longus

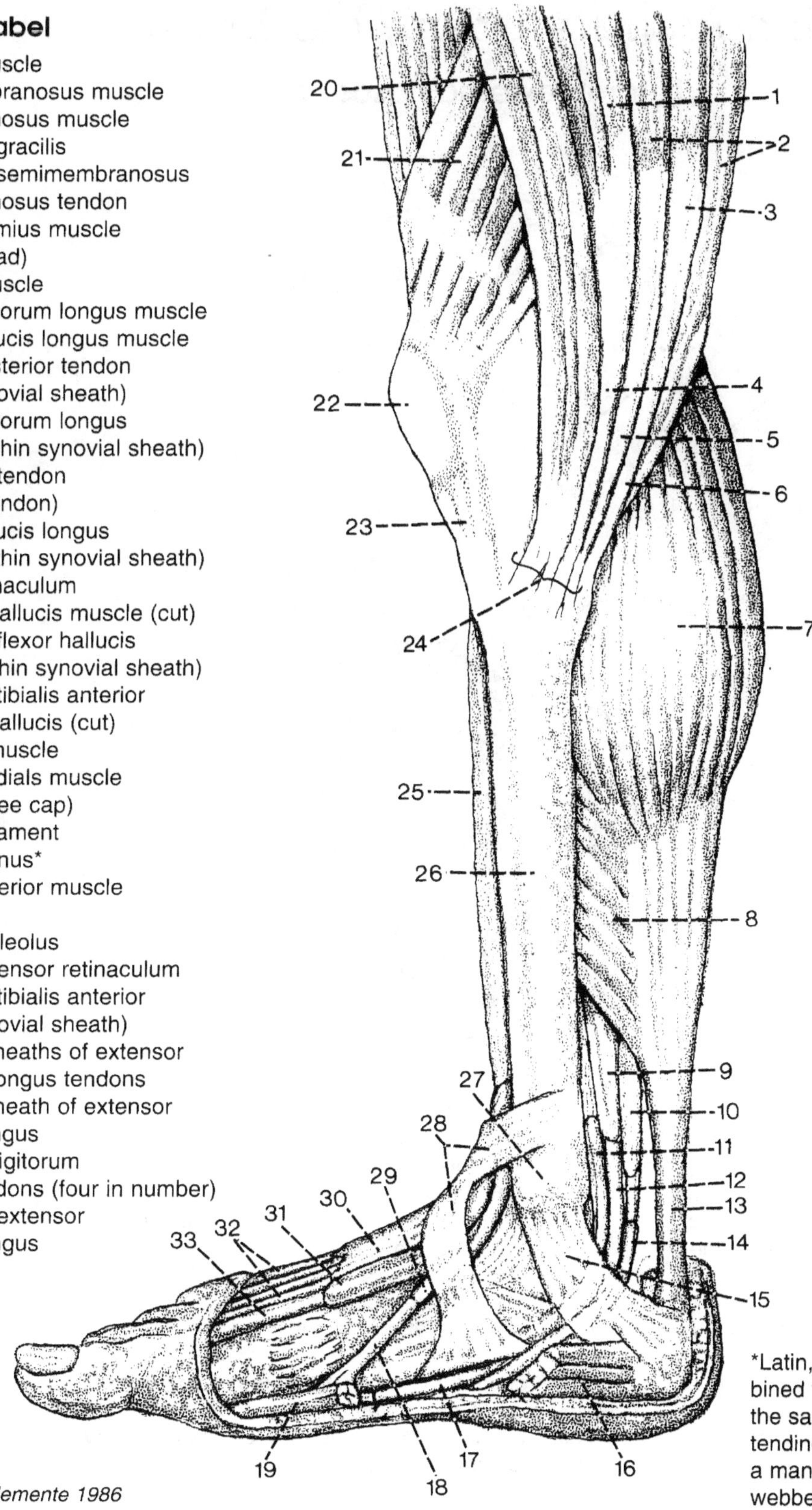

Redrawn from Clemente 1986

*Latin, goose's foot; the combined tendinous insertions of the sartorius, gracilis, and semitendinosus on the medial tibia in a manner resembling the webbed foot of a goose.

LL-9 Right coxal bone (innominate bone, hip bone)

Lateral (external) aspect

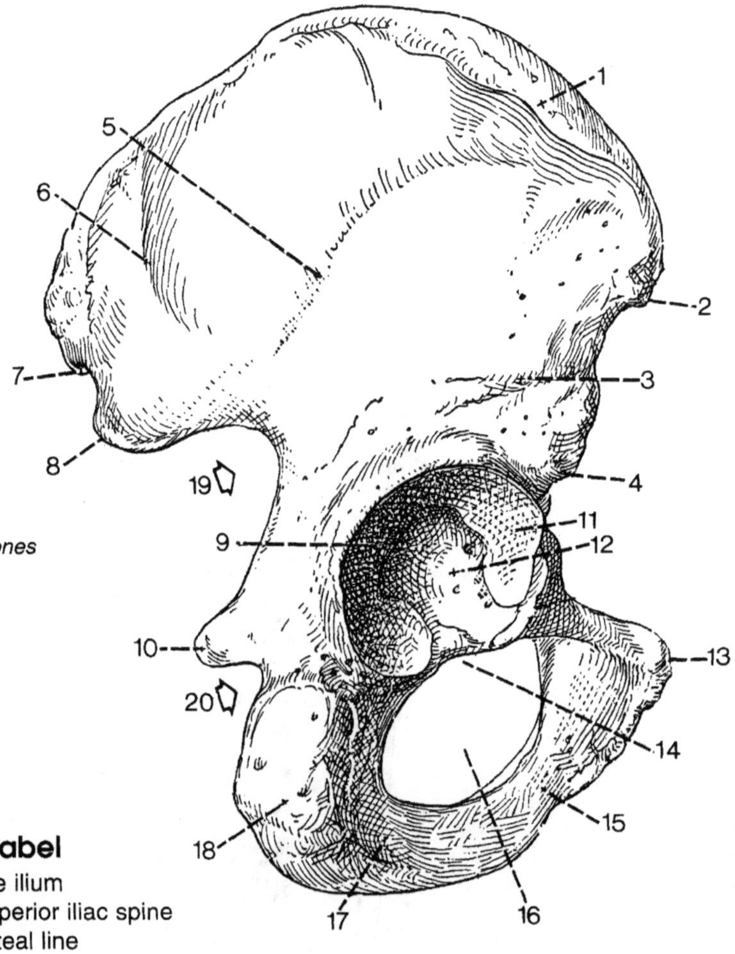

Eycleshymer and Jones

Color and label

1 Crest of the ilium
2 Anterior superior iliac spine
3 Inferior gluteal line
4 Anterior inferior iliac spine
5 Anterior gluteal line
6 Posterior gluteal line
7 Posterior superior iliac spine
8 Posterior inferior iliac spine
9 Acetabulum (socket for the head of the femur)
10 Ischial spine
11 Lunate surface (smooth articular surface)
12 Acetabular fossa (rough nonarticular portion above acetabular notch)
13 Pubic tubercle
14 Acetabular notch
15 Inferior pubic ramus
16 Obturator foramen*
17 Ischial ramus (fused with inferior pubic ramus)
18 Ischial tuberosity
19 Greater sciatic notch
20 Lesser sciatic notch

*The obturator foramen, or "stopped-up foramen" (by muscle and membrane), takes its name from the Latin *obturare*, "to stop up"; the blockage, however, is not complete; the small obturator canal allows the passage of the obturator nerve, artery, and vein.

LL-10 Right hip bone (coxal bone)

Medial (internal) surface

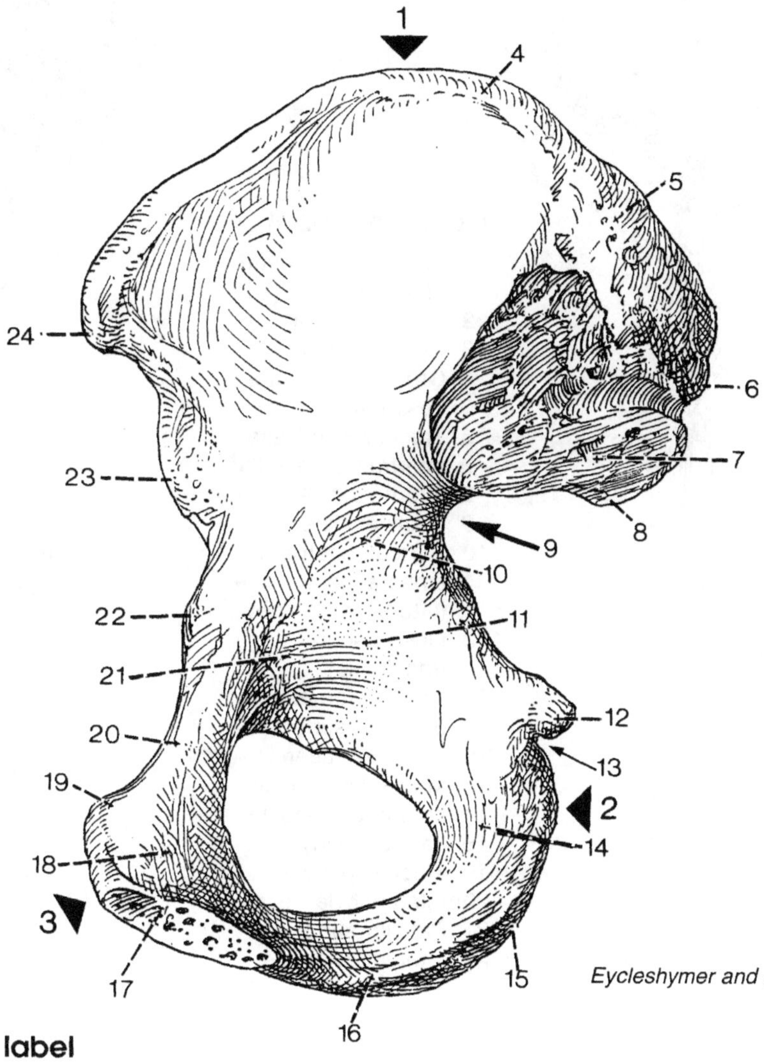

Eycleshymer and Jones

Color and label

1 Ilium
2 Ischium
3 Pubis
4 Iliac crest
5 Iliac tuberosity
6 Posterior superior iliac spine
7 Auricular surface; articulates with sacrum
8 Posterior inferior iliac spine
9 Greater sciatic notch
10 Body of ilium
11 Body of pubis
12 Spine of the ischium (ischial spine)
13 Lesser sciatic notch
14 Ramus of ischium
15 Ischial tuberosity
16 Inferior pubic ramus
17 Symphysial surface of pubis; articulates with opposite pubis in the pubic symphysis.
18 Superior pubic ramus
19 Pubic tubercle
20 Pecten pubis (*pecten*, Latin, comb, comb-like)
21 Body of pubic bone
22 Iliopectineal eminence
23 Anterior inferior iliac spine
24 Anterior superior iliac spine

LL-11 The right femur

Anterior aspect

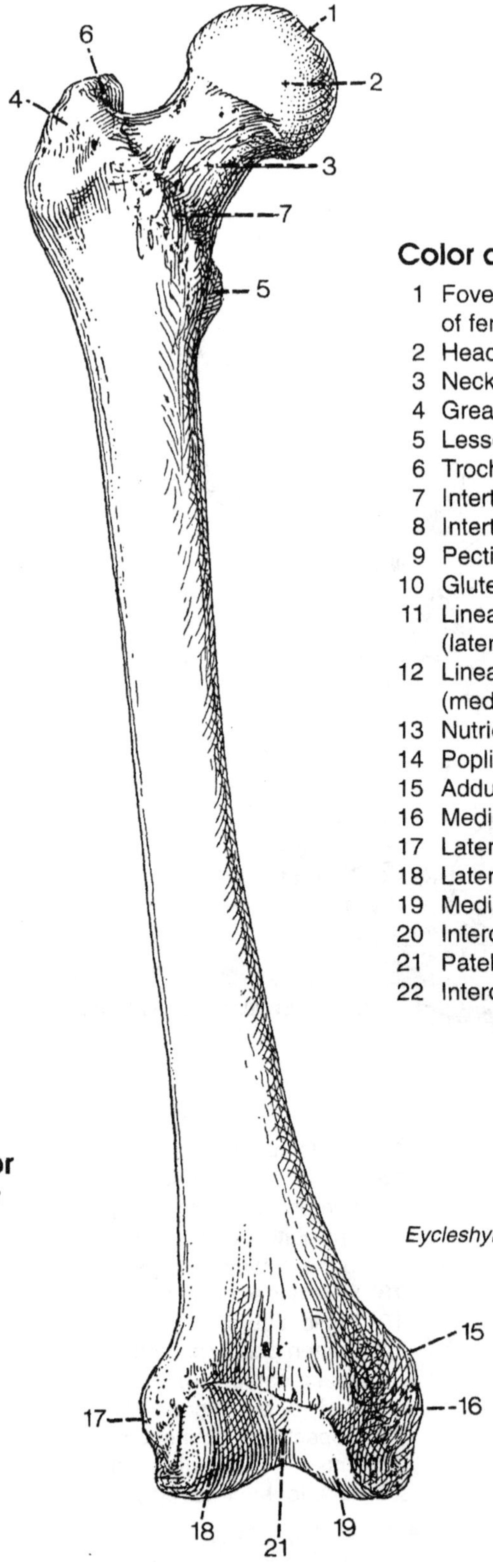

Anterior aspect

Color and label

1 Fovea (pit) of head of femur
2 Head of femur
3 Neck of femur
4 Greater trochanter
5 Lesser trochanter
6 Trochanteric fossa
7 Intertrochanteric line
8 Intertrochanteric crest
9 Pectineal line
10 Gluteal tuberosity
11 Linea aspera (lateral lip)
12 Linea aspera (medial lip)
13 Nutrient foramen
14 Popliteal surface
15 Adductor tubercle
16 Medial epicondyle
17 Lateral epicondyle
18 Lateral condyle
19 Medial condyle
20 Intercondylar fossa
21 Patellar surface
22 Intercondylar line

Eycleshymer and Jones

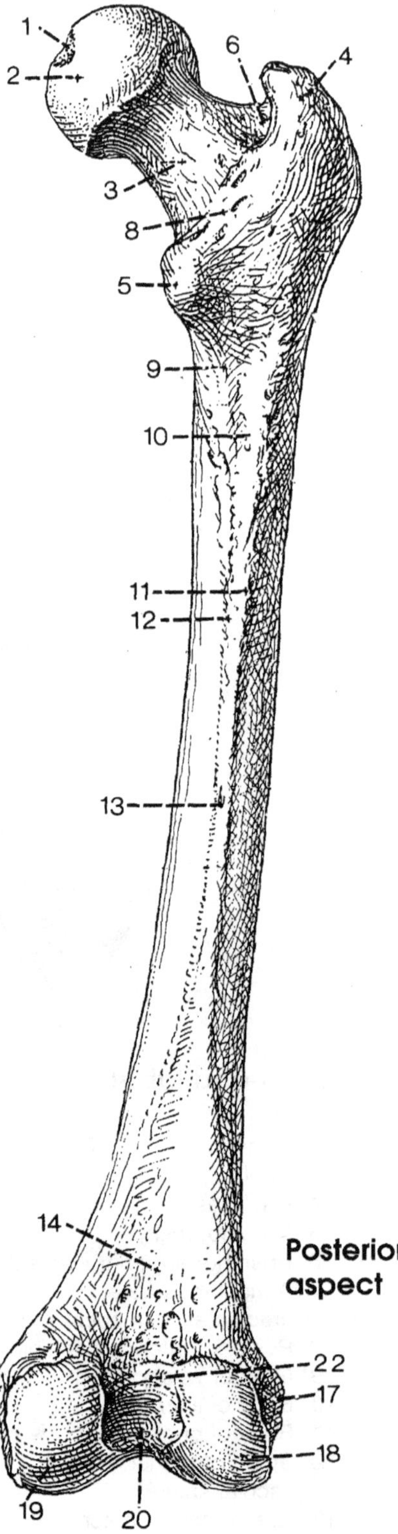

Posterior aspect

LL-12 Right tibia and fibula

Anterior aspect

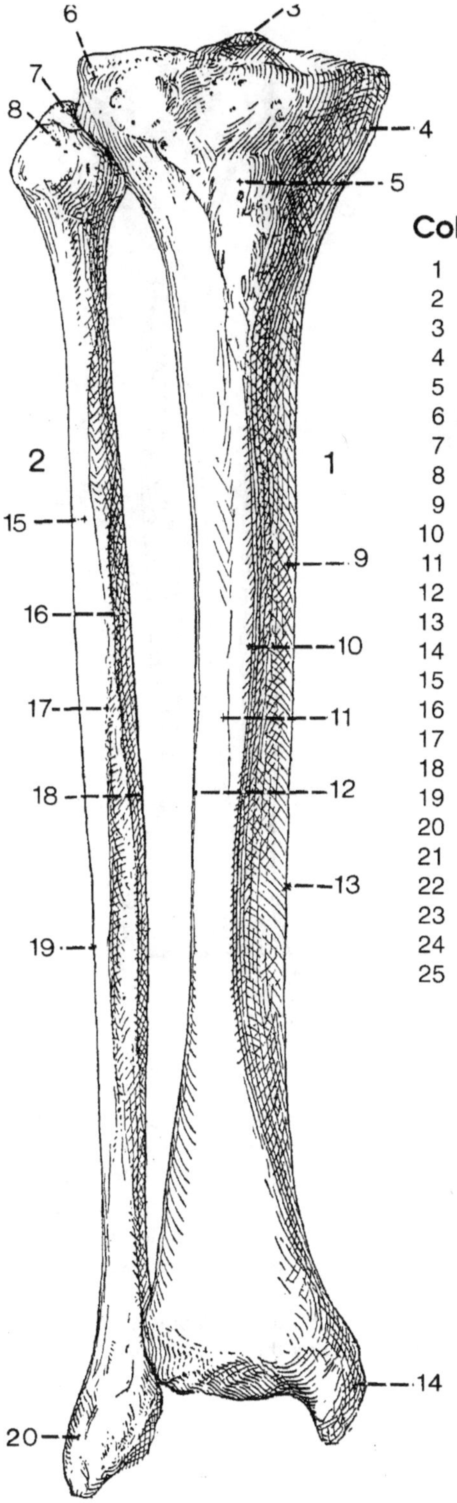

Posterior aspect

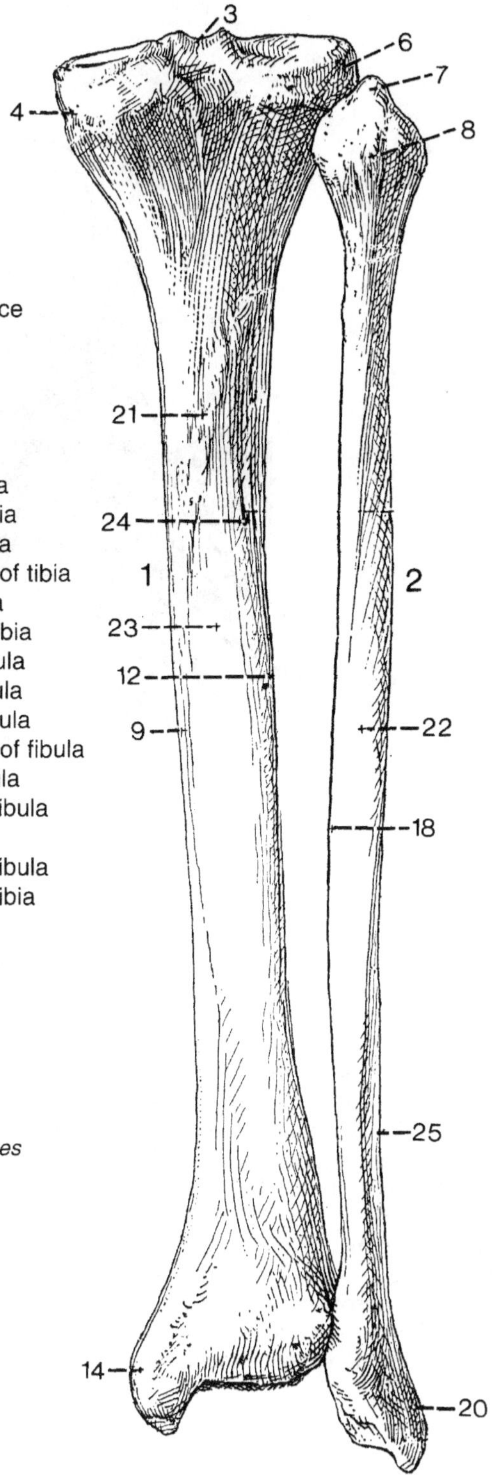

Color and label

1 Tibia
2 Fibula
3 Intercondylar eminence
4 Medial condyle
5 Tibial tuberosity
6 Lateral condyle
7 Apex of fibular head
8 Head of fibula
9 Medial surface of tibia
10 Anterior margin of tibia
11 Lateral surface of tibia
12 Interosseous margin of tibia
13 Medial margin of tibia
14 Medial malleolus of tibia
15 Lateral surface of fibula
16 Medial surface of fibula
17 Anterior margin of fibula
18 Interosseous margin of fibula
19 Lateral margin of fibula
20 Lateral malleolus of fibula
21 Popliteal line of tibia
22 Posterior surface of fibula
23 Posterior surface of tibia
24 Nutrient foramen
25 Lateral crest of fibula

Eycleshymer and Jones

Fibula and tibia:
Etymological cartoon

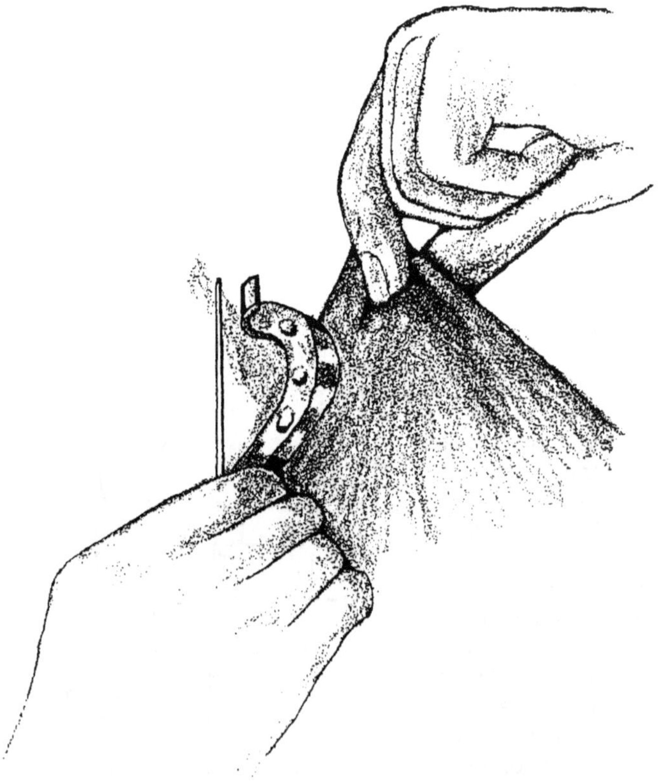

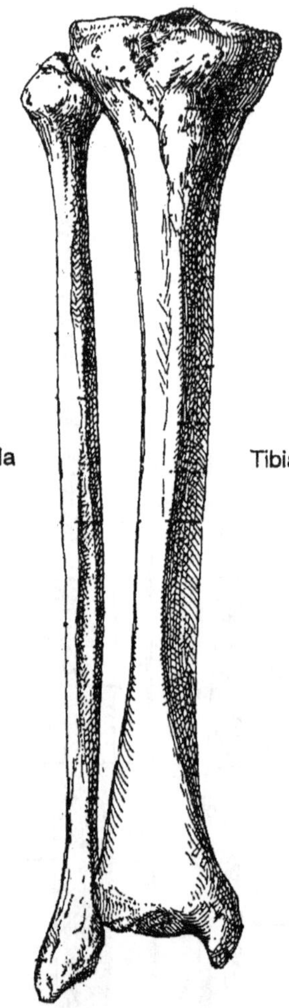

Fibula means a "clasp, brooch, or buckle" in Latin, specifically the thin, pointed tongue of a clasp, as opposed to the much thicker, and often highly ornate, bar of the clasp. Supposedly the Romans thought that the two bones of the lower leg resembled a clasp, with the outer thin fibula suggesting the tongue and the inner thicker tibia suggesting the bar. So they named the thin outer one *fibula*, and the more stout inner one *tibia*. The term *fibula* probably arose from the verb *figo*, "to fix" or "to fasten." The muscles and structures on the outer side of the lower leg that relate to the fibula were named by English-speaking anatomists, not **fibular**, as one might expect, but peroneal, from the Greek word for "brooch," *perone,* which is derived from the verb *peiro*, "to pierce." However, anatomists in countries such as Germany and Switzerland preferred to name these lateral muscles, nerves, and blood vessels **fibular**. So depending on where one studies anatomy, one will learn the outer lower leg muscles and related structures as either **fibular** or **peroneal**. As for remembering which bone is the tibia and which is the fibula, the fibula which is **lateral**, ends with **la** as in **la**teral. The term **tibia** means a "flute" or "pipe" in Latin as well as the shin bone. The ancients probably made flute-like instruments from the shin bones of animals.

LL-13 Bones of the right foot

Viewed from above

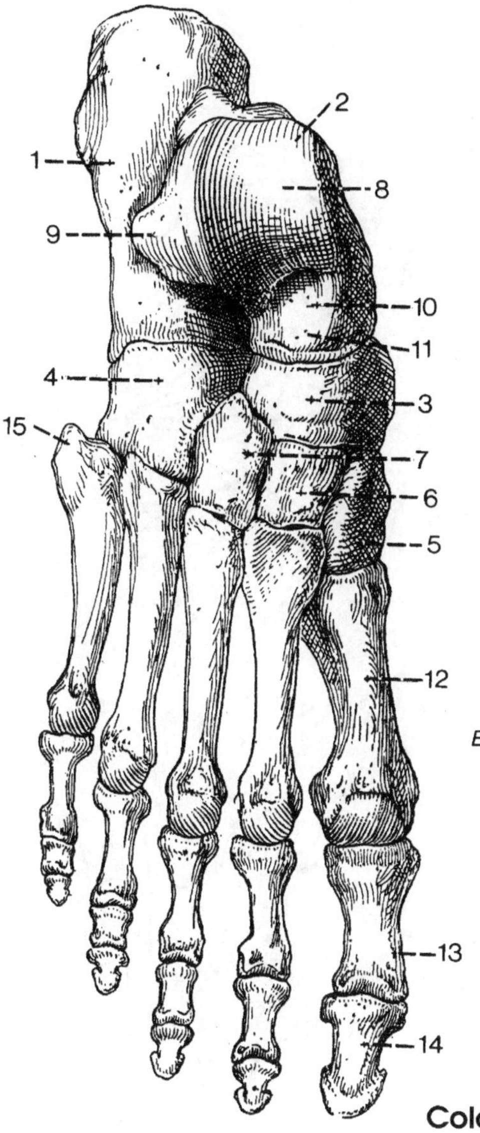

Viewed from below

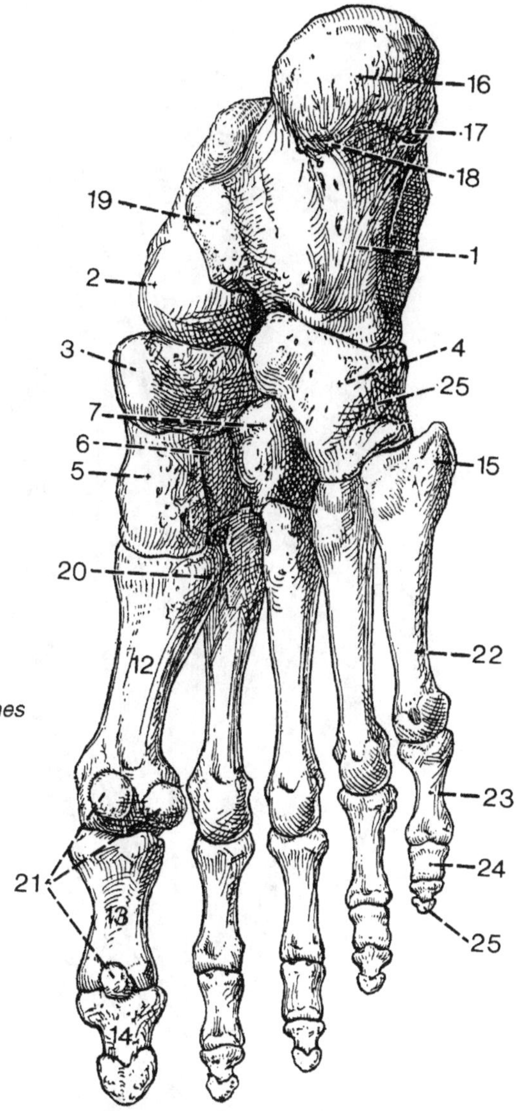

Eycleshymer and Jones

Color and label

1 Calcaneus
2 Talus
3 Navicular
4 Cuboid
5 Medial cuneiform
6 Intermediate cuneiform
7 Lateral cuneiform
8 Trochlea (Latin, pully) of talus
9 Lateral process of talus
10 Neck of talus
11 Head of talus
12 First metatarsal
13 Proximal phalanx of big toe (*hallux*, Latin)
14 Distal phalanx of big toe
15 Tuberosity of fifth metatarsal
16 Calcaneal tuber (Latin, swelling, protuberance)
17 Lateral process of calcaneal tuber
18 Medial process of calcaneal tuber
19 Sustentaculum tali (support of talus) of calcaneus
20 Tuberosity of first metatarsal
21 Sesamoid bones
22 Fifth metatarsal
23 Proximal phalanx of fifth toe
24 Middle phalanx of fifth toe
25 Distal phalanx of fifth toe

LL-14 Lumbar muscles

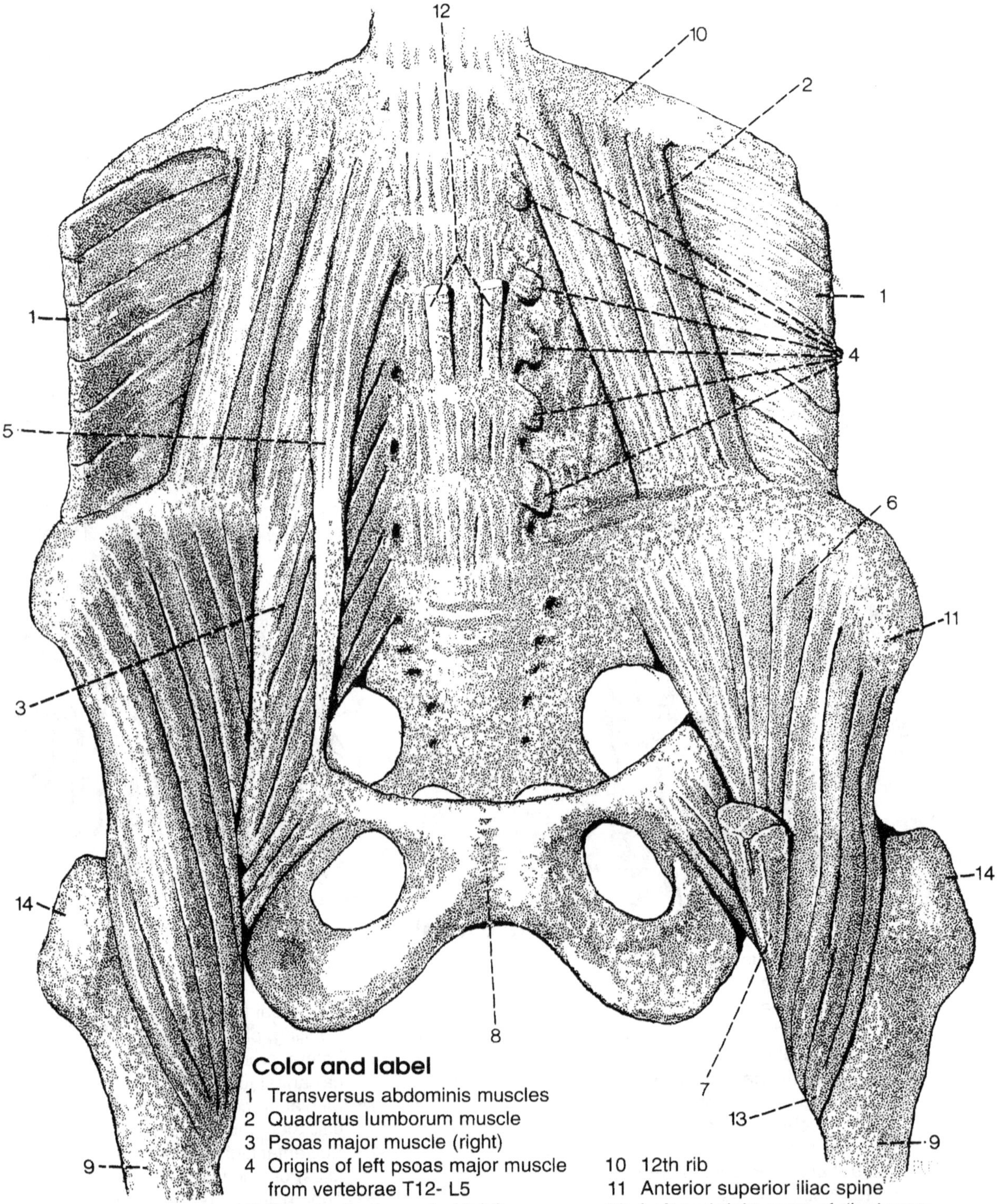

Color and label

1 Transversus abdominis muscles
2 Quadratus lumborum muscle
3 Psoas major muscle (right)
4 Origins of left psoas major muscle from vertebrae T12- L5
5 Psoas minor muscle (right)
6 Iliacus muscle
7 Tendon of psoas major inserting on lesser trochanter
8 Pubic symphysis
9 Femur
10 12th rib
11 Anterior superior iliac spine
12 Left and right crura of diaphragm
13 Insertion of the compound iliopsoas muscle (psoas major + iliacus) onto the lesser trochanter of the femur
14 Greater trochanter

Redrawn from Spalteholz and Spanner

LL-15 Arteries of the right thigh

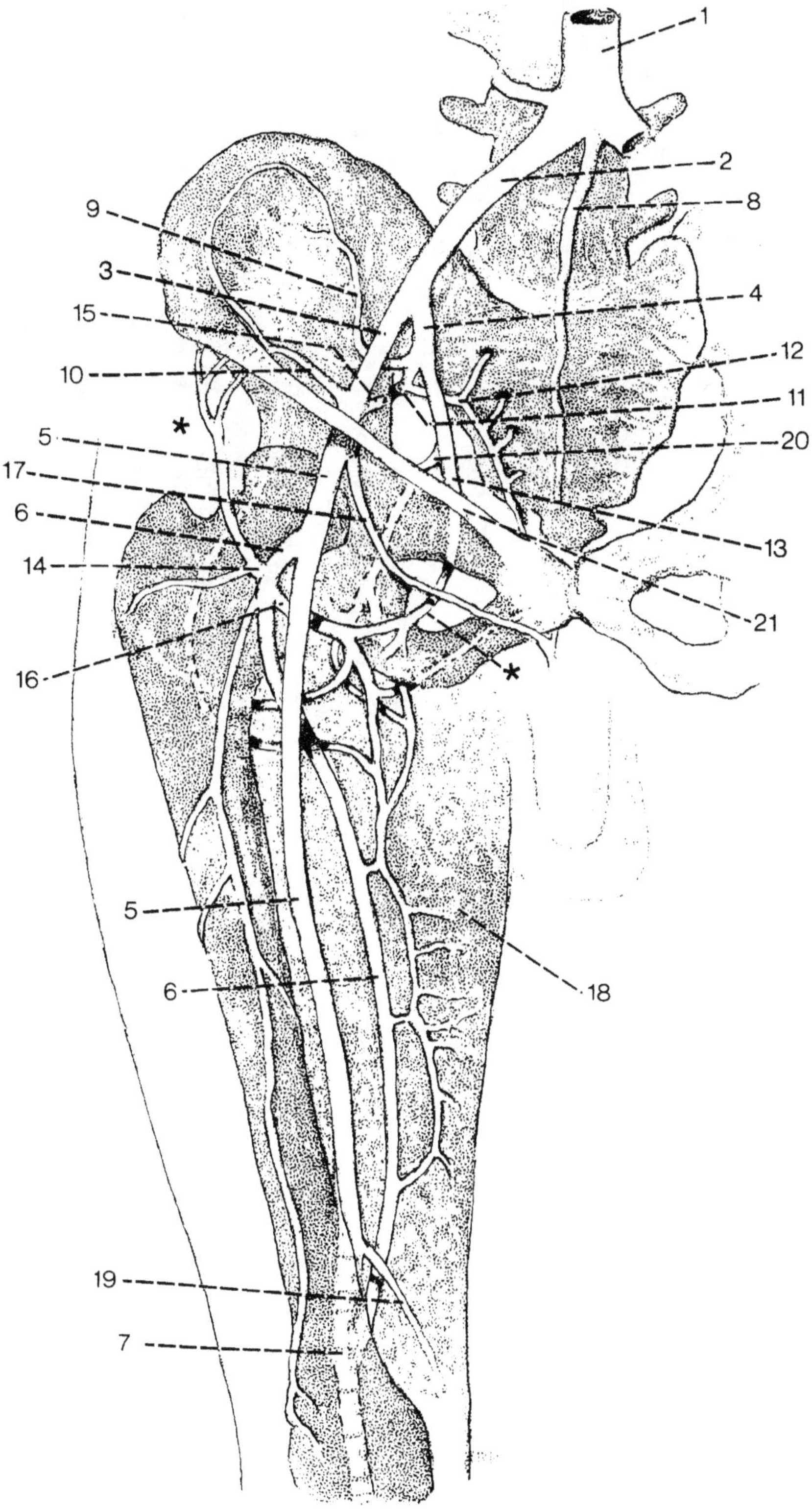

Redrawn from Eycleshymer and Jones

Color and label

1 Abdominal aorta
2 Right common iliac artery
3 External iliac artery
4 Internal iliac artery
5 Femoral artery; the external iliac artery becomes the femoral artery below the inguinal ligament.
6 Deep femoral artery
7 Popliteal artery (posterior to the femur); the femoral artery becomes the popliteal artery below the adductor hiatus. The names of the accompanying veins (not shown) undergo similar changes.
8 Median sacral artery
9 Iliolumbar artery
10 Deep iliac circumflex artery
11 Superior gluteal artery
12 Lateral sacral artery
13 Obturator artery
14 Lateral femoral circumflex artery (*anastomosis between 10 and 14 is exaggerated in thickness to illustrate collateral circulation in case of blockage of the upper femoral artery)
15 Inferior epigastric artery (cut)
16 Medial femoral circumflex artery (*anastomosis between 13 and 16 is exaggerated in thickness to show possible collateral circulation)
17 External pudendal artery
18 Perforating branches of deep femoral artery
19 Descending genicular artery
20 Inferior gluteal artery
21 Inguinal artery

LL-16 Nerves of the lumbar plexus

Color and label

1 Subcostal nerve (T12)
2 Iliohypogastric nerve
3 Ilioinguinal nerve
4 Anterior scrotal branches of ilioinguinal nerve (labial in female)
5 Genitofemoral nerve
6 Genital branch of genitofemoral nerve
7 Femoral branch of genitofemoral nerve
8 Lateral femoral cutaneous nerve
9 Obturator nerve; note that both the obturator and the femoral nerve arise from lumbar nerves L2, L3, L4.
10 Anterior branch of obturator nerve
11 Posterior branch of obturator nerve
12 Femoral nerve
13 Saphenous nerve (branch of femoral nerve)
14 Muscular branches of the femoral nerve; the femoral nerve supplies all the muscles in the anterior compartment of the thigh.
15 Anterior cutaneous branches of the femoral nerve
16 Lumbosacral trunk; carries fibers from L4 and L5 to sacral plexus.
17 Sacral nerves S1-S5
18 Sacral plexus
19 Twelfth rib
20 Right testis
21 Inguinal canal (schematic)

N L1 - L5, lumbar nerves
L1 - L5, lumbar vertebrae

Redrawn from Spalteholz and Spanner

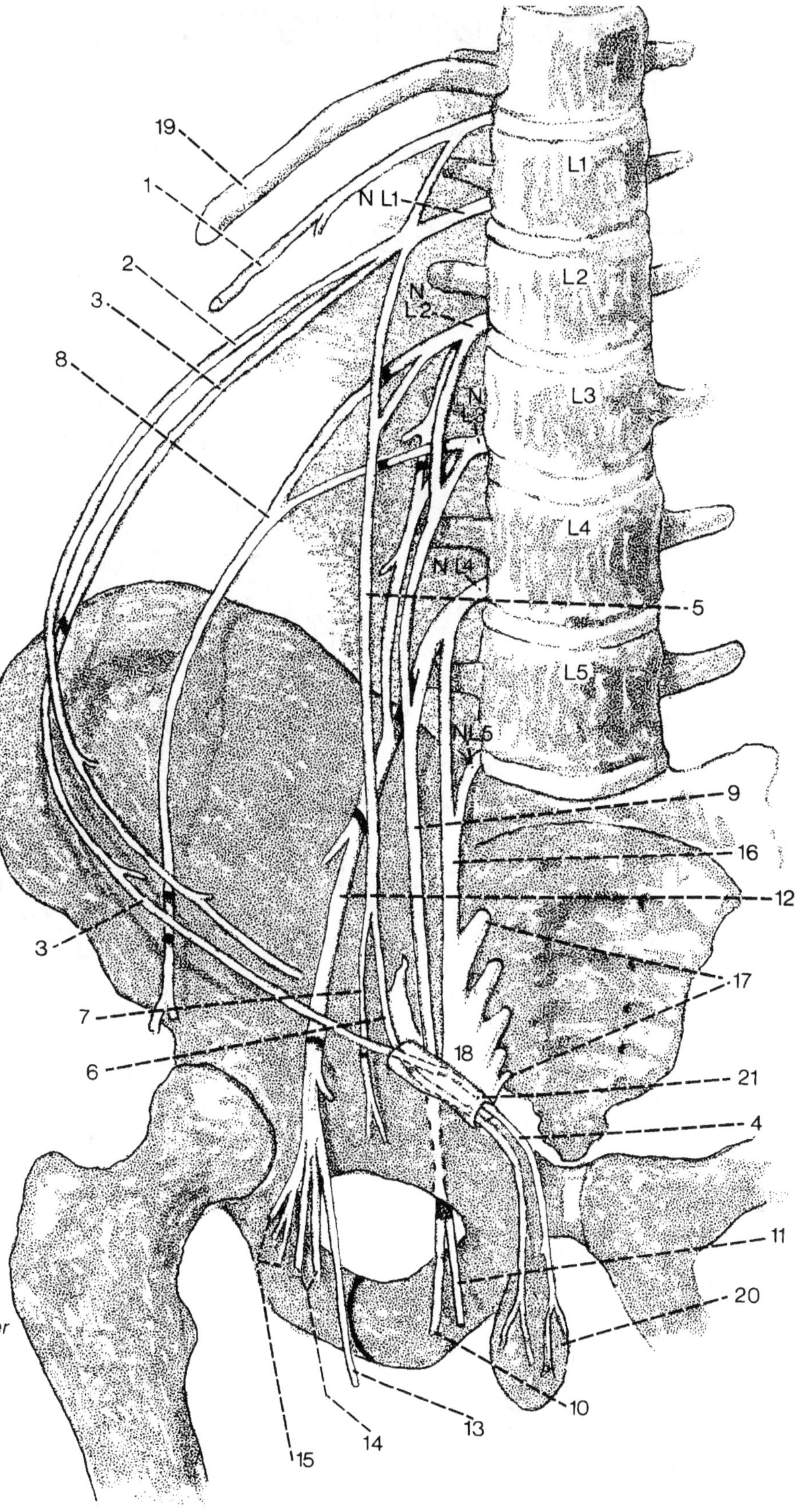

LL-17 Motor distribution of the femoral nerve I

The following muscles are innervated by the femoral nerve except where otherwise indicated. Small portions of these muscles are indicated on the figure's right.

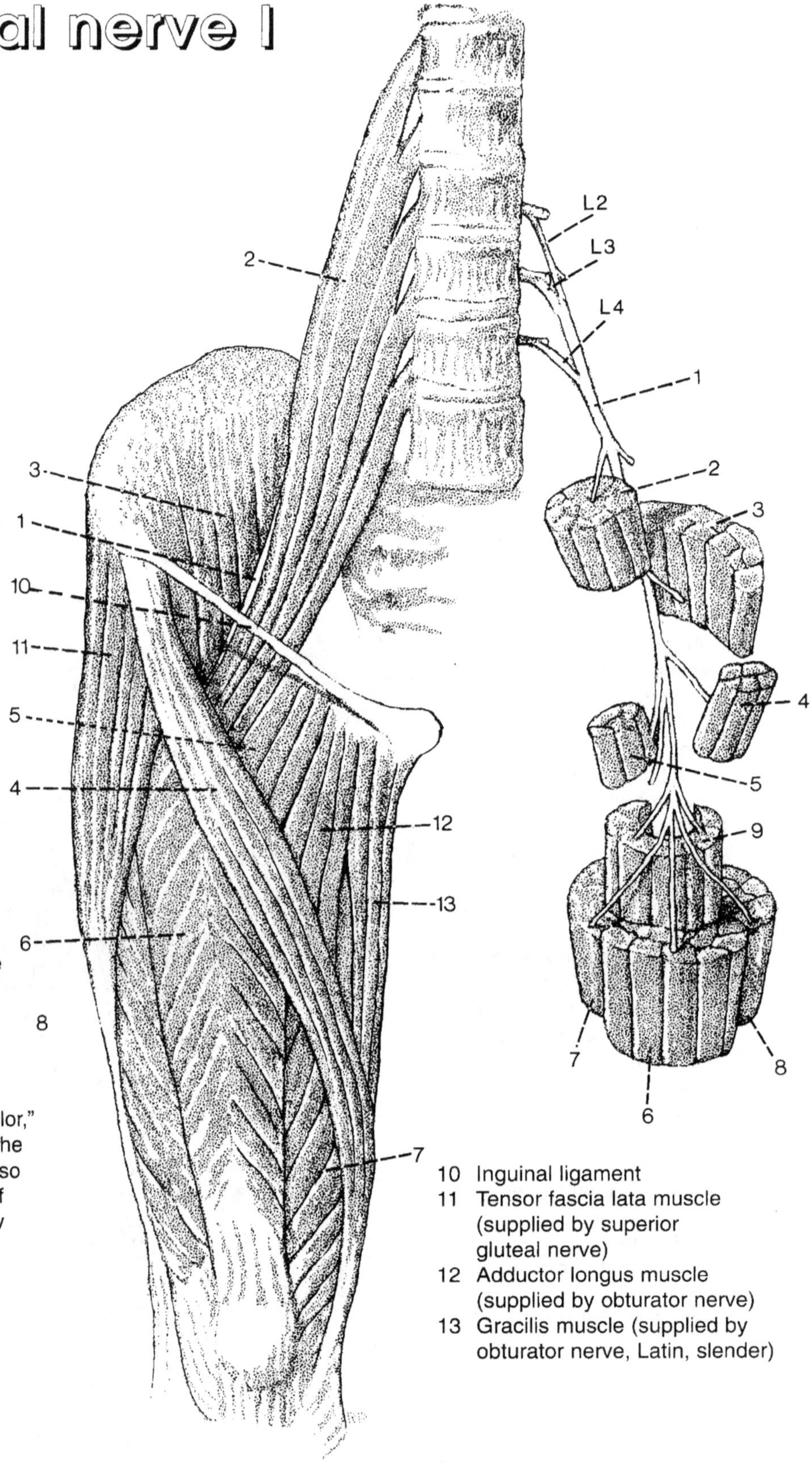

Color and label

1 Femoral nerve; its roots, L2,L3,L4 pass through the substance of the psoas major muscle, which must be removed (left side) for the roots to be seen.
2 Psoas major muscle
3 Iliacus muscle
4 Sartorius muscle (Latin, "of the tailor," so named because it both flexes the knee and rotates the leg outward so that the ankle rests on the knee of the other leg, a postion favored by tailors while sewing clothes)
5 Pectineus muscle
6 Rectus femoris muscle
7 Vastus medialis muscle
8 Vastus lateralis muscle
9 Vastus intermedius muscle; note that the vastus intermedius is covered by the other three muscles (6,7,8) of the quadriceps femoris.
10 Inguinal ligament
11 Tensor fascia lata muscle (supplied by superior gluteal nerve)
12 Adductor longus muscle (supplied by obturator nerve)
13 Gracilis muscle (supplied by obturator nerve, Latin, slender)

LL-18 Motor distribution of the femoral nerve, II

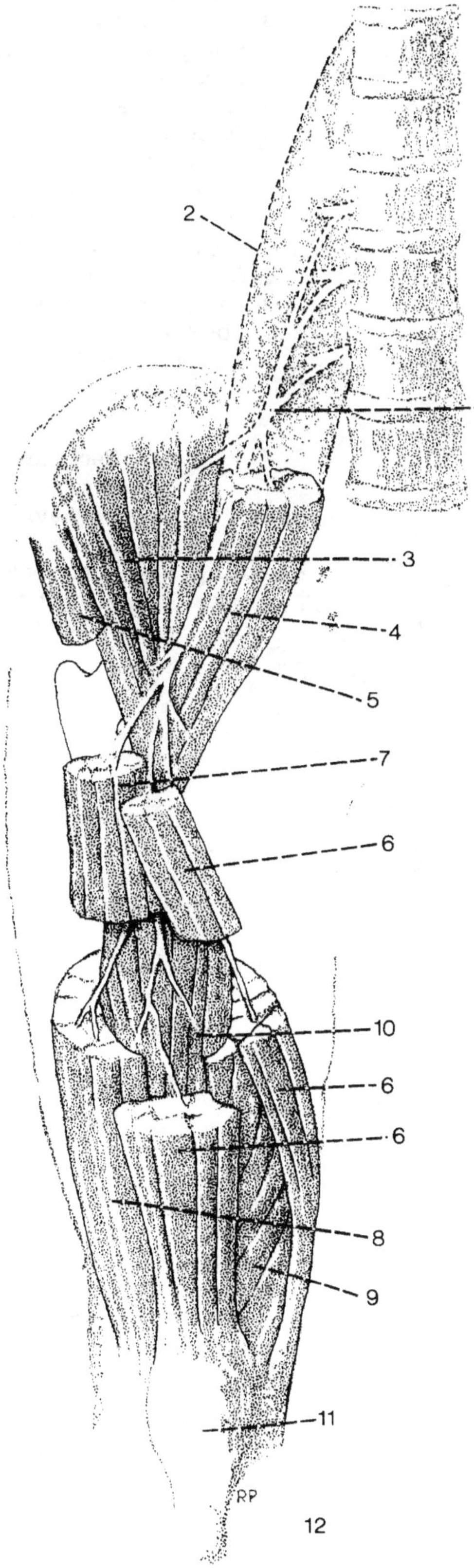

Color and label

1 Femoral nerve formed by the fibers from lumbar nerves L2, L3, L4
2 Outline of psoas major muscle; notice that the femoral nerve and other nerves of the lumbar plexus arise deep within the substance of the psoas major.
3 Iliacus muscle; it inserts by a tendon in common with the psoas major on the lesser trochanter, thus forming the iliopsoas muscle, which flexes the hip.
4 Psoas major muscle
5 Sartorius muscle; origin on the anterior superior iliac spine (cut)
6 Sartorius muscle (a portion)
7 Rectus femoris muscle (cut)
8 Vastus lateralis muscle (cut)
9 Vastus medialis muscle (cut)
10 Vastus intermedius muscle (cut); the three vastus muscles and the rectus femoris form the quadriceps femoris, which means "four-headed muscle of the thigh."
11 Patella (knee cap); notice that the patella lies within the tendon of the quadriceps femoris; it is the largest sesamoid bone in the body; the actual insertion of the quadriceps is on the tibial tuberosity by means of the patellar ligament.
12 Tibial tuberosity

LL-19 Deep dissection of right thigh I

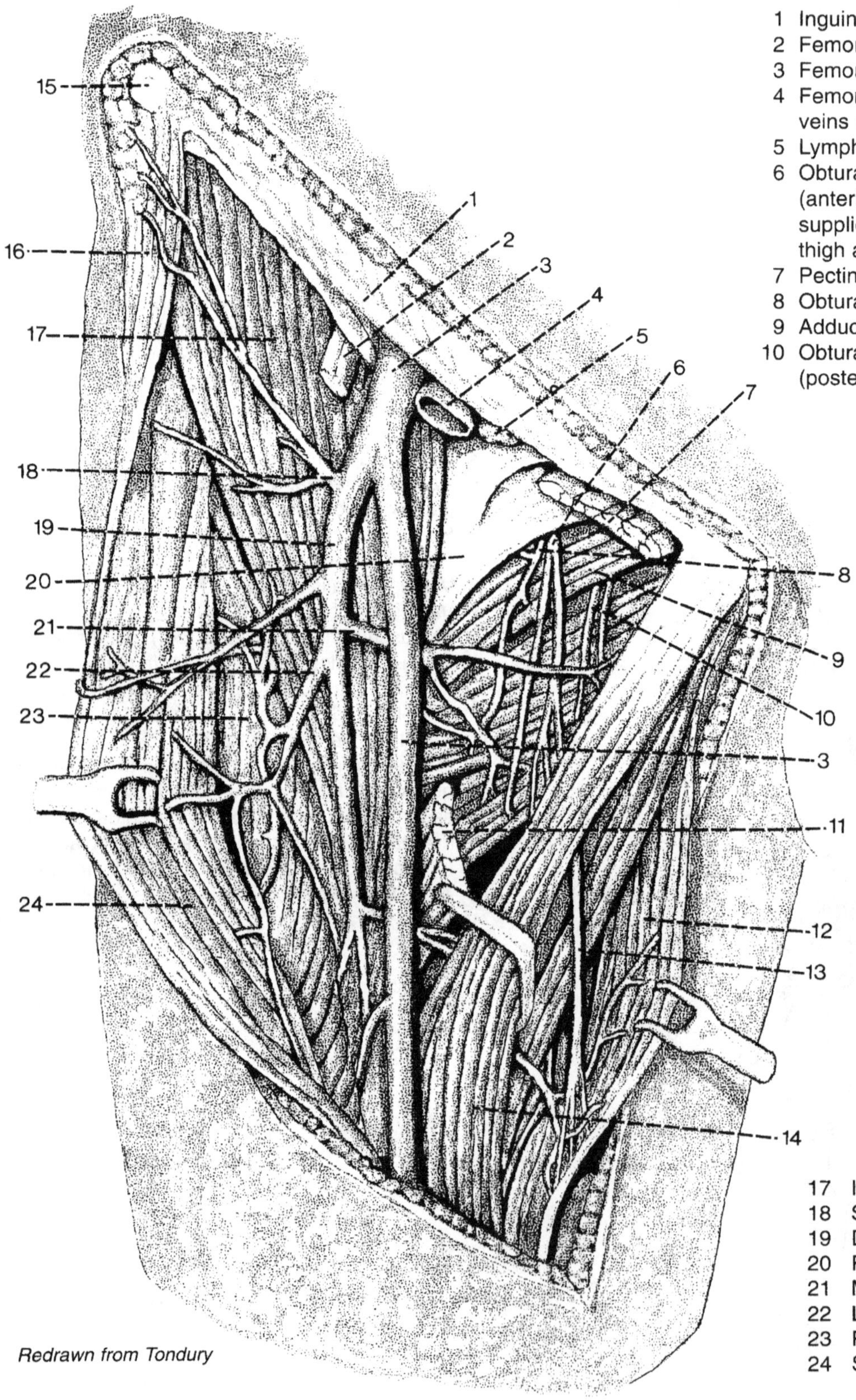

Redrawn from Tondury

Color and label

1 Inguinal ligament
2 Femoral nerve
3 Femoral artery
4 Femoral vein (cut; additional veins not shown)
5 Lymph node
6 Obturator nerve (anterior branch); supplies the medial thigh adductor muscles.
7 Pectineus muscle (cut)
8 Obturator artery
9 Adductor brevis muscle
10 Obturator nerve (posterior branch)
11 Pectineus muscle (cut)
12 Gracilis muscle
13 Obturator nerve (anterior ramus)
14 Adductor longus muscle
15 Anterior superior iliac spine
16 Tensor fascia lata muscle
17 Iliopsoas muscle
18 Superficial circumflex iliac artery
19 Deep femoral artery
20 Pubofemoral ligament
21 Medial circumflex femoral artery
22 Lateral circumflex femoral artery
23 Rectus femoris muscle
24 Sartorius muscle (pulled laterally)

LL-20 Deep dissection of right thigh II

Slightly rotated outward

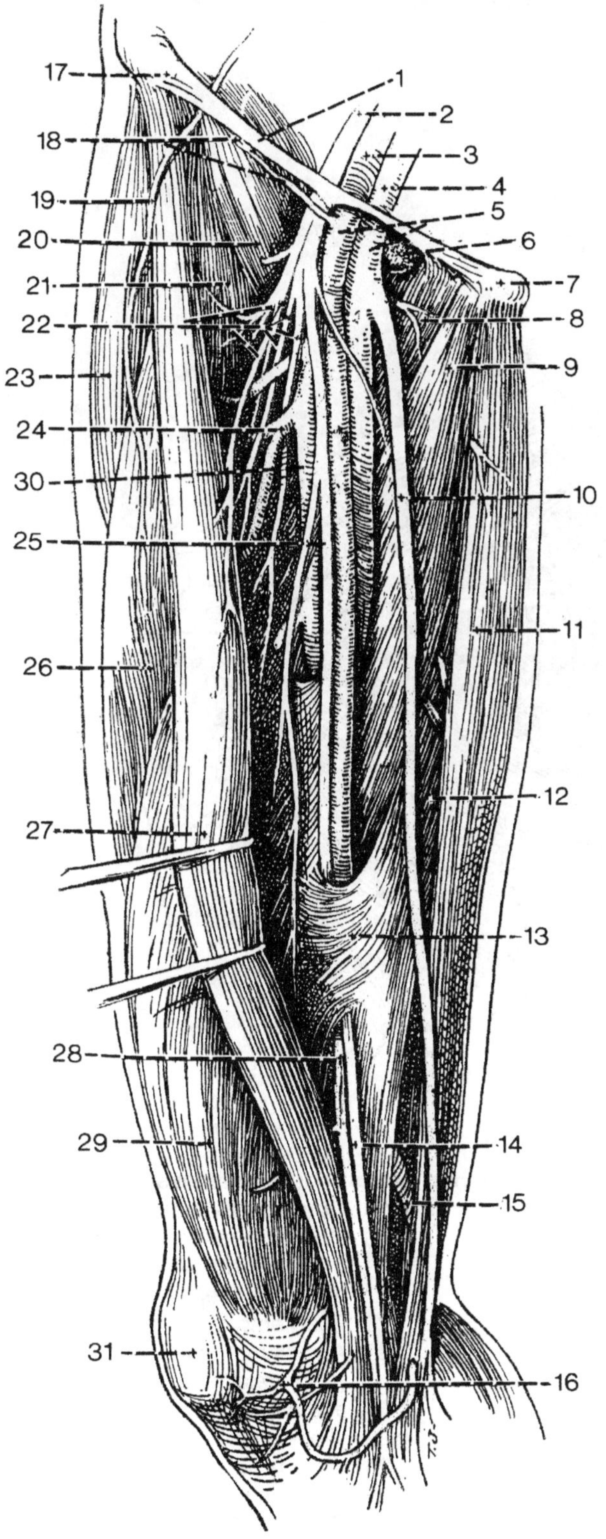

Eycleshymer and Jones

Color and label

1 Inguinal ligament
2 Femoral nerve
3 External iliac artery
4 External iliac vein
5 Femoral artery and vein; note that the **external iliac** artery and vein become the **femoral** artery and vein below the inguinal ligament.
6 Lymph gland
7 Pubic tubercle
8 Pectineus muscle
9 Adductor longus muscle
10 Great saphenous vein (Gk. *saphenes*, visible or clear)
11 Gracilis muscle (L. slender)
12 Adductor magnus muscle
13 Anterior wall of adductor canal (old name, Hunter's canal); a tunnel under the aponeurosis of the adductor magnus transmitting the femoral vessels, deep lymphatics, and the saphenous nerve.
14 Saphenous nerve
15 Popliteal artery; a continuation of the femoral artery extending from the opening in the adductor magnus, across the floor of the popliteal fossa, to the lower border of the popliteus muscle where it ends by dividing into the anterior and posterior tibial arteries.
16 Medial inferior genicular artery
17 Anterior superior iliac spine
18 Superficial circumflex iliac artery (off femoral artery)
19 Lateral femoral cutaneous nerve
20 Iliopsoas muscle
21 Rectus femoris muscle
22 Motor branches of femoral nerve to muscles
23 Tensor fascia lata muscle; inserts on iliotibial tract
24 Lateral femoral circumflex artery (off deep femoral)
25 Saphenous nerve
26 Rectus femoris muscle
27 Sartorius muscle
28 Medial superior genicular artery
29 Vastus medialis muscle
30 Deep femoral artery
31 Patella

LL-21 Dissection of structures deep to inguinal ligament

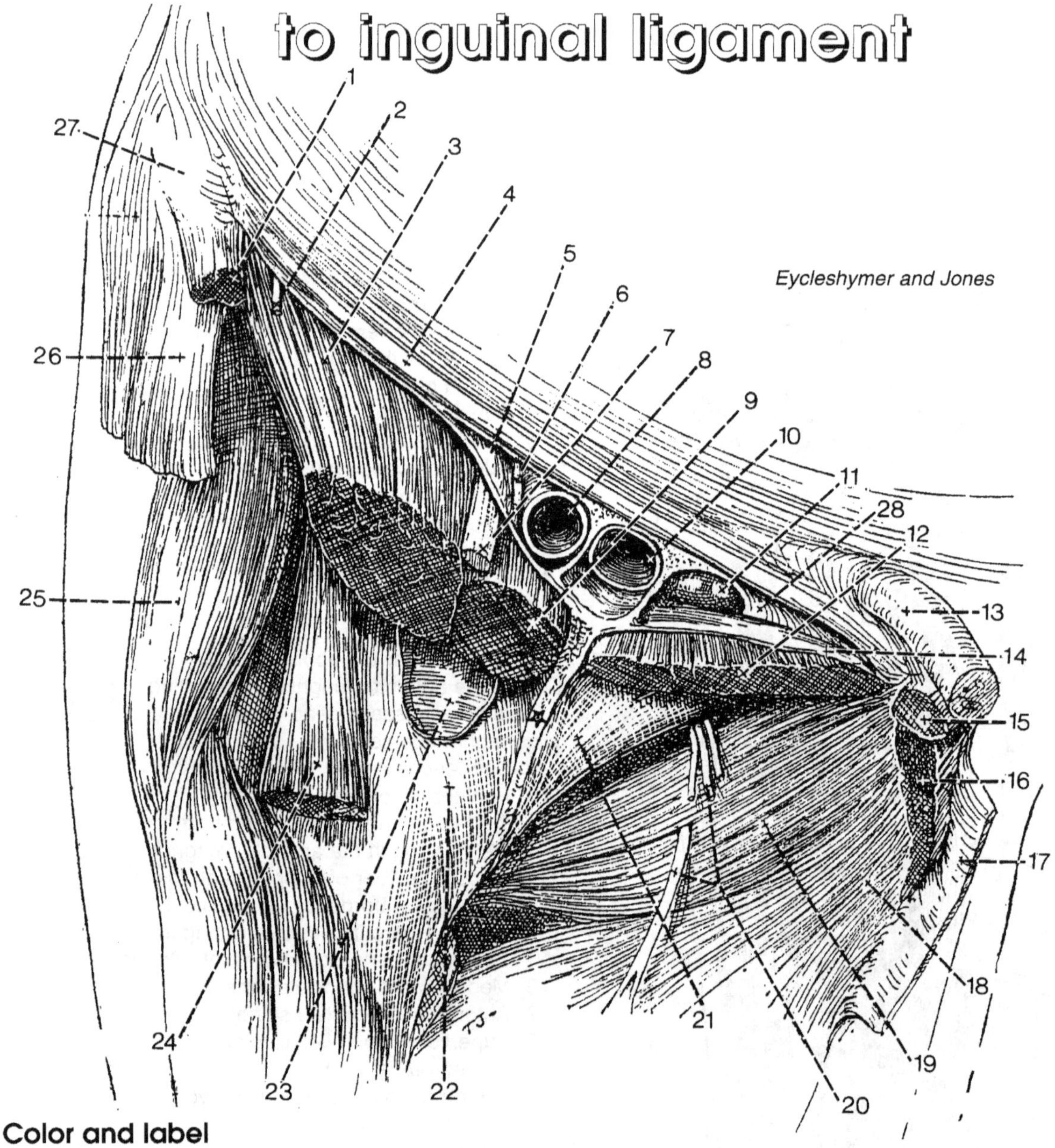

Color and label

1 Sartorius muscle (cut near origin on anterior superior iliac spine)
2 Lateral femoral cutaneous nerve
3 Iliacus muscle
4 Inguinal ligament (old name, Poupart's ligament)
5 Iliopectineal arch; a septum between the inguinal ligament and the iliopectinal eminence of the hip bone that divides the space beneath the inguinal ligament into the lateral muscular lacuna (space) and the medial vascular lacuna. Also iliopectineal septum.
6 Femoral branch of genitofemoral nerve
7 Femoral nerve
8 Femoral artery
9 Psoas major muscle
10 Femoral vein
11 Lymph gland
12 Pectineus muscle (cut near its origin on the pecten of the pubic bone)
13 Spermatic cord
14 Pectineal fascia
15 Adductor longus muscle (cut near origin)
16 Adductor brevis (cut near origin)
17 Gracilis muscle (origin, cut)
18 Adductor magnus muscle
19 Obturator externus muscle
20 Obturator nerve; anterior branches (above) posterior branches (below)
21 Pubofemoral ligament
22 Articular capsule of hip joint (also coxal joint, iliofemoral joint, acetabulofemoral joint)
23 Iliopectineal bursa
24 Rectus femoris muscle (cut)
25 Gluteus medius muscle
26 Tensor fascia lata
27 Anterior superior iliac spine
28 Lacunar ligament (at medial end of inguinal ligament)

LL-22 Iliopsoas muscle and femoral nerve

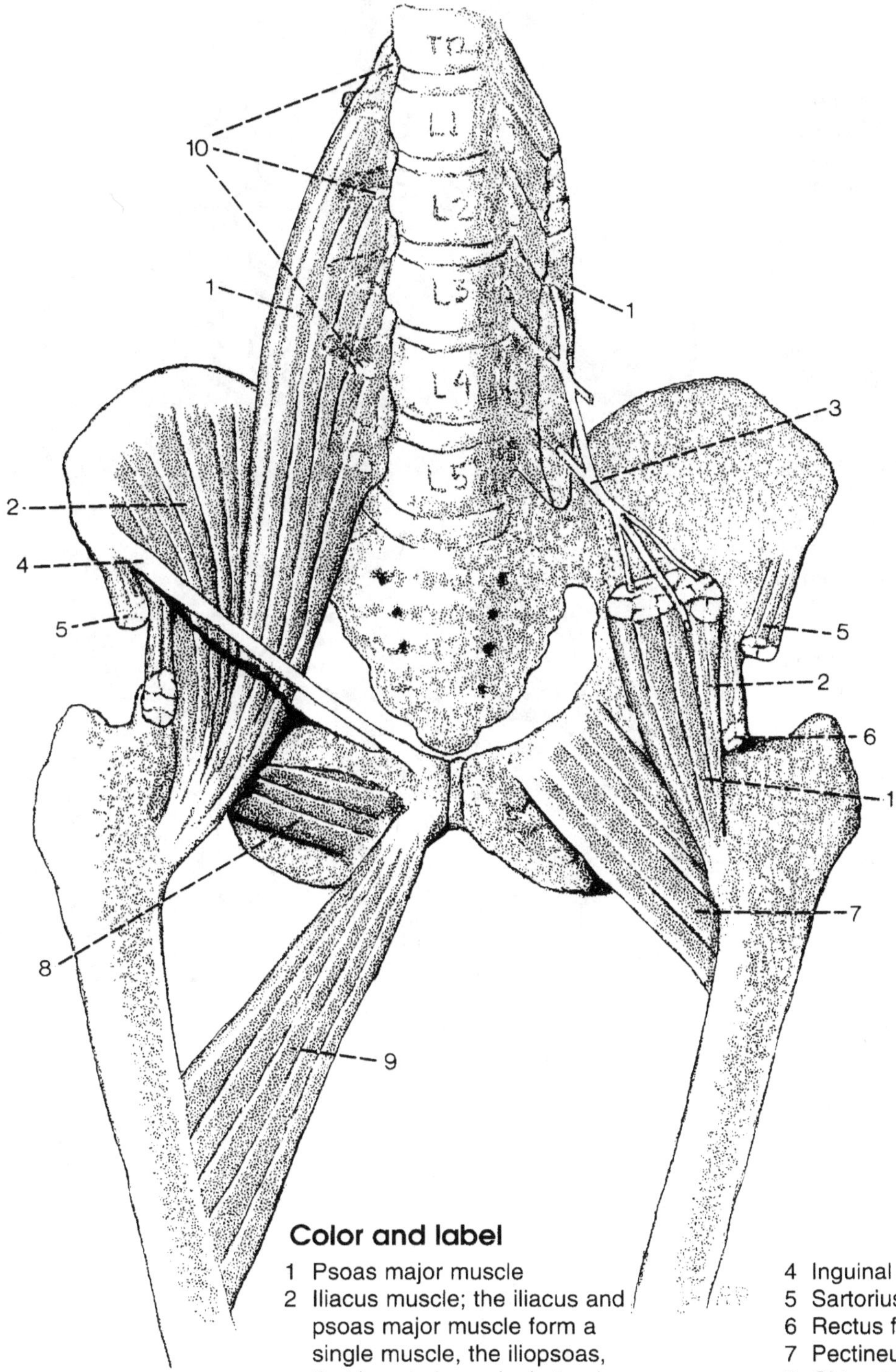

Color and label

1 Psoas major muscle
2 Iliacus muscle; the iliacus and psoas major muscle form a single muscle, the iliopsoas, that inserts by a single tendon on the lesser trochanter of the femur.
3 Femoral nerve; note it forms within the psoas major from the anterior rami of lumbar nerves L2, L3, L4; the psoas major is cut on the left.
4 Inguinal ligament
5 Sartorius (cut)
6 Rectus femoris muscle (cut)
7 Pectineus muscle
8 Obturator externus muscle
9 Adductor longus muscle
10 Origin of psoas major on the transverse processes of the lumbar vertebral and the intervertebral discs

LL-23 Medial thigh muscles and obturator nerve

Color and label

1 Obturator nerve; note that the obturator nerve, like the femoral nerve, is formed by fibers from the anterior rami of lumbar nerves L2, L3, L4.
2 Anterior branch of obturator nerve; note that this branch passes deep to the pectineus and adductor longus, and in front of the obturator externus which it often penetrates, and the adductor brevis; it supplies the adductor brevis, adductor longus, and gracilis muscles.
3 Pectineus muscle (cut on left side)
4 Obturator externus muscle
5 Adductor brevis and its insertion on the **posterior** femur; note that it lies deep to, and is largely covered by, the pectineus and the adductor longus muscles.
6 Adductor longus and its insertion on the **posterior** femur (cut on left side)
7 Adductor magnus muscle (oblique part); the adductor magnus is really a double muscle; this part is innerveted by the posterior branch of the obturator nerve.
8 Adductor magnus muscle (vertical part); this part is innervated by the tibial division of the sciatic nerve; note this part's insertion on the adductor tubercle.
9 Gracilis muscle (cut on left)
10 Tendineus hiatus; opening in the tendon of the adductor magnus for the passage of the femoral vessels from the femoral canal to the popliteal fossa

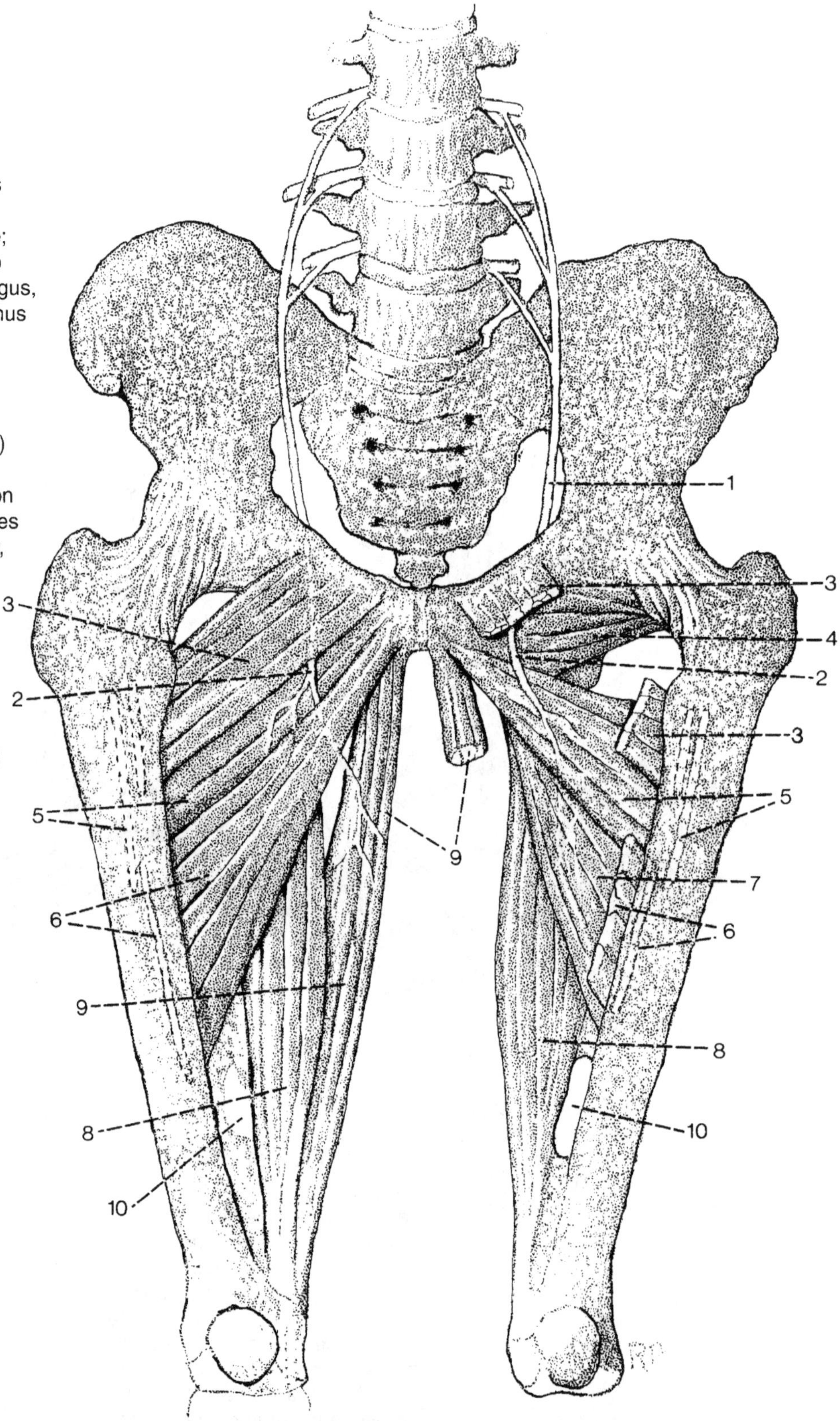

LL-24 Adductor magnus and obturator nerve

Color and label

1 Obturator nerve; it arises within the psoas major muscle (removed) from the anterior rami of lumbar nerves L2, L3, L4; it divides into an anterior branch and posterior branch, which both pass through the obturator foramen.
2 Anterior branch of obturator nerve (cut)
3 Posterior branch of obturator nerve; note its passing through the obturator externus muscle, which it also supplies.
4 Adductor magnus muscle (anterior horizontal part); this part of the adductor magnus is sometimes considered a separate muscle, in which case it is called the adductor minimus.
5 Adductor magnus muscle (anterior oblique part); the anterior horizontal and oblique parts of the adductor magnus are supplied by the posterior branch of the obturator nerve.
6 Adductor magnus (posterior vertical part); this part arises from the ischial tuberosity, descends vertically, forms a tendon that inserts on the adductor tubercle of the femur; the vertical part is innervated by the tibial portion of the sciatic nerve.
7 Femoral nerve and artery (a section of each) passing through the tendineus hiatus (also adductor hiatus)
8 Fibrous expansion of adductor magnus tendon
9 Pectineus muscle (cut); usually supplied by the femoral nerve, sometimes by the obturator nerve or accessory obturator nerve.
10 Obturator externus muscle; shown passing behind the femur and inserting into its trochanter fossa
11 Outline of the anterior part of adductor magnus; note its insertion on the posterior femur
12 Accessory obturator nerve; present 10% of the time; notice it passes over the pubis and not through the obturator foramen.
13 Obturator* foramen
14 Insertion of anterior part of obturator magnus on gluteal ridge and linea aspera of the femur
15 Insertion of iliopsoas tendon on lesser trochanter
16 Origin of pectineus

*From the Latin, *obturare*, to obstruct or stop up

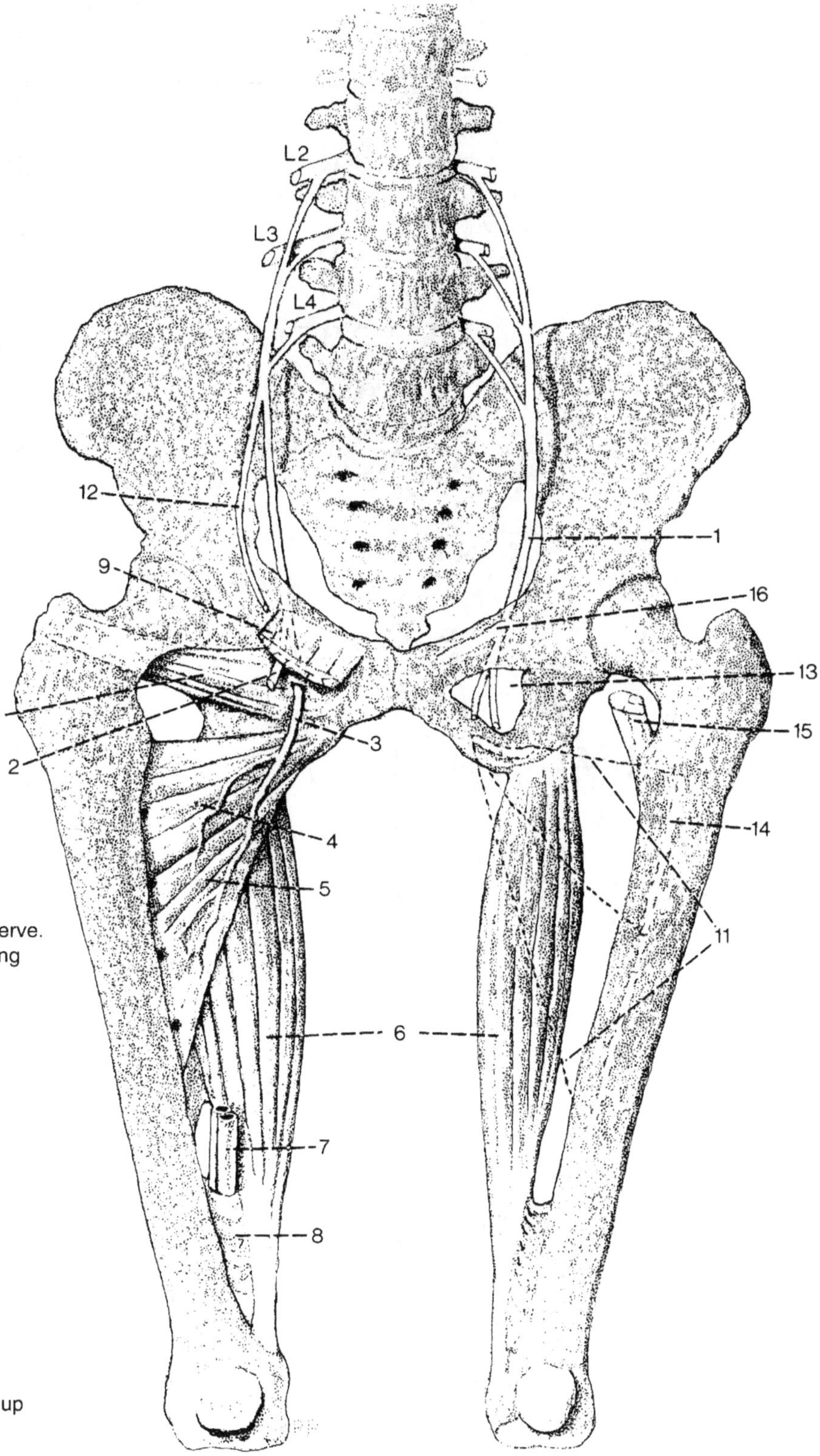

LL-25 Muscles of buttock and posterior thigh

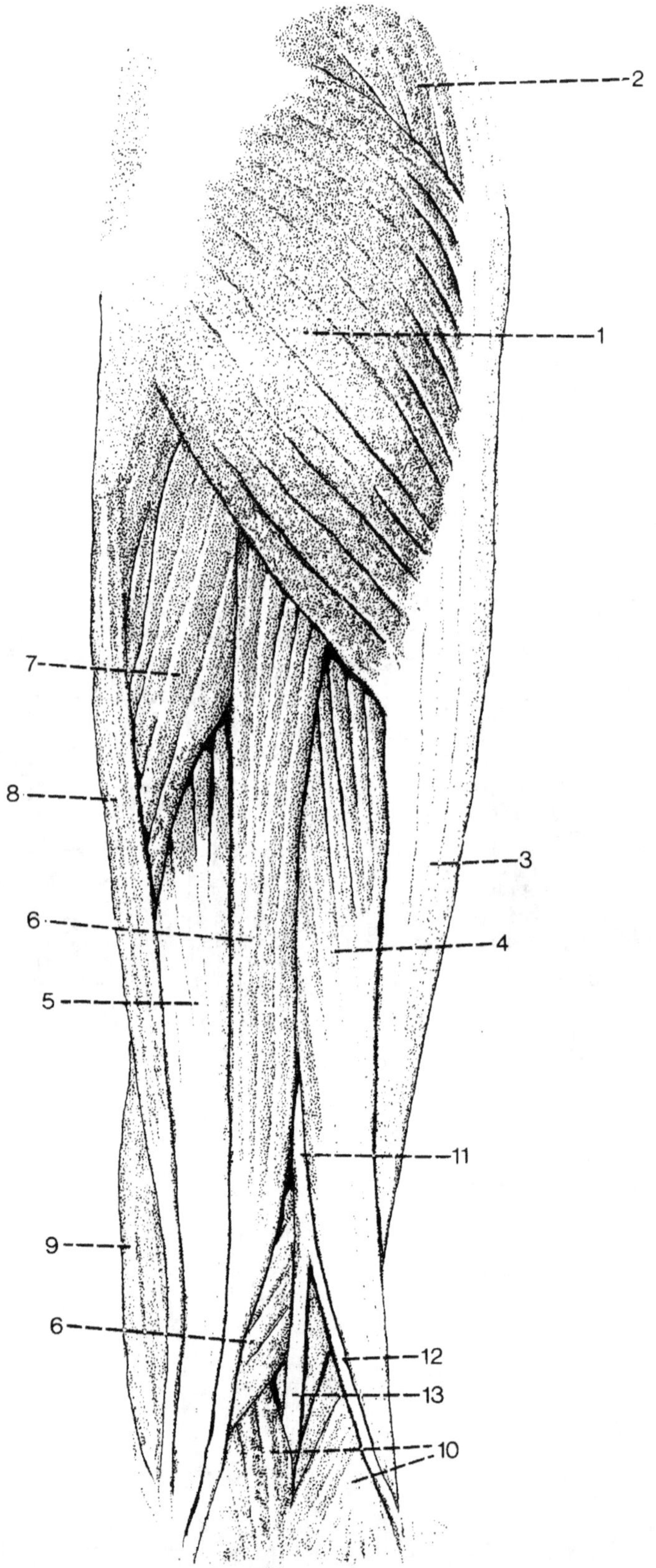

Right thigh

Color and label

1 Gluteus maximus
2 Gluteus medius
3 Iliotibial tract; note that the gluteus maximus inserts mainly on the iliotibial tract
4 Biceps femoris (the lateral hamstring muscle)
5 Semitendinosus (medial hamstring muscle)
6 Semimembranosus
7 Adductor magnus (posterior vertical part)
8 Gracilis
9 Sartorius
10 Medial and lateral heads of gastrocnemius
11 Sciatic nerve; its division into the tibial and common peroneal (fibular) nerves may occur higher in the thigh.
12 Common peroneal (fibular) nerve
13 Tibial nerve

LL-26 Gluteus maximus and iliotibial tract

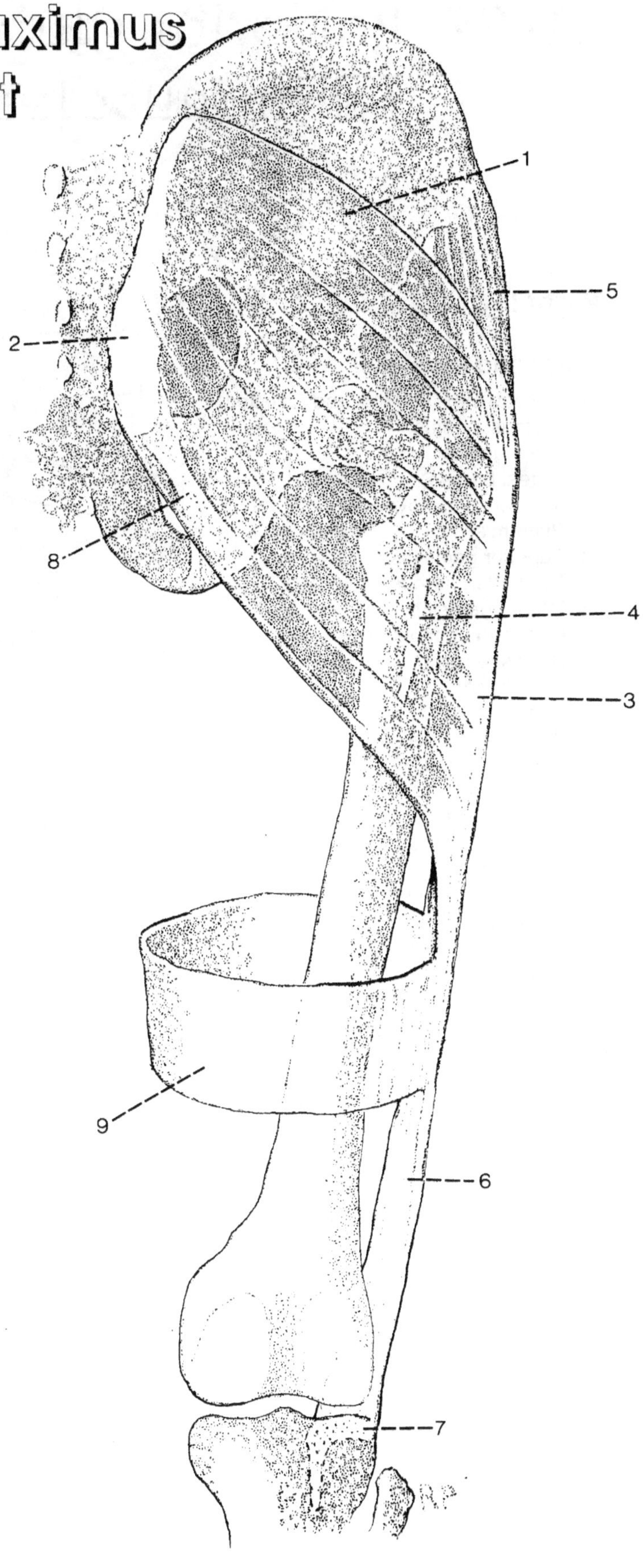

Right leg, posterior view

Color and label

1 Gluteus maximus; largest and most superficial muscle in the gluteal region
2 Origin of gluteus maximus; from ilium and lower part of sacrum; it also arises from the coccyx, aponeurosis of erector spinae, and sacrotuberous ligament (8).
3 Insertion of gluteus maximus on iliotibial tract; besides being a powerful extensor of the thigh at the hip and rotator of the thigh, the gluteus maximus, acting by way of its insertion on the iliotibial tract, braces the fully extended knee (as in standing).
4 Insertion of lower deeper fibers of gluteus maximus on gluteal tuberosity of femur
5 Tensor fascia lata muscle
6 Iliotibial tract (lateral thickened portion of fascia lata)
7 Insertion of iliotibial tract on anterior surface of lateral condyle of tibia
8 Sacrotuberous ligament
9 Small section of fascia lata (deep fascia of the thigh)

LL-27 Posterior gluteal and thigh muscles

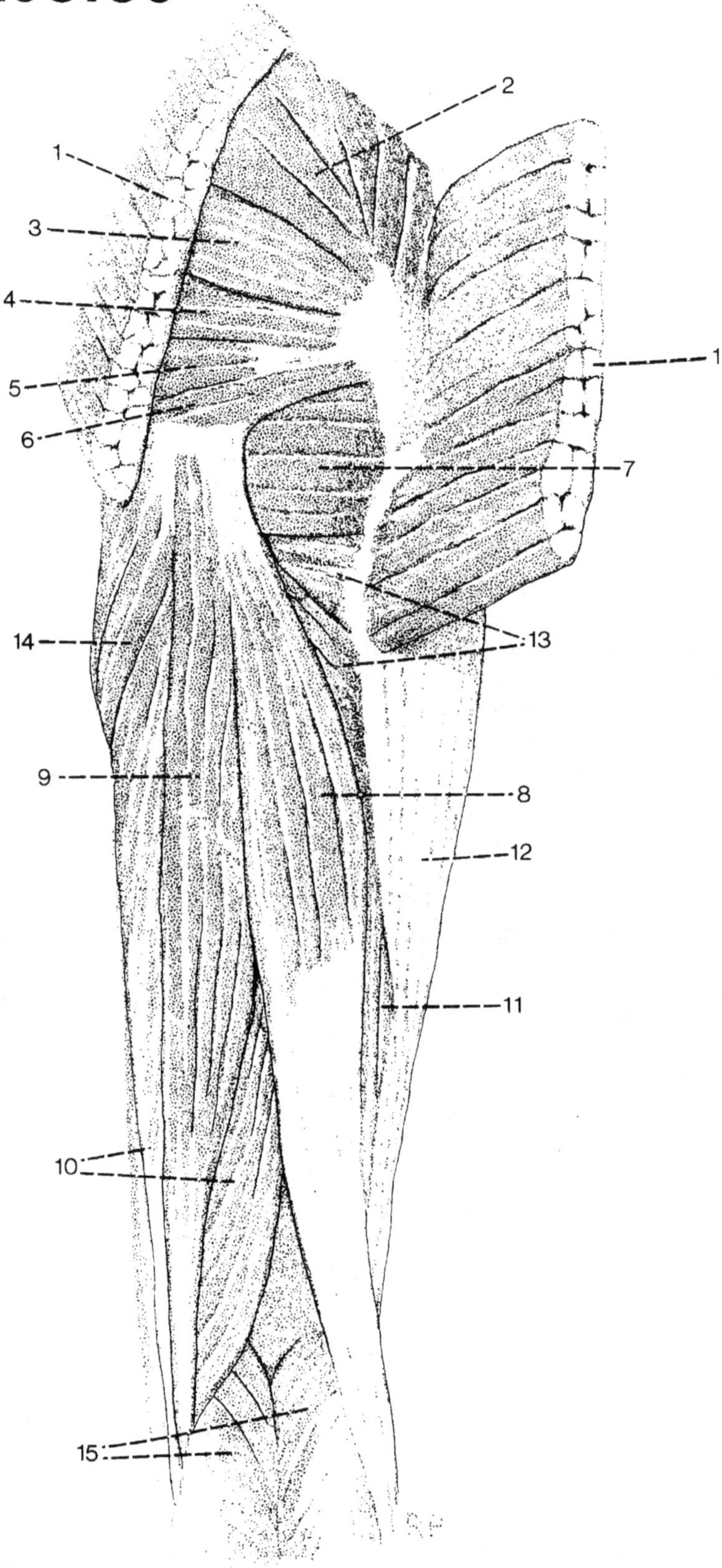

Right leg

Color and label

1 Gluteus maximus (cut and reflected)
2 Gluteus medius; intermuscular gluteal bursae* have been removed
3 Piriformis
4 Superior gemellus
5 Obturator internus
6 Inferior gemellus
7 Quadratus femoris
8 Biceps femoris (long head)
9 Semitendinosus
10 Semimembranosus
11 Biceps femoris (short head)
12 Iliotibial tract
13 Adductor magnus (oblique part)
14 Adductor magnus (vertical part)
15 Gastrocnemius medial and lateral heads

*Bursa (L. a bag or purse): a closed sac or pouch lined with synovial membrane containing synovial fluid formed in areas subject to friction.

LL-28 Posterior muscles of right gluteal region and upper thigh

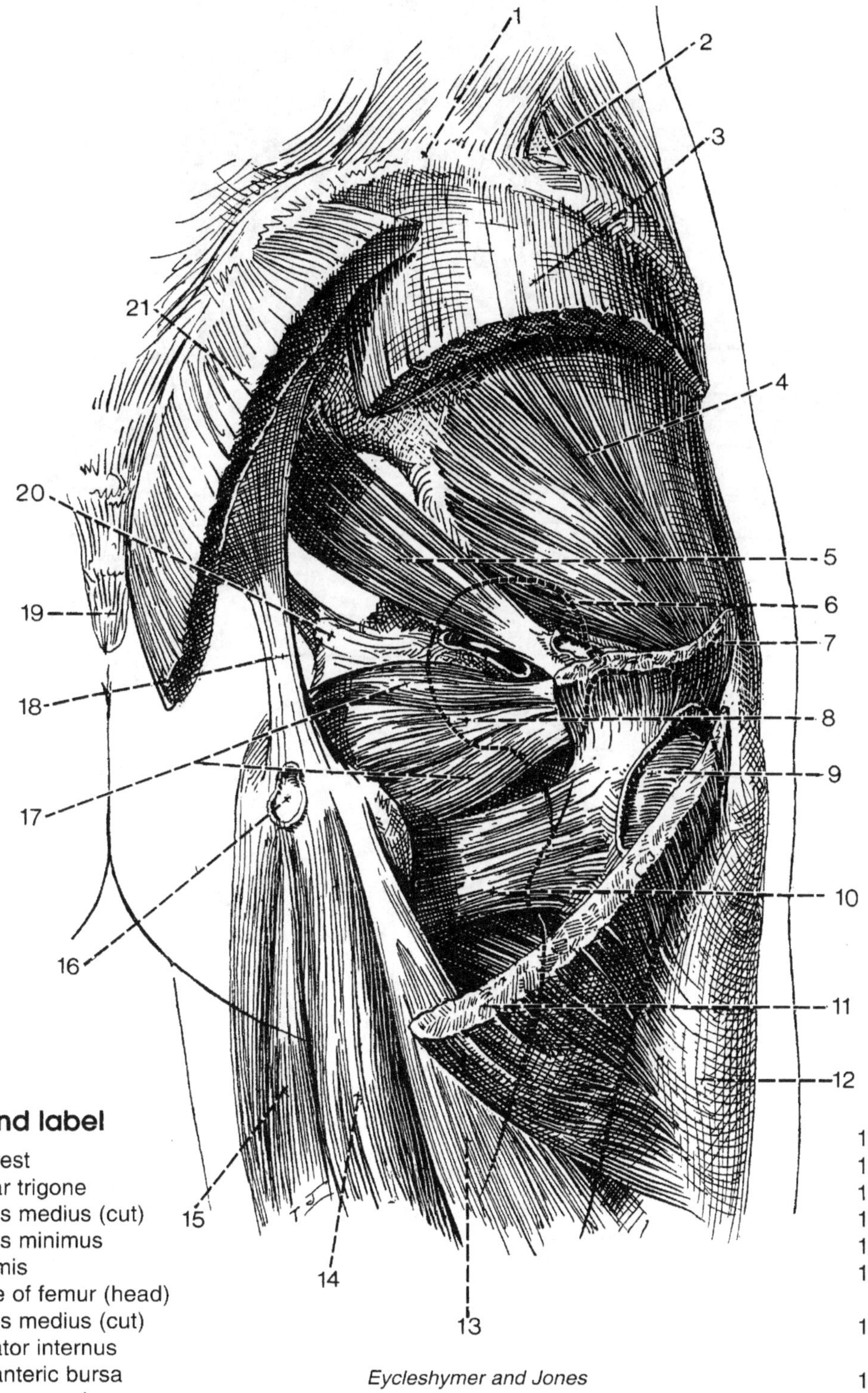

Eycleshymer and Jones

Color and label

1 Iliac crest
2 Lumbar trigone
3 Gluteus medius (cut)
4 Gluteus minimus
5 Piriformis
6 Outline of femur (head)
7 Gluteus medius (cut)
8 Obturator internus
9 Trochanteric bursa of gluteus maximus
10 Quadratus femoris
11 Gluteus maximus (cut)
12 Iliotibial tract
13 Biceps femoris
14 Semitendinosus
15 Semimembranosus
16 Sciatic bursa
17 Gemelli superior and inferior
18 Sacrotuberous ligament
19 Coccyx
20 Spine of the ischium
21 Gluteus maximus (cut)

LL-29 Deep gluteal region

Right leg - posterior aspect

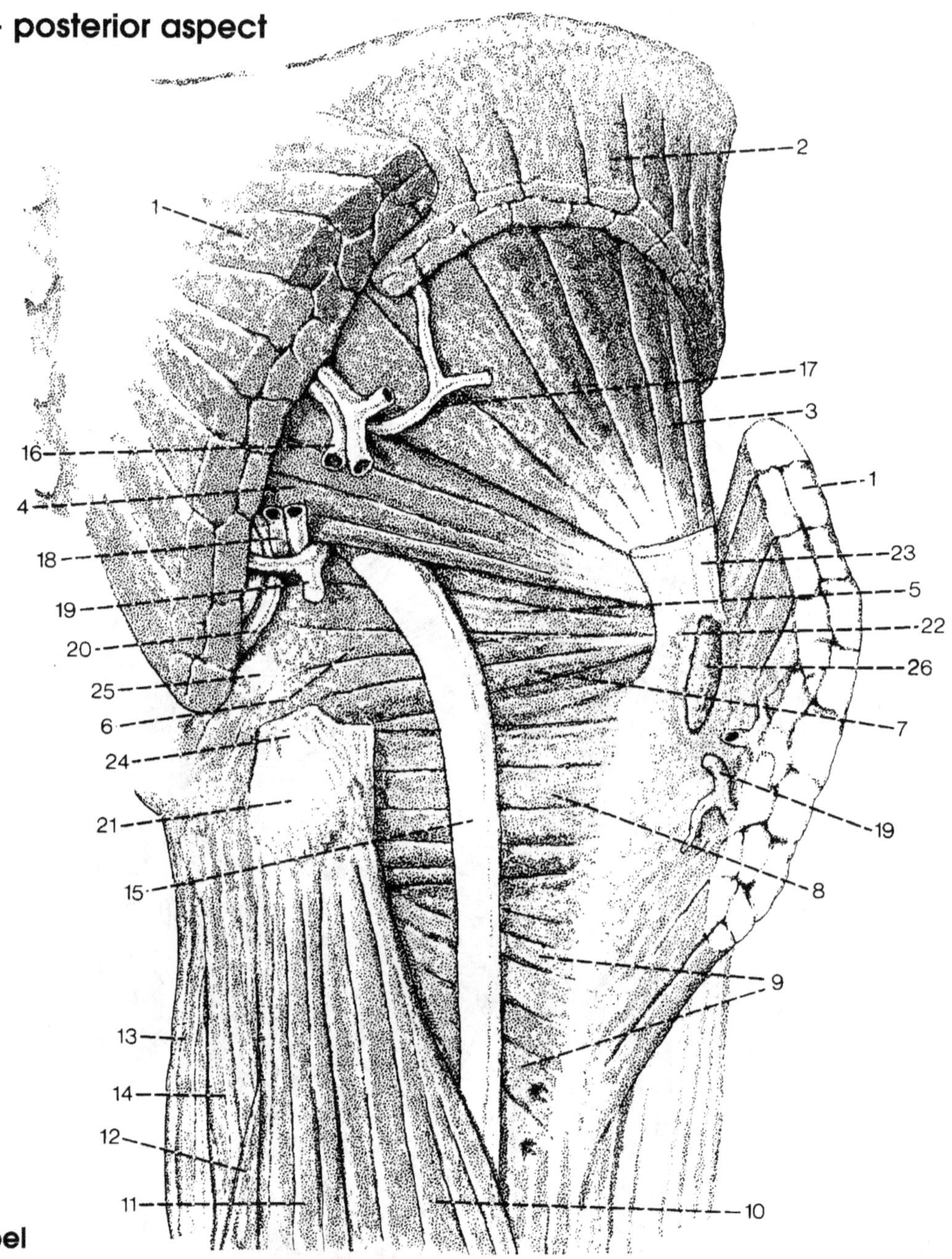

Color and label

1 Gluteus maximus muscle (cut)
2 Gluteus medius muscle (cut)
3 Gluteus minimus muscle (cut)
4 Piriformis muscle
5 Superior gemellus muscle
6 Obturator internus muscle
7 Inferior gemellus muscle
8 Quadratus femoris muscle
9 Adductor magnus (horizontal and oblique parts)
10 Biceps femoris muscle
11 Semitendinosus muscle
12 Semimembranosus muscle
13 Gracilis muscle
14 Adductor magnus muscle (vertical part)
15 Sciatic nerve
16 Superior gluteal artery and vein
17 Superior gluteal nerve (cut; supplies gluteus medius and gluteus minimus)
18 Inferior gluteal artery and vein
19 Inferior gluteal nerve (supplies gluteus maximus)
20 Internal pudendal artery and vein (travel with pudendal nerve; nerve not shown)
21 Ischial tuberosity
22 Greater trochanter of femur
23 Tendon of gluteus medius
24 Sacrotuberous ligament (cut)
25 Bend (genu) in obturator internus muscle on lesser sciatic notch
26 Trochanteric bursa (beneath gluteus maximus)

LL-30 Hamstring muscles and gluteus medius

The hamstring muscles are the semitendinosus, semimembranosus, and biceps femoris. They act both to extend the trunk at the hip joint and flex the knee joint.

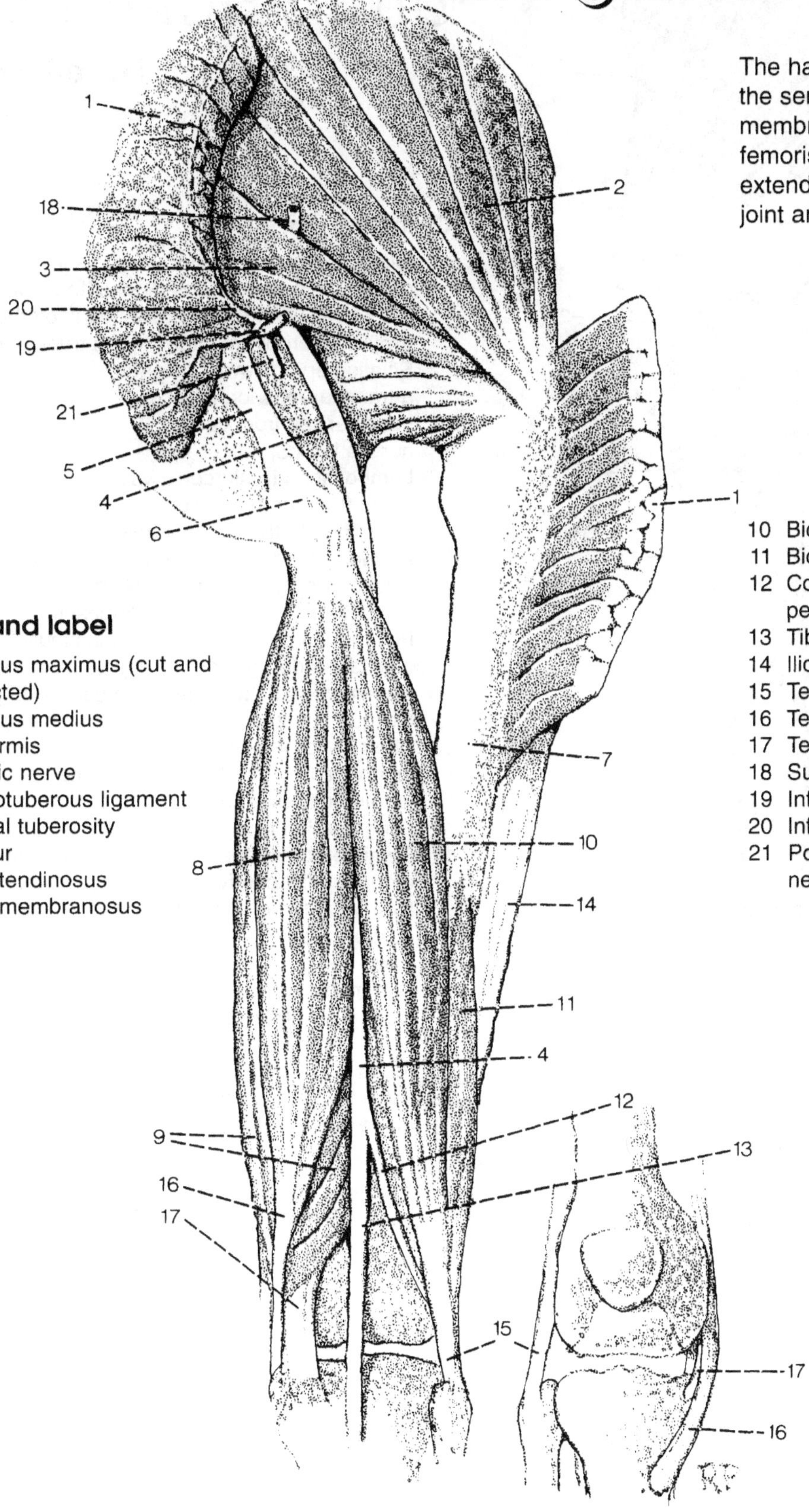

Color and label

1 Gluteus maximus (cut and reflected)
2 Gluteus medius
3 Piriformis
4 Sciatic nerve
5 Sacrotuberous ligament
6 Ischial tuberosity
7 Femur
8 Semitendinosus
9 Semimembranosus
10 Biceps femoris long head
11 Biceps femoris short head
12 Common fibular (common peroneal) nerve
13 Tibial nerve
14 Iliotibial tract
15 Tendon of biceps femoris
16 Tendon of semitendinosus
17 Tendon of semimembranosus
18 Superior gluteal artery (cut)
19 Inferior gluteal artery (cut)
20 Inferior gluteal nerve
21 Posterior femoral cutaneous nerve (cut)

LL-31 Gluteus minimus, semimembranosus, and sciatic nerve

Posterior aspect

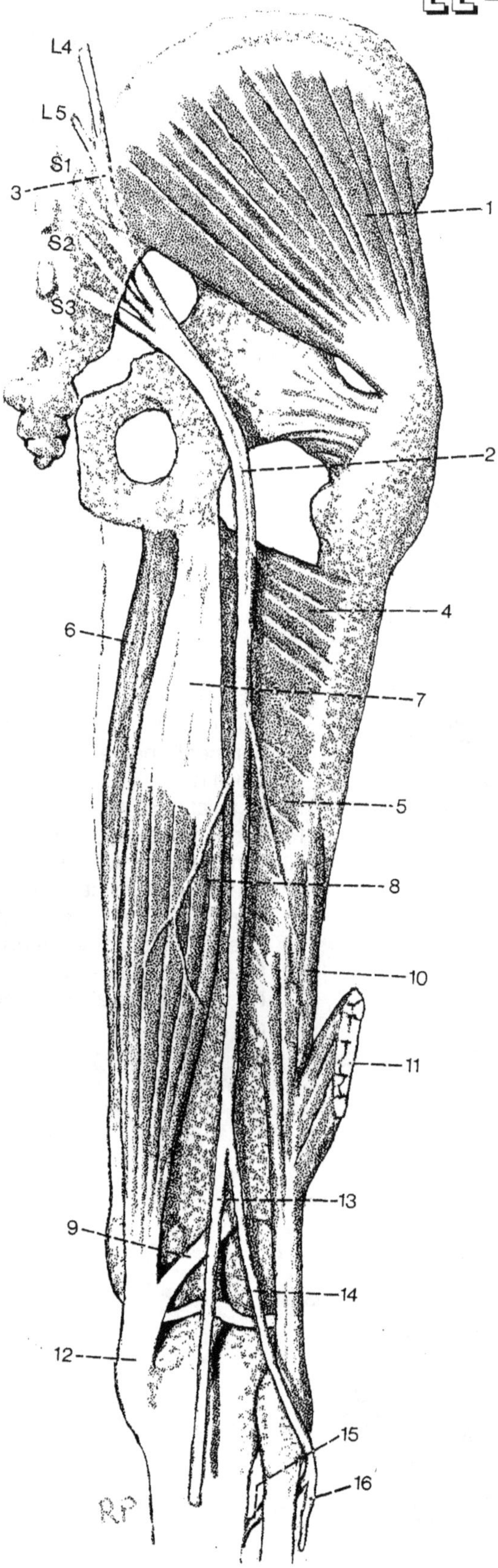

Color and label

1 Gluteus minimus muscle; it works in concert with the gluteus medius to stabilize the pelvis when the opposite leg is off the ground, thereby maintaining the trunk upright.
2 Sciatic nerve (viewed through a transparent sacrum; note how it arises from spinal nerves L4, L5, S1,S2, S3)
3 Lumbosacral trunk; conveys fibers from lumbar nerves L4 and L5 to the sciatic nerve.
4 Adductor magnus muscle (horizontal part)
5 Adductor magnus muscle (oblique part)
6 Adductor magnus muscle (vertical part)
7 Flat tendon of semimembranosus muscle; this flat tendon gives this muscle its name.
8 Semimembranosus muscle (muscular part)
9 Oblique popliteal ligament
10 Short head of biceps femoris muscle; innervated by common peroneal nerve (common fibular nerve)
11 Long head of biceps femoris muscle (cut)
12 Semimembranosus insertion onto the back of the medial condyle of the tibia; also onto the lateral femoral condyle by the oblique popliteal ligament
13 Tibial nerve
14 Common peroneal nerve (common fibular nerve)
15 Deep peroneal nerve (deep fibular nerve)
16 Superficial peroneal nerve (superficial fibular nerve)

LL-32 Deep dissection of the right thigh

Anterior aspect

Color and label

1 Crest of the ilium
2 Gluteus medius muscle (cut)
3 Superior gluteal artery (vein not shown)
4 Superior gluteal nerve
5 Piriformis muscle
6 Inferior gluteal nerve
7 Inferior gluteal artery
8 Gluteus medius muscle (cut); inserting on the greater trochanter
9 Posterior femoral cutaneus nerve
10 Sciatic nerve; largest nerve in the body, consisting of a medial tibial nerve and a lateral common fibular (peroneal) nerve
11 Superior gemellus muscle
12 Obturator internus muscle
13 Inferior gemellus muscle
14 Greater trochanter of femur
15 Quadratus femoris muscle
16 Gluteus maximus (cut); inserting on iliotibial tract
17 Adductor magnus muscle (horizontal part)
18 First perforating branch of deep femoral artery
19 Inferior cluneal nerve* (*clunis*, Latin, the buttocks)
20 Second perforating branch of deep femoral nerve
21 Adductor magnus muscle (oblique part)
22 Branch of common fibular (peroneal) nerve to short head of the biceps femoris muscle
23 Third perforating artery of the deep femoral artery
24 Iliotibial tract
25 Biceps femoris muscle (long head, cut)
26 Popliteal artery (continuation of femoral artery)
27 Popliteal vein (continuation of femoral vein)
28 Tibial nerve
29 Adductor magnus muscle
30 Gracilis muscle
31 Short head of biceps femoris muscle
32 Common fibular (peroneal) nerve

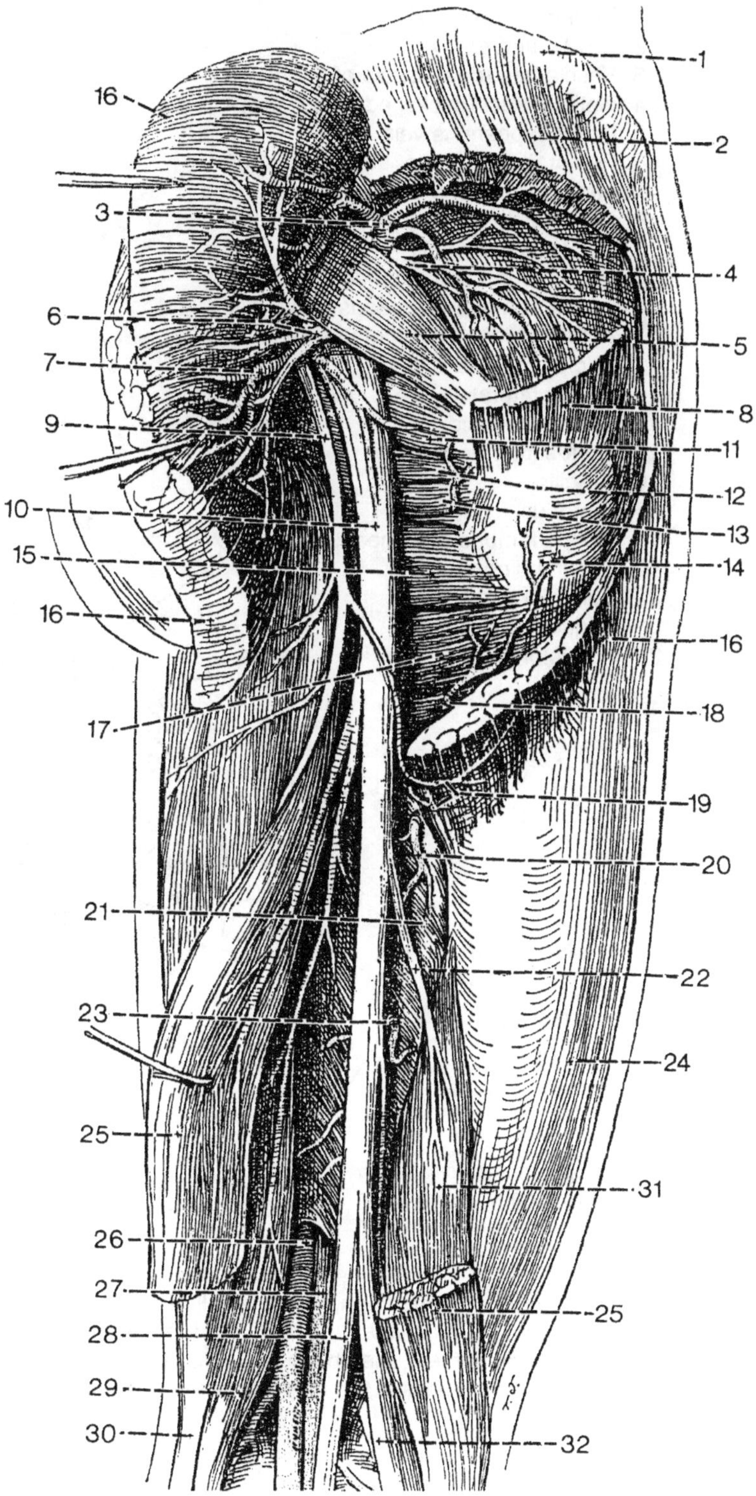

*Inferior cluneal nerves are branches of the posterior femoral cutaneous nerve supplying the skin of the lower half of the gluteal region.

Eycleshymer and Jones with modification

LL-33 Cross section of right thigh

Middle of right thigh

Color and label

1 Femur
2 Sciatic nerve
3 Fascia lata (deep fascia of thigh)
4 Iliotibial tract (thickened fascia lata)
5 Great saphenous vein
6 Femoral artery, vein, and saphenous nerve in adductor canal
7 Deep femoral artery and vein
8 Perforating vessels
9 Posterior femoral cutaneous nerve
10 Lateral femoral cutaneous nerve
11 Anterior branch of obturator nerve
12 Rectus femoris
13 Vastus lateralis
14 Vastus medialis
15 Vastus intermedius
16 Gracilis
17 Sartorius
18 Biceps femoris, long head
19 Semitendinosus
20 Semimembranosus
21 Adductor magnus
22 Adductor longus

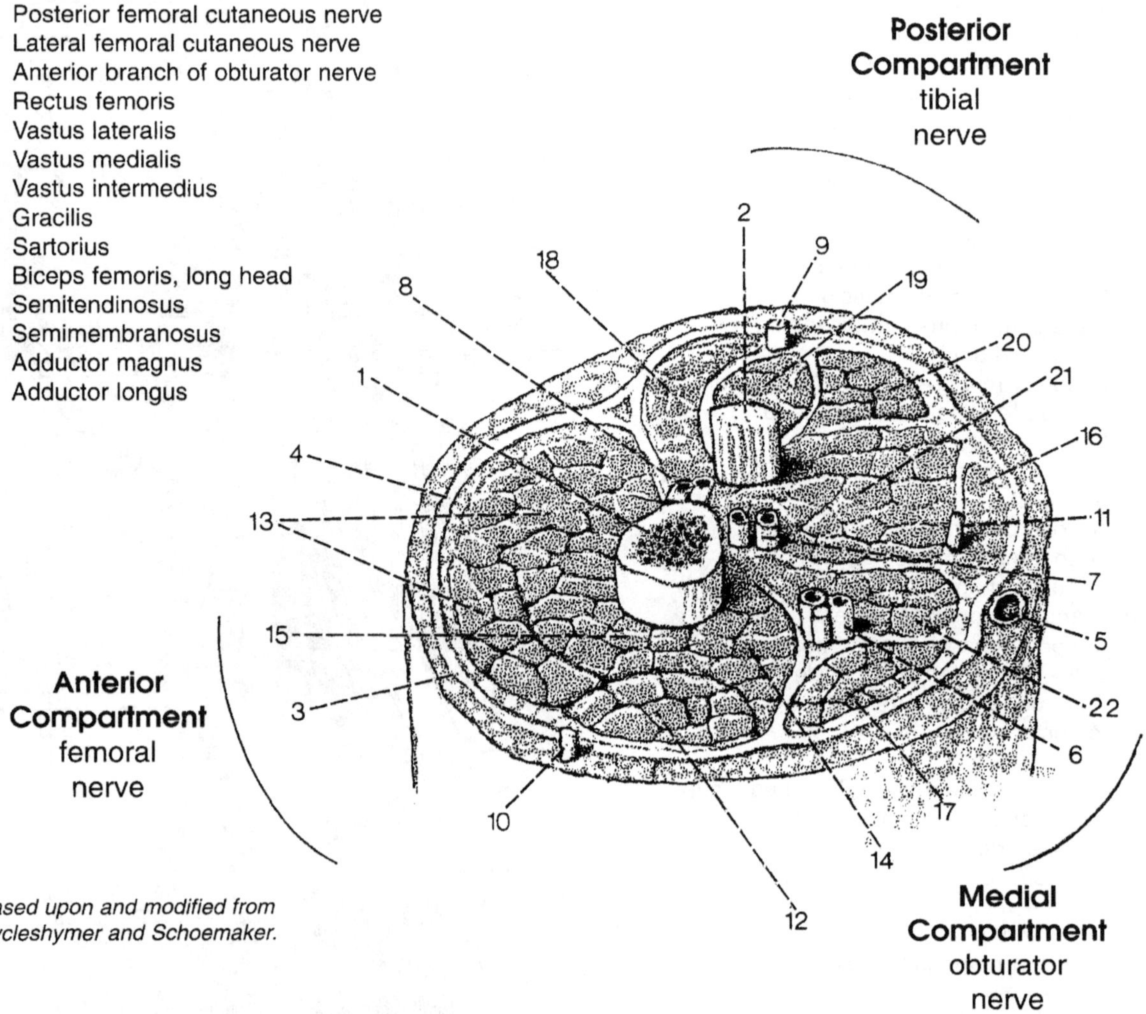

Based upon and modified from Eycleshymer and Schoemaker.

Notice that the deep fascia of the thigh, which is called the fascia lata, sends septa internally that divide the thigh into three compartments, a medial, an anterior, and a posterior compartment. The femoral nerve innervates the muscles of the anterior compartment, the obturator nerve supplies the muscles of the medial compartment, and the tibial portion of the sciatic nerve supplies the muscles of the posterior compartment.

LL-34 Deep structures of the leg and popliteal fossa

Gastrocnemius and soleus removed showing course of popliteal artery and tibial nerve

Color and label

1 Sciatic nerve
2 Biceps femoris
3 Common fibular nerve
4 Tibial nerve
5 Gastrocnemius lateral head (cut)
6 Sural artery and nerve
7 Lateral superior genicular artery
8 Semimembranosus
9 Popliteal artery (vein not shown)
10 Gracilis muscle
11 Gastrocnemius medial head (cut)
12 Artery and nerve to gastrocnemius
13 Medial superior genicular artery
14 Popliteus muscle
15 Soleus muscle (cut)
16 Fibular (peroneal) artery
17 Flexor hallucis longus muscle
18 Fibular (peroneus) longus muscle
19 Fibular (peroneus) brevis muscle
20 Sural nerve
21 Lateral malleolar artery
22 Flexor digitorum longus muscle
23 Tibialis posterior muscle
24 Posterior tibial artery
25 Calcaneal (Achilles) tendon (cut)

Eycleshymer and Jones

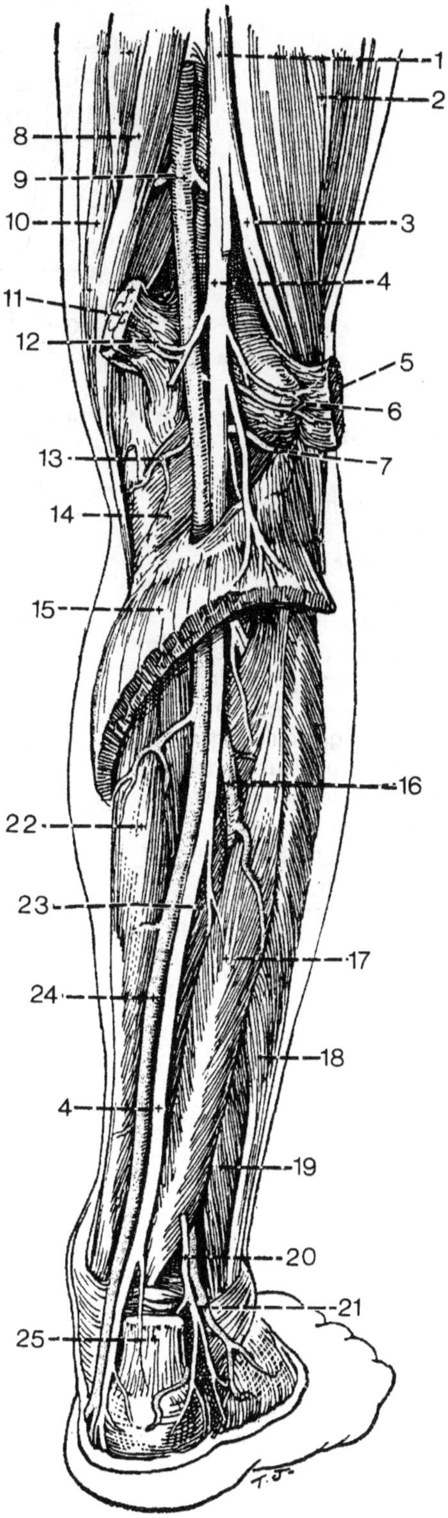

LL-35 Deep dissection of lower leg*

Posterior aspect

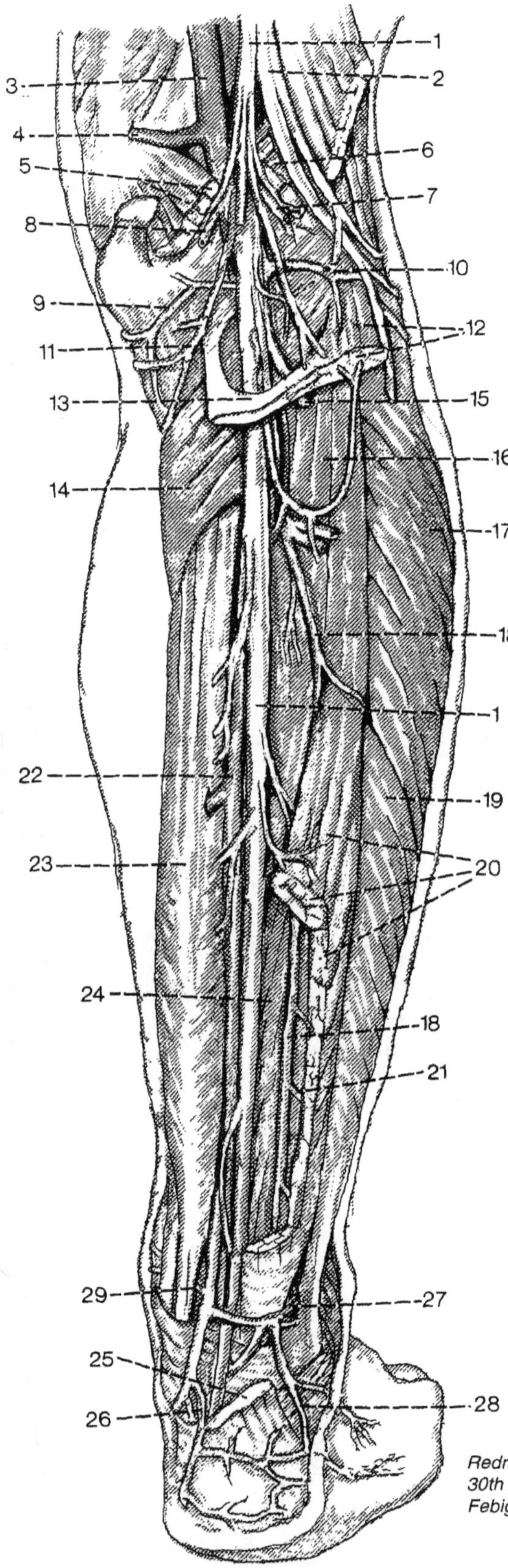

Color and label

1 Tibial nerve
2 Common fibular (peroneal) nerve
3 Popliteal artery
4 Medial superior genicular artery
5 Gastrocnemius muscle (medial head; cut)
6 Gastrocnemius (lateral head; cut)
7 Lateral sural nerve and artery
8 Medial sural artery and nerve
9 Medial inferior genicular artery
10 Lateral inferior genicular artery
11 Medial sural cutaneous nerve
12 Soleus muscle (cut)
13 Tendinous arch (part of soleus)
14 Popliteus muscle
15 Anterior tibial artery
16 Tibialis posterior muscle
17 Peroneus (fibularis) longus muscle
18 Peroneal (fibular) artery
19 Peroneus (fibularis) brevis muscle
20 Flexor hallucis longus muscle; partially dissected to reveal the underlying peroneal artery
21 Perforating branch of the peroneal artery
22 Posterior tibial artery
23 Flexor digitorum longus muscle
24 Tibialis posterior
25 Calcaneal (Achilles) tendon
26 Medial calcaneal artery
27 Lateral malleolar artery
28 Lateral calcaneal artery
29 Medial malleolar artery

*In anatomy the term **leg** designates just that portion of the lower limb below the knee and above the foot. The **thigh** designates the upper portion extending from the hip to the knee.

Redrawn from Clemente, Gray's Anatomy, 30th American ed. Philadelphia, Lea & Febiger, 1985

LL-36 Deep dissection of popliteal region

Right leg

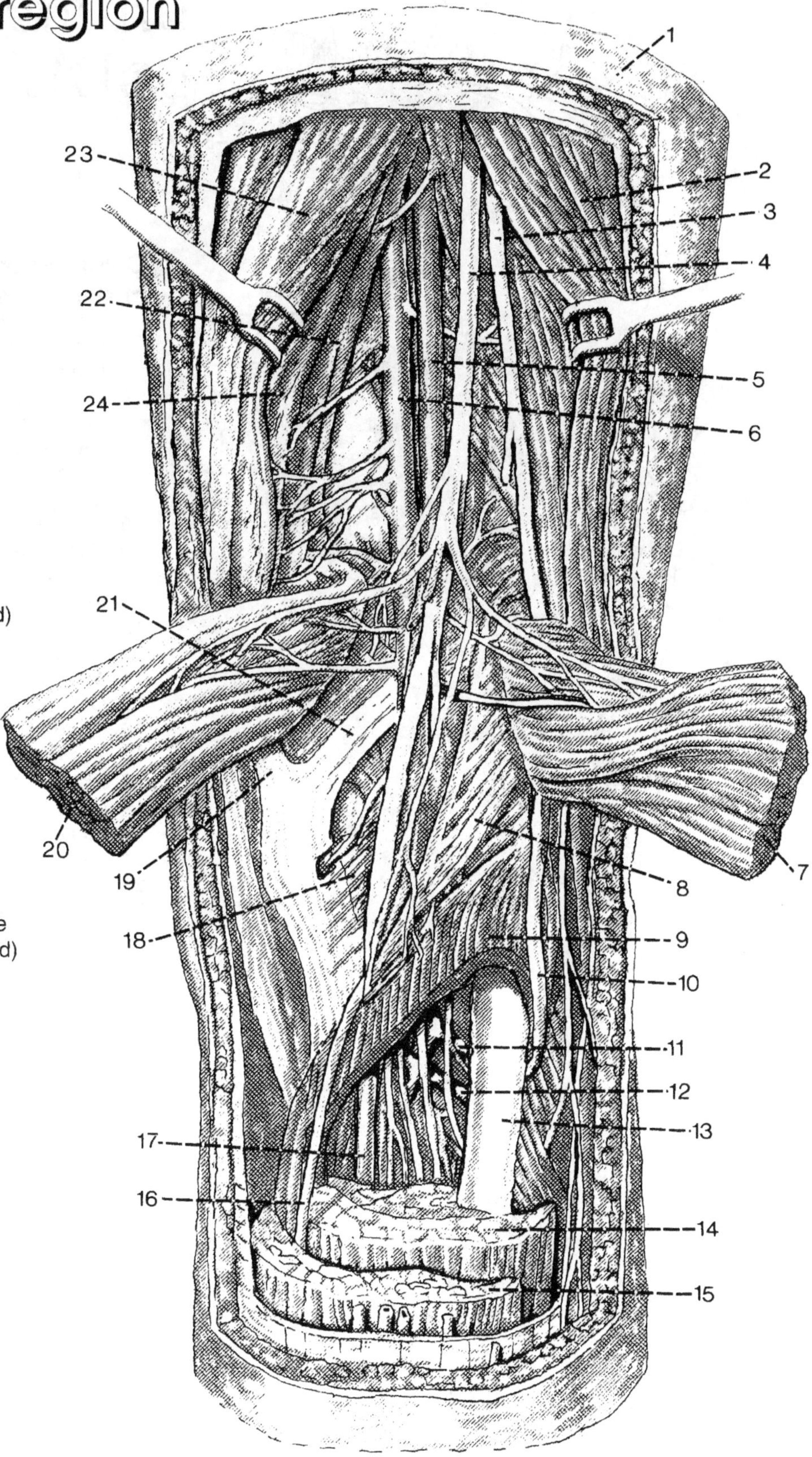

Color and label

1 Fascia lata (deep fascia of thigh)
2 Biceps femoris (long head)
3 Common fibular (peroneal) nerve
4 Tibial nerve
5 Popliteal artery
6 Popliteal vein
7 Gastrocnemius muscle (lateral head)
8 Plantaris muscle
9 Soleus muscle (cut)
10 Common fibular (peroneal) nerve
11 Anterior tibial artery
12 Anterior tibial vein
13 Fibula
14 Soleus muscle
15 Gastrocnemius muscle
16 Tendon of plantaris muscle
17 Tibial nerve
18 Popliteus muscle
19 Tendon of semimembranous muscle
20 Gastrocnemius muscle (medial head)
21 Oblique popliteal ligament
22 Adductor magnus muscle
23 Semitendinosus muscle
24 Semimembranosus muscle

Redrawn from Tondury

LL-37 Muscle attachments on the anterior pelvis and femur

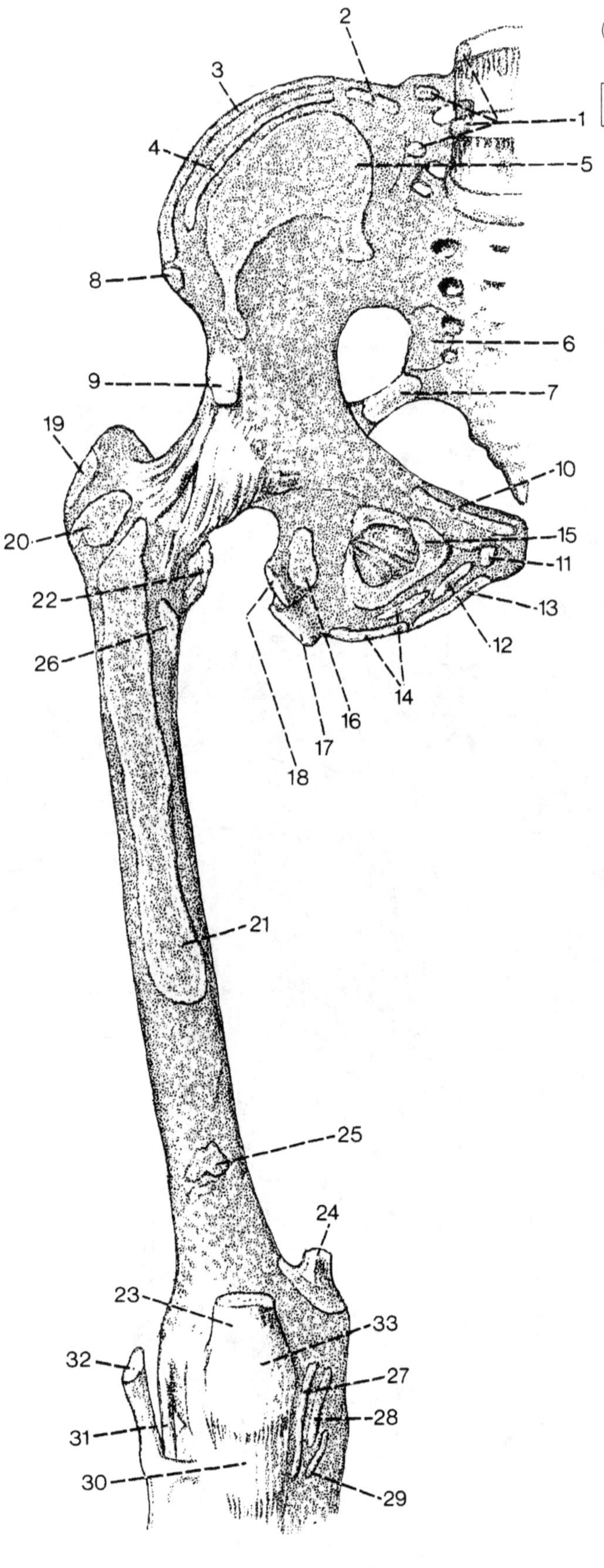

Color the origins (O) RED and the insertions (I) BLUE

1 Psoas major (O)
2 Quadratus lumborum (O)
3 Internal abdominal oblique (O)
4 Transversus abdominis (O)
5 Iliacus (O)
6 Piriformis (O)
7 Coccygeus (O) on sacrospinous ligament
8 Sartorius (O)
9 Rectus femoris (O) straight head
10 Pectineus (O)
11 Adductor longus (O)
12 Adductor brevis (O)
13 Gracilis (O)
14 Adductor magnus (O)
15 Obturator externus (O)
16 Quadratus femoris (O)
17 Semimembranosus (O)
18 Biceps femoris (O)
19 Gluteus minimus (I)
20 Vastus lateralis (O)
21 Vastus intermedius (O)
22 Iliopsoas (I)
23 Quadriceps femoris (I)
24 Adductor magnus (I)
25 Articularis genu (O)
26 Vastus medialis (O)
27 Sartorius (I)
28 Gracilis (I)
29 Semitendinosus (I)
30 Patellar ligament (I)
31 Fibular collateral ligament
32 Biceps femoris (I)
33 Patella

After Clemente

LL-38 Muscle attachments on the posterior pelvis and femur

Color the origins (O) RED and the insertions (I) BLUE

1 External abdominal oblique (I)
2 Gluteus medius (O)
3 Gluteus minimus (O)
4 Gluteus maximus (O) arising on posterior sacroiliac ligament and sacrotuberous ligament
5 Tensor fascia lata (O)
6 Piriformis (O)
7 Rectus femoris oblique head (O)
8 Gemellus superior (O)
9 Gemellus inferior (O)
10 Obturator internus (O)
11 Levator ani (pubococcygeus) (O)
12 Deep transverse perineus (in male) (O)
13 Piriformis (I)
14 Obturator internus with two gemelli (I)
15 Gluteus medius (I)
16 Gluteus minimus (I)
17 Obturator externus (I)
18 Quadratus femoris (I)
19 Iliopsoas (I)
20 Vastus medialis (O)
21 Pectineus (I)
22 Adductor brevis (I)
23 Gluteus maximus (I)
24 Vastus lateralis (O)
25 Vastus intermedius (O)
26 Adductor longus (I)
27 Adductor magnus (I) (anterior oblique part)
28 Biceps femoris short head (O)
29 Plantaris (O)
30 Gastrocnemius (lateral and medial heads) (O)
31 Biceps femoris (I)
32 Semimembranosus (I) *(inserts by three tendons)*
33 Sartorius (I)
34 Gracilis (I)
35 Semitendinosus (I)
36 Semitendinosus (O)
37 Biceps femoris (O)
38 Adductor magnus (I) (posterior vertical part)

After Clemente

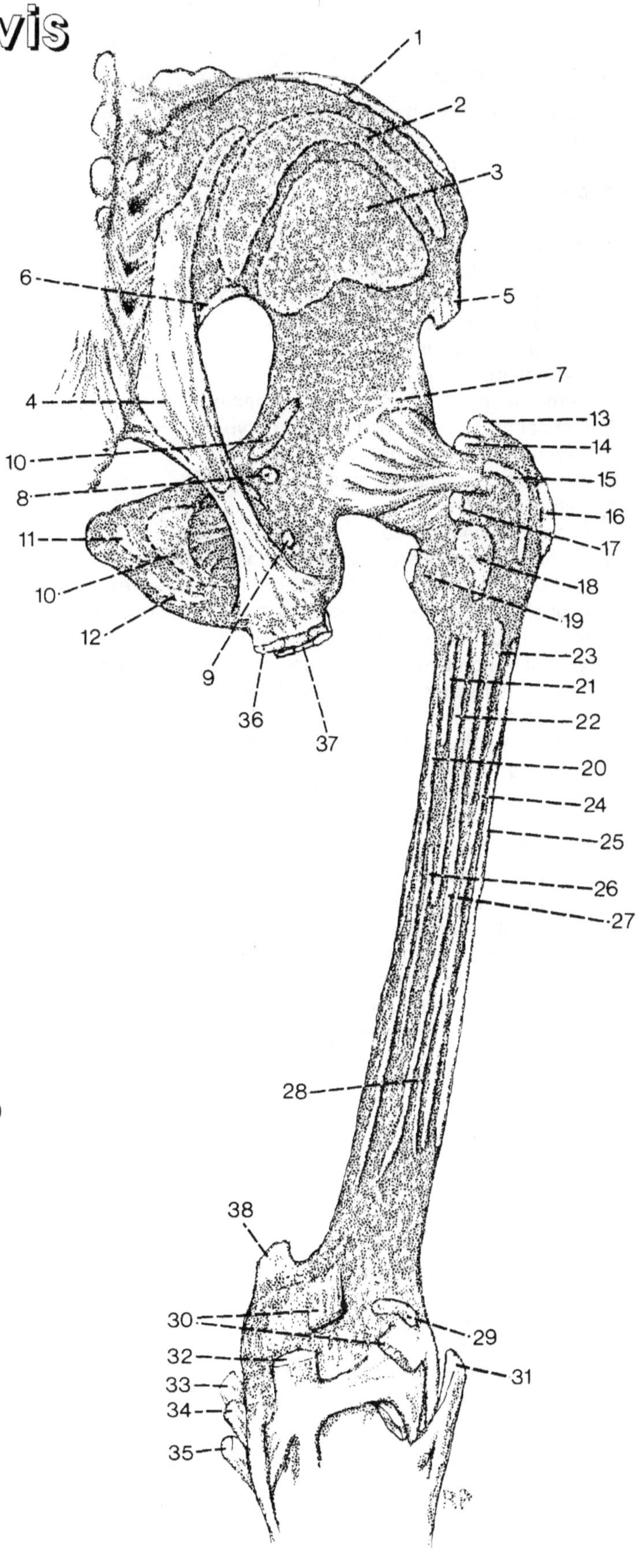

LL-39 Lumbosacral plexus

Right

Color and label

T12, subcostal nerve (twelfth thoracic nerve, ventral ramus)
L1-L5, ventral rami of lumbar nerves 1-5
S1-S5, ventral rami of sacral nerves 1-5
Co, coccygeal nerve

1 Rami to intertransversarii muscle
2 Rami to quadratus lumborum muscle
3 Iliohypogastric nerve
4 Ilioinguinal nerve
5 Lateral cutaneous branch
6 Genitofemoral nerve
7 Femoral branch of genitofemoral nerve
8 Genital branch of genitofemoral nerve
9 Ramus to psoas minor muscle
10 Ramus to psoas major muscle
11 Femoral nerve
12 Branch to iliacus muscle (of femoral nerve)
13 Anterior cutaneous branch (of femoral nerve) and branch to sartorius muscle (of femoral nerve)
14 Branch to quadriceps femoris muscle (of femoral nerve)
15 Saphenous nerve (of femoral nerve)
16 Medial femoral cutaneous branch (of femoral nerve)
17 Branch to pectineus muscle (of femoral nerve)
18 Branch to pectineus and psoas major muscles
19 Accessory obturator nerve *(present in about 10% of legs examined)*
20 Obturator nerve
21 Lumbosacral trunk
22 Superior gluteal nerve
23 Rami to piriformis muscle
24 Peroneal nerve (common peroneal nerve)
25 Inferior gluteal nerve
26 Tibial nerve *(the tibial nerve and the common peroneal nerve usually combine to form the largest nerve in the body, the sciatic nerve)*
27 Branch of tibial nerve to adductor magnus (posterior part), semimembranosus, semitendinosus, and long head of biceps femoris muscles
28 Branch to quadratus femoris and gemellus inferior muscles
29 Branch to obturator internus and gemellus superior muscles
30 Posterior femoral cutaneous nerves
31 Inferior cluneal nerve
32 Perineal nerve and dorsal nerve of penis (clitoris)
33 Inferior rectal nerve
34 Branch to levator ani muscle
35 Branch to coccygeus muscle
36 Anococcygeal nerves
37 Lateral femoral cutaneous nerve

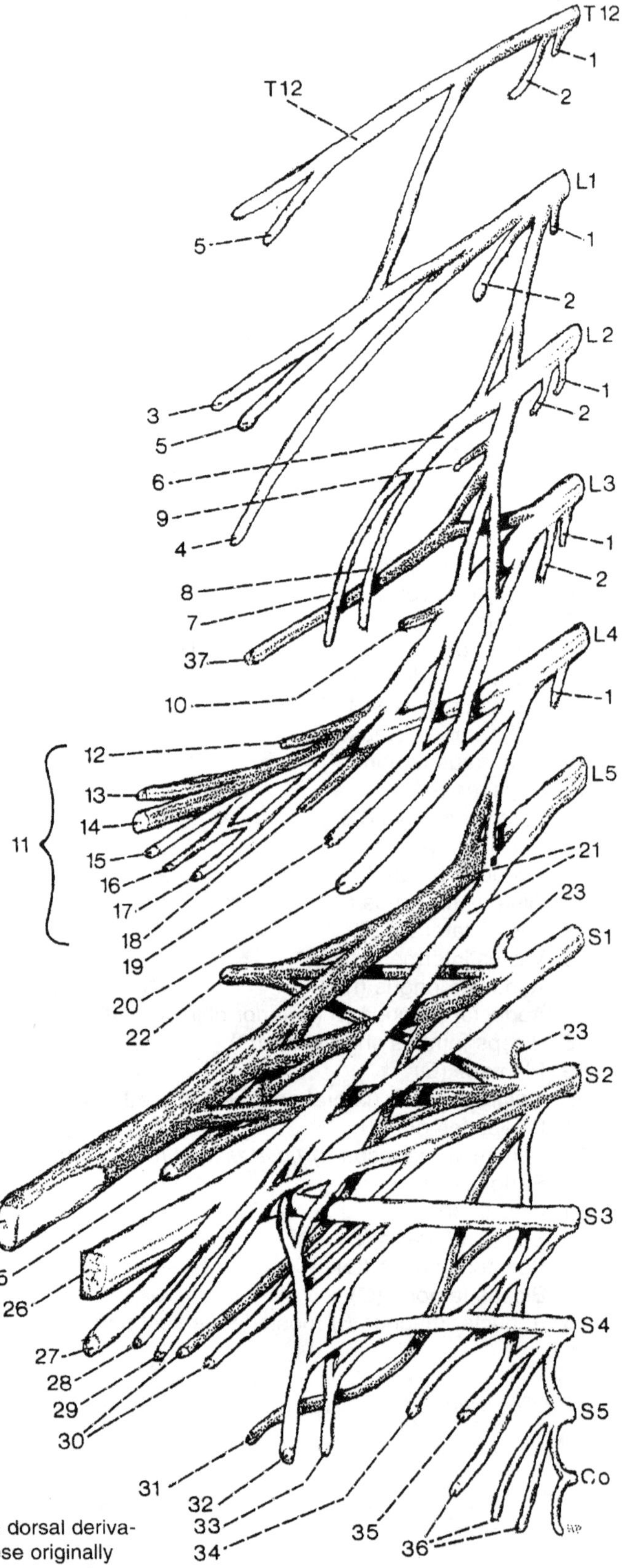

After Spalteholz and Spanner (Eisler)

The shaded nerves are dorsal derivatives of the plexus. These originally innervated dorsal extensor muscles.

LL-40 Gastrocnemius

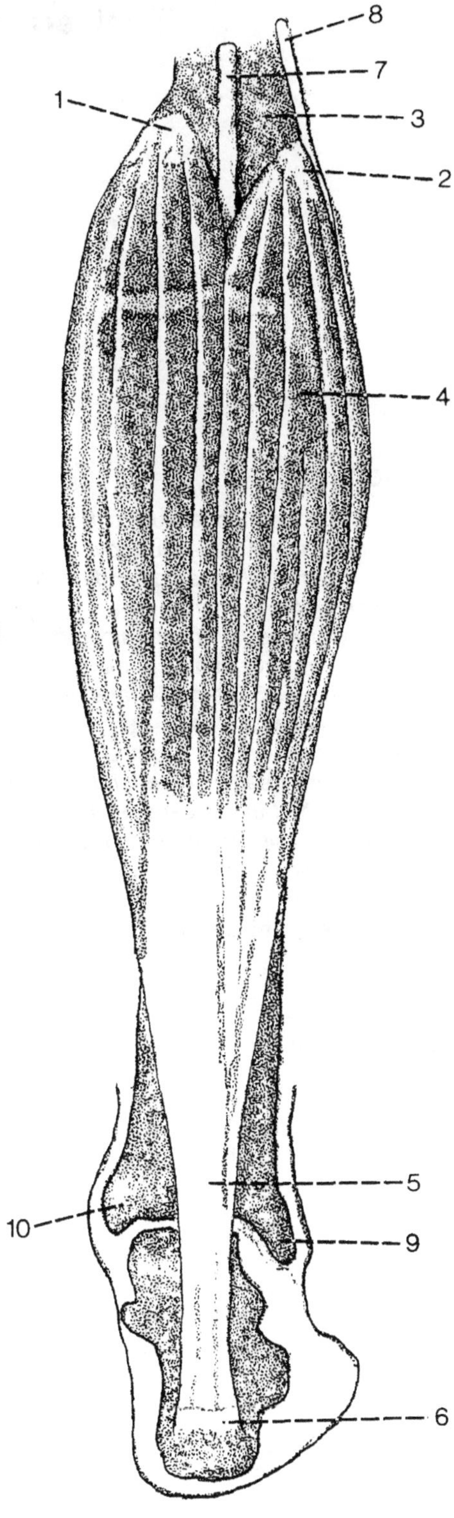

Color and label

1 Gastrocnemius (origin of medial head on femur)
2 Gastrocnemius (origin of lateral head on femur)
3 Femur
4 Gastrocnemius
5 Tendo calcaneus (Achilles tendon)
6 Insertion of gastrocnemius and soleus (triceps surae) on calcaneus
7 Tibial nerve
8 Common peroneal nerve (common fibular nerve)
9 Fibula (lateral malleolus)
10 Tibia (medial malleolus)

LL-41 Soleus, gastrocnemius, and plantaris

Right leg, posterior view

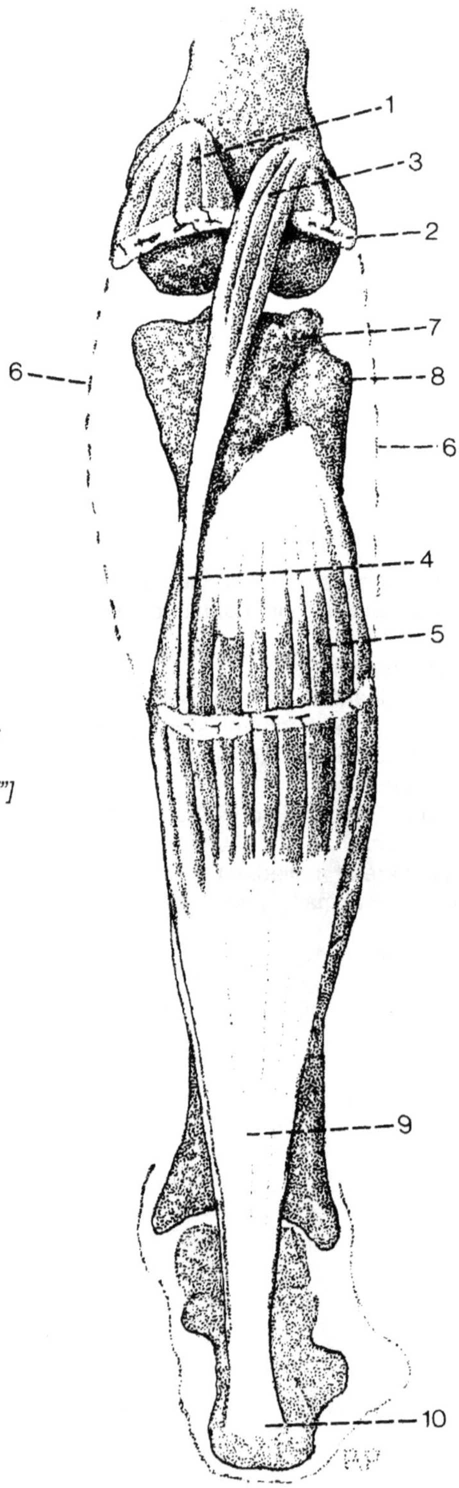

Color and label

1 Medial head of gastrocnemius *(cut)*
2 Lateral head of gastrocnemius *(cut)*
3 Plantaris *(this muscle is small and almost insignificant in the human)*
4 Tendon of plantaris *(long and thin and easily mistaken for a nerve; it may combine with the tendo calcaneous or insert separately on the tubercle of the calcaneus)*
5 Soleus *(it, along with the two heads of the gastrocnemius, inserts by the tendo calcaneus on the tubercle of the calcaneus; the term triceps surae [Latin for "three heads of the calf"] refers to the two heads of the gastrocnemius and the soleus)*
6 Outline of the gastrocnemius
7 Tibia
8 Fibula
9 Tendo calcaneus
10 Insertion of tendo calcaneus

LL-42 Flexor digitorum longus and flexor hallucis longus

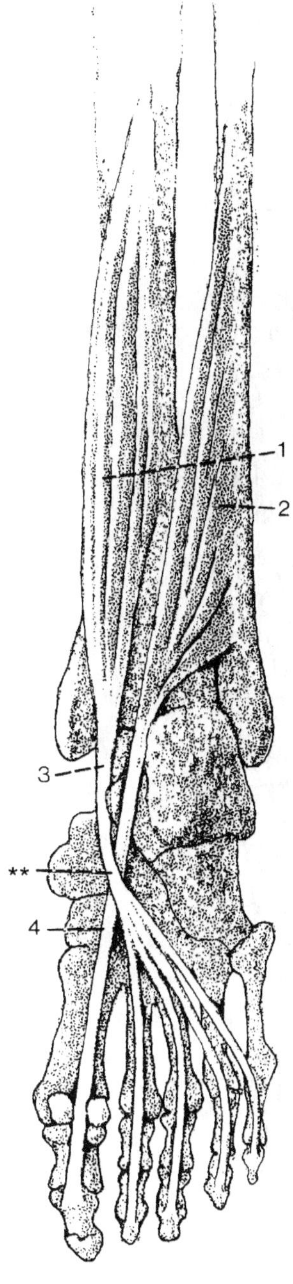

Posterior view of right leg and plantar view of foot

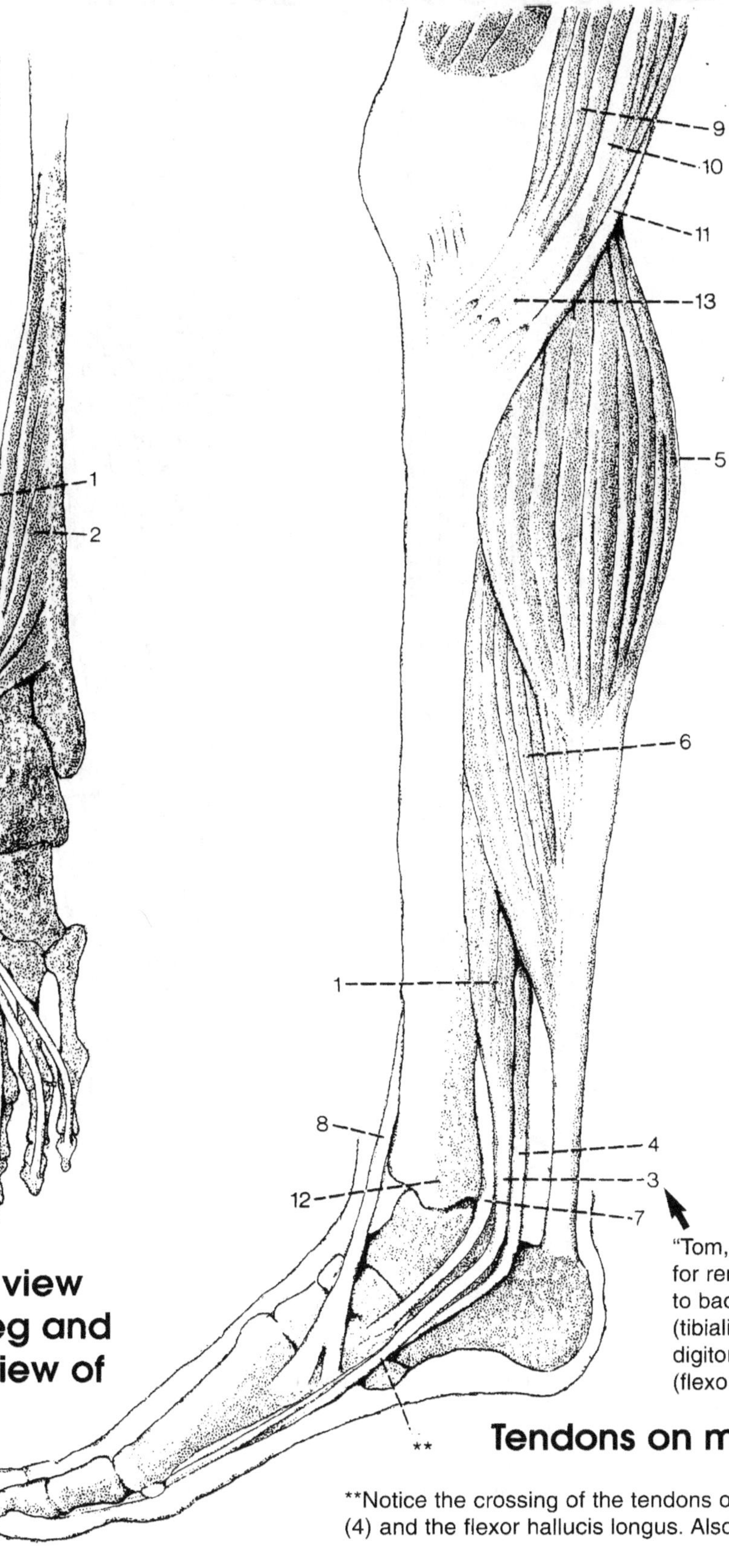

Color and label

1 Flexor digitorum longus muscle
2 Flexor hallucis longus muscle
3 Tendon of flexor digitorum longus
4 Tendon of flexor hallucis longus
5 Gastrocnemius muscle
6 Soleus muscle
7 Tendon of tibialis posterior
8 Tendon of tibialis anterior
9 Sartorius muscle
10 Gracilis muscle
11 Semitendinosus
12 Medial malleolus
13 Pes anserinus "goose's foot"

The tendinous expansions of these 3 muscles (9, 10, 11) on the medial surface of the tibial tuberosity suggested the webbed foot of a goose to the ancient anatomists.

"Tom, Dick, and Harry"; a mnemonic for remembering the order (from front to back) of these 3 tendons: "Tom" (tibialis posterior, 7), "Dick" (flexor digitorum longus, 3), and "Harry" (flexor hallucis longus, 4)

Tendons on medial side of right foot

**Notice the crossing of the tendons of the flexor digitorum (3) longus (4) and the flexor hallucis longus. Also at * in far left figure.

LL-43 Deep muscles in the posterior leg compartment

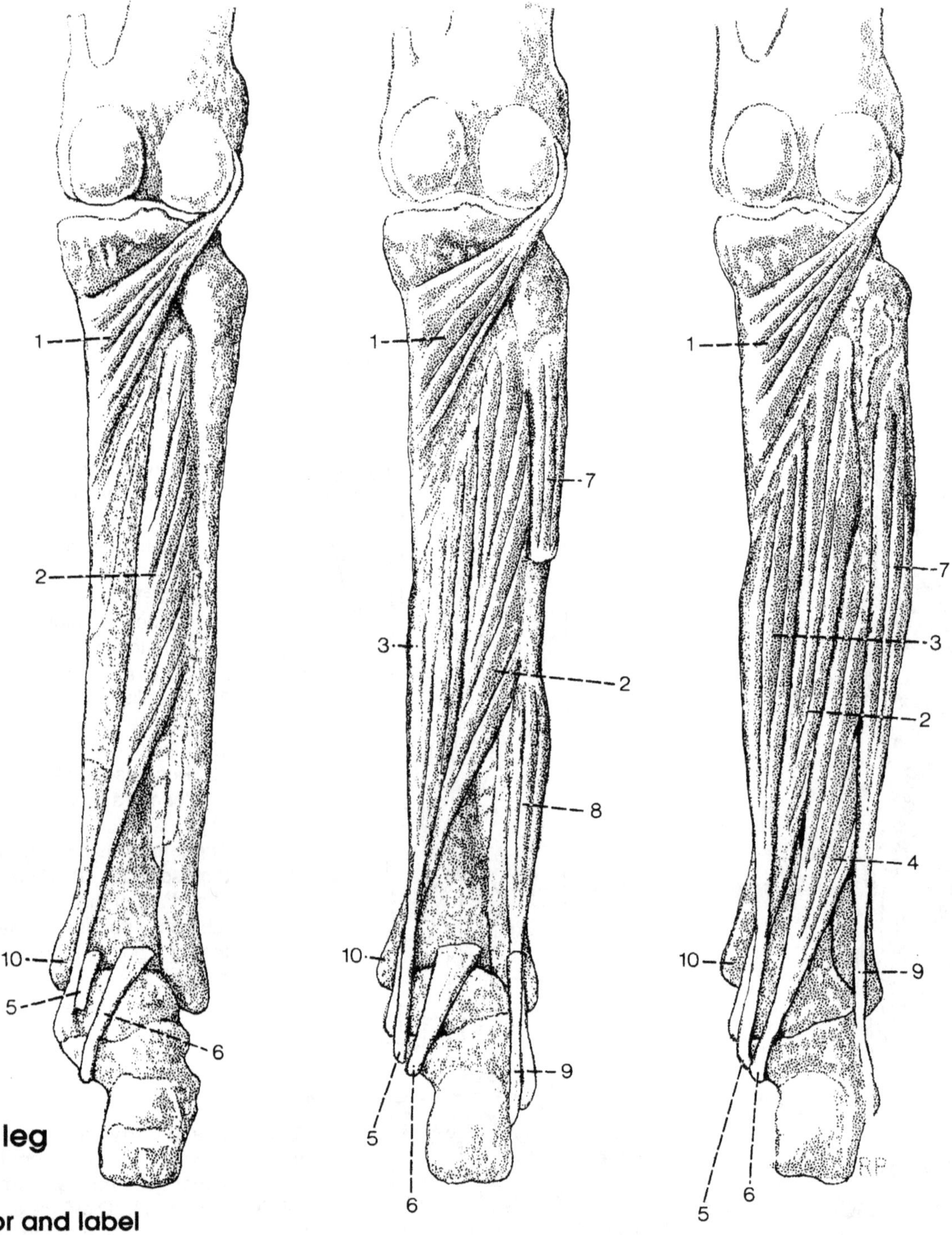

Right leg

Color and label

1 Popliteus
2 Tibialis posterior
3 Flexor digitorum longus
4 Flexor hallucis longus
5 Tendon of flexor digitorum longus
6 Tendon of flexor hallucis longus
7 Peroneus longus (lateral compartment)
8 Peroneus brevis (lateral compartment)
9 Tendon of peroneus longus
10 Medial malleolus

LL-44 Flexor hallucis longus

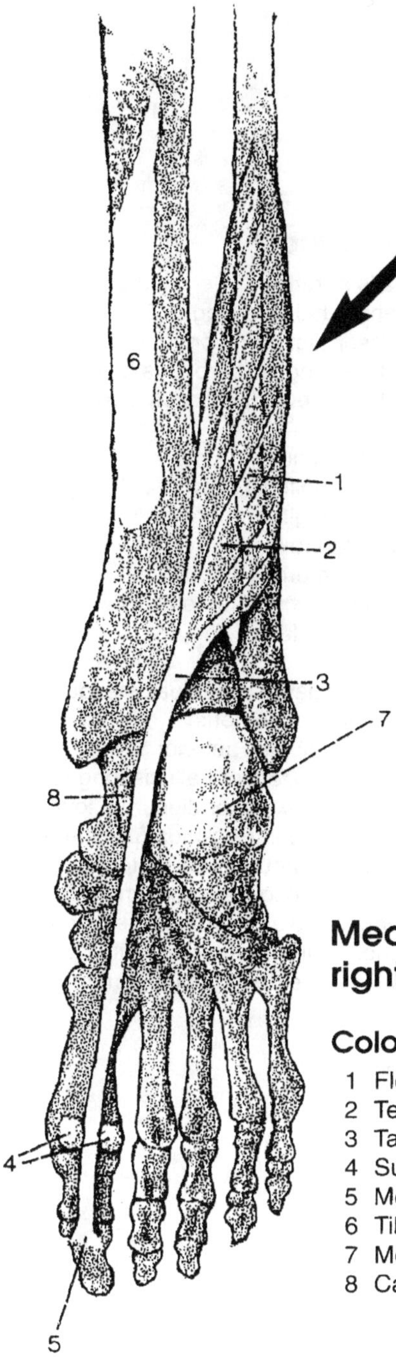

Posterior view of right leg
Foot is plantarflexed

Color and label

1 Origin of flexor hallucis longus on fibula
2 Flexor hallucis muscle
3 Tendon of flexor hallucis longus
4 Medial and lateral sesamoid bones *(in tendons of flexor hallucis brevis [not shown])*
5 Insertion of flexor hallucis longus tendon on distal phalanx of big toe (hallux)
6 Origin of flexor digitorum longus on tibia
7 Tubercle of calcaneus
8 Sustentaculum tali with groove for tendon of flexor hallucis longus

Medial view of right leg

Color and label

1 Flexor hallucis longus muscle
2 Tendon of flexor hallucis longus
3 Talus
4 Sustentaculum tali
5 Medial sesamoid bone
6 Tibia
7 Medial malleolus
8 Calcaneus

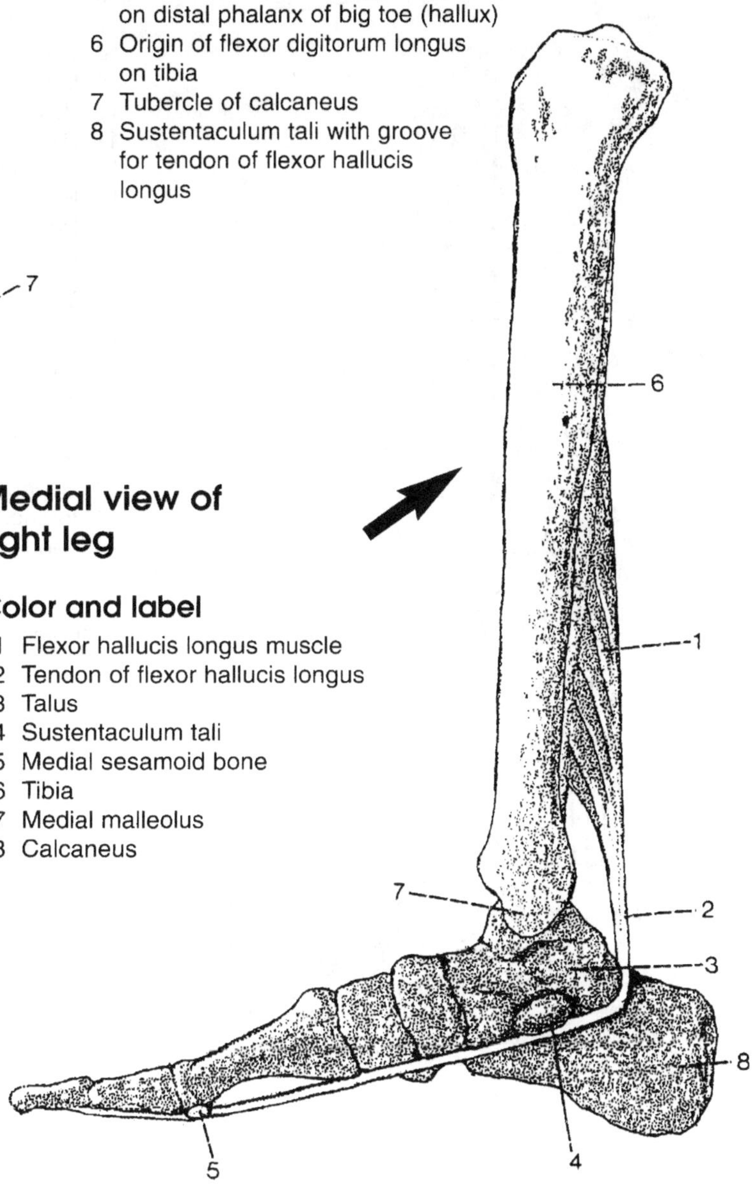

LL-45 Muscles of lateral leg

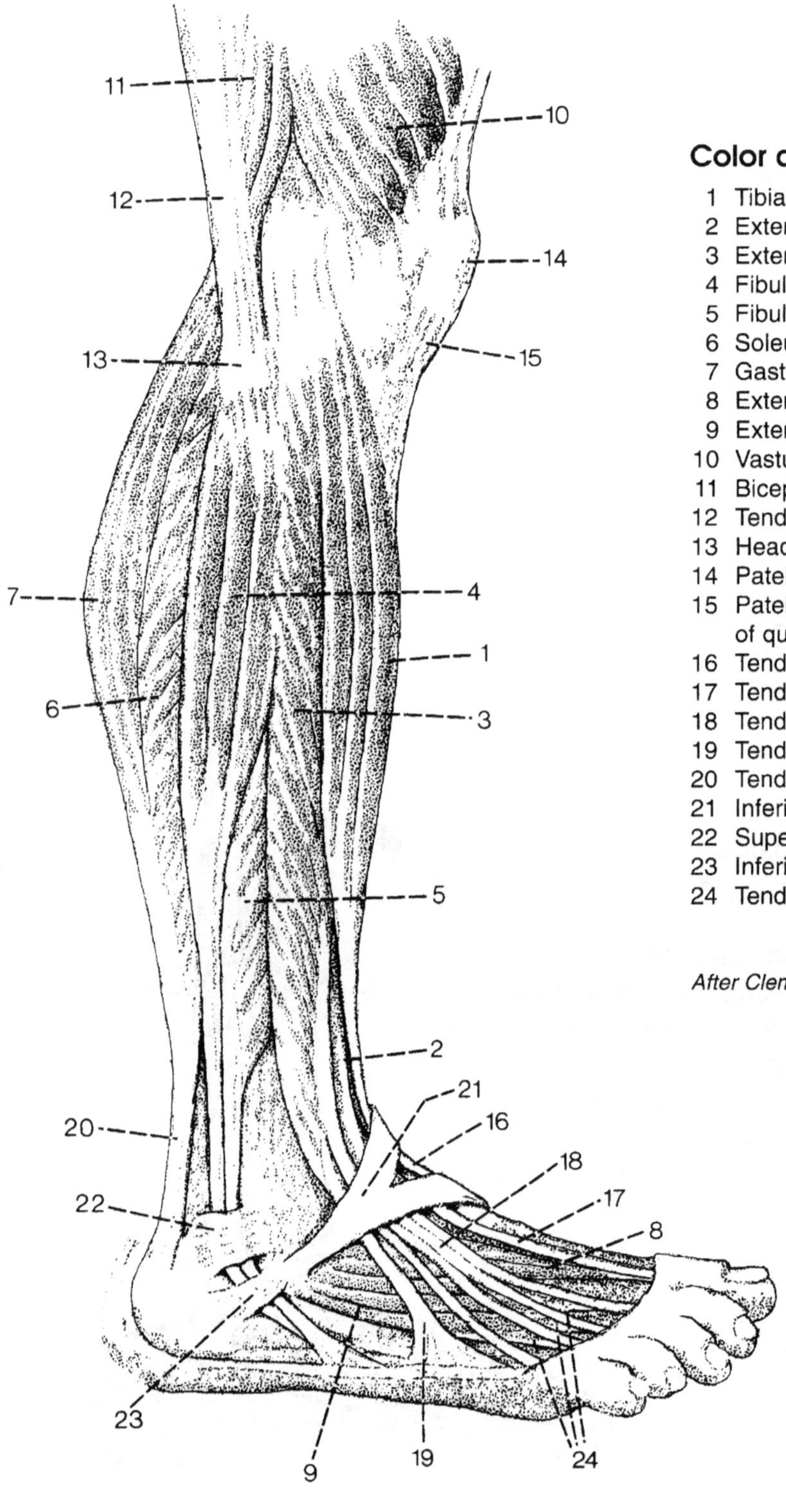

Color and label

1 Tibialis anterior
2 Extensor hallucis longus
3 Extensor digitorum longus
4 Fibularis longus (peroneus longus)
5 Fibularis brevis (peroneus brevis)
6 Soleus
7 Gastrocnemius
8 Extensor hallucis brevis
9 Extensor digitorum brevis
10 Vastus lateralis
11 Biceps femoris
12 Tendon of biceps femoris
13 Head of fibula
14 Patella
15 Patellar "ligament" (actually tendon of quadriceps femoris)
16 Tendon of tibialis anterior
17 Tendon of extensor hallucis longus
18 Tendons of extensor digitorum longus
19 Tendon of fibularis tertius (peroneus tertius)
20 Tendo calcaneus (Achilles tendon)
21 Inferior extensor retinaculum
22 Superior fibular (peroneal) retinaculum
23 Inferior fibular (peroneal) retinaculum
24 Tendons of extensor digitorum brevis

After Clemente

LL-46 Anterior dissection of right leg

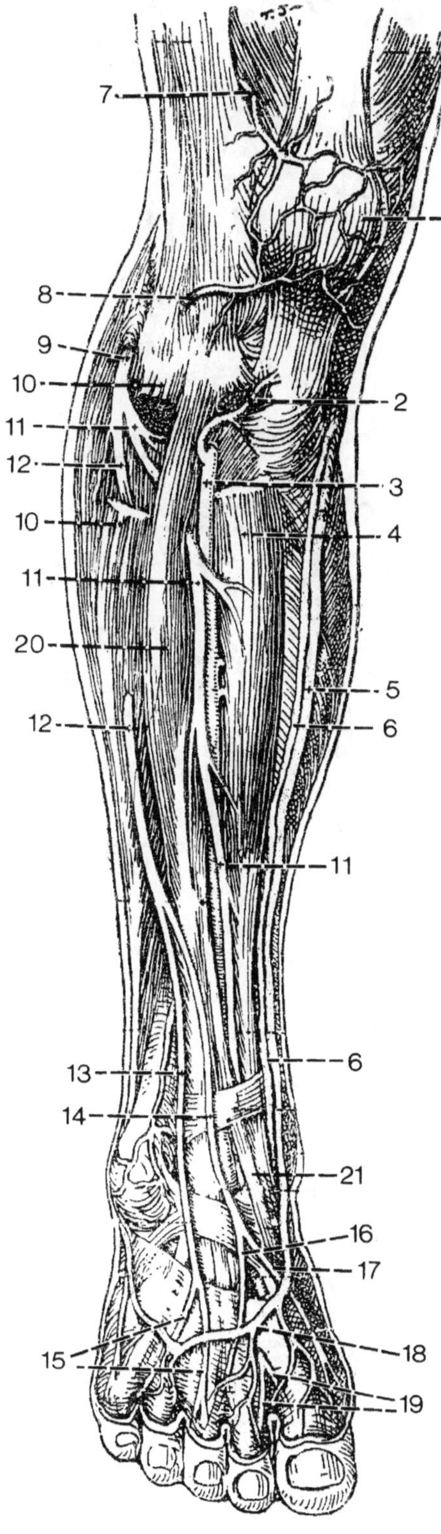

Color and label

1 Patella (knee cap); embedded in the tendon of the quadratus femoris; largest sesamoid bone in the body
2 Anterior recurrent tibial artery
3 Anterior tibial artery
4 Anterior tibialis muscle
5 Great saphenous vein
6 Saphenous nerve (branch of femoral nerve)
7 Superior lateral genicular artery
8 Inferior lateral genicular artery
9 Common peroneal (fibular) nerve
10 Peroneus (fibularis) longus muscle (section removed to show deep peroneal nerve)
11 Deep peroneal (fibular) nerve
12 Superficial peroneal (fibular) nerve
13 Intermediate dorsal cutaneus nerve
14 Medial dorsal cutaneus nerve
15 Dorsal cutaneus rami of superficial peroneal nerve
16 Lateral branch of medial dorsal cutaneus nerve
17 Medial branch of medial dorsal cutaneus nerve
18 Dorsal venous arch of foot
19 Dorsal digital rami of deep peroneal (fibular) nerve; to adjacent skin between toes I and II

Eycleshymer and Jones

LL-47 Muscle attachments on the anterior leg*

Right leg

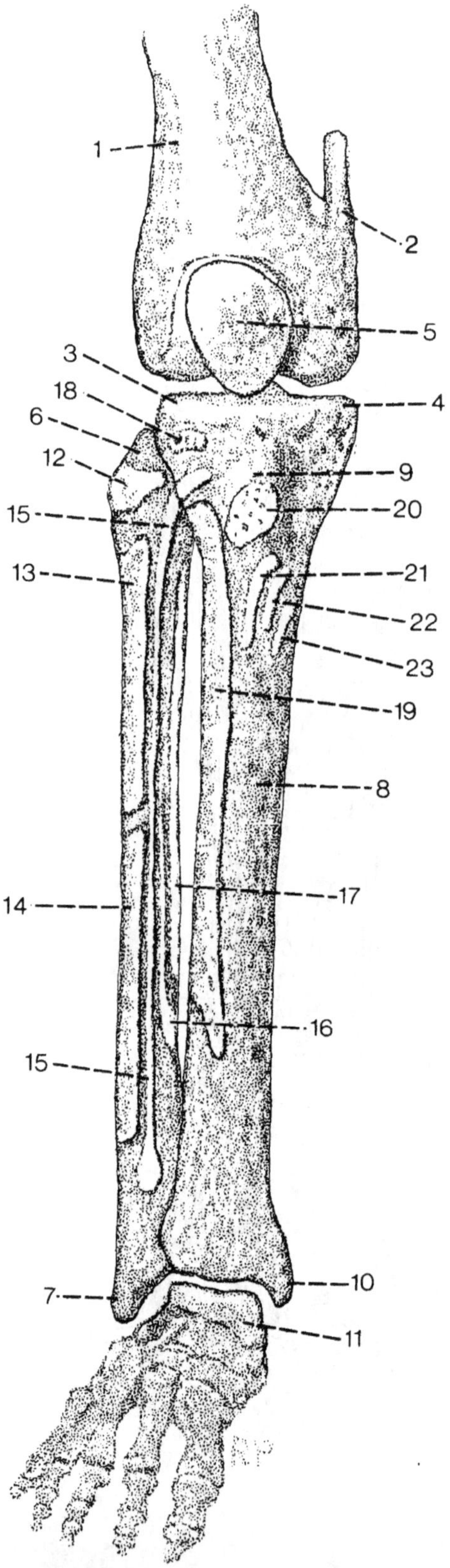

Color and label

1 Femur
2 Adductor tubercle and insertion of vertical part of adductor magnus
3 Lateral tibial condyle
4 Medial tibial condyle
5 Patella
6 Head of fibula
7 Lateral malleolus
8 Tibia
9 Tibial tuberosity
10 Medial malleolus
11 Talus

Color the origins (O) RED and the insertions (I) BLUE

12 Biceps femoris (I)
13 Peroneus longus (fibularis longus) (O)
14 Peroneus brevis (fibularis brevis) (O)
15 Extensor digitorum longus (O)
16 Extensor hallucis longus (O)
17 Tibialis posterior (O)
18 Iliotibial tract (I)
19 Tibialis anterior (O)
20 Quadriceps femoris (patellar "ligament") (I)
21 Sartorius (I)
22 Gracilis (I)
23 Semitendinosus (I)

*In anatomical terminology the lower leg (from knee to ankle) is the leg, and the upper leg (from hip to knee) is the thigh.

LL-48 Muscle attachments

Right leg

Label and color the origins (O) RED and the insertions (I) BLUE

1 Medial and lateral femoral condyles
2 Tendon of vertical part of adductor magnus (I)
3 Gastrocnemius (medial head) (O)
4 Gastrocnemius (lateral head) (O)
5 Intercondylar eminence
6 Medial tibial condyle
7 Lateral tibial condyle
8 Tibia
9 Fibula
10 Lateral malleolus
11 Medial malleolus
12 Head of fibula
13 Talus
14 Calcaneus
15 Semimembranosus (I)
16 Tibial collateral ligament
17 Popliteus (O)
18 Soleus (O)
19 Flexor digitorum longus (O)
20 Tibialis posterior (O)
21 Flexor hallucis longus (O)
22 Peroneus brevis (fibularis brevis) (O)
23 Biceps femoris (I)
24 Fibular collateral ligament
25 Popliteus (I)
26 Groove for tendon of flexor hallucis longus
27 Insertion of tendo calcaneus (gastrocnemius and soleus) (I)
28 Plantaris (O)

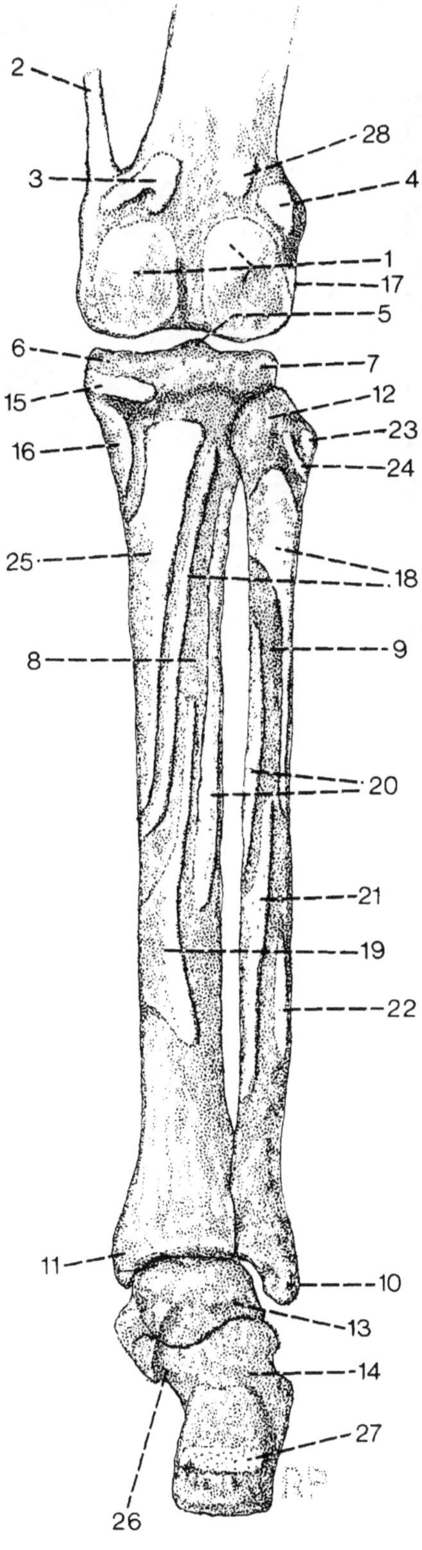

LL-49 Bones of foot, medial aspect

Right foot

Color and label

1 Calcaneus
2 Talus
3 Navicular bone
4 Medial cuneiform bone
5 Intermediate cuneiform bone
6 First metatarsal bone
7 Proximal phalanx of big toe (hallux)
8 Distal phalanx of big toe
9 Sesamoid bones (in tendons of flexor hallucis brevis)
10 Medial malleolus (tibia)
11 Medial malleolar surface of talar trochlea
12 Tuberosity of calcaneus
13 Sustentaculum tali (of calcaneus)
14 Medial process of calcaneal tuberosity

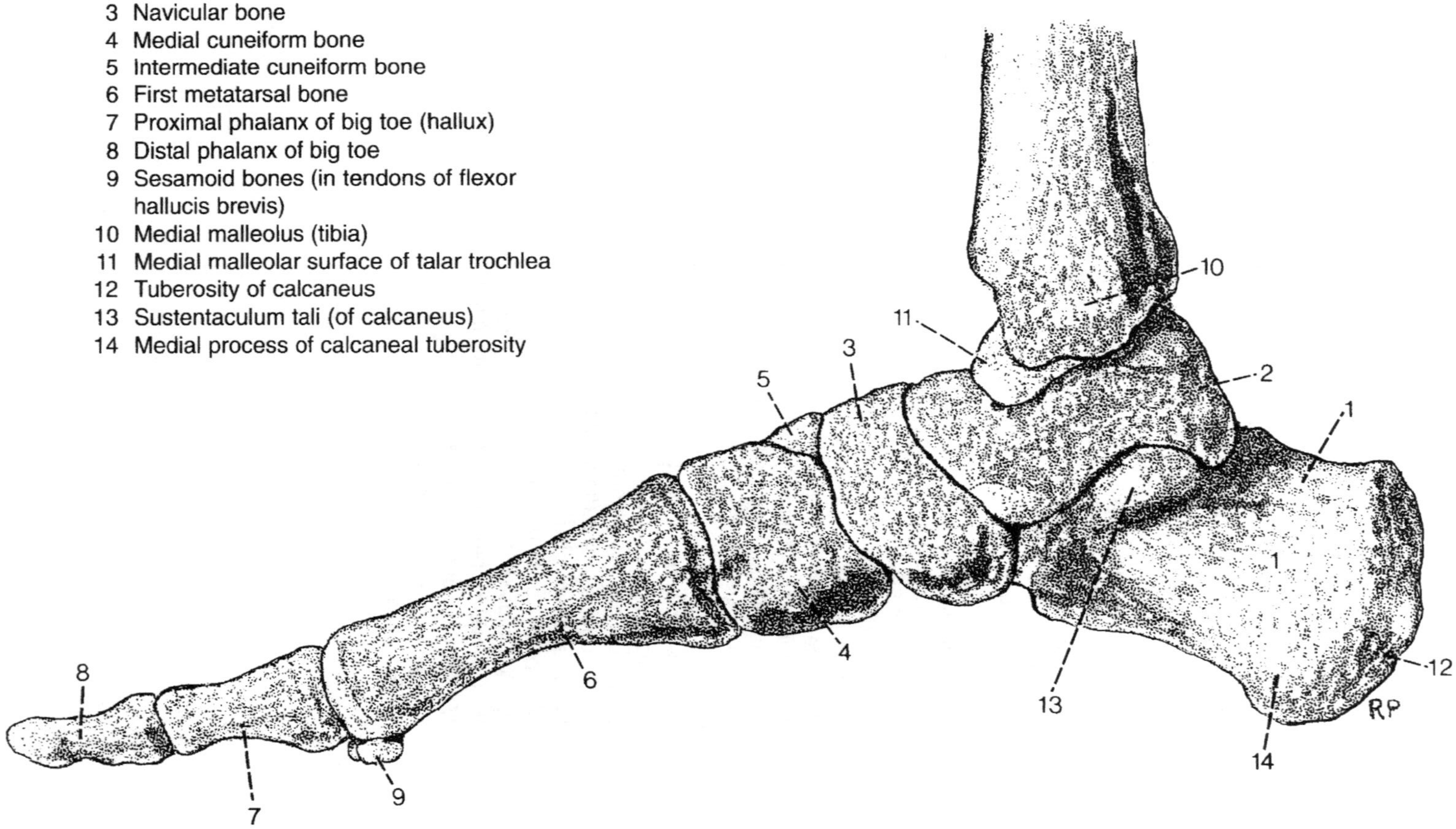

Pedigree
Etymological cartoon

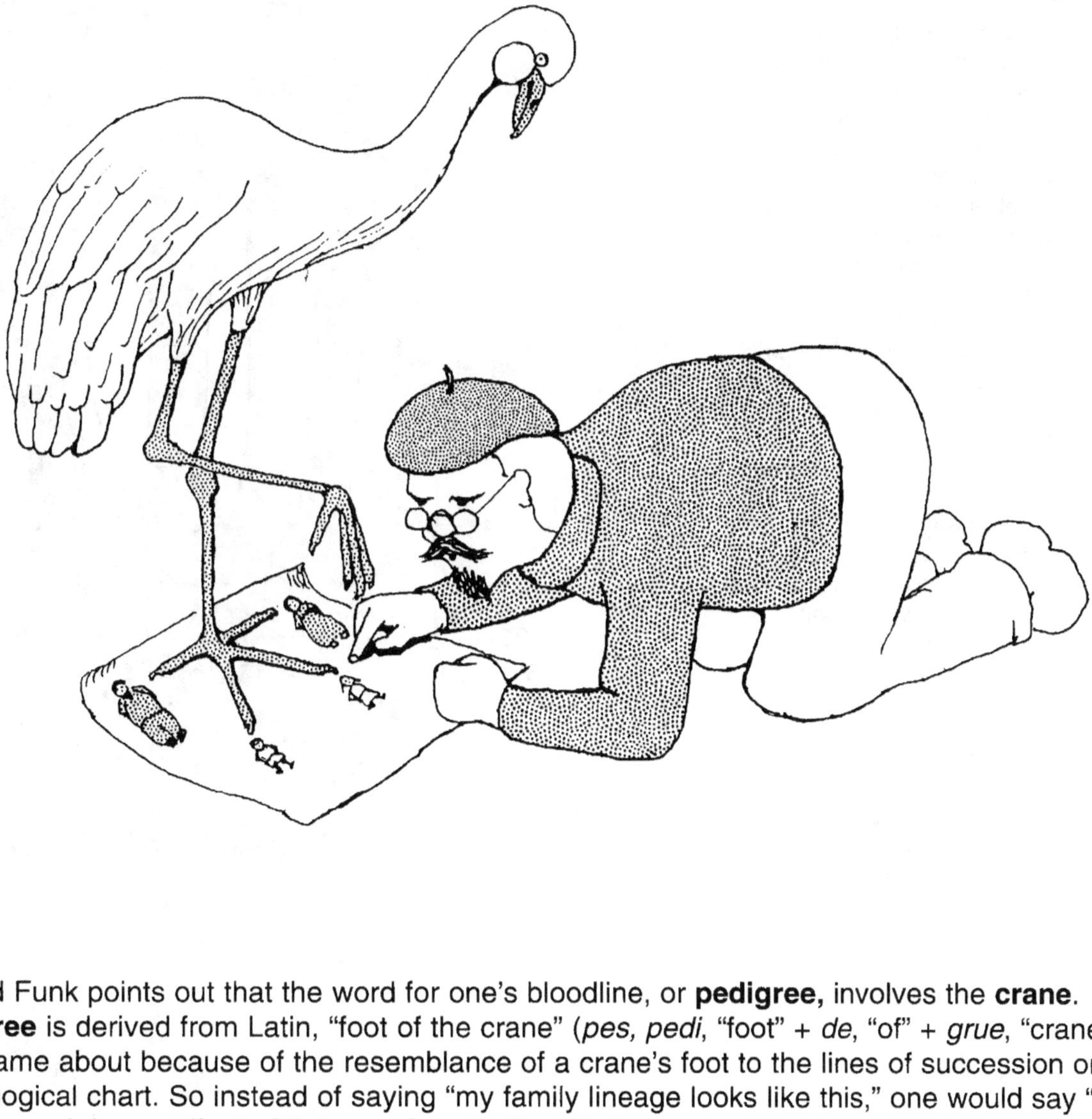

Wilfred Funk points out that the word for one's bloodline, or **pedigree,** involves the **crane**. **Pedigree** is derived from Latin, "foot of the crane" (*pes, pedi*, "foot" + *de*, "of" + *grue*, "crane.") This came about because of the resemblance of a crane's foot to the lines of succession on a genealogical chart. So instead of saying "my family lineage looks like this," one would say "my family's *ped de grue* (foot of the crane) looks like this."

LL-50 Bones of foot, inferior aspect

Plantar (inferior) aspect of the right foot

Color and label

1 Calcaneus (heel bone)
2 Calcaneal tuber (Latin, a swelling or protuberance)
3 Lateral process of calcaneal tuber
4 Medial process of calcaneal tuber
5 Sustentaculum tali (Latin, support of the talus)
6 Groove for the tendon of the flexor hallucis longus muscle
7 Head of talus (caput tali)
8 Cuboid bone
9 Tuberosity of cuboid bone
10 Navicular bone
11 Tuberosity of navicular bone
12 Medial cuneiform bone
13 Intermediate cuneiform bone
14 Lateral cuneiform bone
15 Tuberosity of first metatarsal bone
16 Groove for tendon of peroneus longus
17 Tuberosity of fifth metatarsal bone
18 Proximal phalanx of big toe
19 Distal phalanx of big toe; note that the big toe has only two phalanges
20 Medial and lateral sesamoid bones
21 Body of first metatarsal bone (of big toe or hallux)
22 Head of first metatarsal
23 Base of fifth metatarsal
24 Body of fifth metatarsal
25 Head of fifth metatarsal

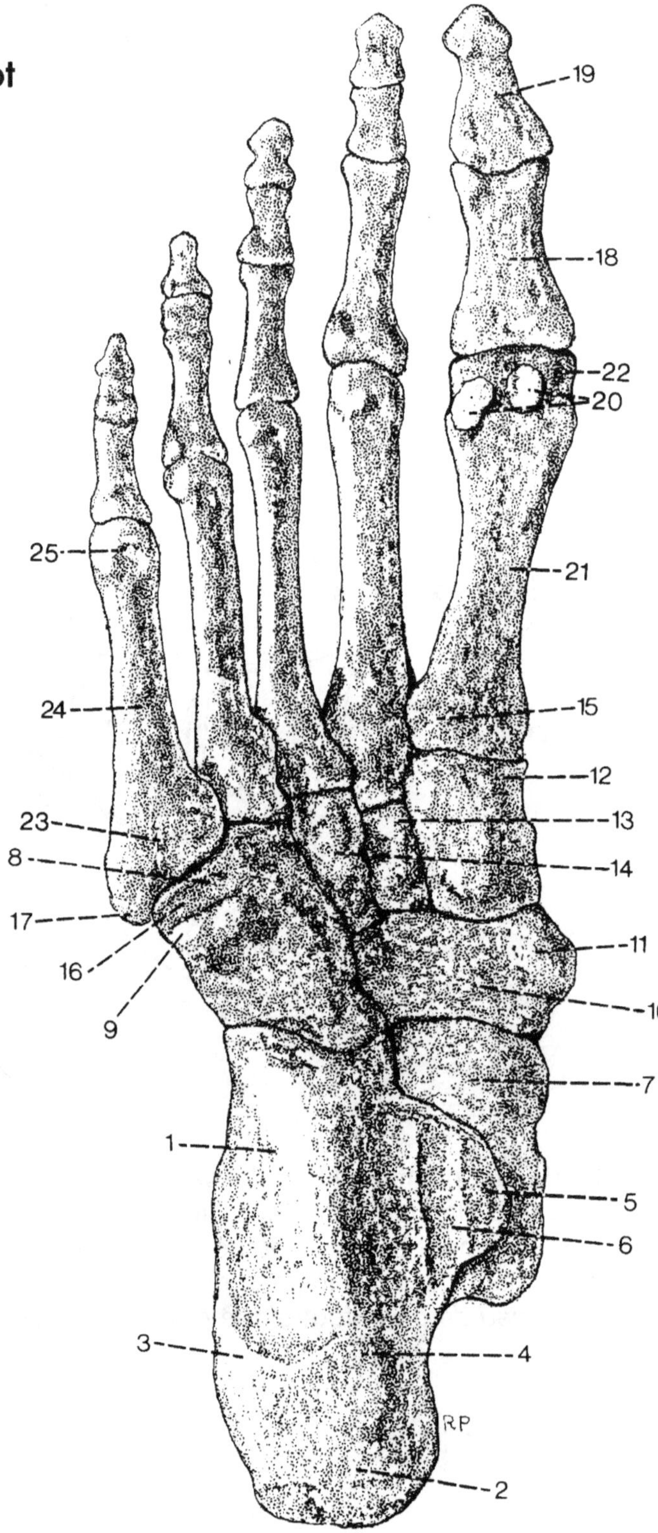

LL-51 Plantar arteries

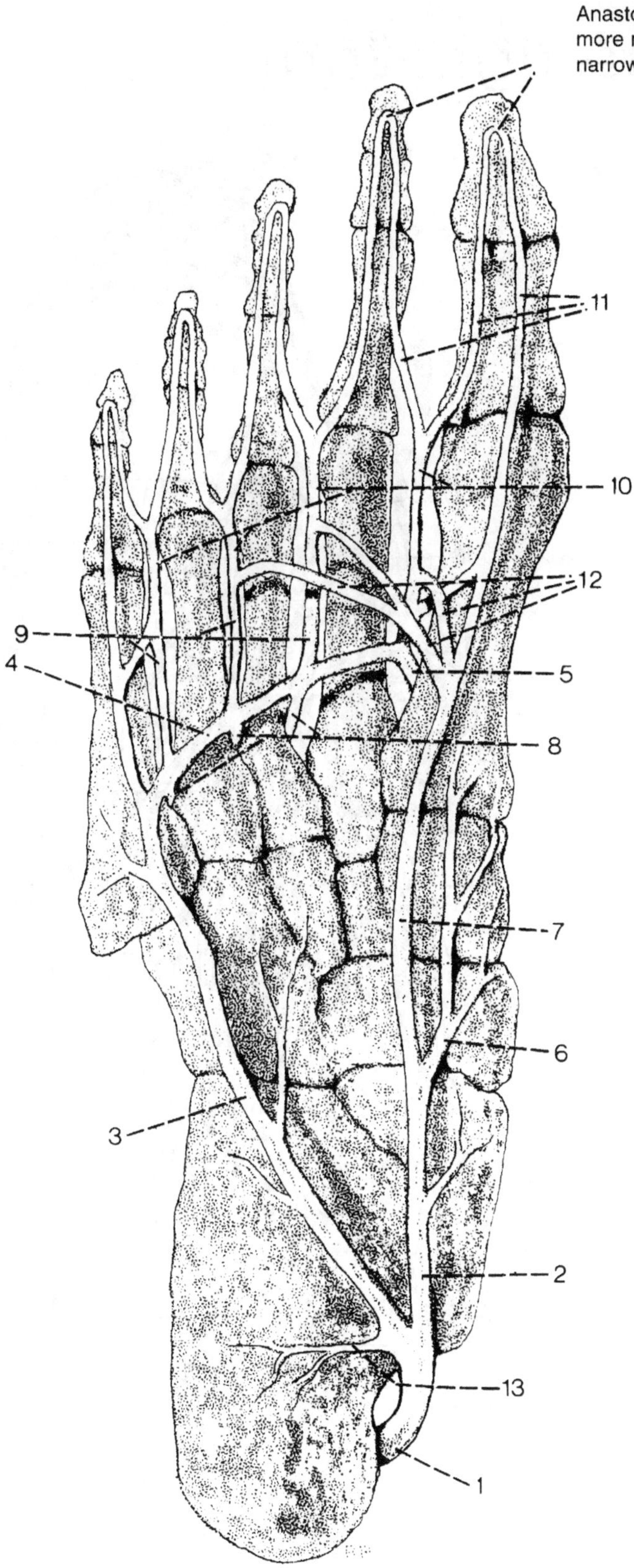

Color and label

1 Posterior tibial artery (note it divides into medial and lateral plantar arteries)
2 Medial plantar artery
3 Lateral plantar artery
4 Deep plantar arch
5 Deep plantar artery (from dorsalis pedis artery)
6 Deep branch of medial plantar artery
7 Superficial branch of medial plantar artery
8 Perforating branches of plantar arch
9 Plantar metatarsal arteries
10 Common plantar digital arteries
11 Proper plantar digital arteries
12 Communicating branches
13 Calcaneal branch

After Hollinshead

LL-52 Plantar dissection of the right foot

Flexor digitorum brevis cut and largely removed

Color and label

1 Plantar aponeurosis (mainly lateral part)
2 Flexor digitorum brevis muscle (cut)
3 Lateral plantar artery (veins not shown)
4 Lateral plantar nerve
5 Abductor digiti minimi muscle
6 Quadratus plantae muscle
7 Deep (profundus) branch of lateral plantar nerve
8 Superficial branches of lateral plantar nerve
9 Flexor digiti minimi muscle
10 Plantar arch
11 Lumbrical muscles (arising on tendons of flexor digitorum longus)
12 Adductor hallucis (transverse head)
13 Tendons of flexor digitorum longus muscle
14 Tendons (cut) of flexor digitorum brevis
15 Fibrous tendon sheaths
16 Central part of plantar aponeurosis (cut)
17 Posterior tibial artery
18 Medial plantar artery
19 Medial plantar nerve
20 Abductor hallucis muscle (cut)
21 Tendon of flexor hallucis longus
22 Common plantar digital nerves
23 Flexor hallucis brevis muscle
24 Common plantar digital arteries
25 Proper plantar digital nerves
26 Proper plantar digital arteries

Redrawn from Tondury

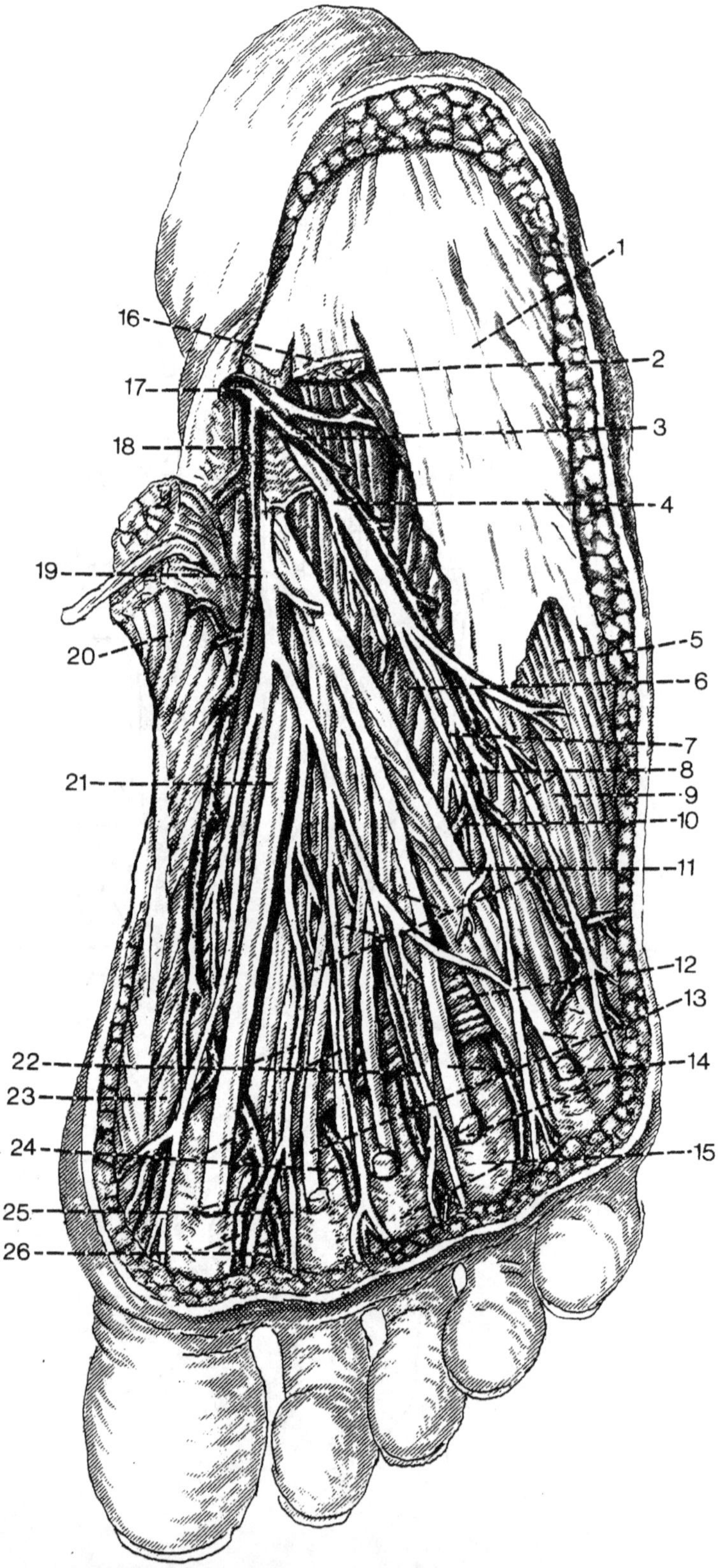

LL-53 Arteries of right knee joint

Viewed from behind

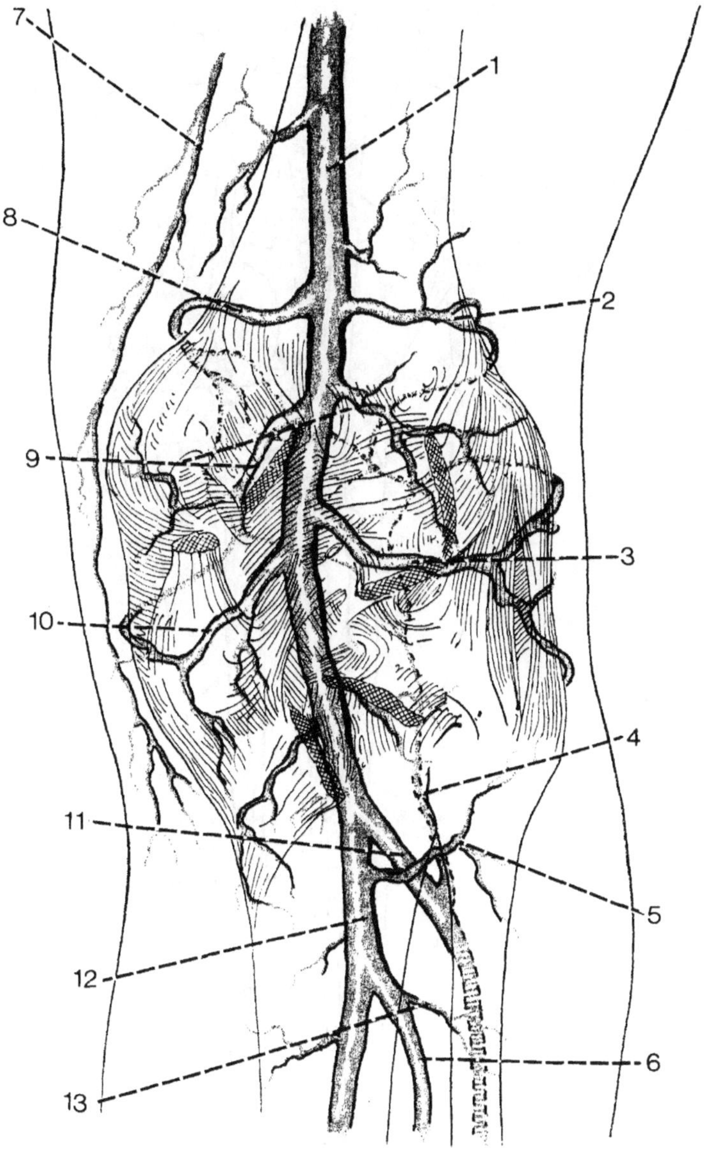

Eycleshymer and Jones

Color and label

1 Popliteal artery (a continuation of the femoral artery); note that the popliteal artery ends by dividing into the anterior and posterior tibial arteries
2 Lateral superior genicular artery
3 Lateral inferior genicular artery
4 Anterior recurrent tibial artery
5 Fibular branch
6 Fibular (peroneal) artery
7 Supreme genicular artery
8 Medial superior genicular artery
9 Sural arteries
10 Medial inferior genicular artery
11 Anterior tibial artery
12 Posterior tibial artery
13 Fibular nutrient artery (enters the bone)

Veins are not shown here. Veins accompanying the arteries (venae comitantes) have the same name as the artery and are often doubled (two veins accompany a single artery).

LL-54 Arteries of the posterior leg

Right leg, posterior aspect

Color and label

1 Femoral artery
2 Popliteal artery
3 Descending genicular artery
4 Anterior tibial artery
5 Posterior tibial artery
6 Fibular (peroneal) artery
7 Lateral malleolar artery
8 Calcaneal artery
9 Lateral superior genicular artery
10 Medial superior genicular artery
11 Lateral inferior genicular artery
12 Medial inferior genicular artery
13 Anterior tibial recurrent artery
14 Fibular (peroneal) circumflex artery
15 Tibial collateral ligament
16 Fibular collateral ligament
17 Dorsalis pedis artery (seen through talis)
18 Interosseous membrane
19 Descending branch of lateral femoral circumflex artery

Not shown are the veins that accompany the arteries (*venae comitantes*, Latin, "veins that run with"). These are often doubled.

After Hollinshead

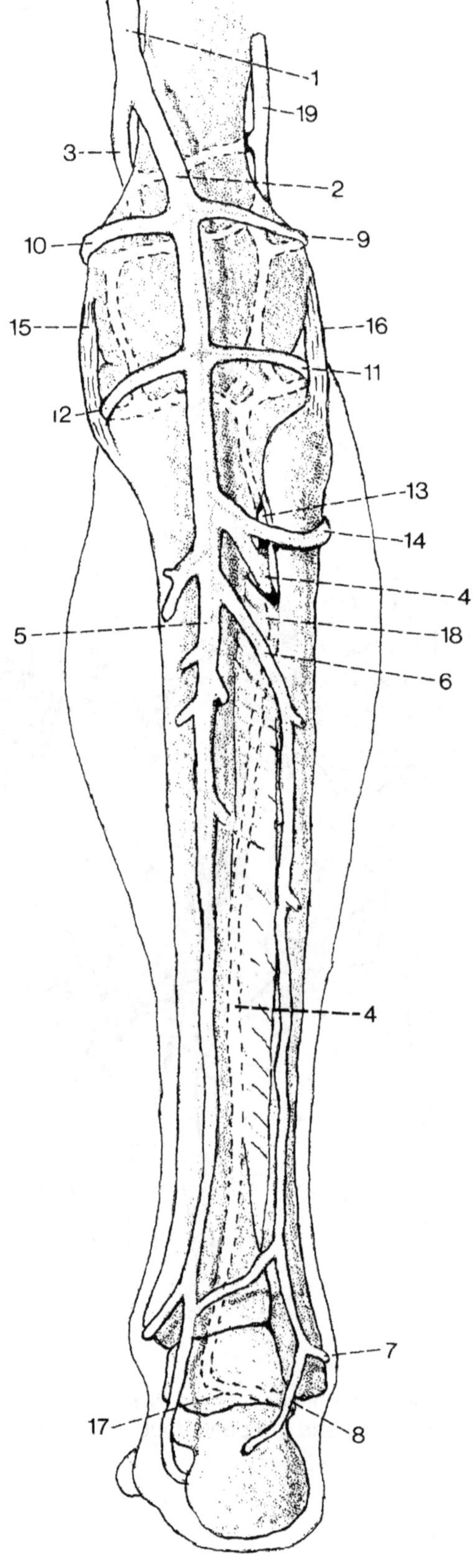

LL-55 Motor distribution of the common fibular (peroneal) nerve

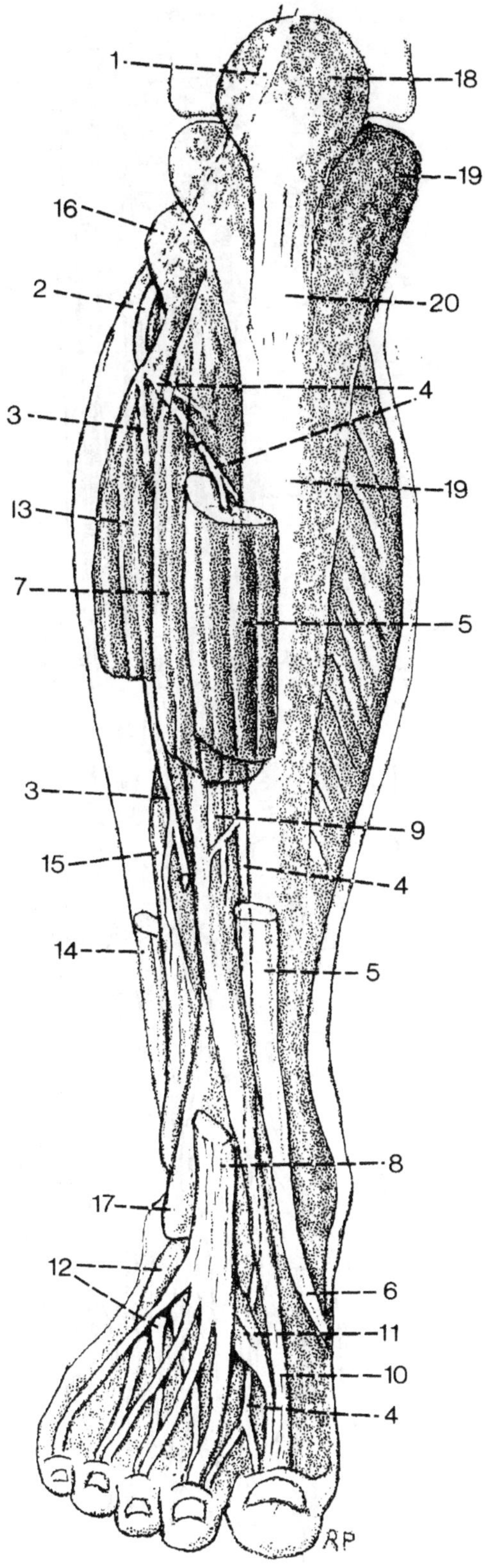

Color and label

1 Common fibular (peroneal) nerve (posterior to knee joint)
2 Common fibular (peroneal) nerve; external to neck of fibula. Note the exposed and vulnerable position of the common fibular nerve.*
3 Superficial fibular (peroneal) nerve; supplies fibularis (peroneus) longus and brevis; these two muscles evert (turn the sole outward) the foot.
4 Deep fibular (peroneal) nerve; innervates the muscles of the anterior compartment: the extensor digitorum longus, the extensor hallucis longus, and the tibialis anterior; these muscles dorsiflex the foot (raise the foot up).
5 Tibialis anterior muscle
6 Tendon of tibialis anterior
7 Extensor digitorum longus muscle
8 Tendon of extensor digitorum
9 Extensor hallucis longus muscle
10 Tendon of extensor hallucis longus
11 Extensor hallucis brevis muscle
12 Extensor digitorum brevis muscle
13 Fibularis (peroneus) longus muscle
14 Tendon of fibularis longus
15 Fibularis (peroneus) brevis muscle
16 Head of fibula
17 Lateral malleolus
18 Patella (knee cap)
19 Tibia
20 Tibial tuberosity

*Damage to this nerve will result in **foot-drop,** in which the foot cannot be dorsiflexed (anterior compartment muscles paralyzed) or everted (lateral compartment muscles paralyzed).

LL-56 Foot: anterior-superior aspect

Left foot

Color and label

1 Tibia
2 Fibula
3 Interosseous membrane
4 Inferior extensor retinaculum
5 Medial malleolus
6 Lateral malleolus (and arterial rete from lateral malleolar artery)
7 Tibialis anterior muscle and tendon
8 Tendon of extensor hallucis longus
9 Extensor digitorum longus muscle
10 Tendon of extensor digitorum longus
11 Extensor hallucis brevis muscle
12 Extensor digitorum brevis muscle (number 3 of 4 brevis muscles)
13 Deep fibular (peroneal) nerve
14 Anterior tibial artery
15 Abductor hallucis muscle
16 Fibularis (peroneus) brevis muscle
17 Fibularis (peroneus) longus muscle and tendon
18 Tibial nerve (divided) and posterior tibial artery and vein (also divided)
19 Superficial fibular (peroneal) nerve (divided into two)
20 Medial dorsal cutaneous branch of superficial fibular nerve
21 Intermediate dorsal cutaneous branch of superficial fibular nerve
22 Lateral dorsal cutaneous nerve (continuation of sural nerve)
23 Dorsal pedal digital nerves
24 Deep fibular (peroneal) nerve innervating skin between toes 1 and 2
25. Dorsal pedis artery (continuation of anterior tibial artery)
26 Dorsal digital nerves
27 First dorsal metatarsal artery
28 Lateral tarsal artery
29 Tendo calcaneus (Achilles tendon)
30 Soleus muscle
31 Tibialis posterior muscle
32 Flexor digitorum longus muscle
33 Flexor hallucis longus muscle

Because a good part of the world uses fibular, whereas in the United States peroneal is used, both terms peroneal and fibular are used here.

Based on and slightly modified from a Somso muscle

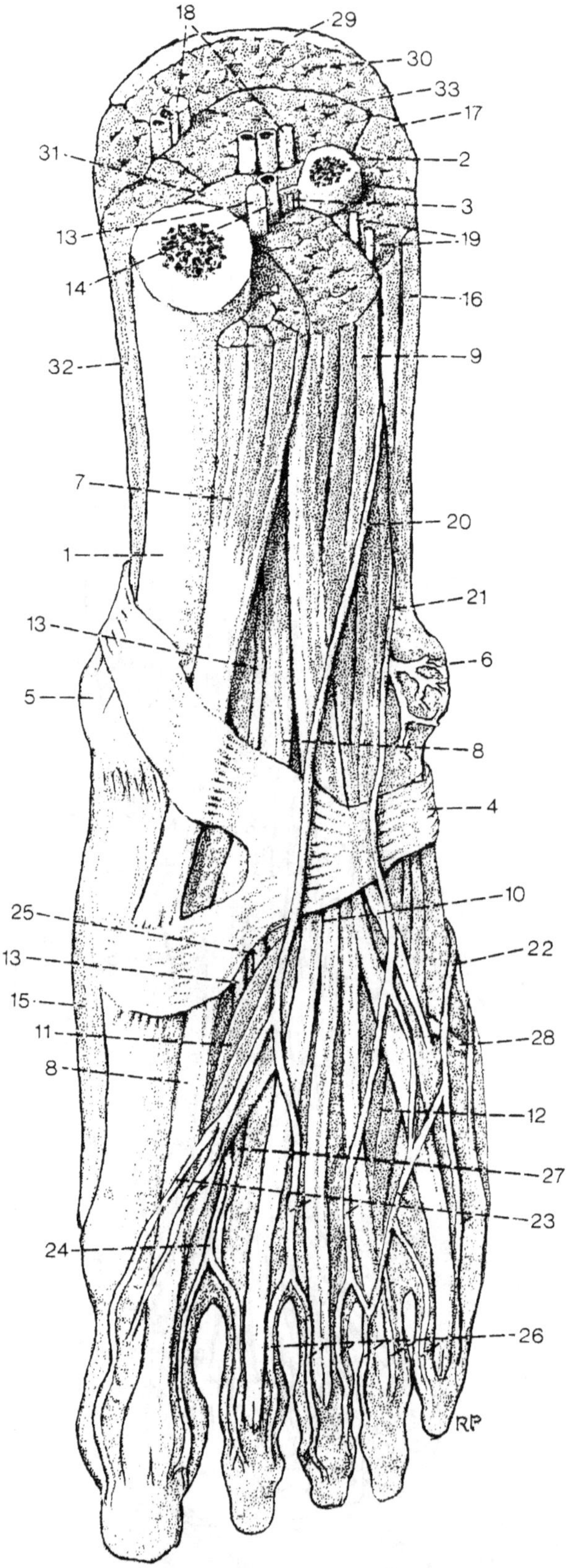

LL-57 Dorsum of the foot

Deep dissection

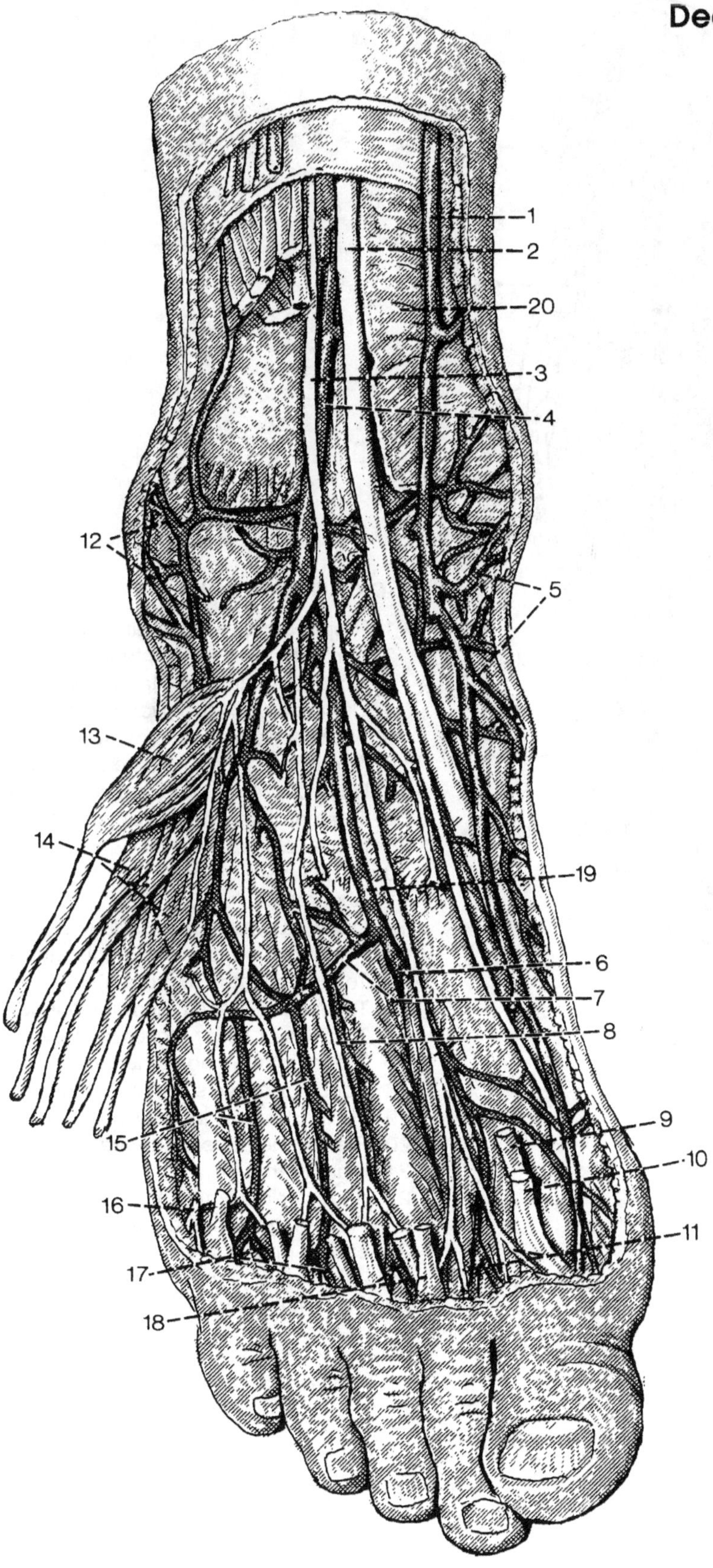

Color and label

1 Great saphenous vein
2 Tendon of tibialis anterior muscle
3 Deep fibular (peroneal) nerve (note its terminal branches supply skin between first and second toes)
4 Anterior tibial artery
5 Medial malleolar arterial and venous network (rete)
6 Deep plantar artery
7 Arcuate artery
8 Dorsal digital nerves
9 Tendon of extensor hallucis longus (cut)
10 Tendon of extensor hallucis brevis (cut)
11 Proper dorsal digital nerves
12 Lateral malleolar vascular plexus
13 Extensor hallucis brevis muscle (cut and pulled laterally)
14 Extensor digitorum brevis muscles (to toes 2-5) (cut and pulled aside)
15 Dorsal metatarsal arteries
16 Proper dorsal digital nerves
17 Dorsal digital arteries
18 Tendons of extensor digitorum brevis (more superficial) and extensor digitorum longus (deeper) to the second toe
19 Dorsalis pedis artery (continuation of anterior tibial artery)
20 Superior extensor retinaculum (one half removed)

Redrawn from Tondury

LL-58 Deep dissection of plantar foot

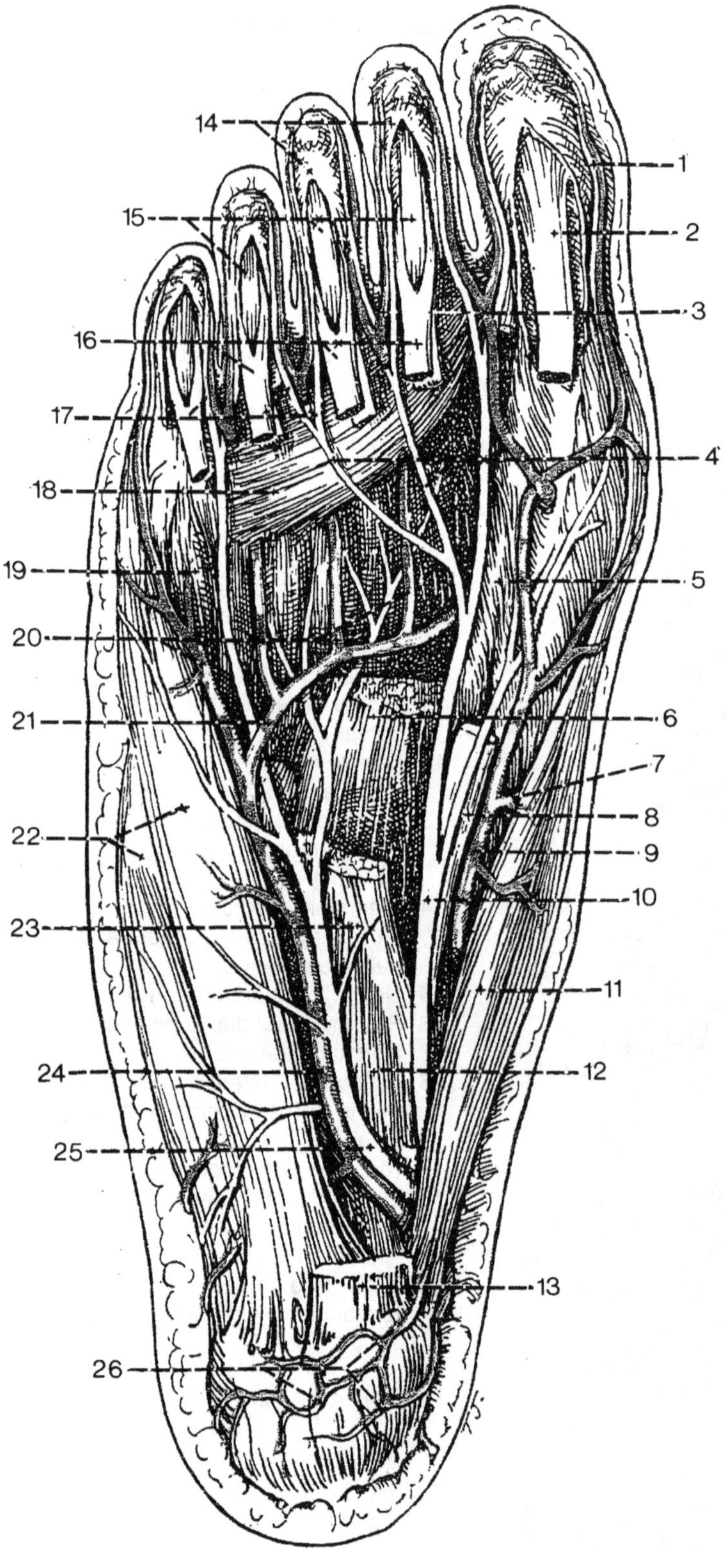

Color and label

1 Proper digital arteries and nerves
2 Flexor hallucis longus tendon
3 Common plantar digital artery
4 Common plantar digital nerves
5 Flexor hallucis brevis muscle
6 Adductor hallucis oblique head (cut)
7 Deep branch of medial plantar artery
8 Tendon of flexor hallucis longus (cut)
9 Medial plantar artery
10 Medial plantar nerve
11 Abductor hallucis muscle
12 Quadratus plantae muscle (cut)
13 Flexor digitorum brevis pedis muscle
14 Tendon sheaths (cut open)
15 Tendons of flexor digitorum longus
16 Tendons of flexor digitorum brevis
17 Proper plantar digital nerves
18 Adductor hallucis transverse head
19 Flexor digiti minimi muscle
20 Plantar metatarsal arteries
21 Plantar arch
22 Abductor digiti minimi muscle
23 Flexor digitorum longus muscle
24 Lateral plantar artery
25 Lateral plantar nerve
26 Calcaneal network

Eycleshymer and Jones

LL-59 Plantar muscles I

And related structures of the left foot

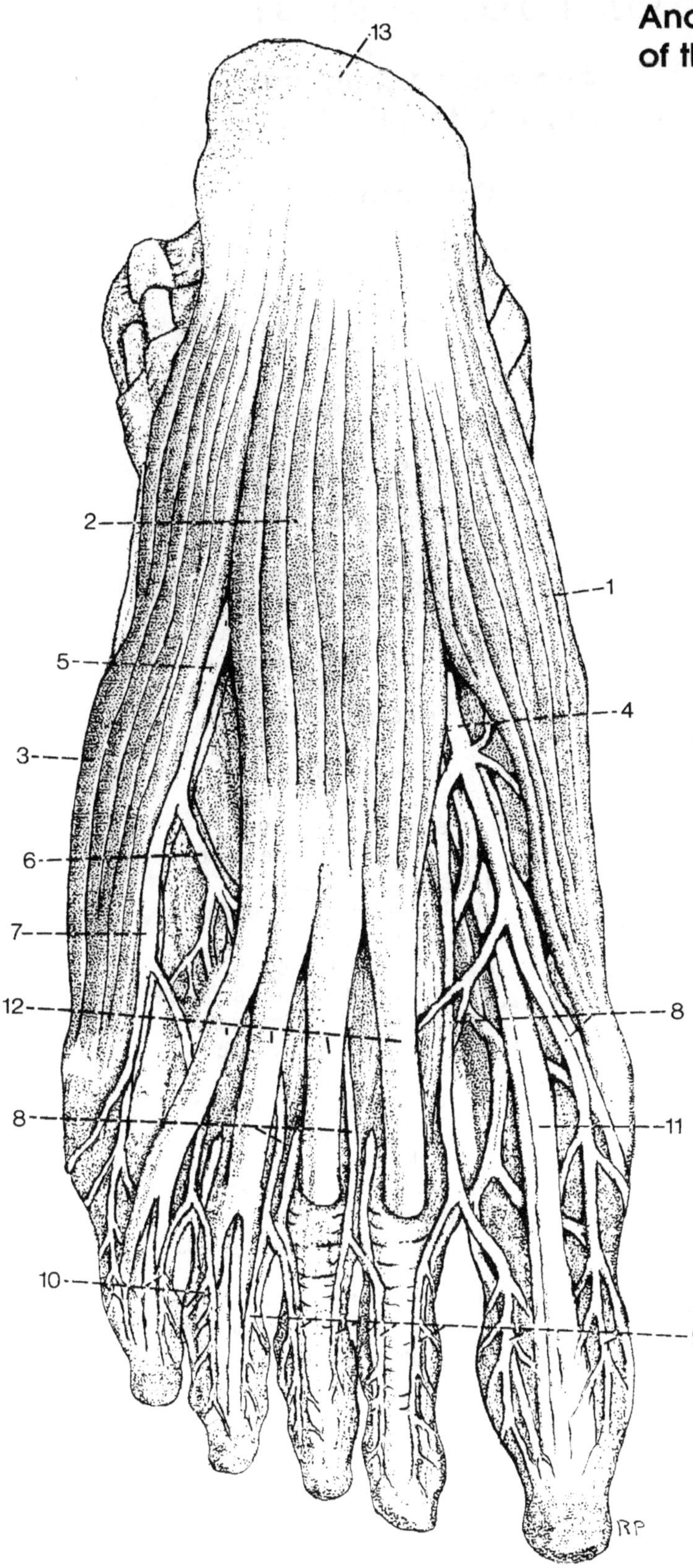

Color and label

1 Abductor hallucis*
2 Flexor digitorum brevis*
3 Abductor digiti minimi*
4 Medial plantar nerve; the tibial nerve ends by dividing into the medial plantar nerve and the lateral plantar nerve; the medial, the larger of the two plantar nerves, corresponds to the median nerve in the hand; it is accompanied by the medial plantar artery and vein (not shown).
5 Lateral plantar nerve; it corresponds to the ulnar nerve in the hand; it supplies the remaining 12 plantar muscles; it is accompanied by the lateral plantar artery and vein (not shown).
6 Deep branch of lateral plantar nerve
7 Superficial branch of lateral plantar nerve
8 Common plantar digital nerves
9 Proper plantar digital nerve (branches of medial plantar nerve)
10 Proper digital nerves (branches of lateral plantar nerve)
11 Tendon of flexor hallucis longus
12 Tendons of flexor digitorum brevis
13 Calcaneus

* Supplied by medial plantar nerve

Based on a Somso model

Both the abductor hallucis and abductor digiti minimi rather than abduct, as their names imply, more importantly support and maintain the arches of the foot.

LL-60 Plantar muscles II

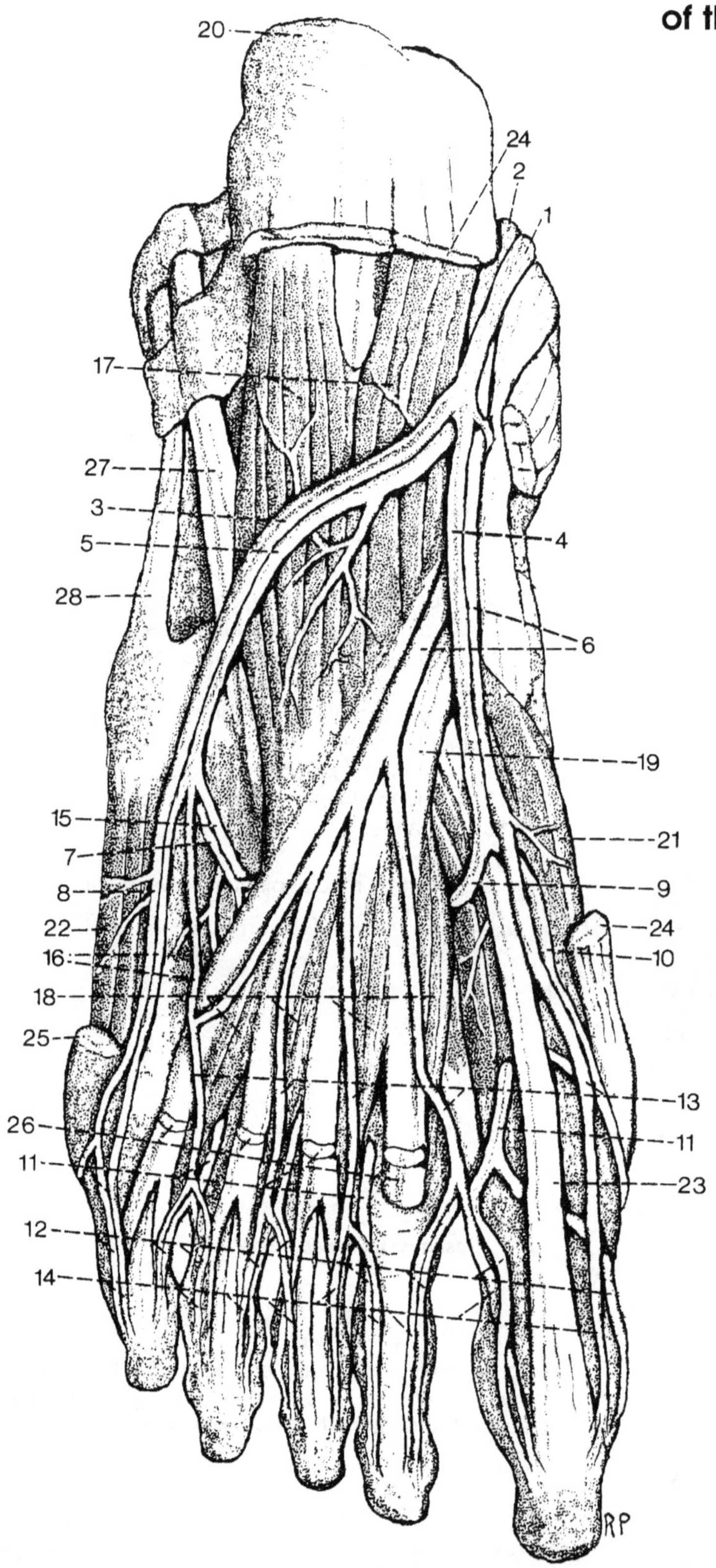

And related structures of the left foot

Color and label

1 Posterior tibial artery
2 Tibial nerve
3 Lateral plantar artery
4 Medial plantar artery
5 Lateral plantar nerve
6 Medial plantar nerve (divided into two branches)
7 Deep plantar arch
8 Superficial branch of lateral plantar artery
9 Deep branch of medial plantar artery
10 Superficial branch of medial plantar artery
11 Plantar metatarsal arteries
12 Proper plantar digital arteries
13 Common plantar digital nerves
14 Proper plantar digital nerves
15 Deep branch of lateral plantar nerve
16 Superficial branches of lateral plantar nerve
17 Quadratus plantae muscle*
18 Lumbrical muscles*
19 Tendon of flexor digitorum longus muscle*
20 Calcaneal tuberosity
21 Flexor hallucis brevis muscle
22 Flexor digiti minimi muscle
23 Tendon of flexor hallucis longus muscle
24 Abductor hallucis muscle (cut; origin and insertion only)
25 Abductor digiti minimi (cut)
26 Tendons (2-5) of flexor digitorum brevis (cut)
27 Tendon of peroneus (fibularis) longus muscle
28 Tendon of peroneus (fibularis) brevis inserting on tuberosity of fifth metatarsal

* Second layer of plantar muscles

Based on and modified from a Somso model

LL-61 Plantar muscles III

And related structures of the left foot

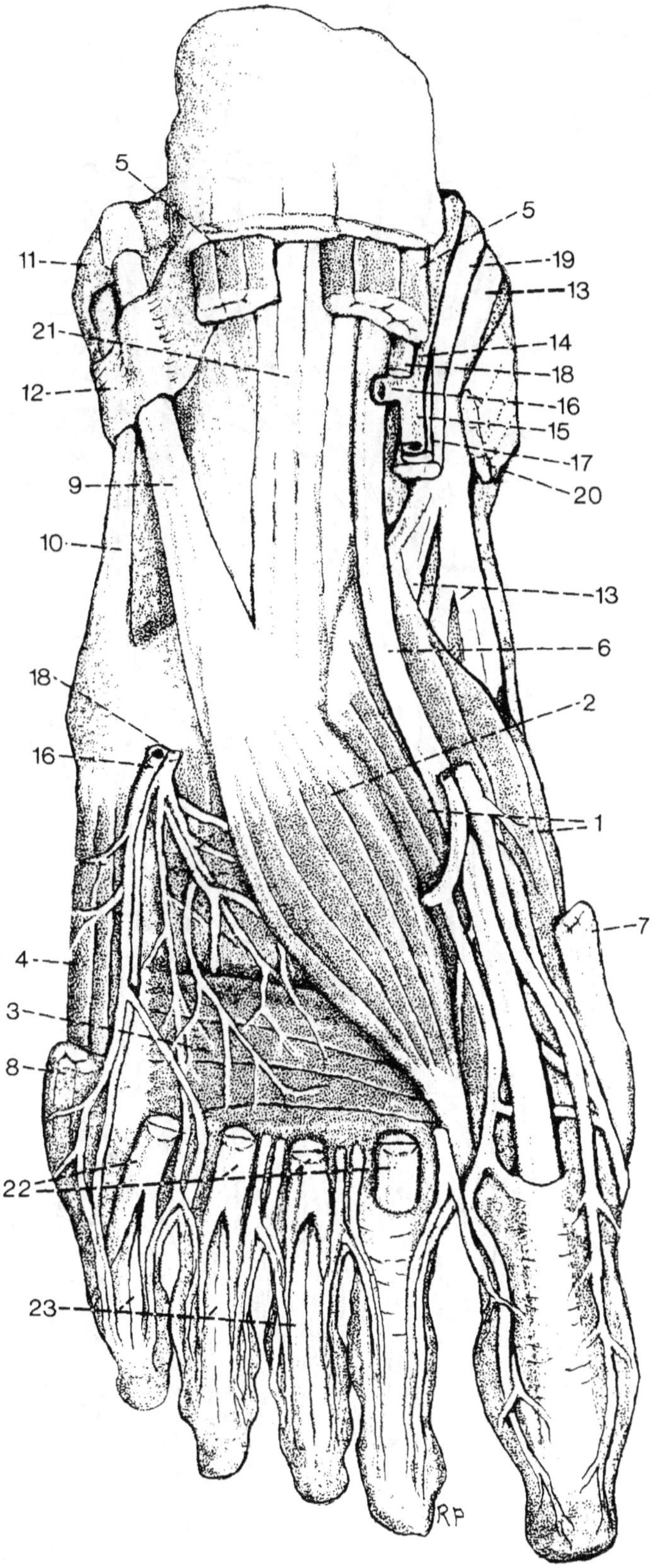

Color and label

1 Flexor hallucis brevis* muscle
2 Adductor hallucis* oblique head
3 Adductor hallucis* transverse head
4 Flexor digiti minimi*
5 Quadratus plantae (cut)
6 Tendon of flexor hallucis longus
7 Abductor hallucis (cut)
8 Abductor digiti minimi (cut)
9 Tendon of peroneus (fibularis) longus
10 Tendon of peroneus (fibularis) brevis
11 Superior fibular retinaculum
12 Inferior fibular retinaculum
13 Tendon of tibialis posterior
14 Posterior tibial artery
15 Medial plantar artery (cut)
16 Lateral plantar artery (cut)
17 Medial plantar nerve (cut)
18 Lateral plantar nerve (cut)
19 Tendon of flexor digitorum longus (cut)
20 Flexor retinaculum (cut)
21 Long plantar ligament
22 Four tendons of flexor digitorum brevis overlying (superficial to) four tendons of flexor digitorum longus (all 8 tendons cut)
23 Tendons 3,4,5 of flexor digitorum longus passing through opened fibrous tendon sheaths to insert on terminal phalanges

* Third layer of plantar muscles

Based on a Somso model

LL-62 Plantar muscles IV

And related structures of the left foot

Color and label

1 Tibial nerve
2 Posterior tibial artery
3 Medial plantar nerve
4 Lateral plantar nerve
5 Medial plantar artery
6 Lateral plantar artery
7 Superficial branch of medial plantar artery
8 Deep branch of medial plantar artery
9 Deep branch of lateral plantar nerve
10 Superficial branch of lateral plantar nerve
11 Deep branch of lateral plantar artery (deep plantar arch)
12 Superficial branch of lateral plantar artery
13 Plantar metatarsal arteries
14 Common plantar digital arteries
15 Proper plantar digital arteries
16 Common plantar digital nerves
17 Proper plantar digital nerves (note these are branches of the medial plantar nerve)
18 Plantar interosseous muscles; (*planta*, Latin, sole); fourth layer of plantar muscles; plantar flexion of the foot is flexion of the ankle that points the foot and toes downwards
19 Dorsal interosseous muscles fourth layer of plantar muscles; (the dorsum of the foot is the superior surface); dorsiflexion of the foot is the flexion of the foot upwards as in walking on the heels.
20 Tendon of tibialis posterior muscle
21 Tendon of fibularis (peroneus) longus muscle

Based on a Somso model

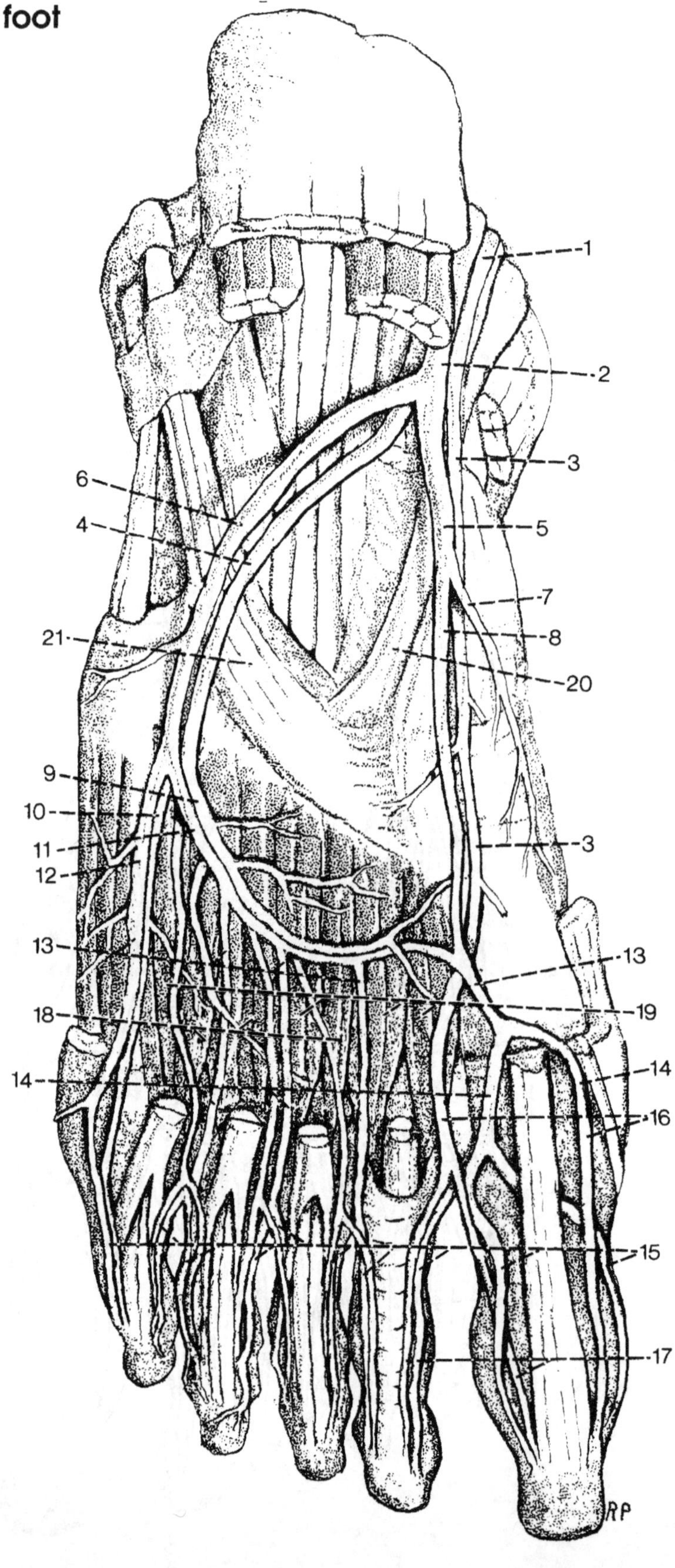

LL-63 Motor distribution of the tibial nerve

Right leg viewed from behind

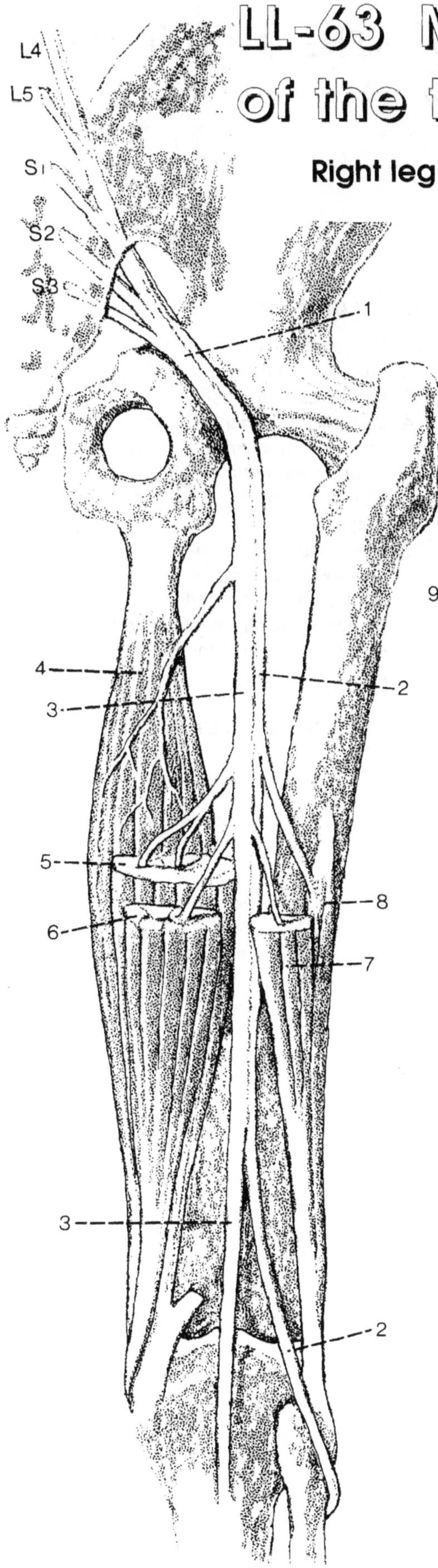

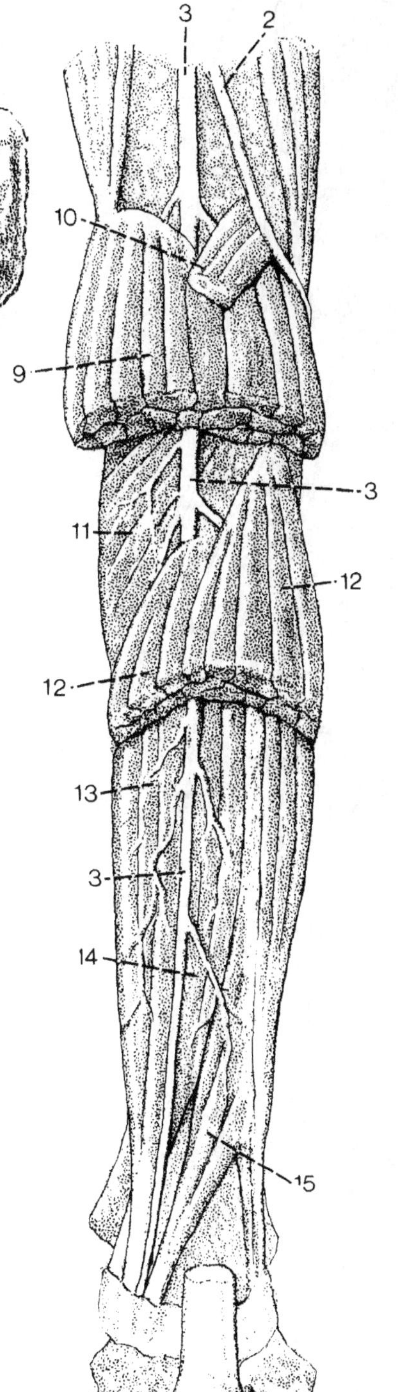

Color and label

1 Sciatic nerve
2 Common fibular (peroneal) nerve
3 Tibial nerve
4 Adductor magnus (vertical part)
5 Semimembranosus
6 Semitendinosus
7 Biceps femoris (long head)
8 Biceps femoris (short head; supplied by common fibular nerve)
9 Gastrocnemius
10 Plantaris
11 Popliteus
12 Soleus
13 Flexor digitorum longus
14 Tibialis posterior
15 Flexor hallucis longus
16 Medial plantar nerve
17 Lateral plantar nerve
18 Abductor hallucis
19 Flexor hallucis brevis
20 Flexor digitorum brevis
21 Medial lumbrical
22 Quadratus plantae
23 Abductor digiti minimi
24 Flexor digiti minimi
25 Lumbricals (three laterals)
26 Plantar interosseous
27 Dorsal interosseous
28 Adductor hallucis

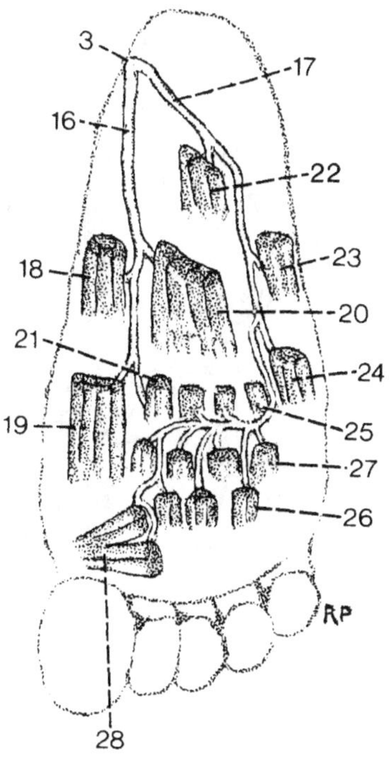

LL-64 Plantar arteries of the right foot

Viewed from below

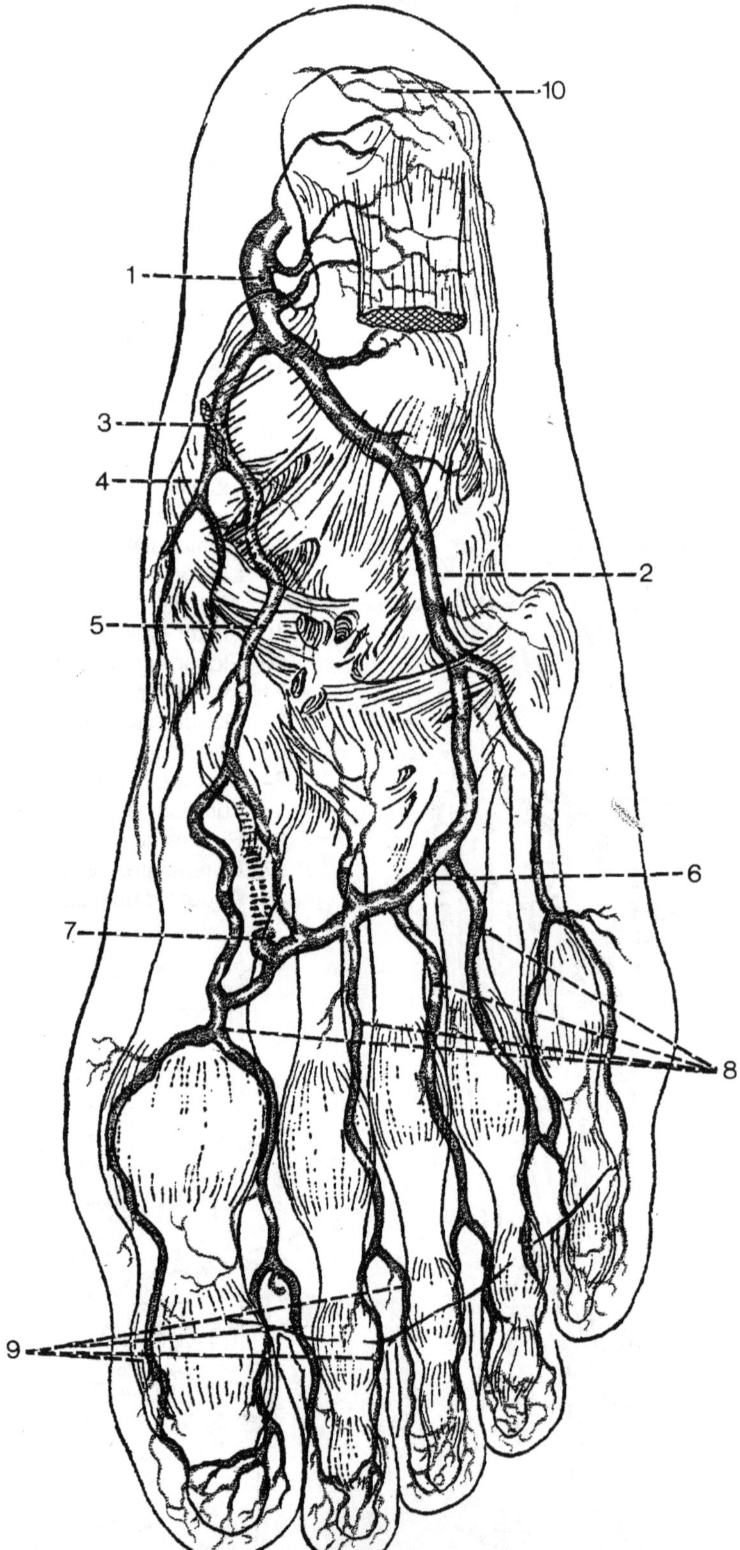

Color and label

1 Posterior tibial artery
2 Lateral plantar artery
3 Medial plantar artery
4 Superficial branch of medial plantar artery
5 Deep branch of medial plantar artery
6 Plantar arch
7 Deep plantar branch of dorsalis pedis artery
8 Plantar metatarsal arteries (common plantar digital arteries)
9 Proper plantar digital arteries
10 Rete* calcaneus

**Rete*, a network or meshwork of arteries or veins

Eycleshymer and Jones

LL-65 Ligaments of the hip joint

Anterior view

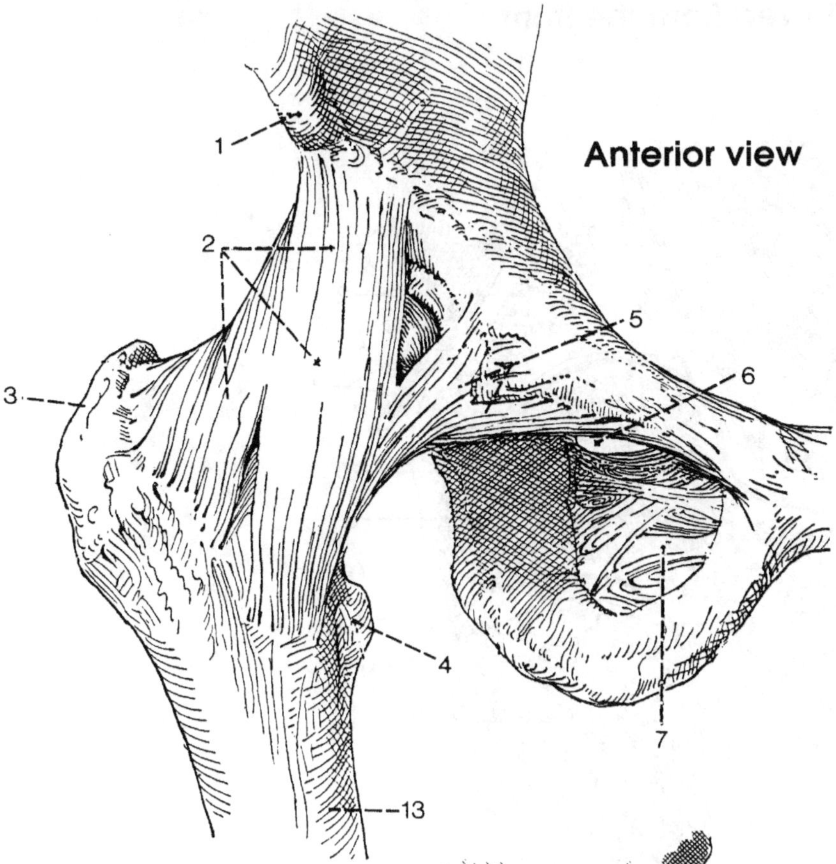

Color and label

1 Anterior inferior iliac spine
2 Iliofemoral ligament
3 Greater trochanter
4 Lesser trochanter
5 Pubofemoral ligament
6 Obturator canal (opening in obturator membrane for obturator nerve artery and vein)
7 Obturator membrane
8 Ischiofemoral ligament (transverse band)
9 Ischiofemoral ligament (spiral band)
10 Neck of femur
11 Ischial tuberosity
12 Obturator foramen
13 Femur

Eycleshymer and Jones

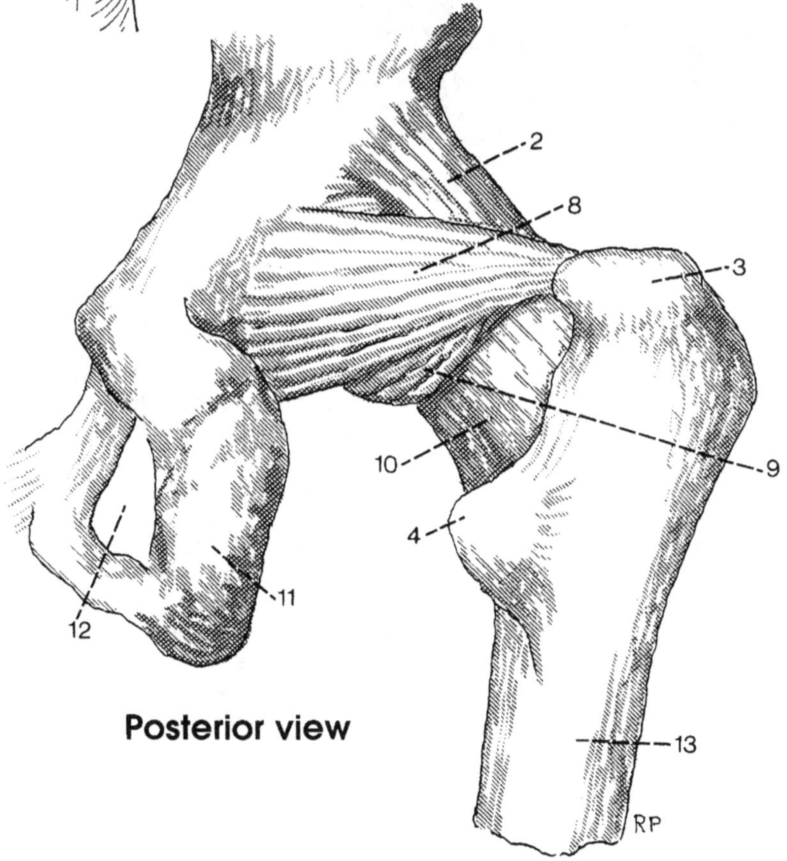

Posterior view

LL-66 Frontal section of right hip joint

Viewed from the front

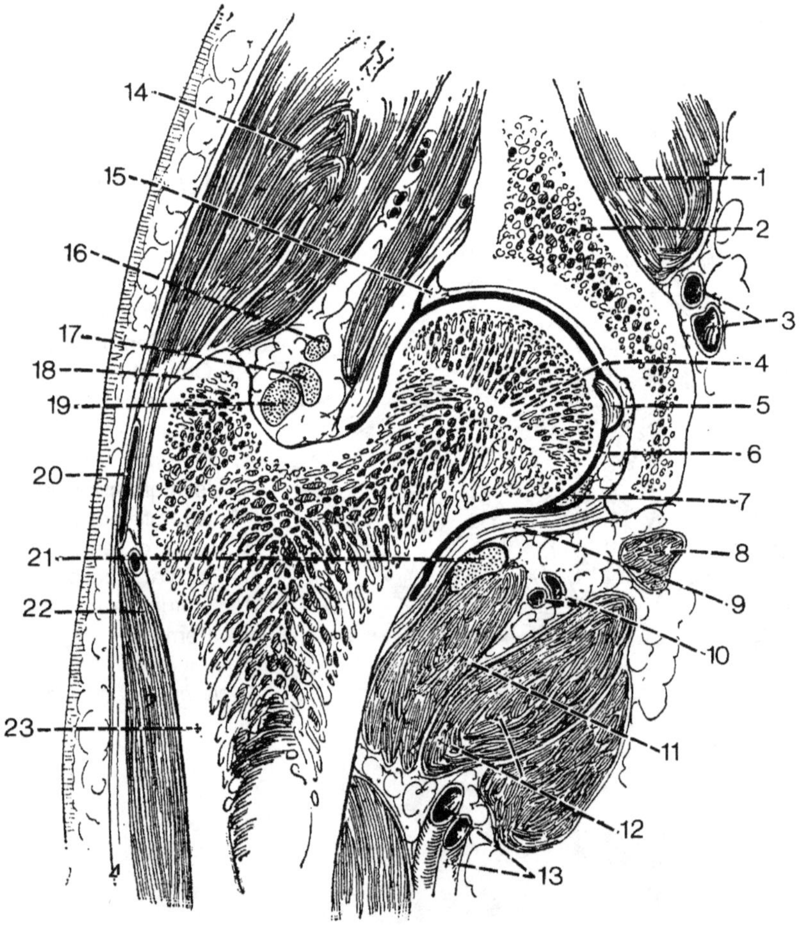

Color and label

1 Iliacus muscle
2 Pelvic bone (ilium)
3 External iliac artery and vein
4 Epiphyseal line in head of femur (remains of growth plate)
5 Ligament of head of femur; attached to fovea (pit) on the head of femur
6 Joint (articular) cavity
7 Transverse acetabular ligament; the acetabular labrum (15) bridges the acetabular notch as the transverse acetabular ligament, thereby forming a complete circle, which closely surrounds the head of the femur and helps hold it in place. (Clemente, 1985)
8 Obturator externus muscle
9 Joint (articular) capsule
10 Medial circumflex femoral artery and vein
11 Iliacus muscle
12 Pectineus muscle
13 Femoral artery and vein
14 Gluteus maximus muscle
15 Acetabular labrum (lip); a fibrocartilaginous rim attached to the margin of the acetabulum, thereby deepening its cavity; it protects bony rim of the cup and smooths its surface. (Clemente, 1985)
16 Tendon of pyramidalis muscle
17 Obturator internus muscle
18 Greater trochanter
19 Obturator externus muscle
20 Bursa between greater trochanter and gluteus maximus
21 Tendon of psoas major
22 Vastus lateralis muscle
23 Femur

Eycleshymer and Jones

LL-67 Right knee joint

Viewed from in front

Knee is flexed in order to show cruciate ligaments

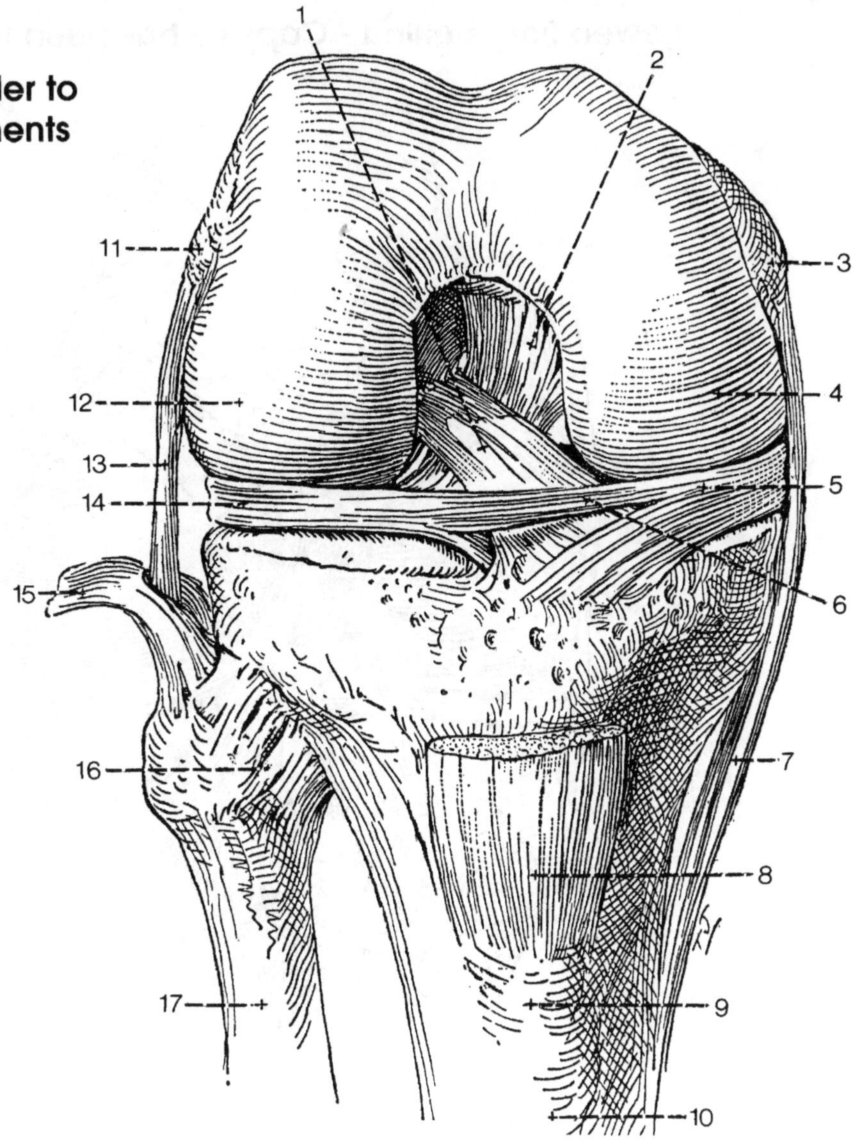

Eycleshymer and Jones

Color and label

1 Anterior ligament
2 Posterior ligament
3 Medial epicondyle of femur
4 Medial condyle of femur
5 Medial meniscus of knee joint; an oval crescent of fibrocartilage situated on the circumferential part of the medial superior articular surface of the tibia
6 Transverse ligament of knee; a fibrous cord of variable thickness connecting the anterior convex margin of the lateral meniscus to the anterior convex margin of the medial meniscus
7 Tibial collateral ligament
8 Patellar ligament; a continuation of the common tendon of the quadriceps femoris (cut); extends from the apex and inferior margins of the patella to insert on the tibial tuberosity
9 Tibial tuberosity
10 Tibia
11 Lateral epicondyle of femur
12 Lateral condyle of femur
13 Fibular collateral ligament
14 Lateral meniscus of knee joint; an oval crescent of fibrocartilage situated on the lateral superior articular surface of the tibia
15 Tendon of biceps femoris; inserting (mainly) on the head of the fibula
16 Anterior ligament of head of fibula
17 Fibula

LL-68 Ligaments of the right knee

Viewed from behind - Capsule has been removed

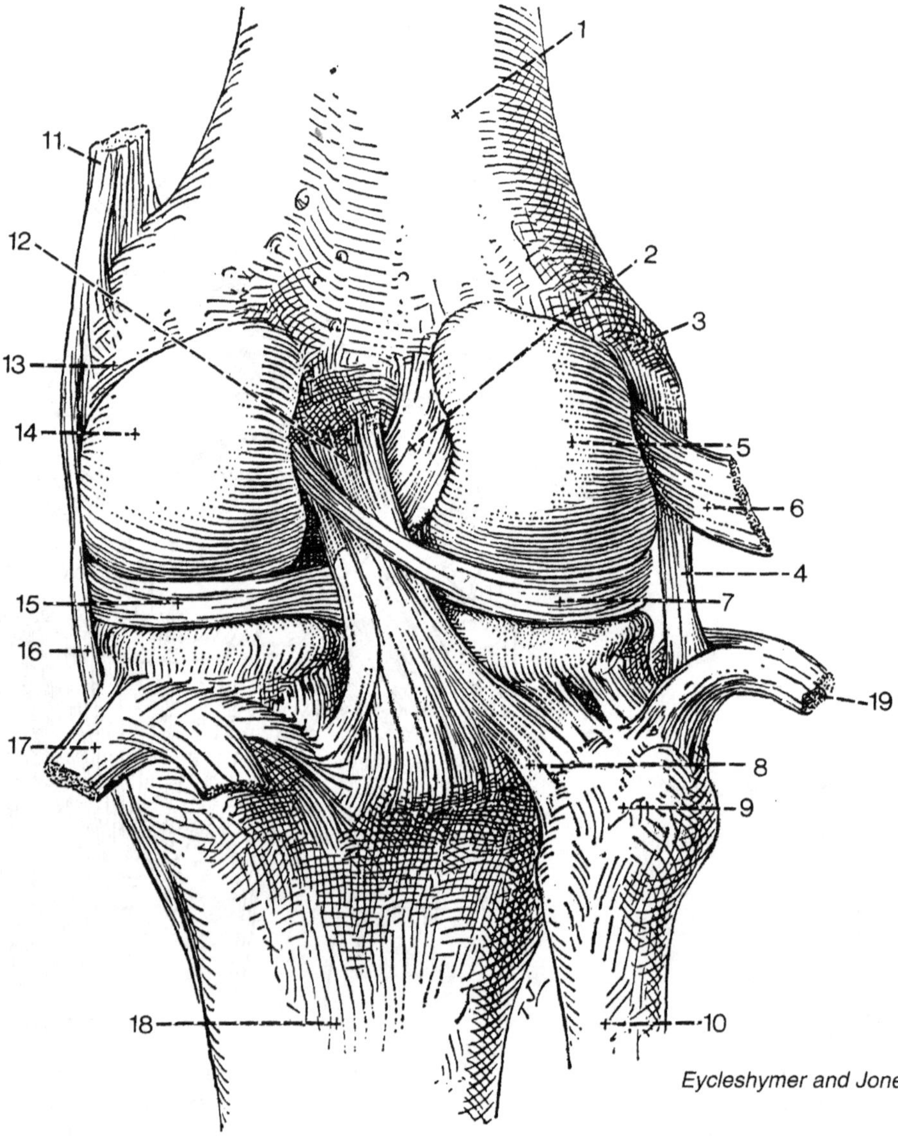

Color and label

1 Femur
2 Anterior cruciate ligament
3 Lateral epicondyle of femur
4 Fibular collateral ligament
5 Lateral condyle of femur
6 Popliteus muscle (cut)
7 Lateral meniscus
8 Posterior ligament of fibular head
9 Head of fibula
10 Fibula
11 Adductor magnus muscle (cut; vertical part)
12 Posterior cruciate ligament
13 Medial epicondyle of femur
14 Medial condyle of femur
15 Medial meniscus
16 Tibial collateral ligament
17 Semimembranosus muscle (cut)
18 Tibia
19 Biceps femoris muscle (cut)

LL-69 Right knee joint

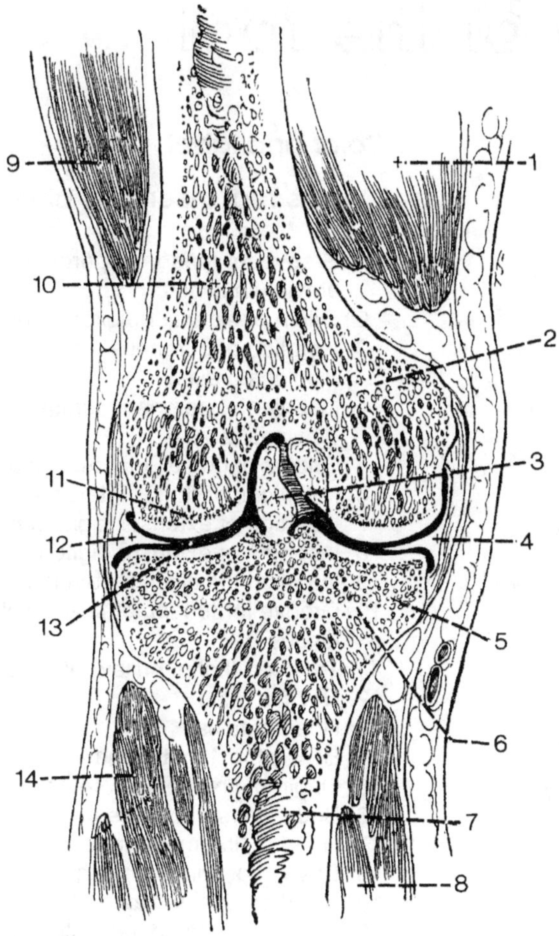

Figure A
Sectioned frontally
Viewed from the front

Color and label

1 Vastus medialis muscle
2 Epiphyseal line of femur (remains of growth plate)
3 Anterior cruciate ligament
4 Medial meniscus
5 Medial condyle of tibia
6 Epiphyseal line of tibia (remains of growth plate)
7 Tibia (shaft)
8 Gastrocnemius (medial head)
9 Vastus lateralis muscle
10 Femur (shaft)
11 Lateral femoral condyle
12 Lateral meniscus
13 Joint cavity
14 Gastrocnemius (lateral head)

Figure B
Superior articular surface of tibia
Viewed from above

Color and label

1 Anterior cruciate ligament
2 Lateral meniscus
3 Posterior cruciate ligament
4 Medial meniscus
5 Transverse ligament of knee
6 Tibial tuberosity

Eycleshymer and Jones

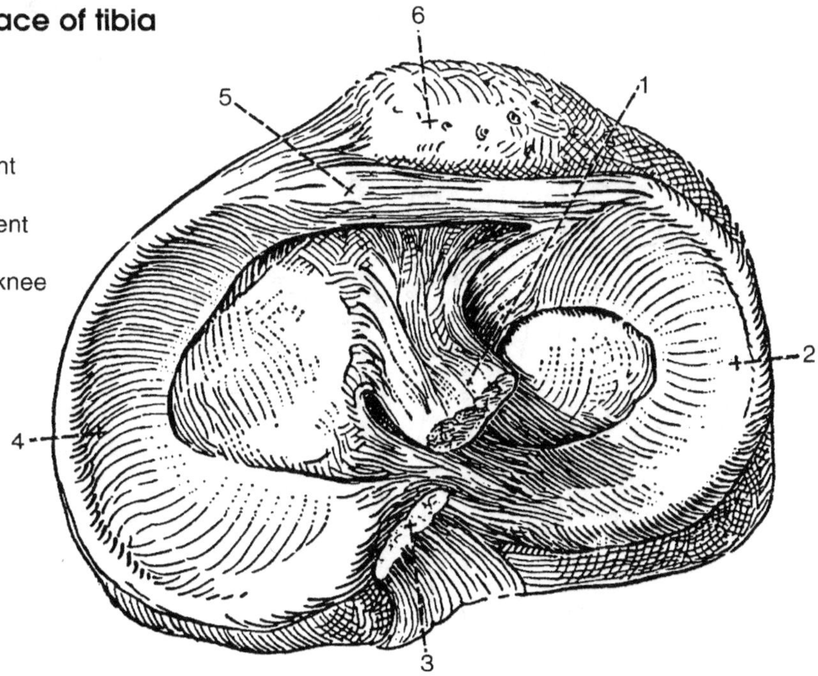

LL-70 Muscle attachments on the dorsum of the foot

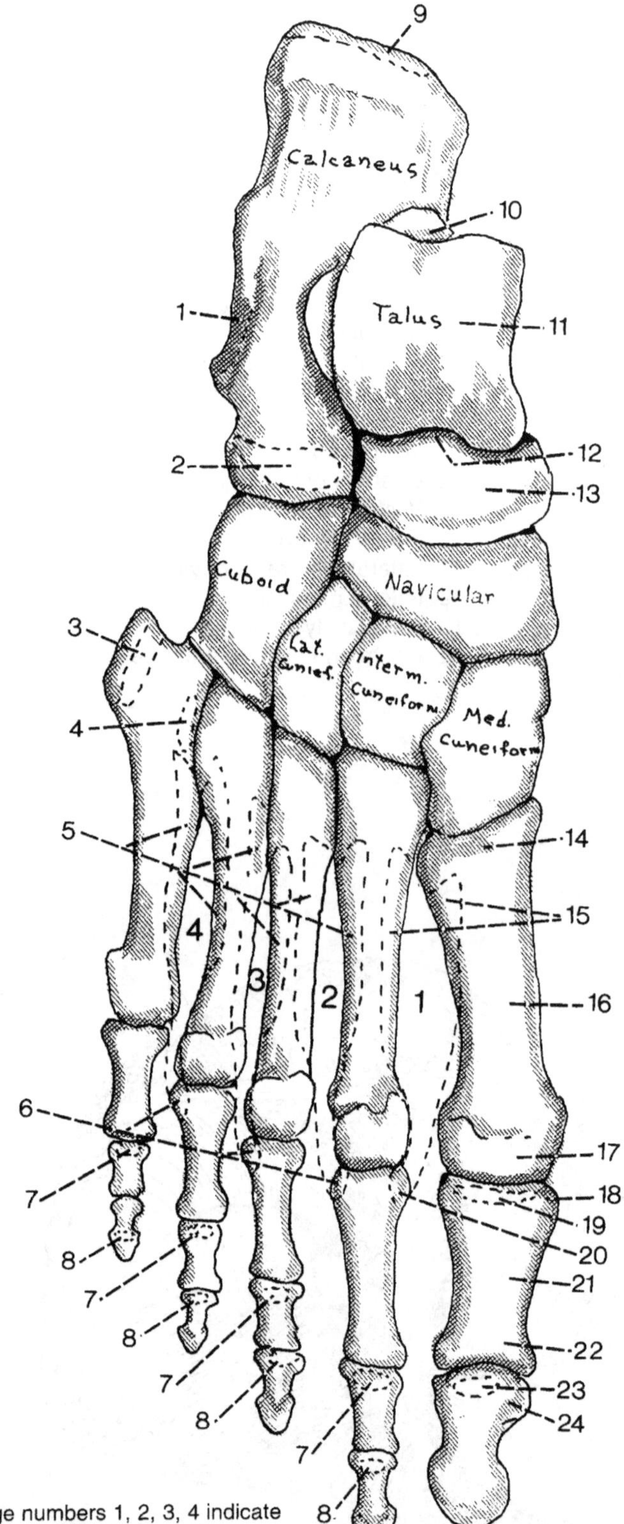

Large numbers 1, 2, 3, 4 indicate dorsal interosseous muscles (shown in inset)

Color and label

Origins red; insertions blue

1 Groove for tendon of peroneus brevis (fibularis brevis)
2 Origin of extensor digitorum brevis
3 Insertion of peroneus brevis (fibularis brevis)
4 Insertion of peroneus tertius (fibularis tertius)
5 Origins of dorsal interossei 2,3,4
6 Insertions of dorsal interossei 2,3,4
7 Insertion of extensor digitorum brevis
8 Insertion of extensor digitorum longus
9 Insertion of calcaneal tendon
10 Groove for tendon of flexor hallucis longus
11 Trochlea (Latin, pulley) of talus
12 Neck of talus
13 Head of talus
14 Base of first metatarsal
15 Origin of first dorsal interosseous
16 Body of first metatarsal
17 Head of first metatarsal
18 Base of proximal phalanx of big toe
19 Insertion of extensor hallucis brevis
20 Insertion of first dorsal interosseous
21 Body of proximal phalanx of big toe
22 Head of proximal phalanx of big toe
23 Insertion of extensor hallucis longus
24 Base of distal phalanx of big toe

After Clemente 1985

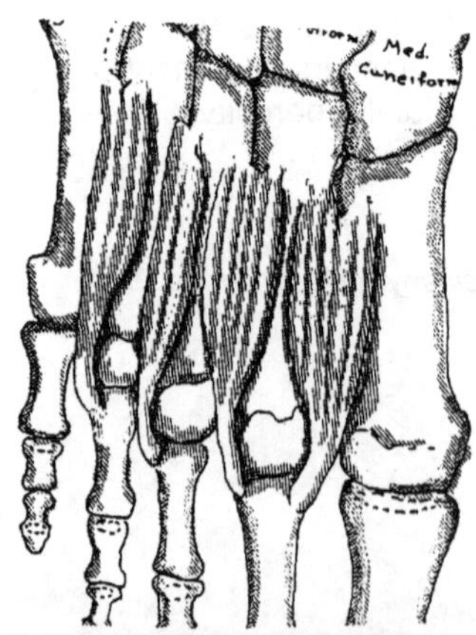

Dorsal interosseous muscles

LL-71 Muscle attachments on plantar surface of right foot

Color and label

Origins red; insertions blue

1 Origin of flexor digitorum brevis and abductor digiti minimi
2 Origin of quadratus plantae (lateral head)
3 Origin of quadratus plantae (medial head)
4 Insertion of tibialis posterior
5 Origin of flexor hallucis brevis
6 Groove for tendon of peroneus longus
7 Origin of flexor digiti minimi
8 Insertion of tibialis posterior
9 Insertion of tibialis posterior (three insertions)*
10 Origins of plantar interossei 1,2,3
11 Insertion of flexor digiti minimi and abductor digiti minimi
12 Insertion of plantar interossei 1,2,3
13 Insertions of flexor digitorum brevis 1,2,3,4
14 Insertions of flexor digitorum longus 1,2,3,4
15 Insertion of flexor hallucis longus
16 Insertion of adductor hallucis and flexor hallucis brevis
17 Insertion of flexor hallucis brevis and abductor hallucis
18 Sesamoid bones
19 Insertion of peroneus (fibularis) longus
20 Insertion of tibialis anterior
21 Origin of abductor hallucis longus
22 Groove on underside of sustentaculum tali for tendon of flexor hallucis longus

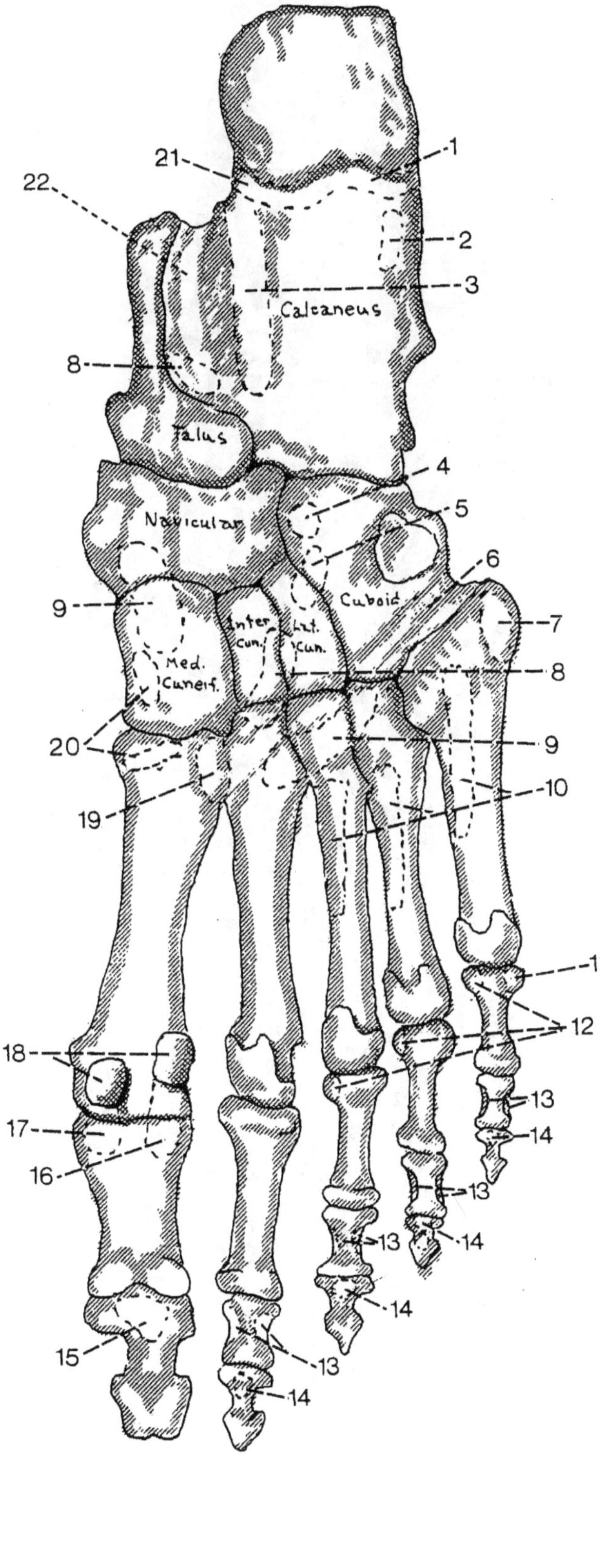

* Notice that the tendons of the tibialis posterior and the peroneus (fibularis) longus divide into several smaller tendons that have multiple insertions on the plantar surface of the foot.

LL-72 Muscles of plantar foot

Right foot inferior aspect

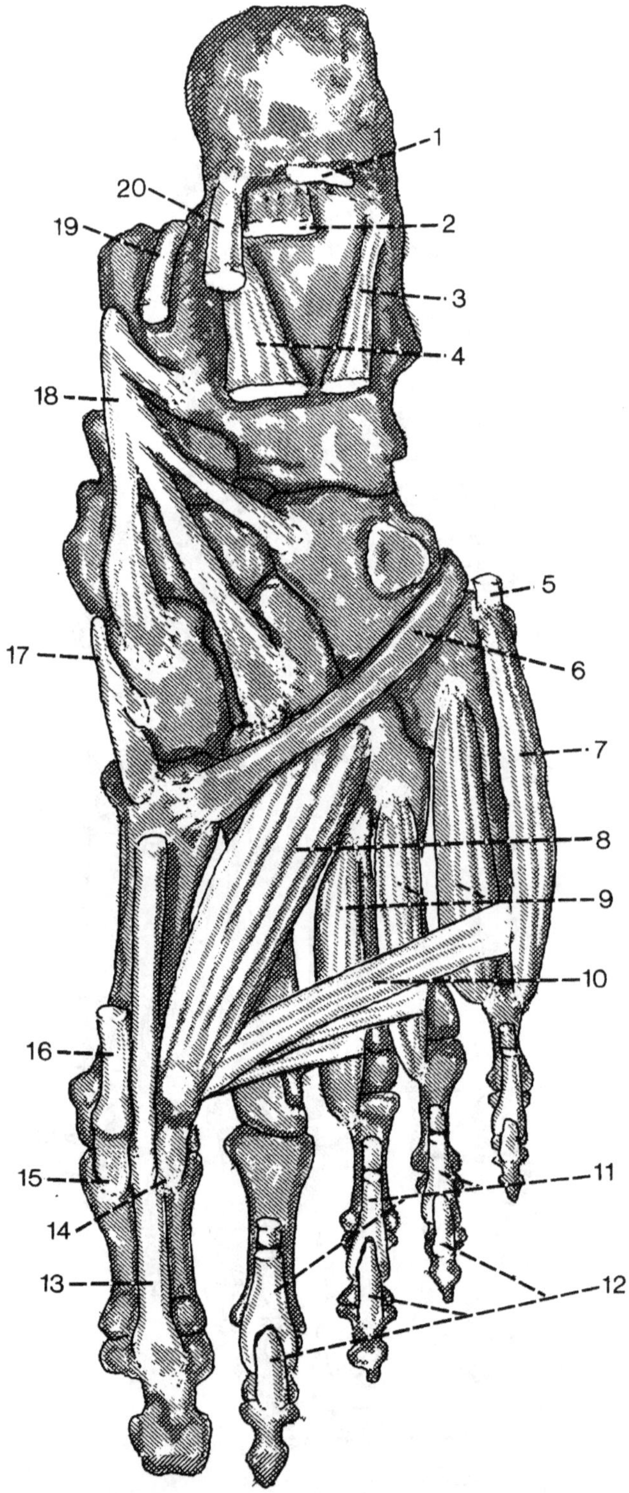

Color and label

1 Origin of flexor digitorum brevis
2 Abductor digiti minimi
3 Quadratus plantae (lateral head)
4 Quadratus plantae (medial head)
5 Insertion of abductor digiti minimi on tuberosity of 5th metatarsal
6 Tendon of peroneus (fibularis) longus
7 Flexor digiti minimi
8 Adductor hallucis (oblique head)
9 Plantar interossei (1st, 2nd, 3rd)
10 Adductor hallucis (transverse head)
11 Tendons (cut) of flexor digitorum brevis to toes 2,3,4
12 Tendons (cut) of flexor digitorum longus to toes 2,3,4
13 Tendon of flexor hallucis longus
14 Insertion of adductor hallucis
15 Insertion of flexor hallucis brevis
16 Tendon of flexor hallucis brevis and abductor hallucis
17 Tendon of tibialis anterior
18 Tendon of tibialis posterior (notice tendon divides into several insertions)
19 Tendon of flexor hallucis longus
20 Origin of abductor hallucis

LL-73 Planes of sections of right foot

Color and label

1 Calcaneus
2 Talus
3 Navicular bone
4 Medial cuneiform bone
5 Intermediate cuneiform bone
6 First metatarsal bone
7 Proximal phalanx of big toe (hallux)
8 Distal phalanx of big toe
9 Sesamoid bones (in tendons of flexor hallucis brevis)
10 Medial malleolus (tibia)
11 Medial malleolar surface of talar trochlea
12 Tuberosity of calcaneus
13 Sustentaculum tali (of calcaneus)
14 Medial process of calcaneal tuberosity

Bones of right foot medial aspect Sectioned through talus and calcaneus

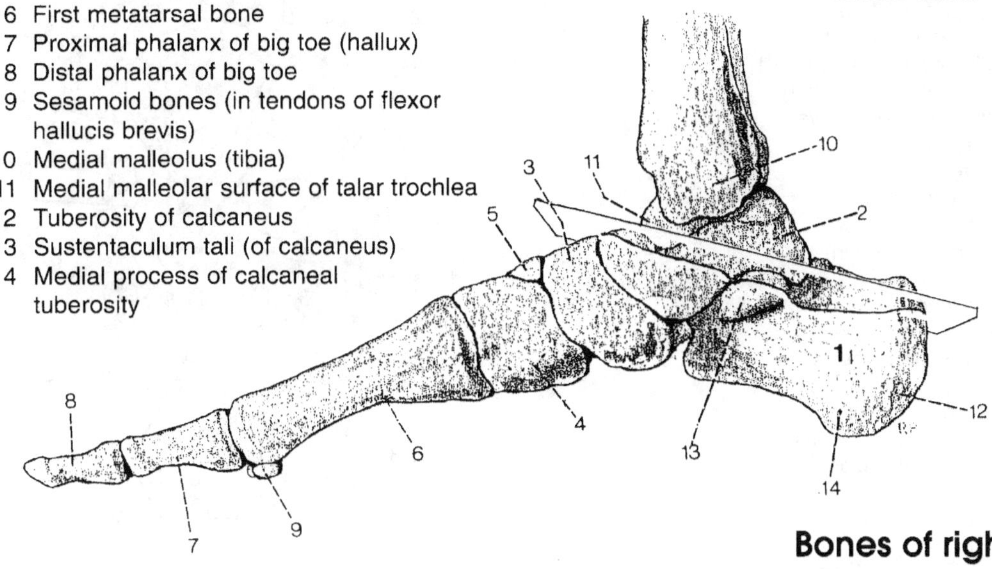

Bones of right foot superior aspect

Sectioned through bases of metatarsal bones

Color and label

1 Talus
2 Calcaneus
3 Navicular
4 Cuboid
5 Medial cuneiform
6 Intermediate cuneiform
7 Lateral cuneiform
8 Tuberosity on base of 5th metatarsal
9 Trochlea of talus

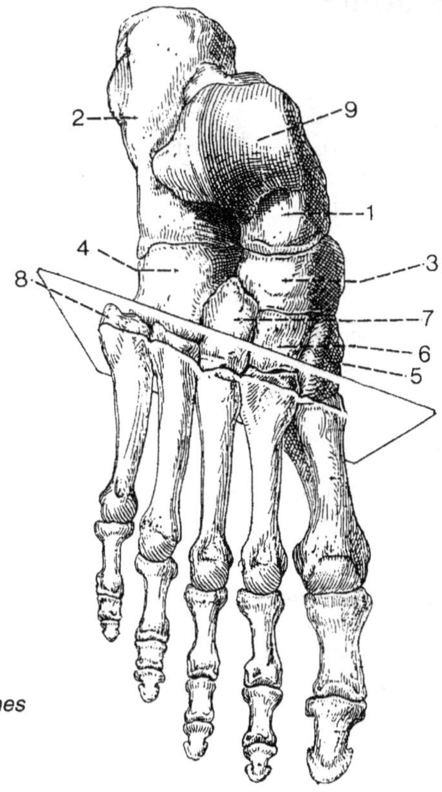

Eycleshymer and Jones

LL-74 Sections of right foot

Looking up from below

Color and label

1 Talus
2 Tendon of extensor hallucis longus
3 Tendon of tibialis anterior
4 Great saphenous vein
5 Talocalcaneal joint
6 Tendon of tibialis posterior ("Tom")
7 Sustentaculum tali (part of calcaneus)
8 Tendon of flexor digitorum longus ("Dick")
9 Tendon of flexor hallucis longus ("Harry")
10 Medial plantar artery, vein, and nerve
11 Lateral plantar artery, vein, and nerve
12 Quadratus plantae muscle (also called flexor accessorius)
13 Calcaneal tuberosity
14 Tendo calcaneus (Achilles tendon)
15 Calcaneus
16 Tendon of peroneus longus
17 Tendon of peroneus brevis
18 Talus, lateral tuberosity (or process)
19 Talocalcaneal joint
20 Extensor digitorum brevis muscle
21 Tendons of extensor digitorum longus
22 Dorsalis pedis artery (continuation of anterior tibial artery)
23 Interosseous talocalcaneal ligament in tarsal sinus

A

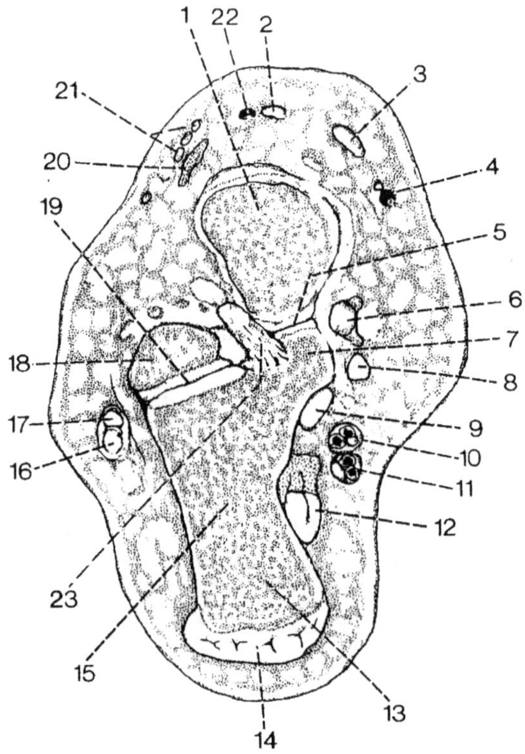

Viewed from the front

Color and label

1 Fifth metatarsal bone
2 Fourth metatarsal bone
3 Third metatarsal bone and interosseous ligament
4 Extensor digitorum brevis muscle
5 Lateral cuneiform (a small piece)
6 Tendon of extensor digitorum longus
7 Second metatarsal bone and interosseous ligament
8 Extensor hallucis brevis muscle
9 Medial cuneiform bone
10 Tendon of extensor hallucis longus
11 First metatarsal bone
12 Tendon of peroneus longus
13 Abductor hallucis muscle
14 Adductor hallucis muscle, oblique head
15 Flexor hallucis brevis muscle
16 Tendon of flexor hallucis longus (note its thickness; the big toe is very important in walking)
17 Medial plantar artery, vein, and nerve
18 Plantar aponeurosis
19 Flexor digitorum brevis muscle and tendons
20 Tendons of flexor digitorum longus muscle
21 Second plantar interosseous muscle and lateral plantar artery, vein, and nerve
22 Third plantar interosseous muscle
23 Flexor digiti minimi muscle
24 Opponens digiti minimi muscle
25 Abductor digiti minimi muscle

B

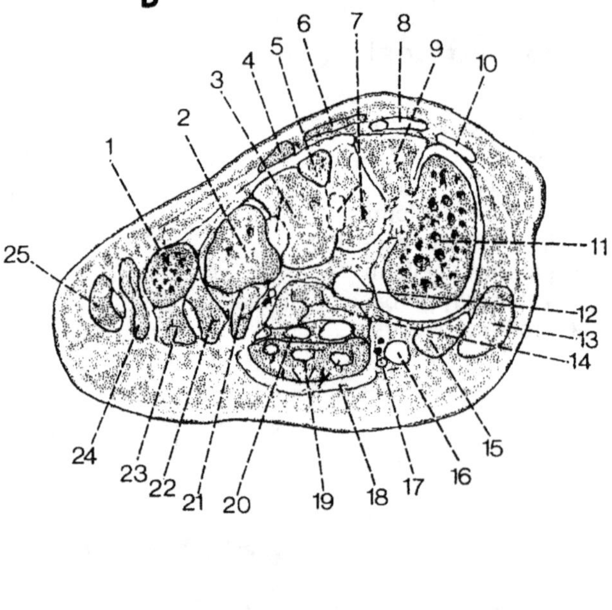

LL-75 Ligaments of right ankle joint and foot

Viewed from the medial side

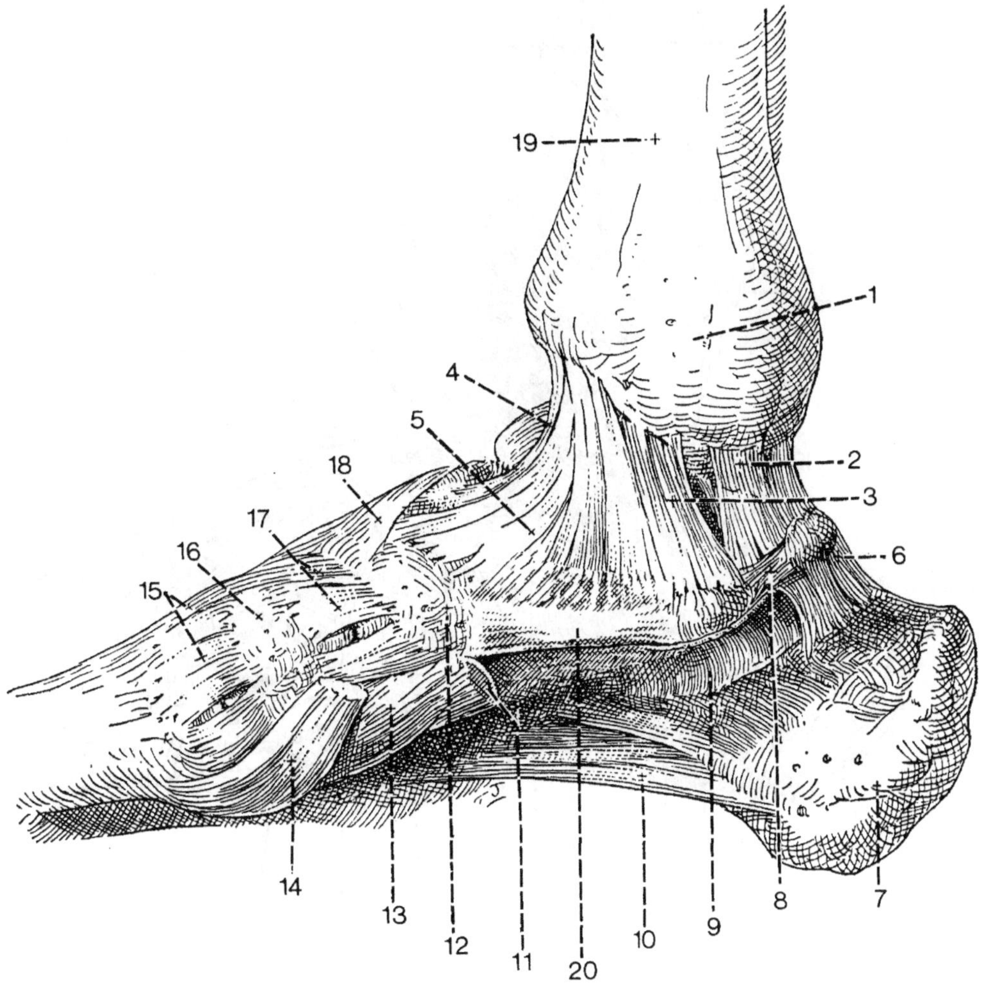

Color and label

1 Medial malleolus
2 Posterior tibiotalar ligament (part of deltoid ligament)
3 Tibiocalcaneal ligament (part of deltoid ligament)
4 Anterior tibiotalar ligament (part of deltoid ligament)
5 Tibionavicular ligament (part of deltoid ligament)
6 Posterior talocalcaneal ligament
7 Calcaneus
8 Medial talocalcaneal ligament
9 Groove for tendon of flexor hallucis longus muscle
10 Long plantar ligament
11 Tendon of tibialis posterior muscle
12 Navicular bone
13 Plantar navicular cuneiform ligament
14 Tendon of tibialis anterior
15 Dorsal tarsometatarsal ligaments
16 Cuneiform bone
17 Dorsal navicular cuneiform ligaments
18 Talonavicular ligament
19 Tibia
20 Plantar calcaneonavicular ligament

Eycleshymer and Jones with modification

LL-76 Ligaments of the ankle joint and foot

Right foot lateral view

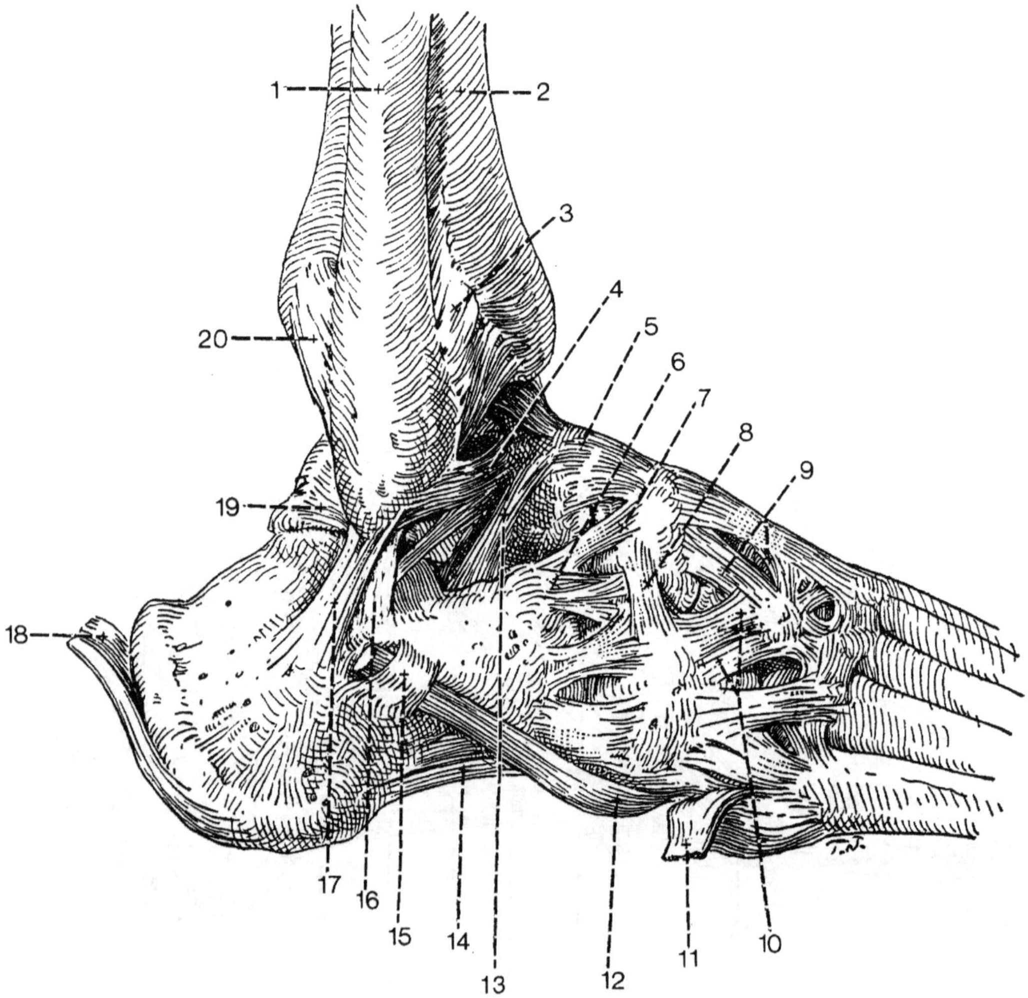

Color and label

1 Fibula
2 Tibia
3 Anterior tibiofibular ligament
4 Anterior talofibular ligament
5 Talonavicular ligament
6 Calcaneocuboid ligament (part of bifurcated ligament)
7 Calcaneonavicular ligament (part of bifurcated ligament)
8 Dorsal cuboideonavicular ligament
9 Dorsal cuneonavicular ligaments
10 Dorsal cuneocuboid ligaments
11 Tendon of fibularis (peroneus) brevis
12 Tendon of fibularis (peroneus) longus
13 Anterior talocalcaneal ligament
14 Long plantar ligament
15 Inferior fibular (peroneal) retinaculum
16 Lateral talocalcaneal ligament
17 Calcaneofibular ligament
18 Calcaneal tendon (Achilles tendon)
19 Posterior talofibular ligament
20 Posterior tibiofibular ligament

Eycleshymer and Jones with modification

LL-77 Ligaments of the foot and ankle

Right foot viewed from behind

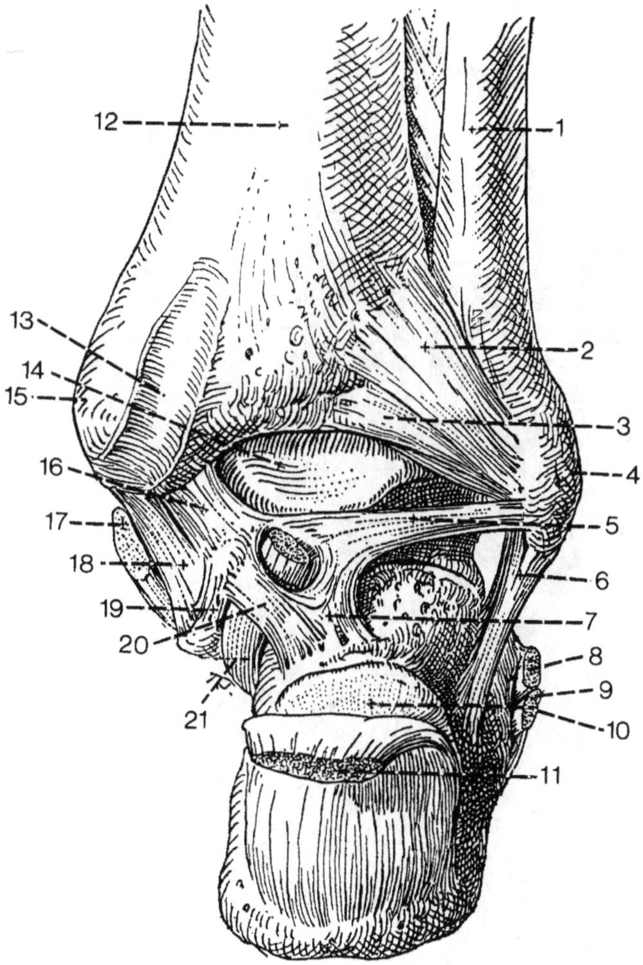

Color and label

1 Fibula
2 Posterior tibiofibular ligament
3 Inferior transverse (tibiofibular) ligament
4 Lateral malleolus
5 Posterior talofibular ligament
6 Calcaneofibular ligament
7 Talocalcaneal ligament
8 Tendon of peroneus (fibularis) brevis
9 Tendon of peroneus (fibularis) longus
10 Calcaneus (tuberosity)
11 Tendon calcaneus (Achilles) (cut and pulled posterior)
12 Tibia
13 Groove for tendon of tibialis posterior
14 Trochlea (pulley, Latin) of talus
15 Medial malleolus
16 Posterior tibiotalar ligament (part of deltoid ligament)
17 Tendon of tibialis posterior ("**Tom**" of "Tom, Dick, and Harry")
18 Tibiocalcaneal ligament (part of deltoid ligament)
19 Medial talocalcaneal ligament
20 Retinaculum for tendon of flexor hallucis longus
21 Tendon of flexor hallucis longus ("**Harry**" of "Tom, Dick, and Harry")

Eycleshymer and Jones with modification

LL-78 Plantar ligaments of the right foot

Viewed from below

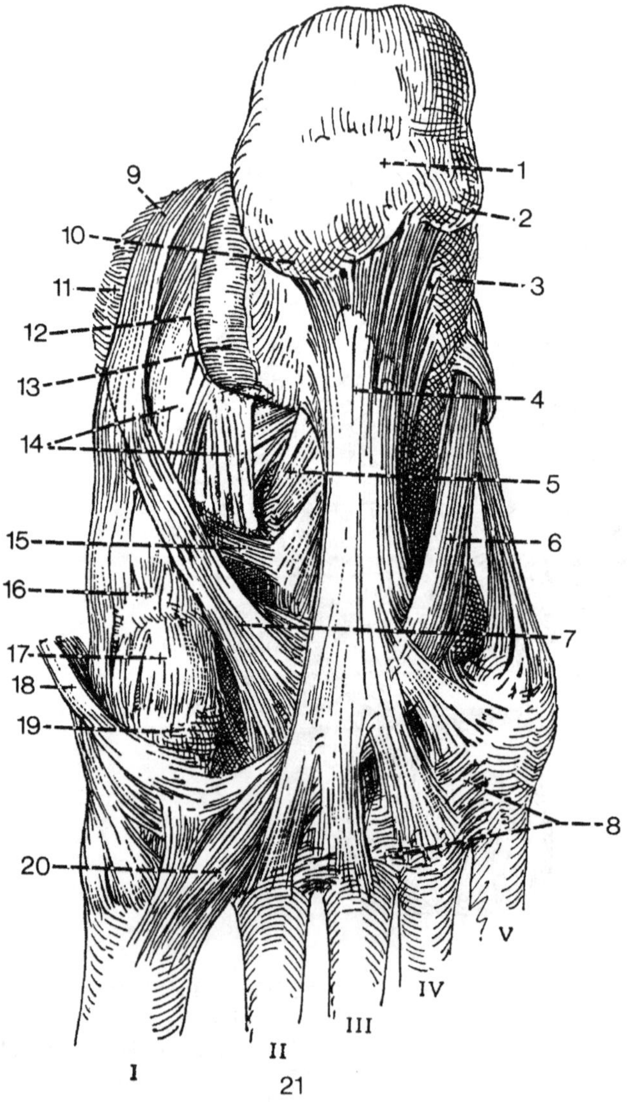

Color and label

1 Calcaneal tuberosity
2 Lateral process of calcaneal tuberosity
3 Calcaneus
4 Long plantar ligament
5 Plantar calcaneocuboid ligament
6 Tendon of peroneus (fibularis) longus muscle
7 Tendon of tibialis posterior muscle
8 Plantar intermetatarsal ligaments
9 Tendon of tibialis posterior muscle
10 Medial process of calcaneal tuberosity
11 Talus
12 Sustentaculum tali ("support for the talus"; shelf-like part of the calcaneus)
13 Sulcus (groove) on underside of sustentaculum tali for flexor hallucis longus tendon
14 Plantar calcaneonavicular ligament
15 Plantar cuboideonavicular ligament
16 Navicular bone
17 Plantar cuneonavicular ligament
18 Tibialis anterior tendon
19 Medial cuneiform bone
20 Peroneus (fibularis) longus tendon
21 Metatarsal bones (with Roman numerals)

Eycleshymer and Jones with modification

LL-79 Frontal section of ankle and foot

Right foot and ankle viewed from the front

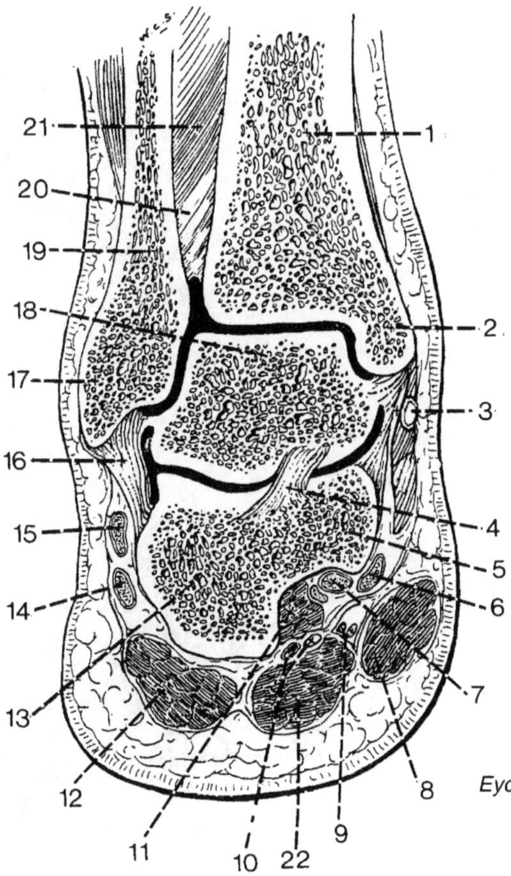

Eycleshymer and Jones

Color and label

1 Tibia
2 Medial malleolus
3 Tendon of tibialis posterior ("Tom")
4 Interosseous talocalcaneal ligament
5 Sustentaculum tali
6 Tendon of flexor digitorum longus ("Dick")
7 Tendon of flexor hallucis longus ("Harry")
8 Abductor hallucis muscle
9 Medial plantar nerve and artery (veins not shown)
10 Lateral plantar nerve and artery
11 Quadratus plantae muscle
12 Abductor digiti quinti muscle
13 Calcaneus
14 Tendon of peroneus (fibularis) longus
15 Tendon of peroneus (fibularis) brevis
16 Calcaneofibular ligament
17 Lateral malleolus
18 Talus
19 Fibula
20 Tibiofibular ligament
21 Interosseous membrane
22 Flexor digitorum brevis muscle

LL-80 Incisions on plantar surface of foot

Cross section of inferior foot

Color and label

1 Flexor hallucis longus tendon
2 Abductor hallucis longus muscle
3 Medial plantar nerve and artery
4 Flexor digitorum brevis muscle
5 Lateral plantar nerve and artery
6 Plantar aponeurosis
7 Plantar arch
8 Abductor digiti minimi muscle

Line X-----X indicates plane of section through foot shown in figure B (viewed from behind).

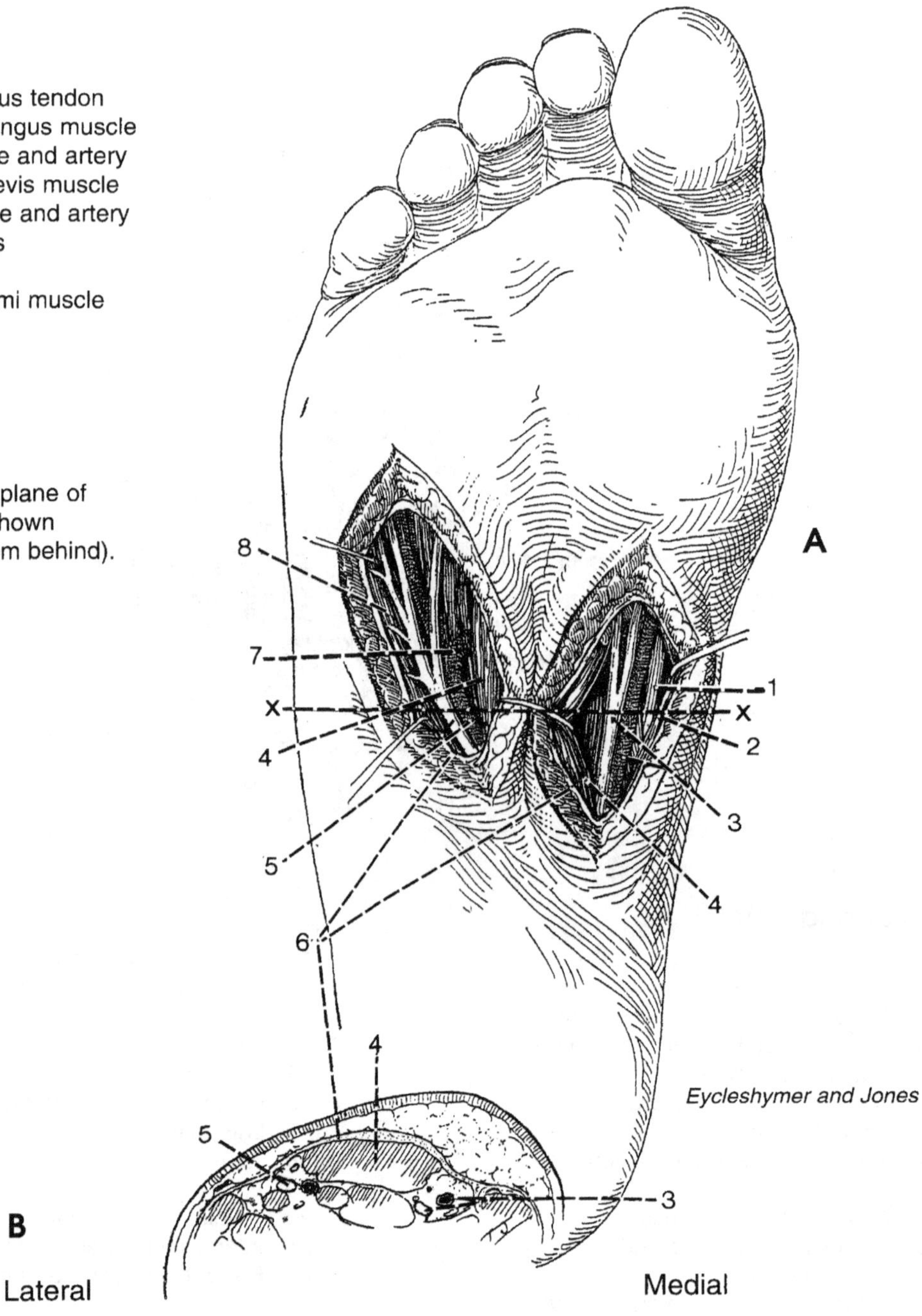

LL-81 Incision in back of medial malleolus

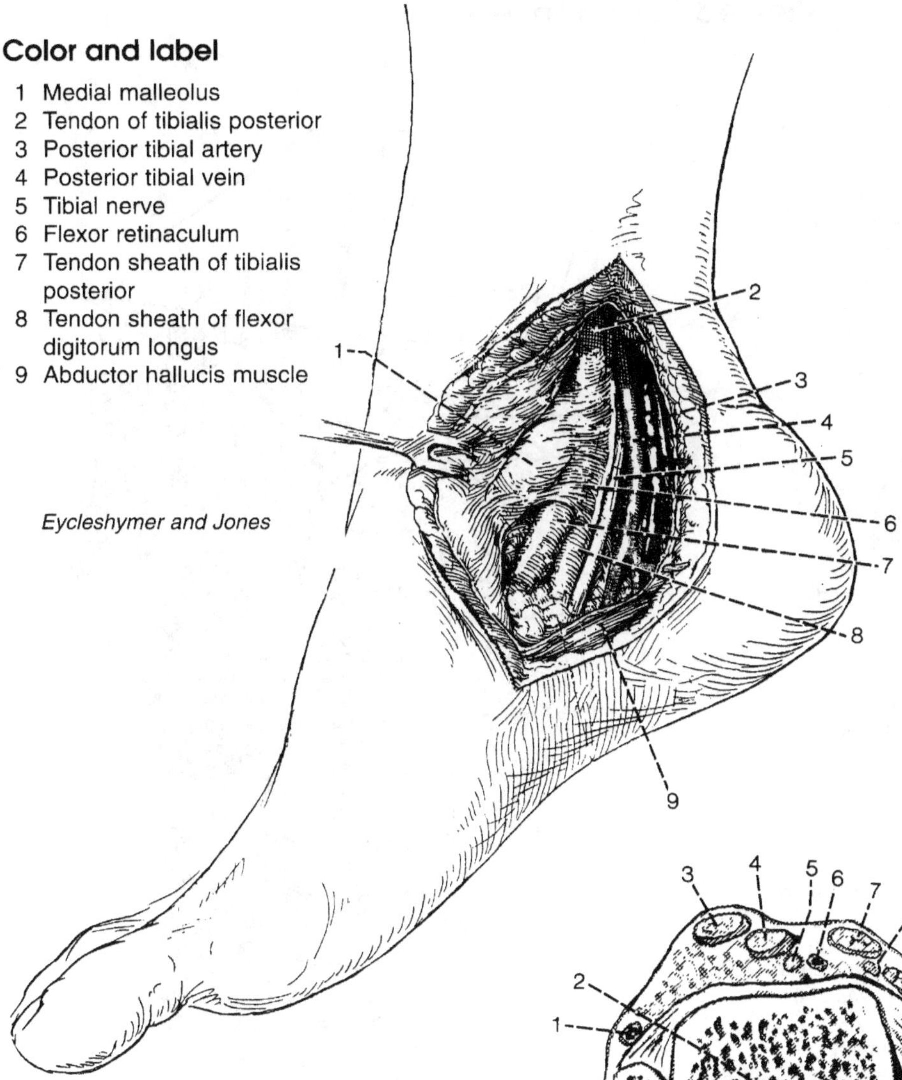

Color and label

1 Medial malleolus
2 Tendon of tibialis posterior
3 Posterior tibial artery
4 Posterior tibial vein
5 Tibial nerve
6 Flexor retinaculum
7 Tendon sheath of tibialis posterior
8 Tendon sheath of flexor digitorum longus
9 Abductor hallucis muscle

Eycleshymer and Jones

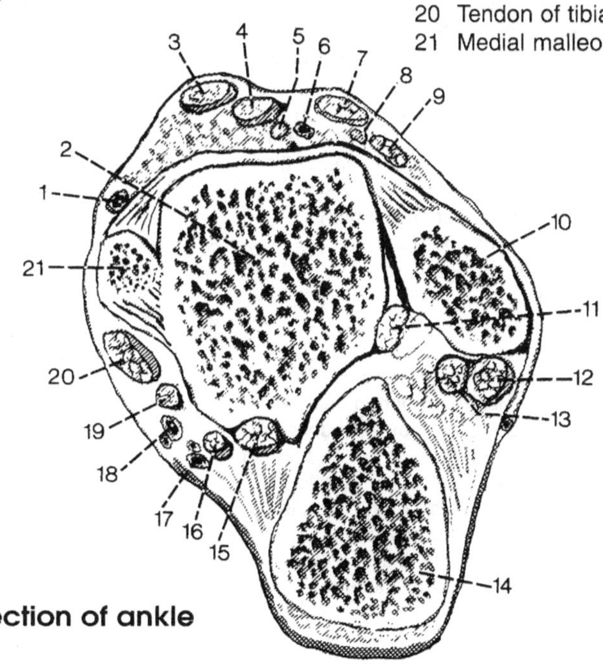

Cross section of ankle

Color and label

1 Great saphenous vein
2 Talus
3 Tendon of tibialis anterior
4 Tendon of extensor hallucis longus
5 Deep fibular (peroneal) nerve
6 Anterior tibial artery
7 Tendon of extensor digitorum longus
8 Superficial fibular (peroneal) nerve
9 Peroneus tertius
10 Lateral malleolus
11 Posterior talofibular ligament
12 Tendon of fibularis (peroneus) longus
13 Tendon of peroneus (fibularis) brevis
14 Calcaneus
15 Tendon of flexor hallucis longus
16 Tibial nerve
17 Lateral plantar artery and vein(s)
18 Medial plantar artery and vein(s)
19 Tendon of flexor digitorum longus
20 Tendon of tibialis posterior
21 Medial malleolus

LL-82 Oblique section of the right foot

Viewed from above

Color and label

1 Tibia
2 Tibialis posterior tendon
3 Fibula
4 Tibiofibular syndesmosis; the fibrous articulation between the triangular surface on the medial aspect of the distal end of the fibula and the fibular notch of the tibia, bound together by the anterior and the posterior tibiofibular ligaments and the interosseous membrane.
5 Calcaneofibular ligament
6 Talocrural articulation; a compound hinge joint in which the malleolar articular surface of the fibula, the inferior and malleolar articular surfaces of the tibia, and the inferior and malleolar articular surfaces of the tibia, and the inferior transverse tibiofibular ligament form a deep socket that receives the body of the talus.
7 Talocalcaneal joint (or articulation)
8 Calcaneus
9 Interosseous talocalcaneal ligament
10 Calcaneocuboid part of bifurcated ligament
11 Calcaneonavicular part of bifurcated ligament
12 Cuboid bone
13 Lateral cuneiform bone
14 Interosseous cuneocuboid ligament
15 Intermetatarsal articulation(s); simple plane joints between the adjacent sides of the bases of the five metatarsal bones
16 Interosseous metatarsal ligaments; strong transverse bands connecting the nonarticular parts of the adjacent surfaces of bases of the lateral four metatarsal bones
17 Interosseous cuneometatarsal ligament
18 Tarsometatarsal articulations (joints)
19 Interosseous cuneiform ligament
20 Medial cuneiform bone
21 Cuneonavicular joint
22 Navicular bone
23 Talocalcaneonavicular joint; a compound, multiaxial joint in which the rounded head of the talus articulates with the posterior concave surface of the navicular bone, while the anterior and middle calcaneal facets on the inferior surface of the neck and head of the talus fit on corresponding articular facets on the upper surface of the calcaneus and on the upper surface of the plantar calcaneonavicular ligament
24 Head of talus
25 Part of deltoid ligament
26 Metatarsal bones

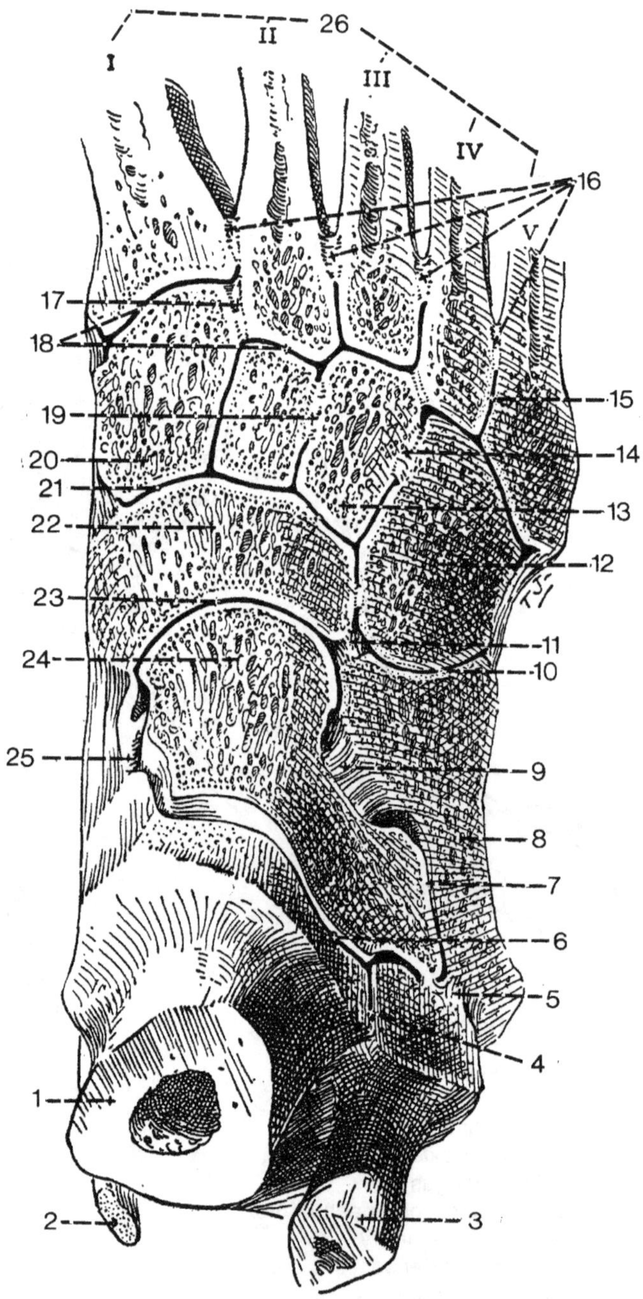

Eycleshymer and Jones

LL-83 Cutaneous nerves of the lower extremity

Anterior aspect

Letters and numbers in the left figure indicate the spinal origin of the nerves distributed to each area. The figure at the right shows the area of distribution of the cutaneous nerves.

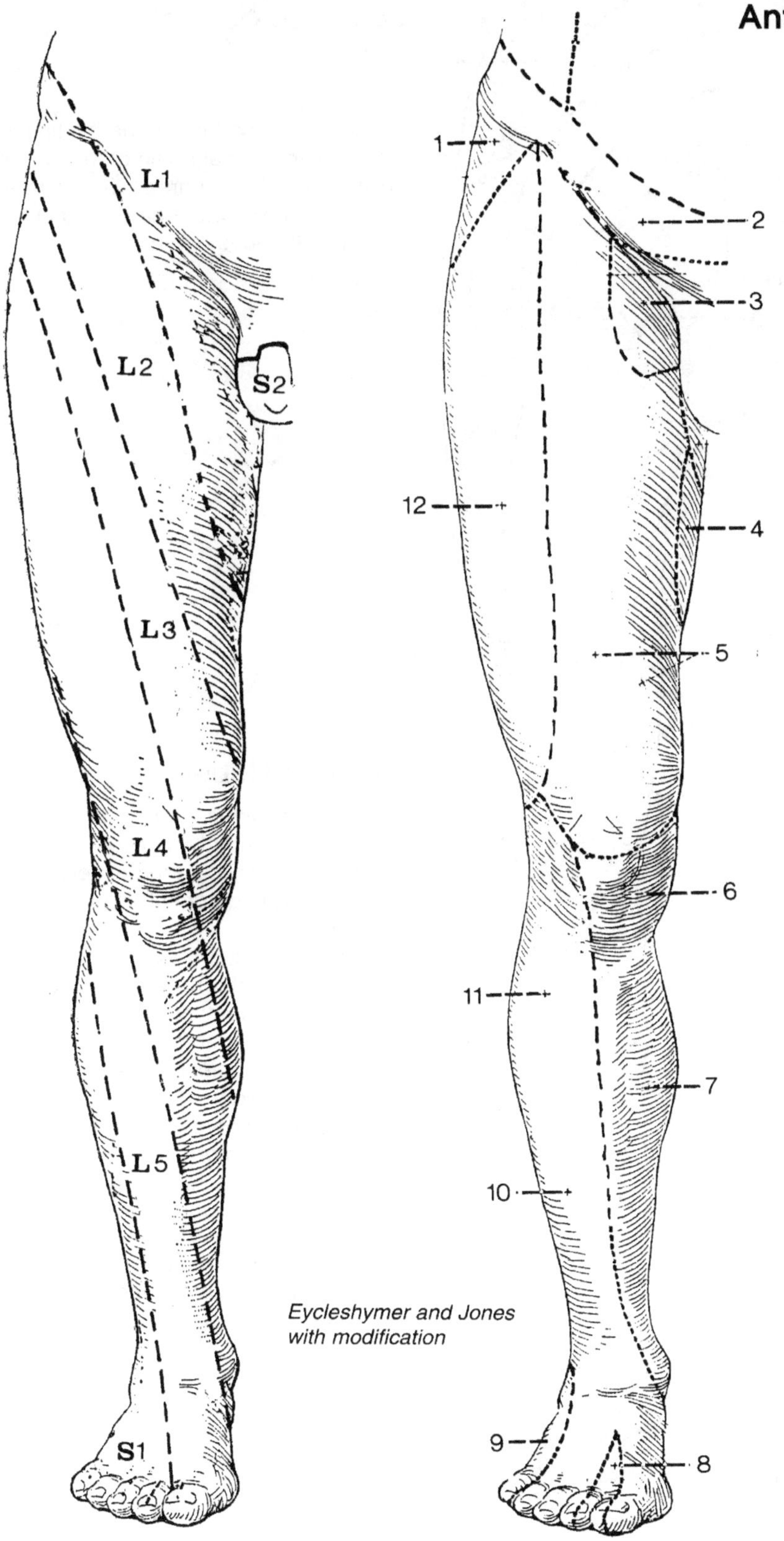

Eycleshymer and Jones with modification

Color and label

1 Lateral cutaneous ramus of subcostal nerve (T 12)
2 Anterior cutaneous ramus of iliohypogastric nerve
3 Ilioinguinal nerve
4 Obturator nerve
5 Anterior cutaneous ramus of femoral nerve
6 Infrapatellar ramus of saphenous nerve (branch of femoral nerve)
7 Saphenous nerve
8 Deep peroneal (fibular) nerve
9 Sural nerve
10 Superficial peroneal (fibular) nerve
11 Lateral sural cutaneous nerve
12 Lateral femoral cutaneous nerve

Remember, there is considerable overlap of sensory innervation between adjacent cutaneous nerves.

LL-84 Cutaneous nerves of the lower extremity

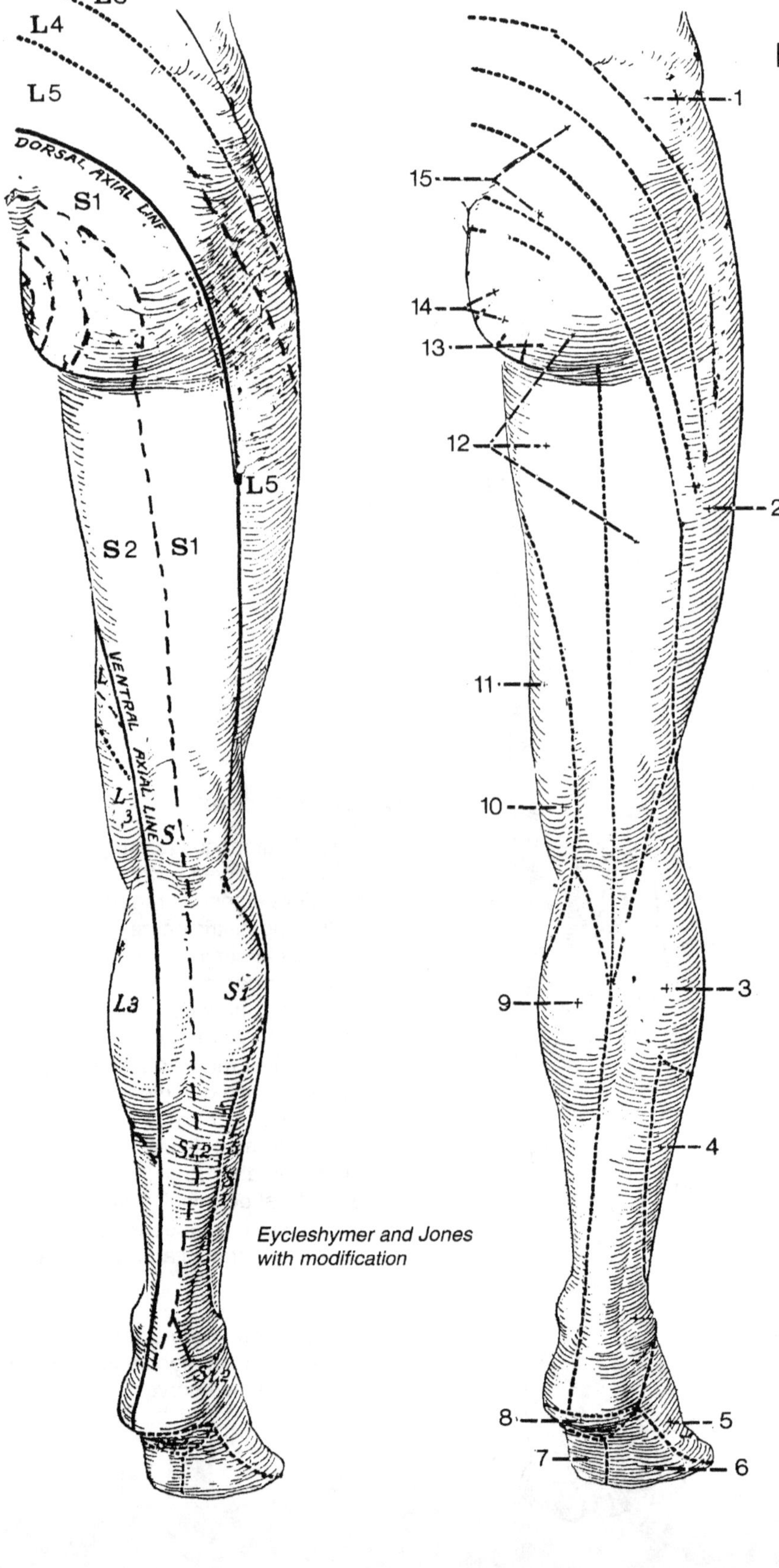

Eycleshymer and Jones with modification

Posterior aspect

Letters and numbers in the left figure indicate the spinal origin of the nerves distributed to each area. The figure at the right shows the area of distribution of the cutaneous nerves.

Color and label

1 Iliohypogastric nerve
2 Lateral femoral cutanous nerve
3 Lateral sural cutaneous nerve
4 Superficial peroneal (fibular) nerve
5 Sural nerve
6 Lateral plantar nerve (tibial nerve)
7 Medial plantar nerve (tibial nerve)
8 Calcaneal rami of tibial nerve
9 Saphenous nerve
10 Anterior cutaneous rami of femoral nerve
11 Obturator nerve
12 Posterior femoral cutaneous nerve
13 Inferior clunial rami of posterior femoral cutaneous nerve
14 Medial inferior clunial nerve (perforating cutaneous nerve)
15 Superior clunial nerves (off L1, L2, L3)

Part VII: Head and Neck

Trigemini
(Triplets)

Trigemini is Latin for "triplets." The trigeminal nerve is named the triplet nerve because it divides into three large nerves, the ophthalmic nerve, the maxillary nerve, and the mandibular nerve.

Gemini means "twins" and *quadrigemini* is "quadruplets."

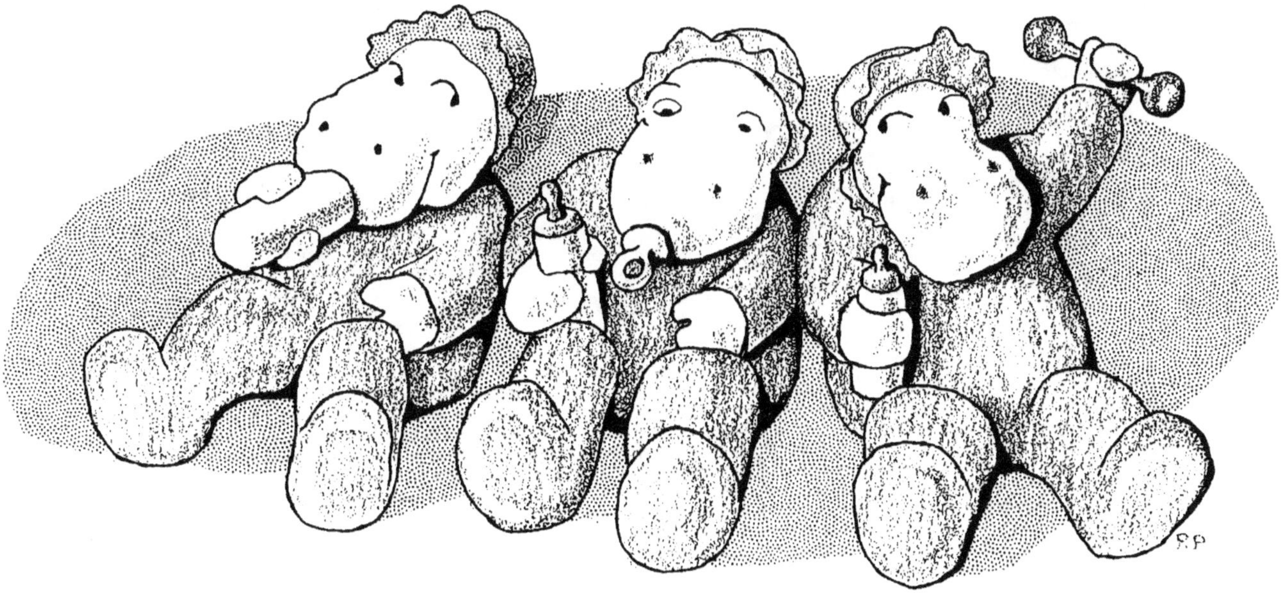

H&N-1 Superficial muscles of the face and neck

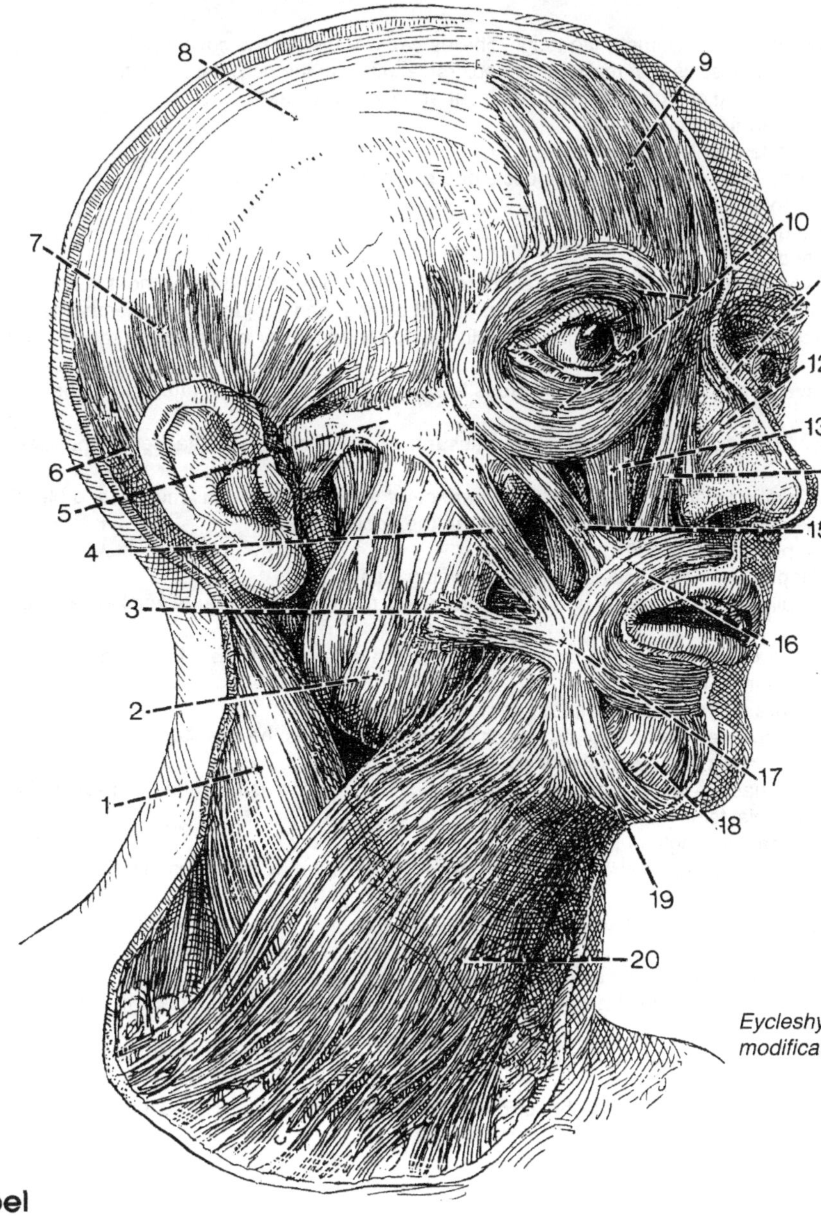

Eycleshymer and Jones with modification

Color and label

1 Sternocleidomastoid
2 Masseter
3 Risorius
4 Zygomaticus major
5 Zygomatic arch (also, zygoma)
6 Occipitalis
7 Superior auricular
8 Galea aponeurotica (also, epicranial aponeurosis)
9 Frontalis (also, frontal belly of occipitofrontalis)
10 Orbicularis oculi (orbital part)
11 Procerus
12 Nasalis (transverse part)
13 Levator labii superioris (also, levator muscle of upper lip)
14 Levator labii superioris alaeque nasi (also, levator muscle of upper lip and ala of nose)
15 Zygomaticus minor
16 Orbicularis oris (marginal part)
17 Modiolus
18 Depressor labii inferioris (also, depressor of lower lip)
19 Depressor anguli oris (also, depressor of angle of mouth)
20 Platysma

H&N-2 Muscles of facial expression

(opposite page)

Color and label

1 Galea aponeurotica (*galea*, L. a helmet); the tough, fibrous cap-like membrane covering the top of the skull anchored on each side by 3 paired muscles that make up the epicranial muscle: the occipitalis, the frontalis, and the temporoparietalis (also called epicranial aponeurosis; cut edge indicated at *).
2 Frontal belly of occipitofrontalis muscle
3 Temporoparietalis muscle (highly variable)
4 Orbicularis oculi muscle (also called orbicular muscle of the eye, sphincter of eye)
4A Orbital part (cut on left side of face)
4B Palpebral part (cut on left side)
4C Origin of medial orbital part
The upper and lower eyelids are each a fold of reinforced skin that consists of (from without inward): skin, areolar tissue, orbicularis oculi muscle, tarsus, orbital septum, tarsal glands, and conjunctiva (a membrane that lines both the inside of the eyelid and the outer surface of the eyeball; the upper and lower eyelids close the eye and wink the eye.
5 Medial palpebral ligament
6 Superior tarsus of eyelid (a plate of condensed fibrous tissue); its orbital margin is attached to the superior orbit by the orbital septum.
7 Inferior tarsus of eyelid (a plate of condensed fibrous tissue); its orbital margin is attached to the lower orbit by the orbital septum.
8 Orbital septum; a thin, fibrous sheath lining the inner surface of the orbicularis oculi muscle and blending with the aponeurosis of the levator palpebrae superioris muscle in the upper eyelid.
9 Tendon of levator palpebrae superioris muscle
10 Corrugator supercilii; produces a vertical furrow, the frowning muscle.
11 Procerus muscle; it pulls down the medial end of the eyebrows, producing transverse wrinkles above the root of the nose.
12 Auricularis anterior; in humans the three auricular muscles of the external ear are rather weak movers of the ears, unlike the auricular muscles in most mammals.
13 Zygomaticus major; pulls the angle of the mouth upward and laterally.
14 Zygomaticus minor; raises the outer part of the upper lip and accentuates the nasolabial fold.
15 Levator labii superioris; raises and everts the upper lip.
16 Levator labii superioris alaeque nasi; its medial part dilates the nostril, and its lateral part raises and everts the upper lip, and elevates the nasolabial fold.
17 Levator anguli oris; raises the angle of the mouth.
18 Masseter; a muscle of mastication; a strong closer of the jaw, innervated by the trigeminal nerve (cranial nerve V)
19 Parotid duct
20 Risorius; pulls the angle of the mouth laterally.
21 Nasalis
21A Transverse part; compresses the nasal septum.
21B Alar part; this part pulls the wings (alae) of the nose downwards and laterally, dilating the nostrils.
22 Depressor septi
23 Orbicularis oris (also called the orbicular muscle of the mouth); it closes the mouth, compresses the lips against the teeth, and protrudes the lips.
23A Marginal part; this part blends with eight surrounding muscles that converge and interlace at the modiolus at each angle of the mouth.
23B Labial part; this part lies within the lips.
24 Depressor anguli oris
25 Depressor labii inferior
26 Mentalis; draws up and wrinkles the skin of the chin, protruding the lower lip.
27 Buccinator; flattens the cheeks, and pulls the angle of the mouth laterally (*buccinator* means trumpeter in Latin)
28 Platysma; a thin broad muscle covering most of the anterior neck; pulls the lower lip and mouth laterally and inferiorly, partially opening the mouth
29 Outline of masseter

The facial muscles of expression (or muscles of facial expression) are unusual in that they insert not on bone, but on the skin of the face. By pulling on the skin, especially that around the eyes and mouth, they are able to express one's feelings and emotions. They are all innervated by the facial nerve, even the platysma which is largely in the neck. At their insertions they tend to blend and intertwine with neighboring facial muscles.

H&N-2 Muscles of facial expression

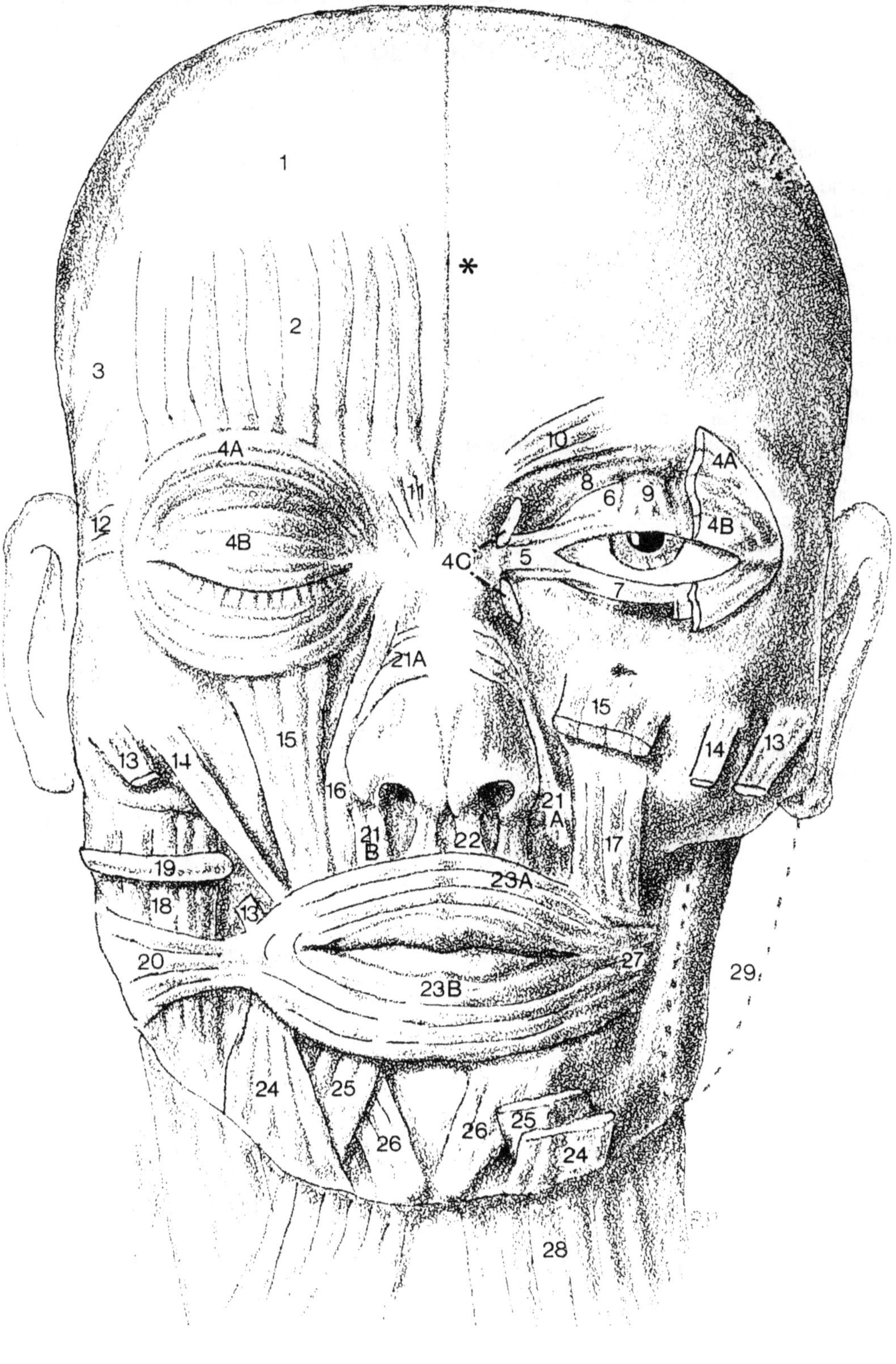

H&N-3 Superficial structures of the lateral head

(opposite page)

Color and label

1 Parotid gland
2 Parotid duct
3 Temporal branches of the facial nerve
4 Zygomatic branches of facial nerve
5 Buccal branches of facial nerve
6 Marginal mandibular branch of facial nerve
7 Cervical branch of facial nerve
8 Transverse facial artery
9 Facial artery and vein
10 Superficial temporal artery and vein
11 Auriculotemporal nerve; a branch of the mandibular nerve (of nerve V)
12 External jugular vein
13 Great auricular nerve
14 Transverse cervical nerves
15 Supraclavicular nerve
16 Lesser occipital nerve
17 Accessory parotid gland
18 Buccal fat pad
19 Accessory nerve (cranial nerve XI)
20 Angular artery and vein
21 Masseter muscle
22 Orbicularis oculi muscle
23 Zygomaticus major muscle
24 Zygomaticus minor muscle
25 Platysma muscle
26 Sternocleidomastoid muscle
27 Trapezius muscle
28 Occipital artery
29 Greater occipital nerve
30 Modiolus (or modiolus labii); a nodular mass of decussating muscles mainly from the upper and lower lips interlacing with other facial muscles such as the buccinator (which has been removed).

H&N-3 Superficial structures of the lateral head

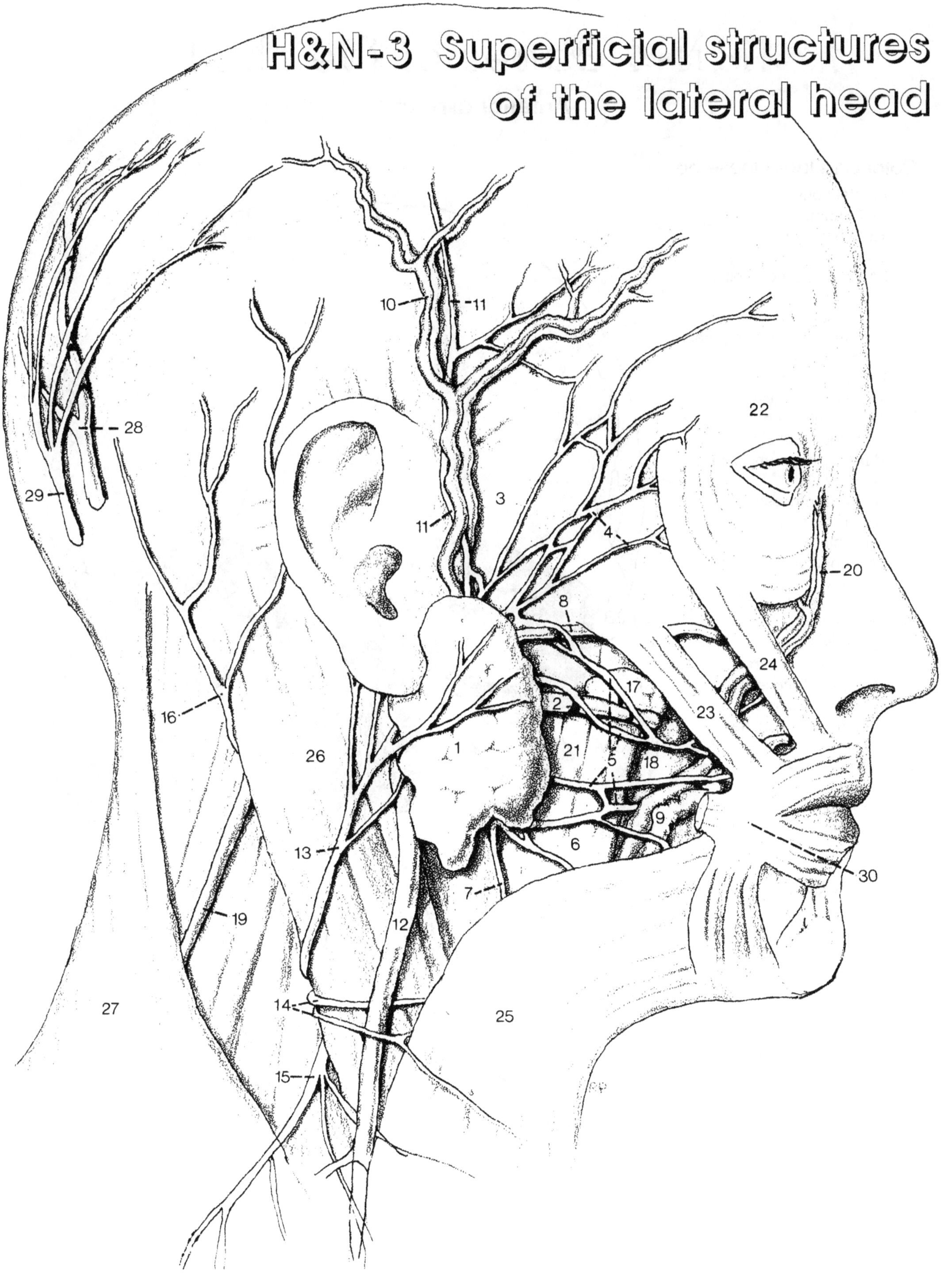

H&N-4 Bones of the skull

Anterior aspect

Color and label these bones

1 Frontal bone
  1A Squamous part
  1B Orbital part
2 Sphenoid bone
  2A Greater wing, orbital surface
  2B Lesser wing
  2C Greater wing, temporal surface
3 Zygomatic bone
  3A Lateral surface
  3B Frontal process
  3C Orbital surface
4 Maxillary bone (maxilla)
  4A Body
  4B Nasal process
  4C Orbital surface
5 Mandible
  5A Mental protuberance
  5B Body
  5C Ramus
6 Nasal bone
7 Temporal bone
  7A Squamous part
  7B Mastoid process
  7C Zygomatic process
8 Inferior nasal concha
9 Lacrimal bone
10 Parietal bone
11 Vomer
12 Ethoid bone
  12A Perpendicular plate
  12B Middle nasal concha

Label these foramina

13 Optic canal
14 Superior orbital fissure
15 Inferior orbital fissure
16 Infraorbital groove
17 Supraorbital foramen (sometimes just a notch)
18 Infraorbital foramen
19 Mental foramen

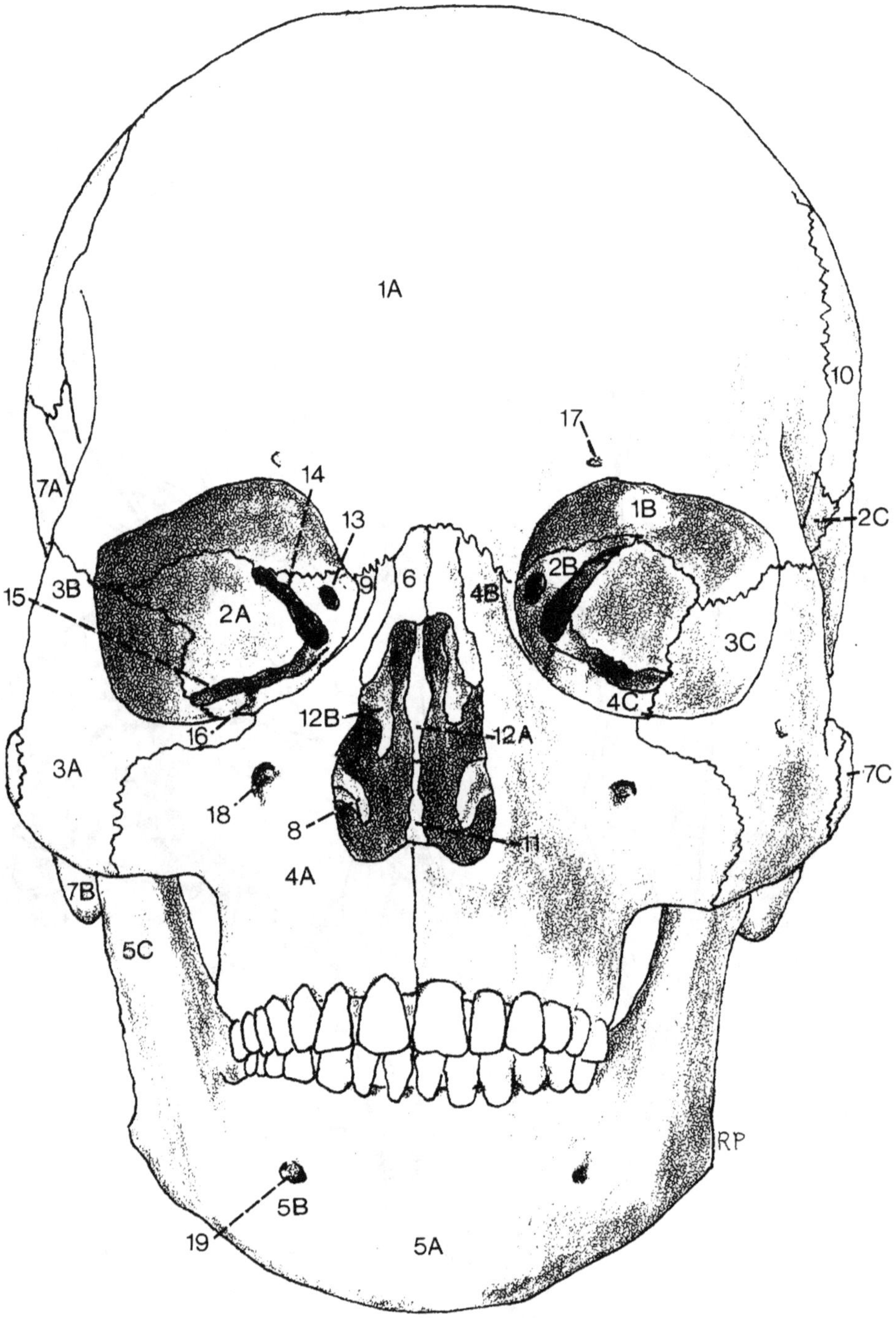

H&N-5 Bones of the skull

Lateral aspect

Color and label

1 Mental protuberance
2 Mental foramen
3 Infraorbital foramen
4 Neck of mandible (head of mandible forms temporomandibular joint with temporal bone)
5 Coronoid process
6 Mastoid process of temporal bone
7 External auditory meatus
8 Lambdoidal suture
9 Squamous suture
10 Coronal suture

S	Sphenoid bone
F	Frontal bone
L	Lacrimal bone
N	Nasal bone
Max	Maxillary bone
P	Parietal bone
O	Occipital bone
T	Temporal bone
Z	Zygomatic bone
E	Ethmoid bone
M	Mandible

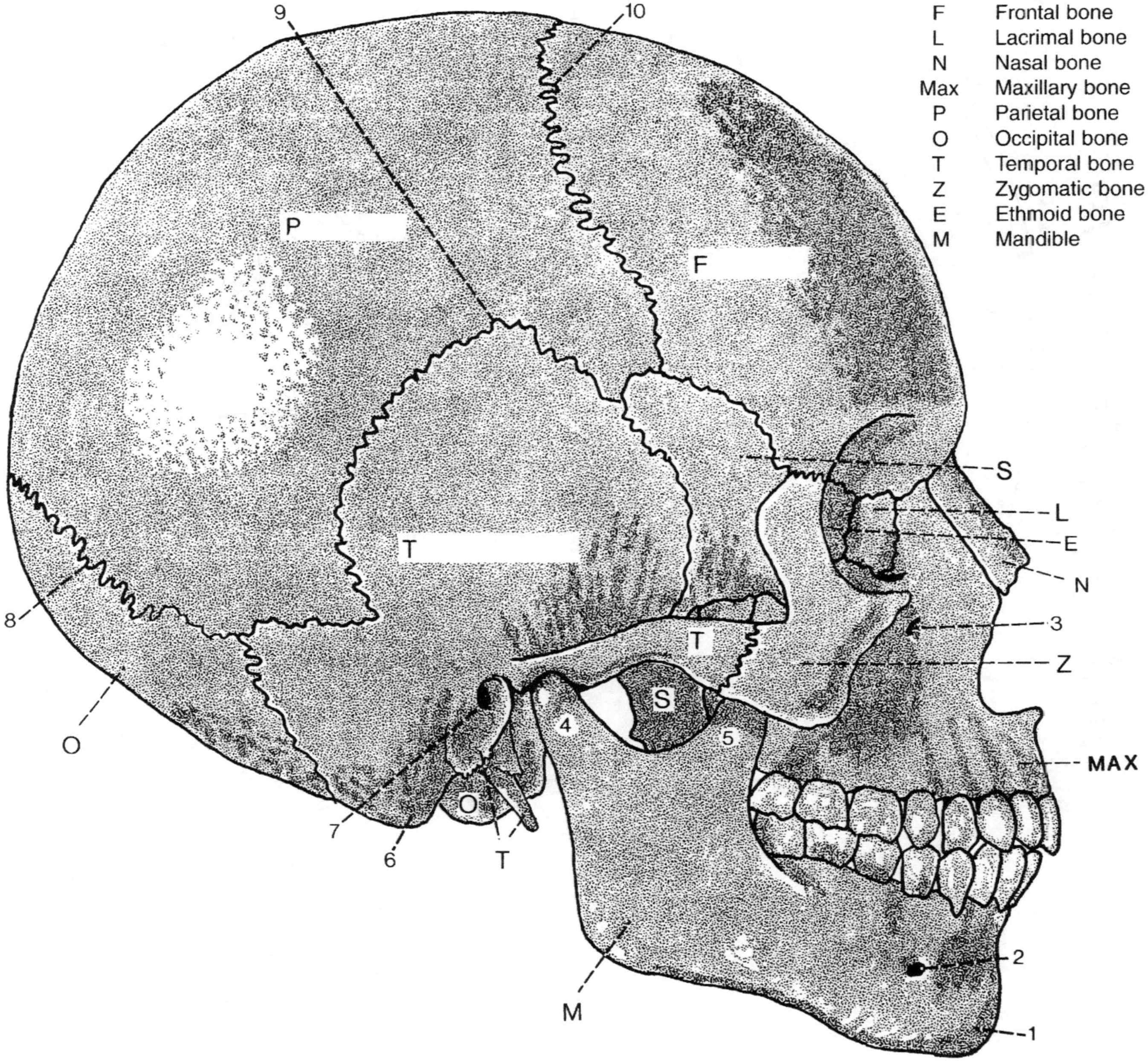

H&N-6 Facial nerve

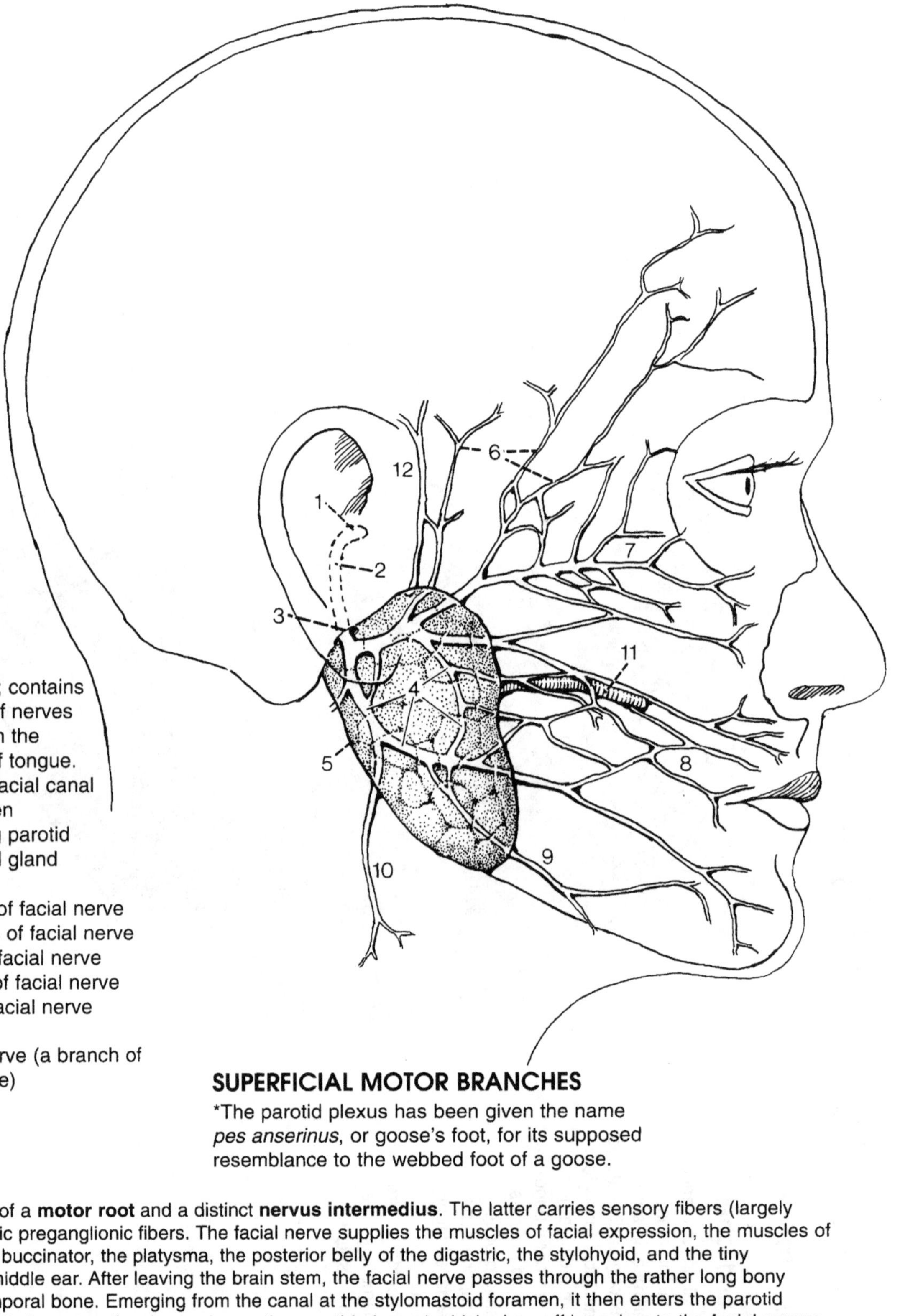

Color and label

1 Geniculate ganglion; contains neuron cell bodies of nerves conveying taste from the anterior two-thirds of tongue.
2 Facial nerve within facial canal
3 Stylomastoid foramen
4 Facial nerve forming parotid plexus within parotid gland
5 Parotid gland
6 Temporal branches of facial nerve
7 Zygomatic branches of facial nerve
8 Buccal branches of facial nerve
9 Mandibular branch of facial nerve
10 Cervical branch of facial nerve
11 Parotid duct
12 Auriculotemporal nerve (a branch of the mandibular nerve)

SUPERFICIAL MOTOR BRANCHES

*The parotid plexus has been given the name *pes anserinus*, or goose's foot, for its supposed resemblance to the webbed foot of a goose.

The facial nerve consists of a **motor root** and a distinct **nervus intermedius**. The latter carries sensory fibers (largely taste) and parasympathetic preganglionic fibers. The facial nerve supplies the muscles of facial expression, the muscles of the scalp and auricle, the buccinator, the platysma, the posterior belly of the digastric, the stylohyoid, and the tiny stapedius muscle in the middle ear. After leaving the brain stem, the facial nerve passes through the rather long bony facial canal within the temporal bone. Emerging from the canal at the stylomastoid foramen, it then enters the parotid gland in which it ramifies, its branches forming a plexus, the parotid plexus,* which gives off branches to the facial expression muscles. The facial nerve's motor branches from the parotid plexus to the facial muscles travel close to the skin. Damage to the facial nerve results in Bell's palsy (unilateral paralysis of facial muscles supplied by the seventh nerve).

H&N-7 Landmarks on the lateral skull

Label these landmarks

1 Mental protuberance
2 Mental foramen
3 Body of mandible
4 Angle of mandible
5 Ramus of mandible
6 Condyloid process
7 Coronoid process
8 Head of mandible
9 Zygomatic arch
10 Mastoid process
11 Styloid process
12 Tympanic part of temporal bone
13 External acoustic opening
14 Squamous part of temporal bone
15 Coronal suture
16 Lambdoid suture
17 Greater wing of sphenoid bone
18 Infraorbital foramen
19 Superior temporal line
20 Inferior temporal line

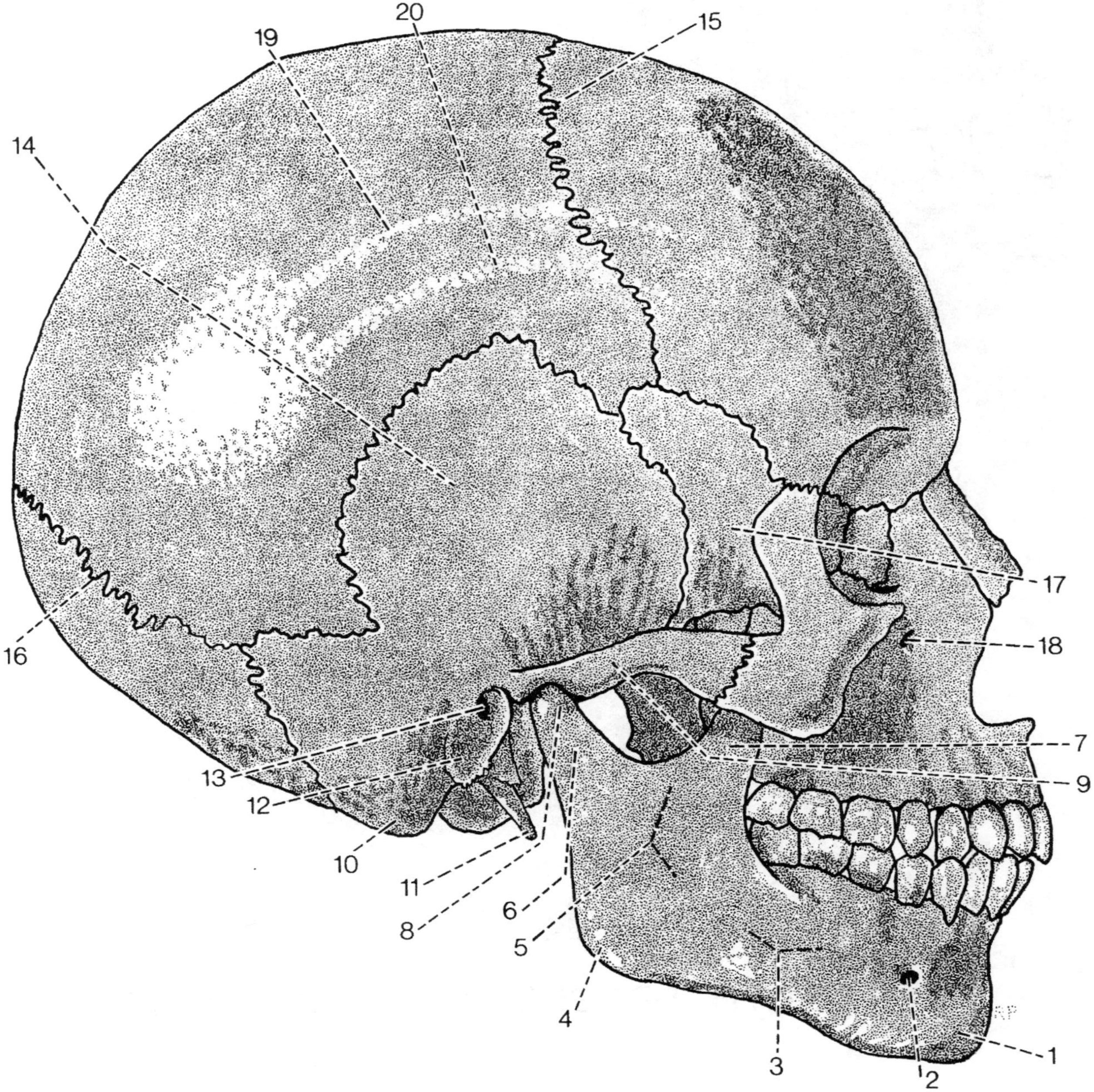

H&N-8 Temporalis and masseter muscles

Color and label

1 Temporalis muscle
2 Masseter muscle
3 Deep part of masseter

The temporalis, masseter, medial and lateral pterygoids are the muscles of mastication (chewing). They are innervated by nerve V, the trigeminal nerve.

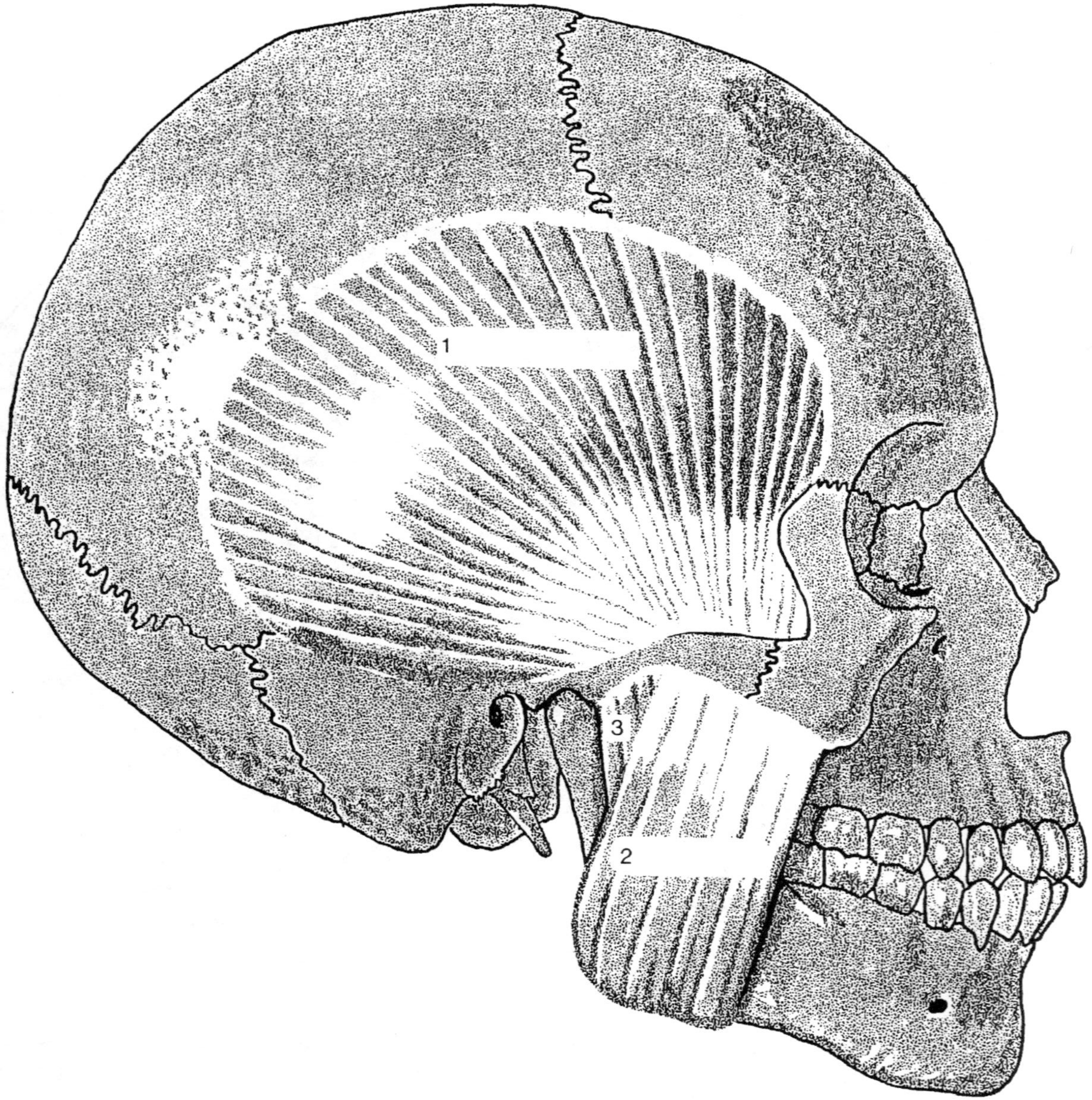

H&N-9 Temporalis muscle

Color and label

1 Temporalis muscle
2 Insertion of temporalis on coronoid process and ramus of mandible
3 Zygomatic arch (cut)
4 Insertion of masseter on ramus and angle of mandible

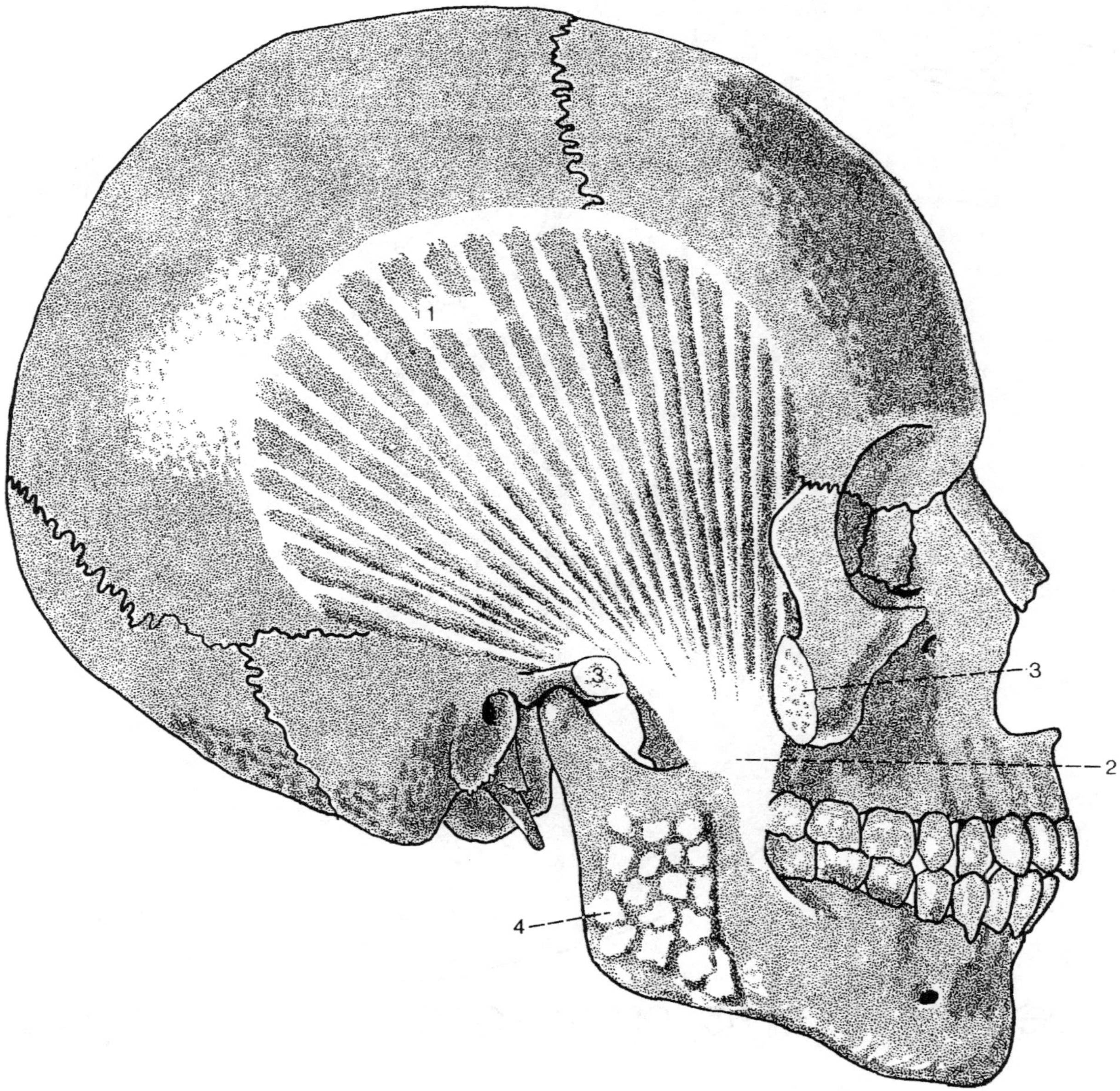

H&N-10 Buccinator and orbicularis oris muscles

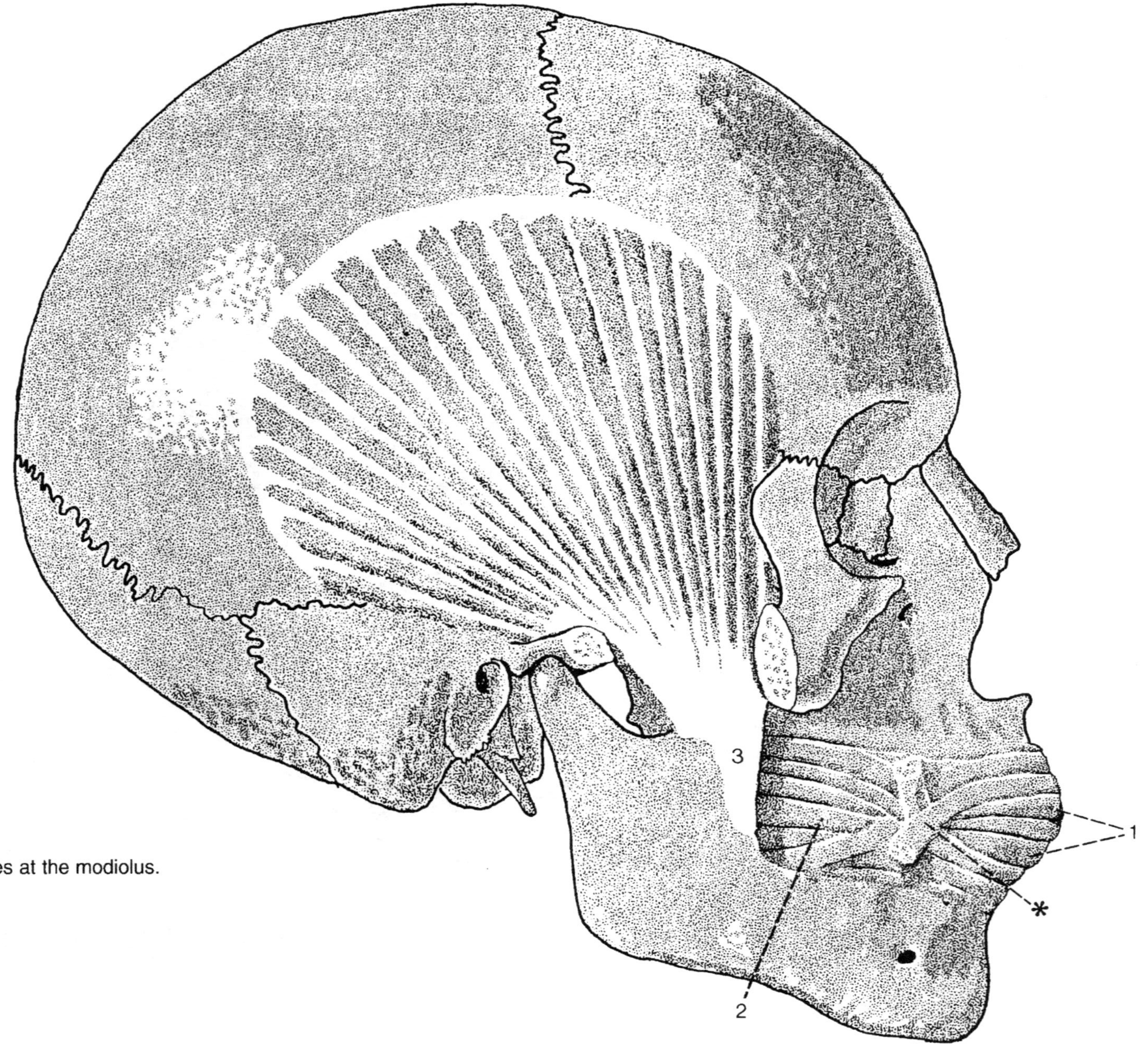

Color and label

1 Orbicalaris oris
2 Buccinator
3 Insertion of temporalis on mandible

*Note the intertwining of muscles at the modiolus.

H&N-11 Median section of skull and mandible

Viewed from the left

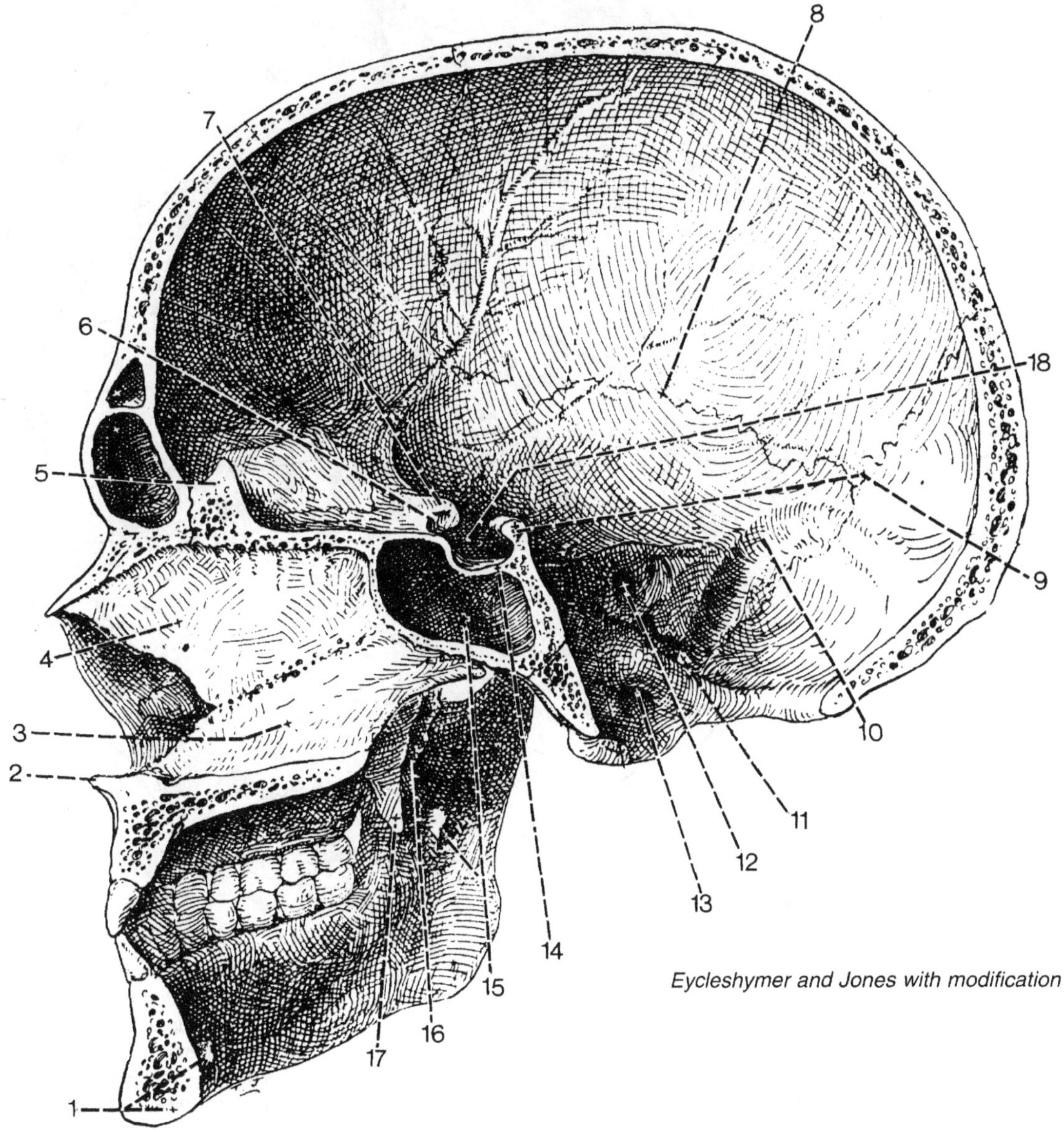

Eycleshymer and Jones with modification

Label these landmarks

1 Mandible and genial tubercle
2 Anterior nasal spine
3 Vomer
4 Perpindicular plate of ethmoid
5 Crista galli (Latin, cock's comb)
6 Optic canal
7 Anterior clinoid process
8 Squamous suture
9 Dorsum sellae
10 Groove for sigmoid sinus
11 Jugular foramen
12 Internal auditory meatus
13 Hypoglossal foramen
14 Sella turcica (Latin, Turkish saddle)
15 Sphenoid sinus
16 Lateral pterygoid plate (part of sphenoid bone)
17 Medial pterygoid plate (part of sphenoid bone)
18 Hypophyseal fossa (site of pituitary gland)

H&N-12 Interior of the skull

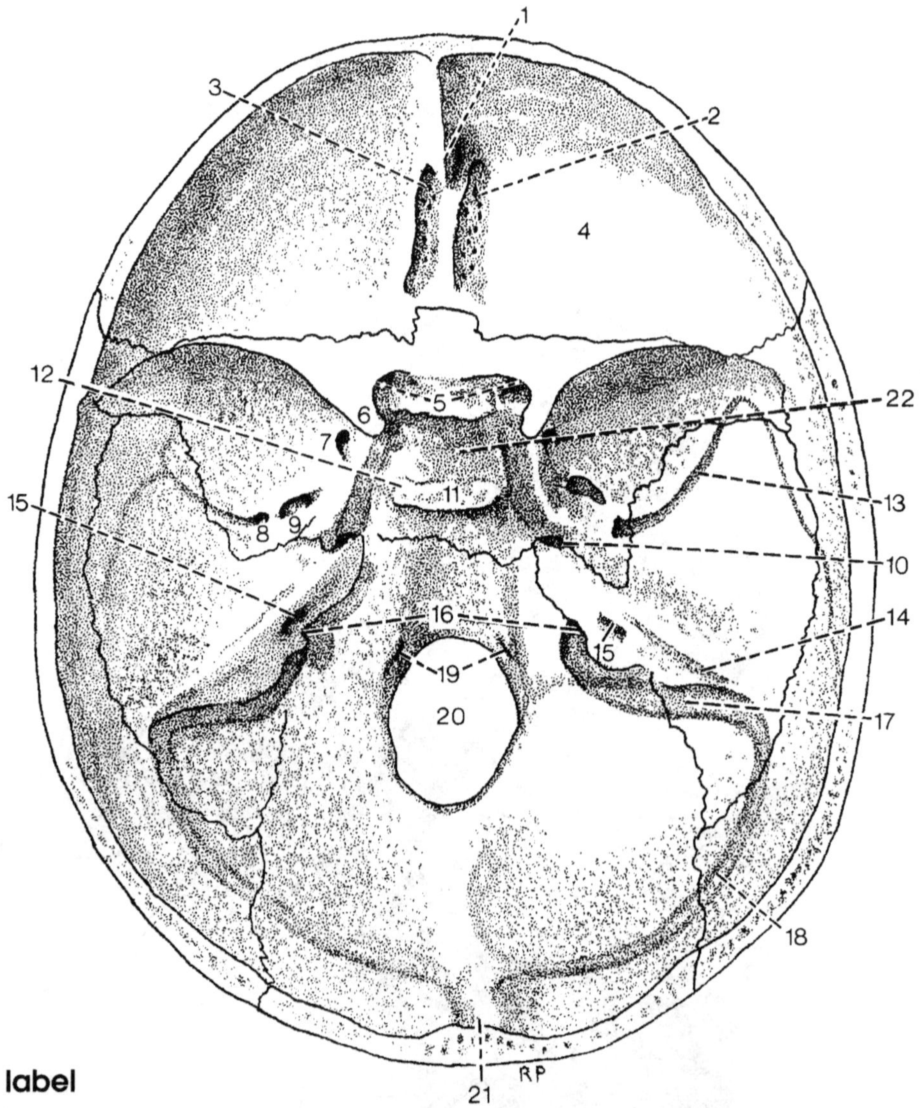

Color and label

1 Crista galli
2 Cribriform plate of ethmoid bone
3 Foramina for olfactory nerve fibers (cranial nerve I)
4 Orbital part of frontal bone
5 Optic canal; transmits optic nerve (cranial nerve II) and ophthalmic artery
6 Anterior clinoid process
7 Foramen rotundum (transmits maxillary branch of trigeminal nerve)
8 Foramen spinosum (transmits the middle meningeal artery and the meningeal branch of the mandibular nerve into the middle cranial fossa)
9 Foramen ovale (also called oval foramen of sphenoid bone; transmits mandibular branch of trigeminal nerve)
10 Foramen lacerum (in life it does not exit, rather it is filled with cartilage)
11 Dorsum sellae
12 Posterior clinoid process
13 Groove for middle meningeal artery
14 Groove for superior petrosal sinus*
15 Internal auditory meatus; passage conveying the facial nerve (cranial nerve VII), the vestibulocochlear nerve (cranial nerve VIII), and the labyrinthine artery
16 Jugular foramen; it transmits the glosspharyngeal nerve, the vagus nerve, the accessory nerve, and the internal jugular vein (continuation of the sigmoid sinus)
17 Sulcus for sigmoid sinus*
18 Sulcus for transverse sinus*
19 Hypoglossal canal
20 Foramen magnum
21 Sulcus for superior sagittal sinus*
22 Hypophyseal fossa (site of pituitary gland)

*These sinuses are dural venous sinuses that drain blood from the brain and bones of the cranium. They are located between two layers of dura mater, are lined with endothelium, and lack valves.

H&N-13 Superficial veins of the head and neck

Color and label

1 Superficial temporal vein
2 Middle temporal vein
3 Transverse facial vein
4 Maxillary vein (runs deep to mandible)
5 Retromandibular vein
6 Posterior auricular vein
7 External jugular vein
8 Anterior jugular vein
9 Posterior external jugular vein
10 Occipital vein
11 Facial vein
12 Submental vein
13 Inferior labial vein
14 Superior labial vein
15 Deep facial vein
16 Parotid ramus
17 External nasal vein
18 Inferior palpebral vein
19 Superior palpebral vein
20 Supratrochlear vein
21 Supraorbital vein
22 Internal jugular vein
23 Superior thyroid vein
24 Angular vein
25 Connection between angular vein and superior ophthalmic vein
26 Sternocleidomastoid muscle
27 Outline of parotid gland
28 Thyroid gland

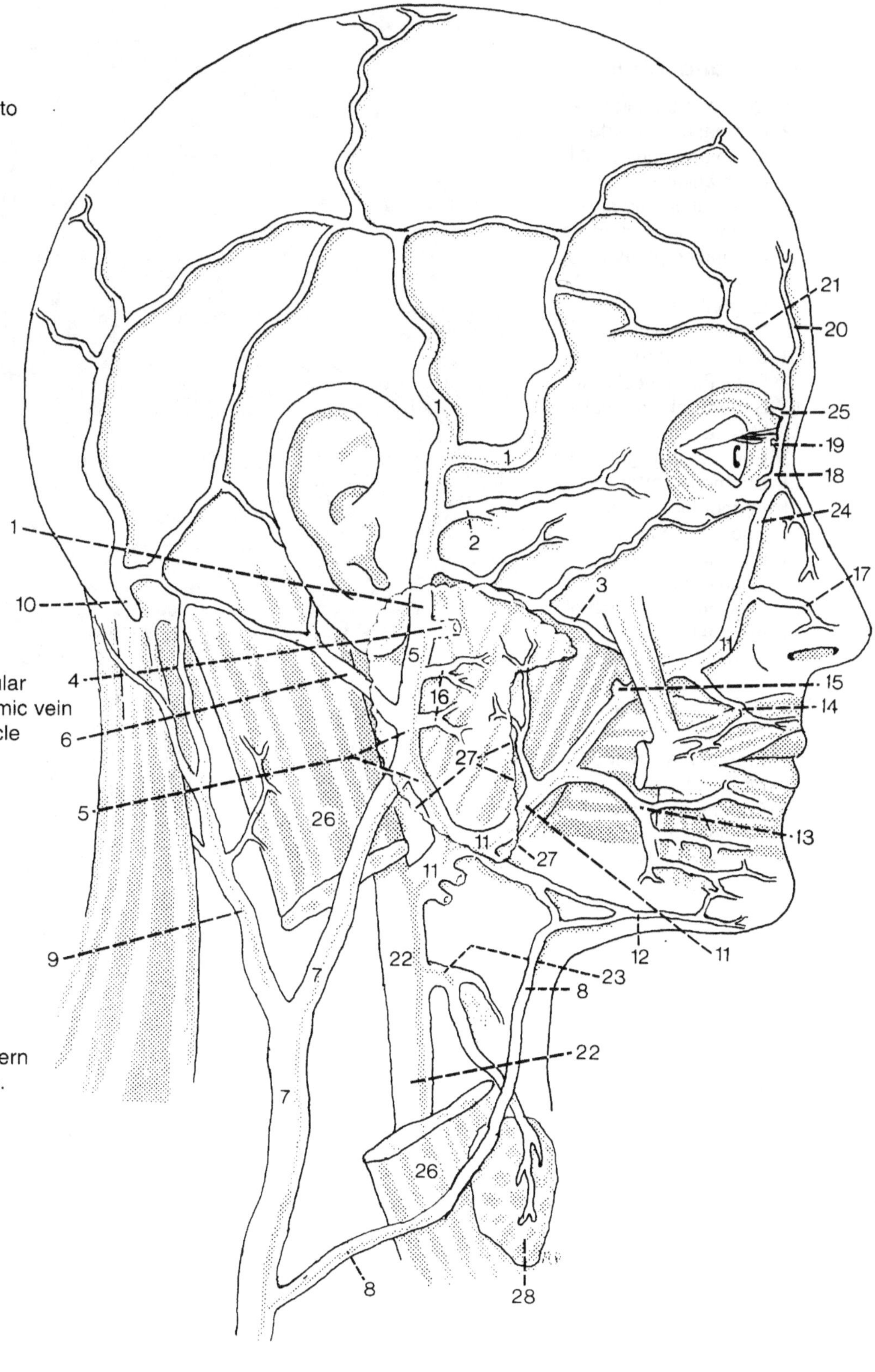

Veins tend to vary in their pattern more than arteries and nerves.

H&N-14 External carotid artery and its branches

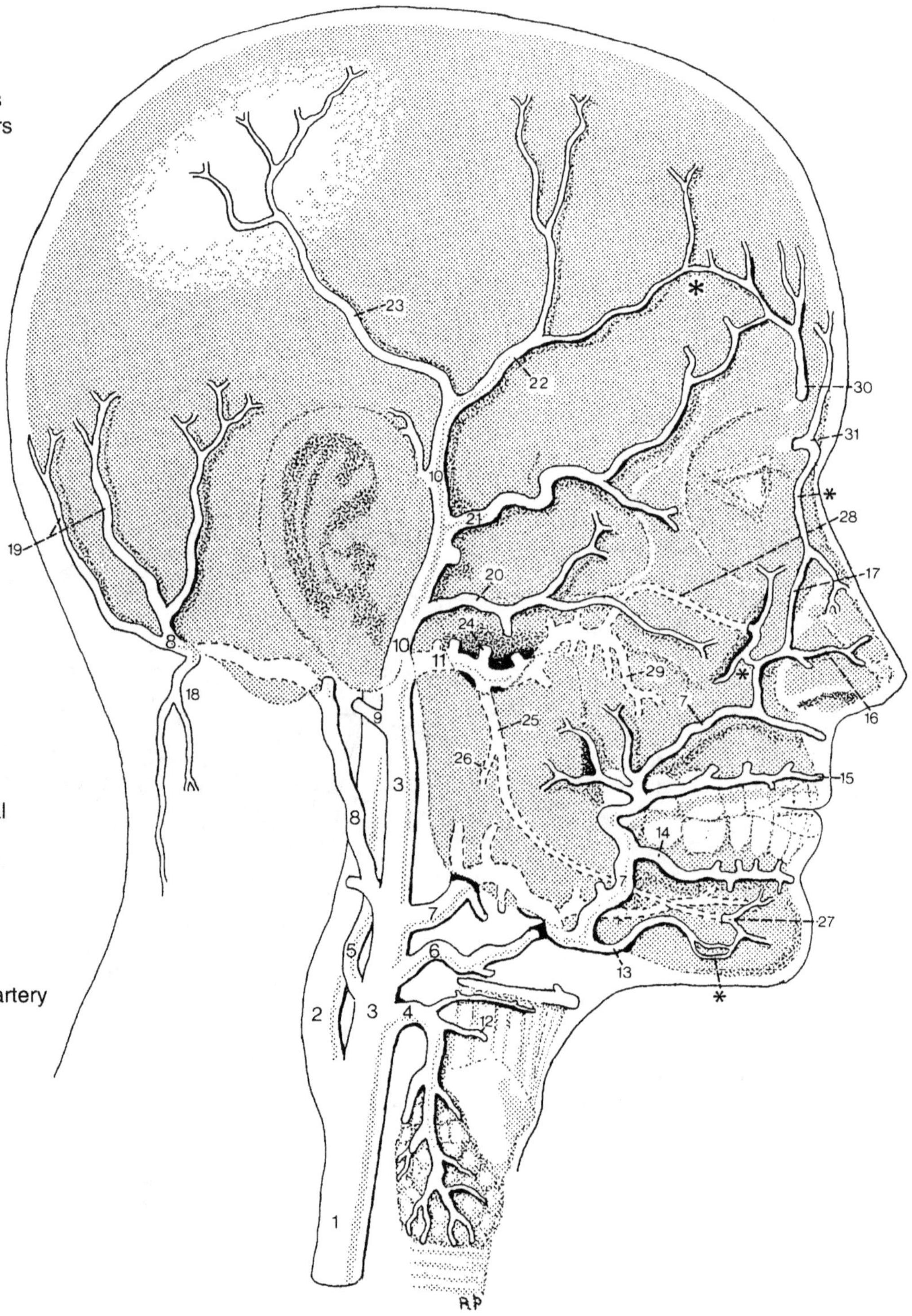

Color and label

1 Common carotid artery
2 Internal carotid artery (gives off no branches until it enters the cranium)
3 External carotid artery
4 Superior thyroid artery
5 Ascending pharyngeal artery
6 Lingual artery
7 Facial artery
8 Occipital artery
9 Posterior auricular artery
10 Superficial temporal artery
11 Maxillary artery
12 Superior laryngeal artery
13 Submental artery
14 Inferior labial artery
15 Superior labial artery
16 Lateral nasal artery
17 Angular artery
18 Descending branch of occipital artery
19 Terminal branches of occipital artery
20 Transverse facial artery
21 Zygomatico-orbital artery
22 Frontal branch of superficial temporal artery
23 Parietal branch of superficial temporal artery
24 Middle meningeal artery
25 Inferior alveolar artery
26 Mylohyoid artery
27 Mental artery
28 Infraorbital artery
29 Posterior superior alveolar artery
30 Supraorbital artery
31 Supratrochlear artery

*Points of anastomoses

Sagitta

Etymological cartoon)

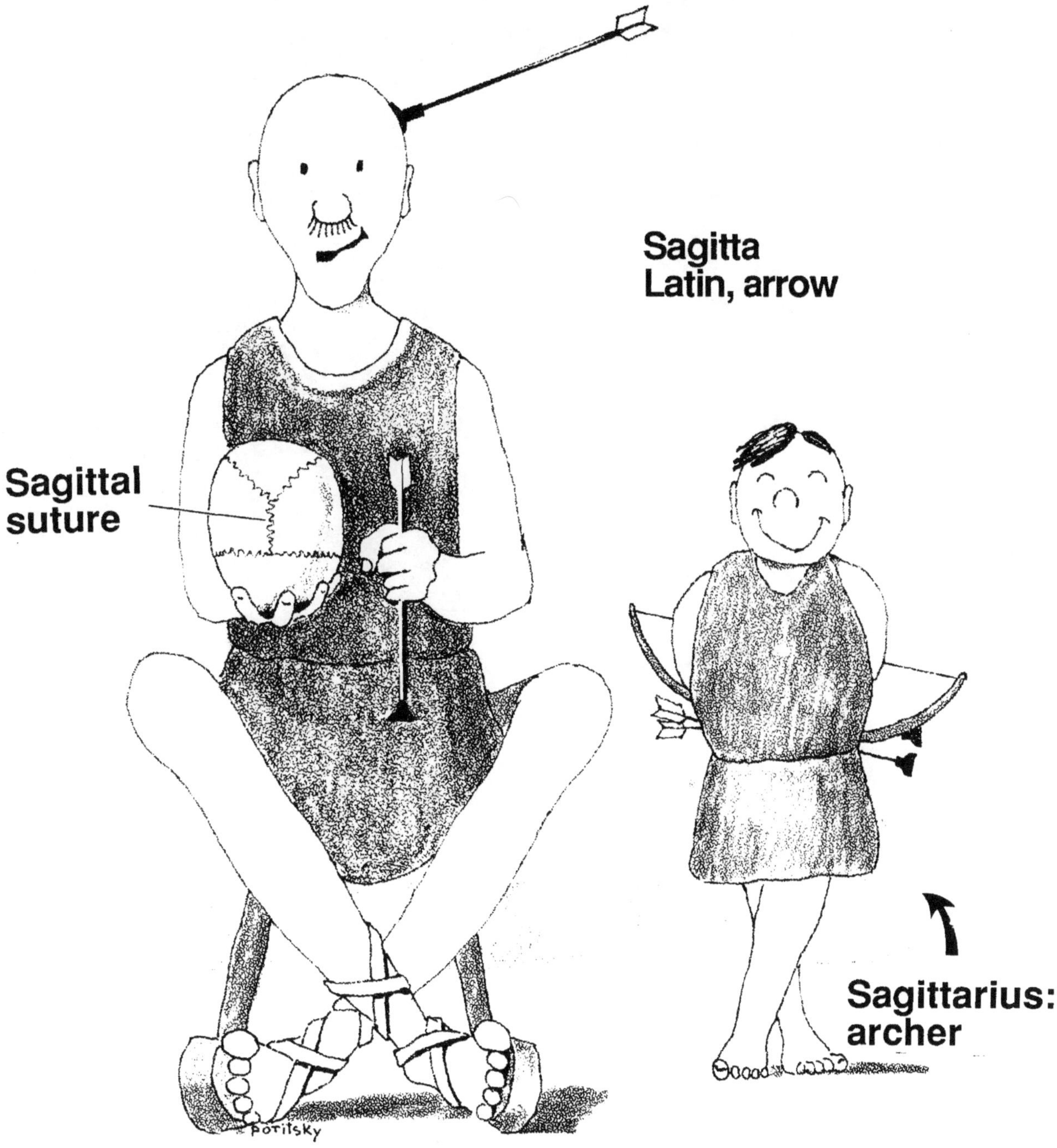

Sagitta is Latin for arrow. The sagittal plane in anatomy takes its name from the sagittal suture on the top of the skull, which runs between the two parietal bones in a front-to-back direction. At the back of the skull the sagittal suture meets the inverted V-shape of the lambdoid suture. With a bit of imagining one can visualize the sagittal suture forming the shaft of an arrow and a portion of the lambdoid forming the feathers.

H&N-15 Cranial dural venous sinuses

Beneath the brain

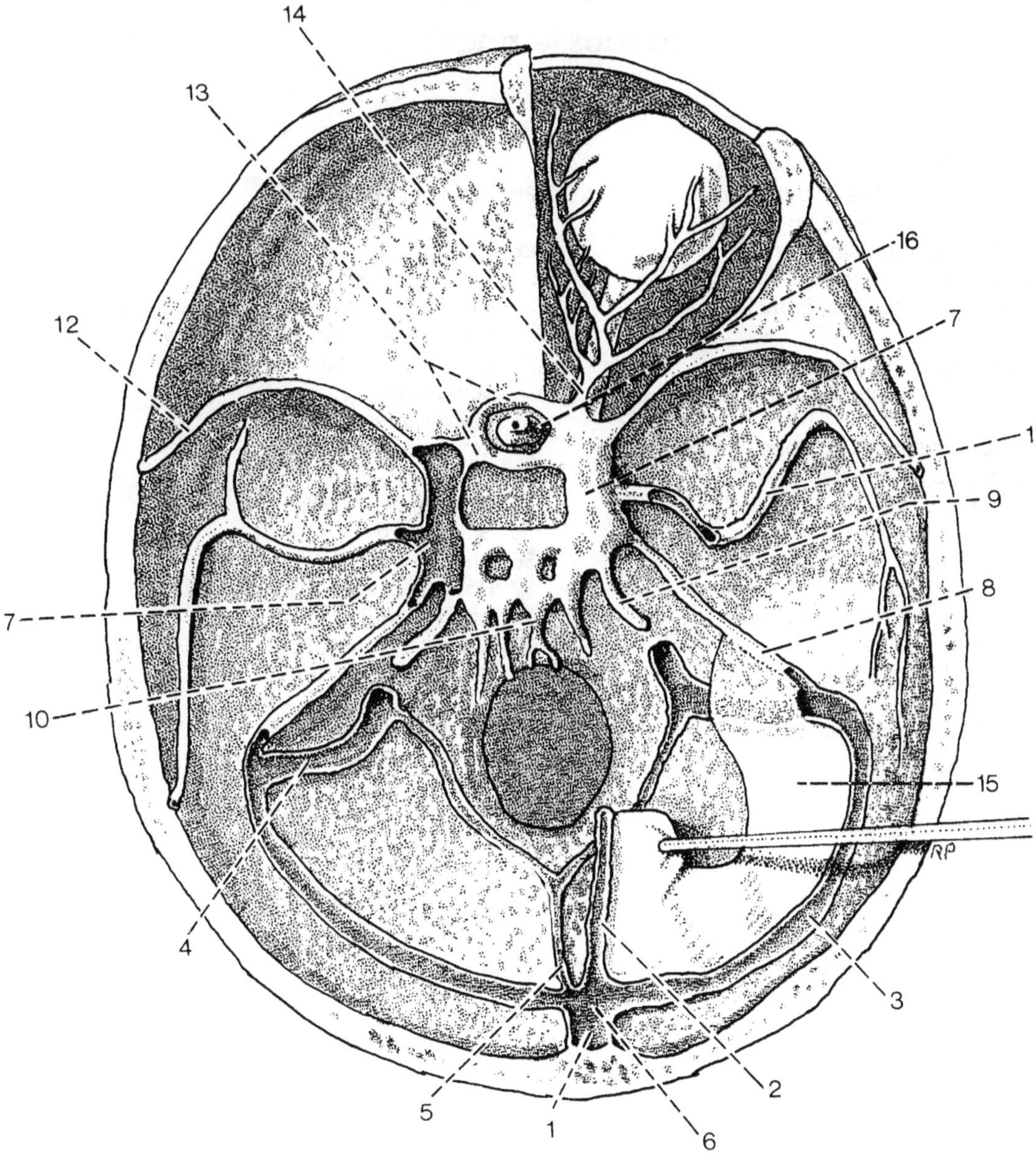

Color and label

1 Superior sagittal sinus (cut open)
2 Straight sinus (cut open)
3 Right transverse sinus (cut open)
4 Sigmoid sinus (cut open)
5 Occipital sinus
6 Confluence of sinuses
7 Cavernous sinus (cut open on left)
8 Superior petrosal sinus
9 Inferior petrosal sinus
10 Basilar venous plexus
11 Middle meningeal vein
12 Sphenoparietal sinus
13 Anterior and posterioir intercavernous sinuses
14 Superior ophthalmic vein
15 Tentorium cerebelli (cut and pulled to the right)
16 Pituitary gland (cut at stalk; also called hypophysis)

H&N-16 Head and neck

Midsagittal aspect

(opposite page)

Color and label

1 Scalp (skin and soft tissue covering the head that bears hair in both sexes)
2 Calavaria (the upper dome-like part of the skull or cranium, comprising the upper parts of the parietal, frontal and occipital bones)
3 Diploe (red bone marrow between the two layers of compact bone of the cranium)
4 Superior sagittal sinus (cut open to show opening of a superior cerebral vein)
5 Falx cerebri (a sickle-shaped fold of dura mater between the two cerebral hemispheres; *falx*, Latin, a sickle or scythe)
6 Inferior sagittal sinus
7 Crista galli (Latin, rooster's comb)
8 Straight sinus
9 Great cerebral vein
10 Confluence of sinuses
11 Opening of right transverse sinus
12 Occipital sinus
13 Falx cerebelli
14 Frontal sinus
15 Corpus callosum
16 Anterior cerebral artery
17 Septum pellucidum
18 Fornix
19 Thalamus and interthalamic adhesion
20 Optic chiasm
21 Pituitary gland (hypophysis)
22 Sphenoidal sinus
23 Mamillary body
24 Midbrain (mesencephalon)
25 Mesencephalic tectum
26 Pineal gland
27 Cerebral aqueduct
28 Cerebellum
29 Fourth ventricle
30 Cisternal magna (an enlargement of the subarachnoid space filled with cerebrospinal fluid under the cerebellum)
31 Basilar artery
32 Left vertebral artery
33 Pons
34 Medulla oblongata
35 Spinal cord
36 Anterior arch of atlas
37 Body and dens of atlas
38 Pharyngeal tonsil
39 Opening of auditory tube (eustachian tube)
40 Nasal pharynx
41 Middle nasa concha
42 Inferior nasal concha
43 Hard palate
44 Soft palate and uvula
45 Mandible
46 Hyoid bone
47 Genioglossus muscle
48 Geniohyoid muscle
49 Mylohyoid muscle
50 Epiglottis
51 Thyroid cartilage
52 Cricoid cartilage (arch and lamina)
53 Trachea
54 Oral pharynx
55 Laryngeal pharynx
56 Esophagus

H&N-16 Head and neck

Midsagittal aspect

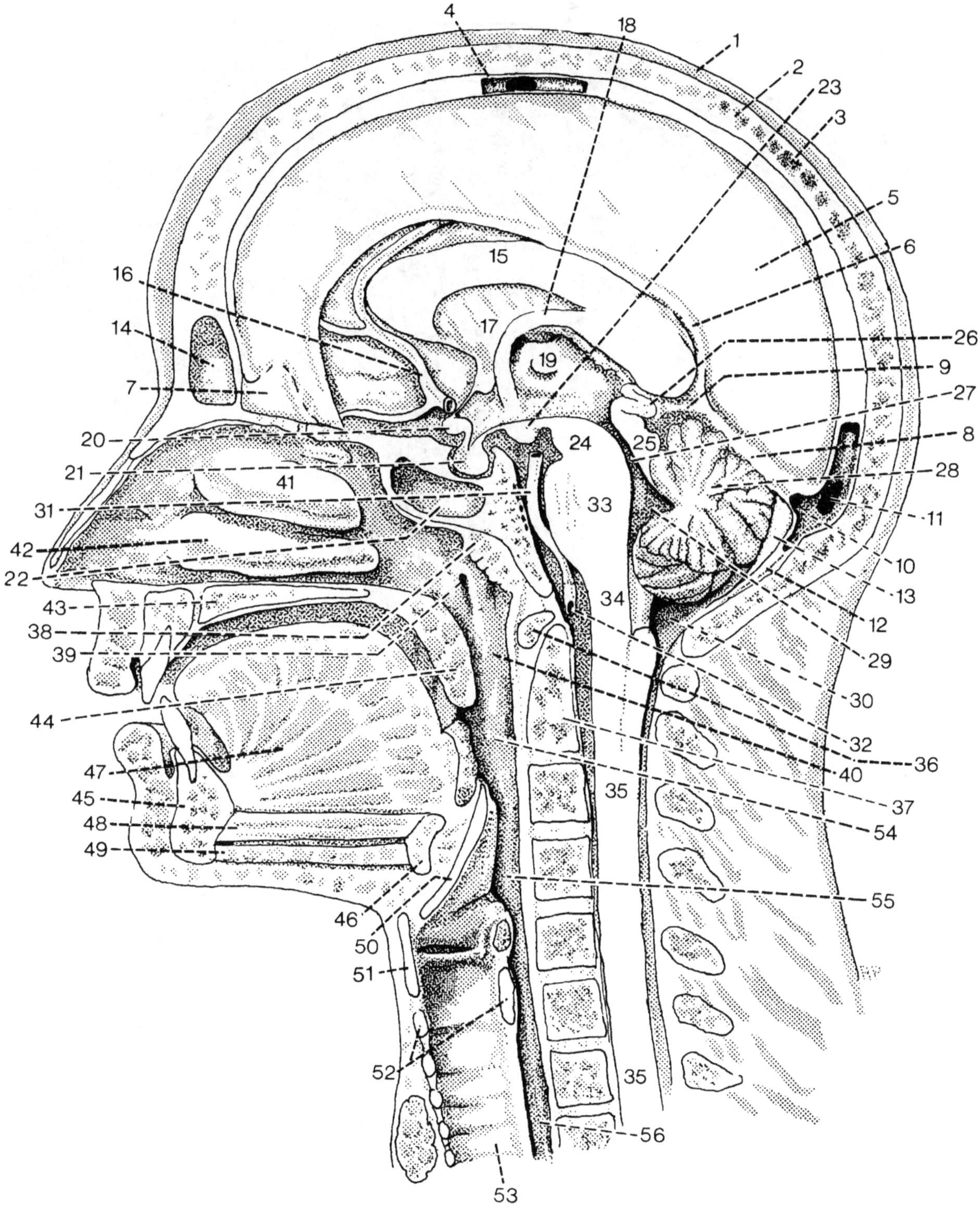

H&N-17 Superior sagittal sinus

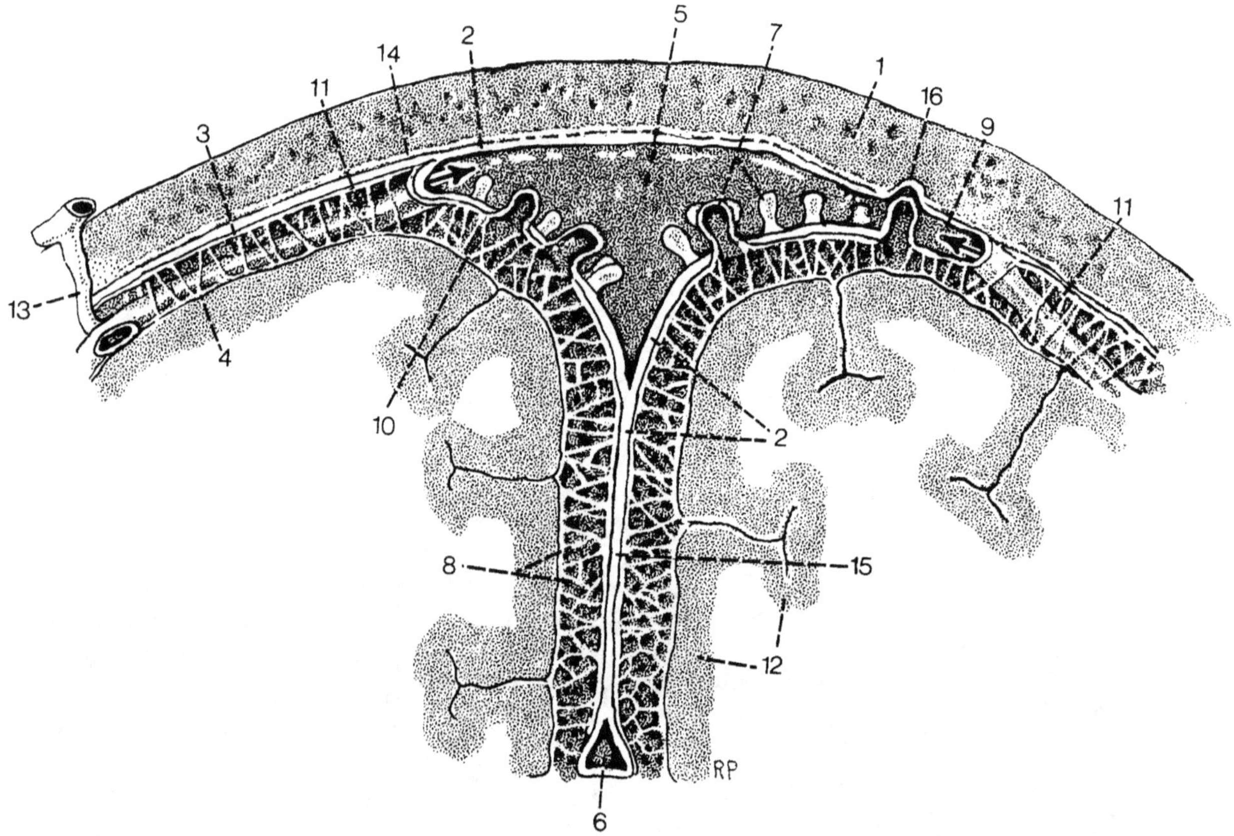

Color and label

1 Bone of skull
2 Dura mater (tough outermost membrane covering the brain and spinal cord)
3 Arachnoid (also called arachnoid membrane); closely applied to the inner surface of the dura mater; middle covering membrane (or meninx, plural, meninges)
4 Pia mater (innermost membrance investing the brain and spinal cord)
5 Superior sagittal sinus (large arched vein; drains blood from the brain, formed by walls of dura mater).
6 Inferior sagittal sinus
7 Arachnoid granulations; hollow finger-like projections into the superior sagittal sinus and its lateral expansions; these contain cerebrospinal fluid from the subarachnoid space which drains into and mixes with the venous blood of the superior sagittal sinus.
8 Arachnoid trabeculae; these form a mesh-work of small fibers that crisscross the subarachnoid space.
9 Lateral lacunae (outpouchings of the superior sagittal sinus)
10 Subarachnoid space (present between arachnoid and pia mater contains cerebrospinal fluid)
11 Superior cerebral vein emptying into superior sagittal sinus
12 Cerebral cortex
13 Emissary vein; these pass completely through the skull; link intracranial venous blood flow with external veins.
14 Periosteum of skull
15 Falx cerebri (*falx*, Latin, a sickle or scythe)
16 Pit on inside of skull caused by arachnoid granulation

H&N-18 Interior of the skull with cranial nerve exits

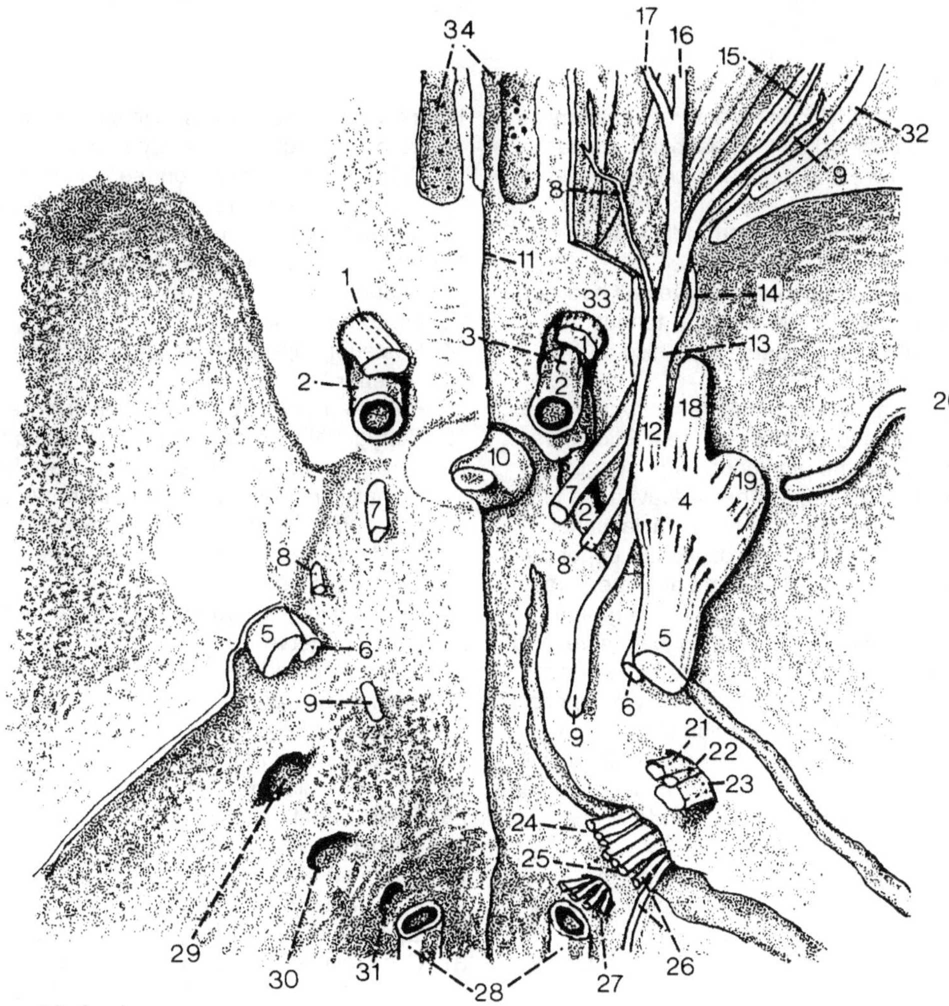

Color and label

1 Optic nerve (cranial nerve II) exiting skull through optic canal
2 Internal carotid artery
3 Ophthalmic artery arising from internal carotid
4 Trigeminal ganglion
5 Sensory root of trigeminal nerve
6 Motor root of trigeminal nerve
7 Oculomotor nerve (cranial nerve III)
8 Trochlear nerve (cranial nerve IV)
9 Abducent nerve (cranial nerve VI)
10 Pituitary gland (*pituita*, Latin, phlegm)*
11 Cut edge of dura mater
12 Ophthalmic nerve
13 Frontal nerve
14 Nasocilliary nerve
15 Lacrimal nerve
16 Supraorbital nerve
17 Supratrochlear nerve
18 Maxillary nerve
19 Mandibular nerve
20 Middle meningeal artery entering skull
21 Facial nerve motor root (cranial nerve VII)
22 Nervus intermedius of facial nerve (cranial nerve VII)
23 Vestibulocochlear nerve (cranial nerve VIII)
24 Glossopharyngeal nerve (cranial nerve IX)
25 Vagus nerve (cranial nerve X)
26 Accessory nerve (cranial nerve XI)
27 Hypoglossal nerve (cranial nerve XII)
28 Vertebral artery (right and left)
29 Internal acoustic meatus
30 Jugular foramen
31 Hypoglossal canal
32 Roof of orbit (cut and removed)
33 Roof of orbit
34 Cribriform plate (of ethmoid bone) with foramina for about 20 olfactory fila; each filum contains bundles of unmyelinated olfactory axons from olfactory receptors in the roof of the nasal cavity; the olfactory fila (not shown) collectively make up the olfactory nerve (cranial nerve I)

* See cartoon. Thalamus means bedroom.

H&N-19 Facial nerve and its branches

Color and label

1 Facial nerve; here lying in the internal auditory meatus accompanied by the vestibulocochlear nerve (not shown) and internal auditory vessels (not shown); taste fibers and parasympathetic fibers travel in the nervus intermedius part of the facial nerve.
2 Geniculate ganglion (contains nerve cell bodies of taste fibers to anterior two-thirds of tongue and some general sensory fibers to the skin of the external ear)
3 Greater petrosal nerve (carries taste fibers to the palate and preganglionic parasympathetic fibers, which synapse in the pterygopalatine ganglion)
4 Chorda tympani nerve; this nerve leaves the facial nerve in its descending part of the facial canal, enters the tympanic cavity, crosses the upper part of the internal surface of the tympanic membrane (hence its name), leaves the skull through the petrotympanic fissure, joins the lingual nerve, and supplies the taste buds on the anterior two-thirds of the tongue. Its preganglionic parasympathetic fibers synapse in the submandibular ganglion.
5 Nerve to stapedius muscle (damage to the facial nerve proximal to this branch will cause stapedius to lose its damping action and sounds will be unusually loud)
6 Lingual nerve (cut; part of the mandibular nerve)
7 Deep petrosal nerve (postganglionic sympathetic fibers from the internal carotid plexus)
8 Nerve of pterygoid canal (note that it consists of the deep petrosal nerve and the greater petrosal nerve)
9 Pterygopalatine ganglion (contains postganglionic parasympathetic neurons whose secretomotor fibers enter the nasal cavity and supply glands and vessels in the nose)
10 Internal carotid plexus (sympathetic nerve fibers from cell bodies in the superior cervical ganglion)
11 Submandibular ganglion (sends postganglionic secretomotor fibers to the submandibular gland and sublingual salivary glands)
12 Maxillary nerve (cut; exiting skull via foramen rotundum)
13 Infraorbital nerve
14 Posterior superior alveolar nerve (to posterior superior teeth)
15 Palatine nerves (descend to supply palate)
16 Pterygopalatine nerves (convey postganglionic parasympathetic secretomotor fibers from ganglion to maxillary nerve to zygomatic nerve to lacrimal nerve to lacrimal gland)
17 Middle superior alveolar nerve (to superior teeth)
18 Zygomatic nerve
19 Communicating branch to lacrimal nerve
20 Lacrimal nerve
21 Internal carotid artery
22 Mastoid process
23 Styloid process
24 Ear drum and malleus
25 Stylomastoid foramen
26 Facial canal
27 Carotid canal
28 Foramen lacerum
29 Medial pterygoid plate
30 Canal and groove for greater petrosal nerve
31 Orbit (eye and muscles removed)
32 Internal acoustic meatus (roof removed)

H&N-19 Facial nerve and its branches

Lateral view of facial nerve with internal auditory meatus and canal exposed, carotid canal opened, and greater wing of sphenoid removed

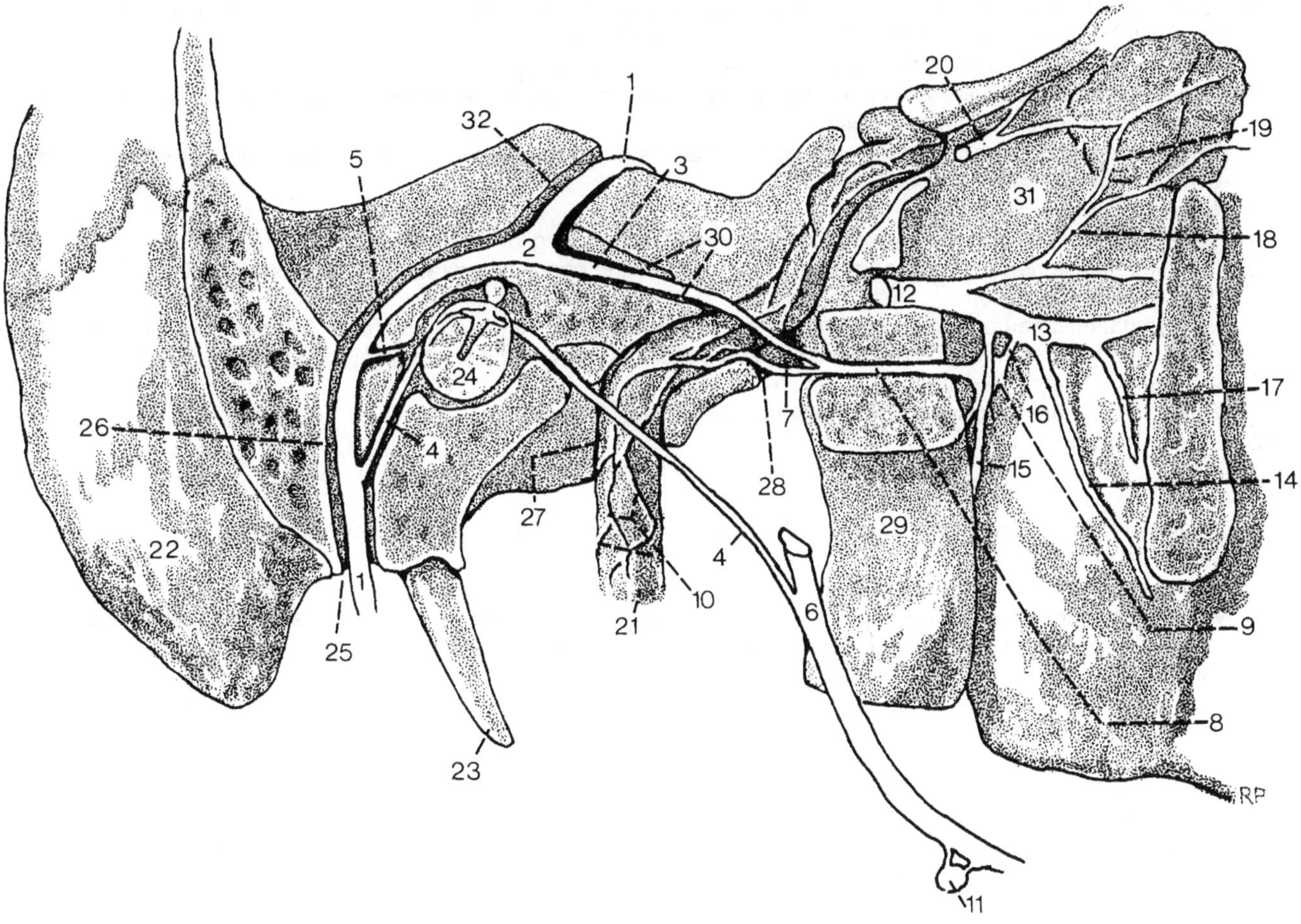

H&N-20 Functional components of the facial nerve

(opposite page)

Color and label these nerve cells and their fibers (axons)

1 Motor neuron to muscles of facial expression (also to platysma, stapedius, stylohyoid, and posterior belly of digastric)
2 Facial motor nucleus
3 Parasympathetic neuron (preganglionic secretomotor) to submandibular ganglion
4 Parasympathetic neuron (preganglionic secretomotor) to pterygopalatine ganglion
5 Superior salivatory ganglion
6 Cell body of neuron carrying taste from the tongue via chorda tympani nerve; note this neuron resides in the geniculate, or "bent", (*genu*, Latin, knee) ganglion of the facial nerve
7 Cell body of neuron carrying taste from the palate via the greater petrosal nerve
8 Neuron in nucleus of solitary tract; this neuron receives taste from incoming neuron taste fiber of neuron 6 and relays it to higher centers (not shown)
9 Neuron in nucleus of solitary tract; this neuron receives taste from incoming neuron taste fiber of neuron 7 and relays it to higher centers (not shown)
10 Nucleus of solitary tract
11 Parasympathetic neuron (postganglionic) in pterygopalatine ganglion secretomotor to lacrimal gland
12 Parasympathetic neuron (postganglionic) in pterygopalatine ganglion secretomotor to nasal glands
13 Pterygopalatine ganglion
14 Parasympathetic neuron (postganglionic) in submandibular ganglion secretomotor to submandibular gland
15 Parasympathetic neuron (postganglionic) in submandibular ganglion secretomotor to sublingual gland
16 Sympathetic neuron (preganglionic) in spinal cord
17 Sympathetic neuron (postganglionic) in superior cervial ganglion
18 Superior cervical ganglion
19 Internal carotid plexus
20 Geniculate ganglion of facial nerve
21 Greater petrosal nerve; note it carries both taste and parasympathetic fibers (parasympathetic root of pterygopalatine ganglion)
22 Deep petrosal nerve
23 Nerve of pterygoid canal; note it consists of taste fibers from the palate (neuron 9), parasympathetic fibers to the palate (neuron 4), and sympathetic fibers (fibers 22) to blood vessels and glands in the nose.
24 Nerve to tiny stapedius muscle in middle ear
25 Chorda tympani; note this nerve is a branch of the intermediate nerve of the facial nerve. It carries incoming taste from the tongue (neuron 6) and outgoing parasympathetic fibers to the submandibular gangion (neuron 3). In this sense, the chorda tympani nerve functions as the parasympathetic root of submandibular ganglion.
26 Facial canal
27 Stylomastoid foramen
28 Maxillary nerve in foramen rotundum (a small portion)
29 Lacrimal nerve (a branch of the ophthalmic nerve); it recieves its parasympathetic secretomotor fibers from nerve 11 in the pterygopalatine ganglion
30 Zygomatic nerve
31 Zygomaticotemporal nerve
32 Communicating branch between zygomaticotemporal nerve and lacrimal nerve
33 Facial nerve exiting stylomastoid foramen
34 Genu (or geniculum) "bend" or "knee" of facial nerve
35 Submandibular ganglion

Each nerve cell (or neuron) diagramatically represents hundred or even thousands of similarly directed neurons.

A **nucleus** is a group of nerve cells in the brain or spinal cord. A similar collection of neurons outside the brain and spinal cord is called **ganglion.**

H&N-20 Functional components of the facial nerve

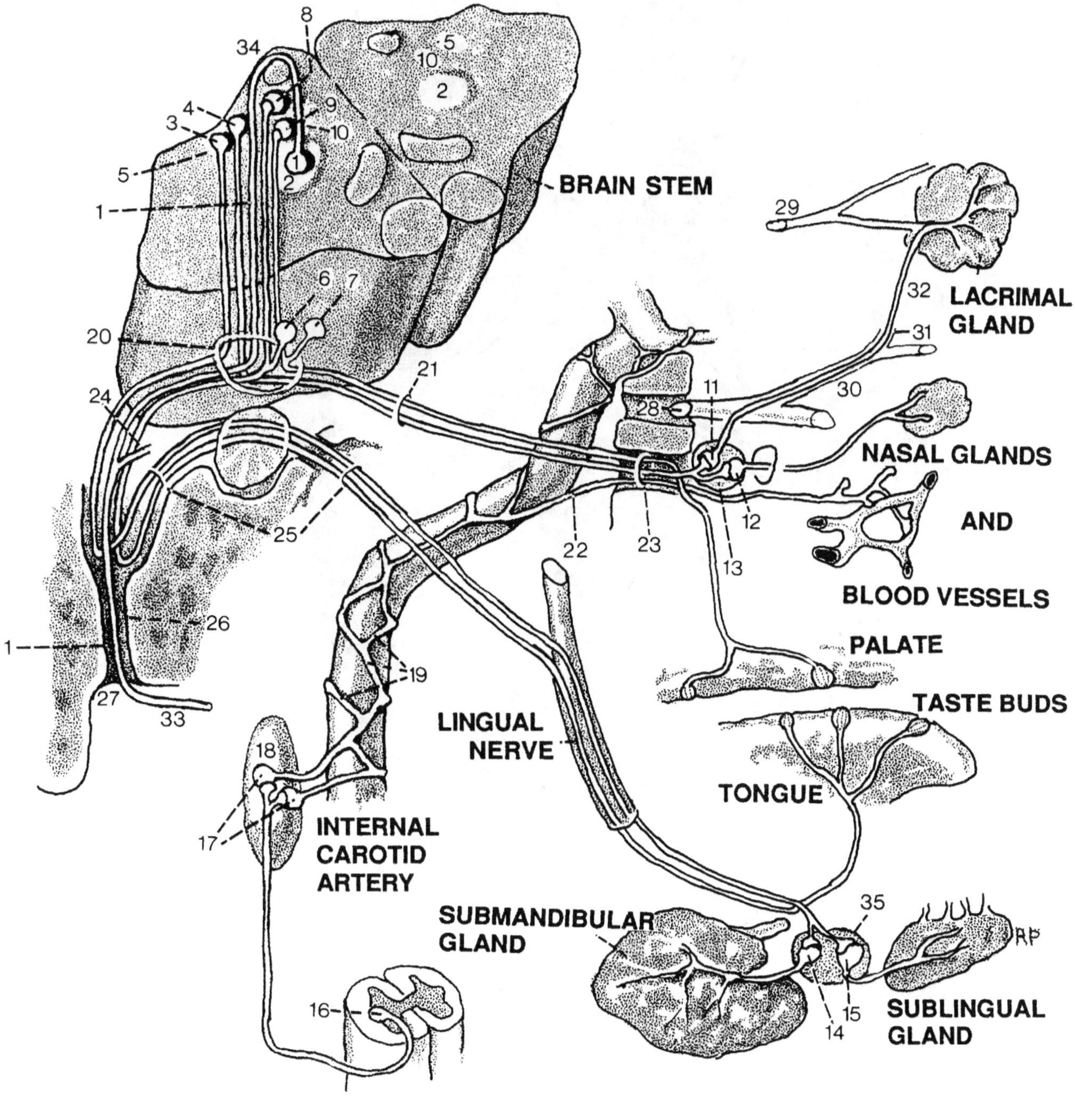

H&N-21 Inferior surface of skull

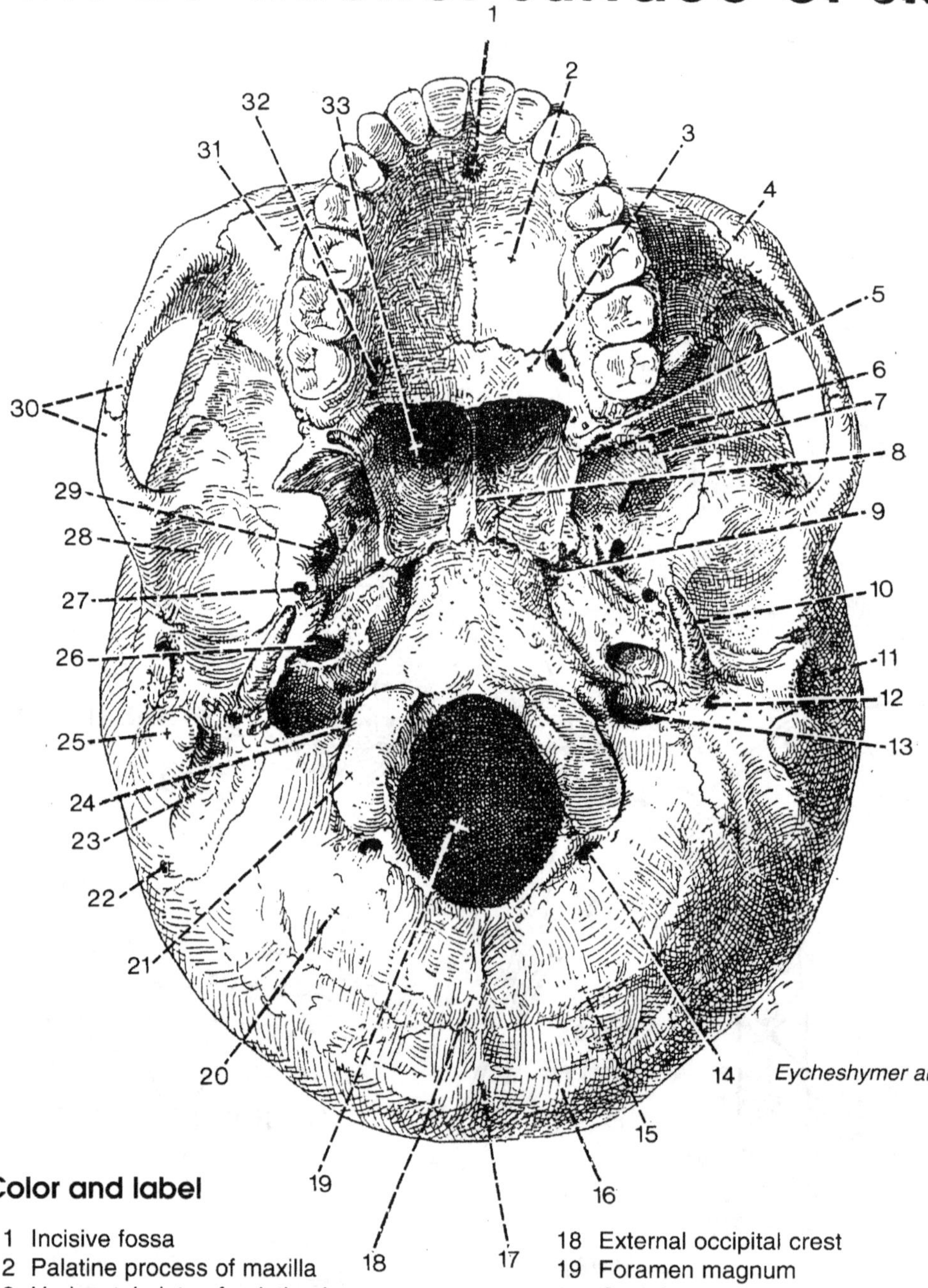

Eycheshymer and Jones

Color and label

1 Incisive fossa
2 Palatine process of maxilla
3 Horizontal plate of palatine bone
4 Zygomatic bone
5 Pterygoid hamulus
6 Medial pterygoid plate
7 Lateral pterygoid plate
8 Vomer
9 Foramen lacerum
10 Stylomastoid process
11 External acoustic meatus
12 Stylomastoid foramen
13 Jugular foramen
14 Condylar foramen
15 Inferior nuchal line
16 Superior nuchal line
17 External occipital protuberance
18 External occipital crest
19 Foramen magnum
20 Occipital bone
21 Occipital condyle
22 Mastoid foramen
23 Mastoid notch
24 Hypoglossal canal
25 Mastoid process
26 Carotid canal
27 Foramen spinosum
28 Mandibular fossa
29 Foramen ovale
30 Zygomatic arch
31 Maxilla
32 Greater and lesser palatine foramina
33 Posterior nasal aperature (choana)

Temporal
Etymological cartoon

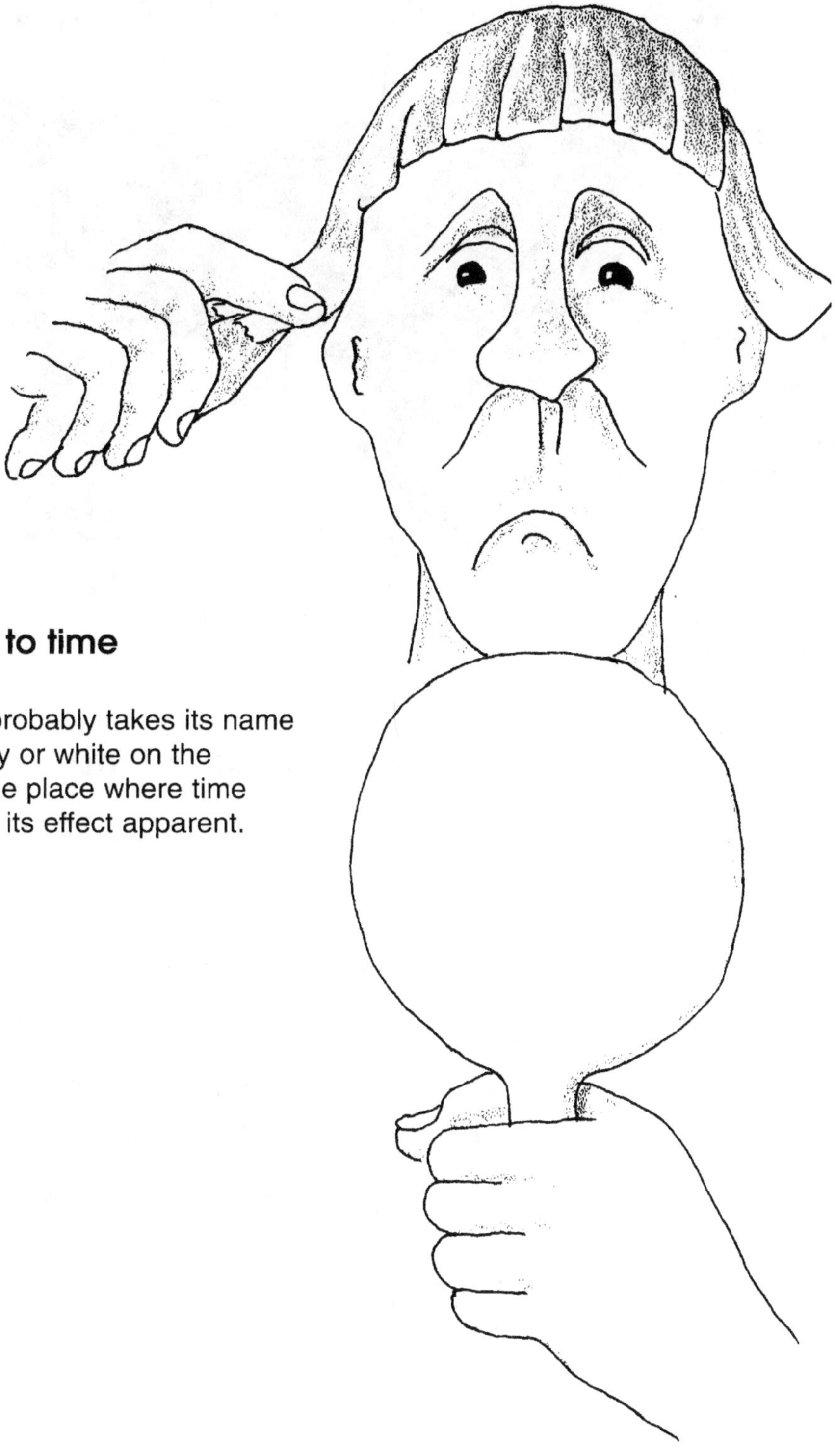

Latin, pertaining to time

The temporal bone probably takes its name from hair turning gray or white on the temples. Thus it is the place where time (tempus) first makes its effect apparent.

H&N-22 Sphenoid bone

Viewed from the front

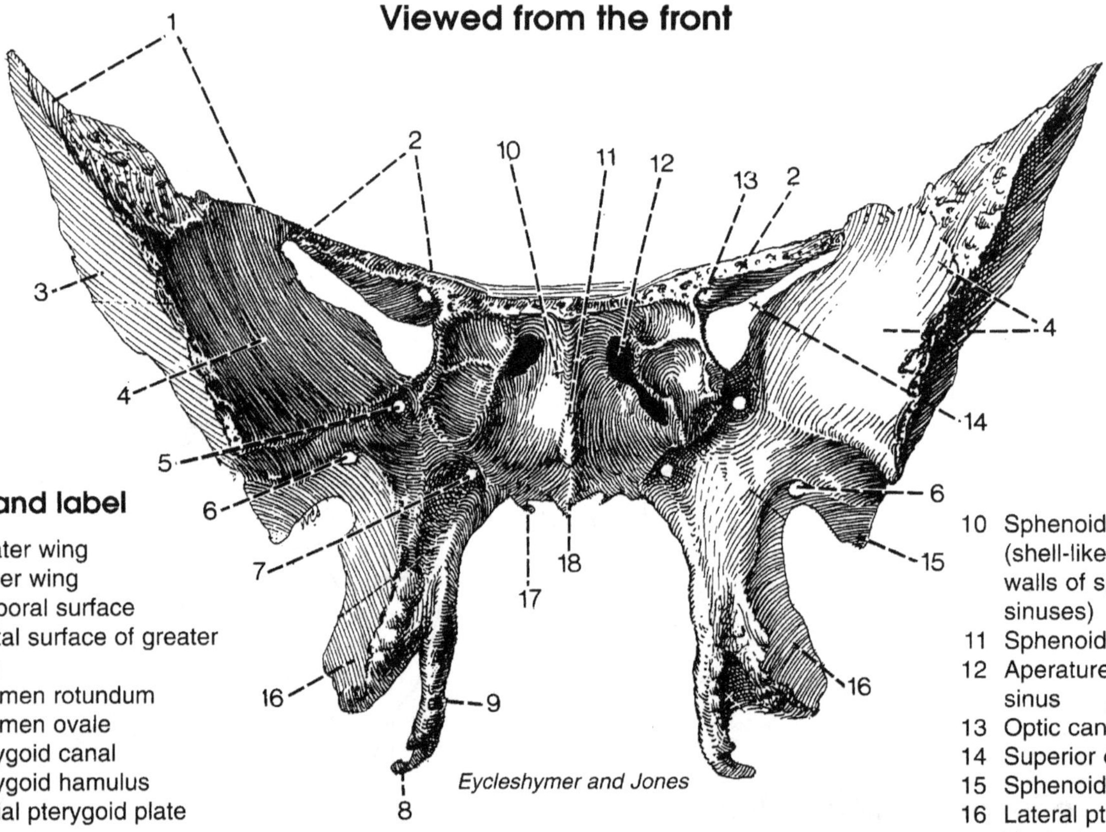

Color and label

1 Greater wing
2 Lesser wing
3 Temporal surface
4 Orbital surface of greater wing
5 Foramen rotundum
6 Foramen ovale
7 Pterygoid canal
8 Pterygoid hamulus
9 Medial pterygoid plate
10 Sphenoid conchae (shell-like anterior walls of sphenoid sinuses)
11 Sphenoidal crest
12 Aperature to sphenoid sinus
13 Optic canal
14 Superior orbital fissure
15 Sphenoidal spine
16 Lateral pterygoid plate
17 Vaginal process
18 Rostrum

Viewed from behind

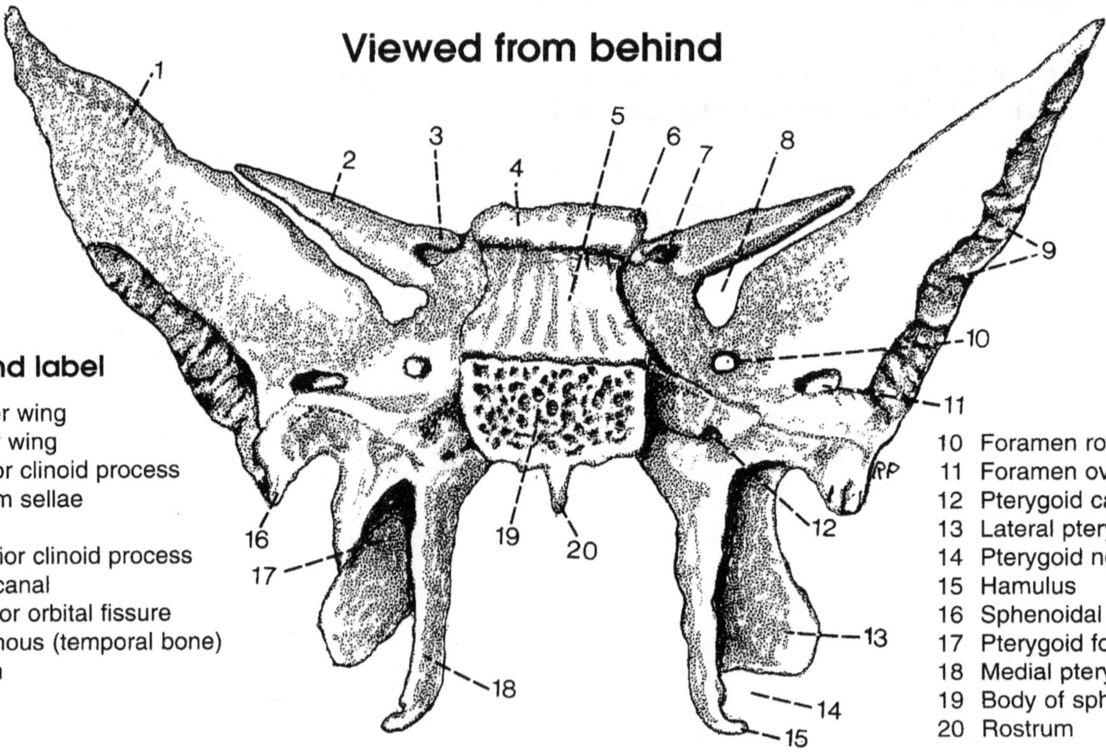

Color and label

1 Greater wing
2 Lesser wing
3 Anterior clinoid process
4 Dorsum sellae
5 Clivus
6 Posterior clinoid process
7 Optic canal
8 Superior orbital fissure
9 Squamous (temporal bone) margin
10 Foramen rotundum
11 Foramen ovale
12 Pterygoid canal
13 Lateral pterygoid plate
14 Pterygoid notch
15 Hamulus
16 Sphenoidal spine
17 Pterygoid fossa
18 Medial pterygoid plate
19 Body of sphenoid bone
20 Rostrum

H&N-23 Temporal bone

External surface viewed from the right

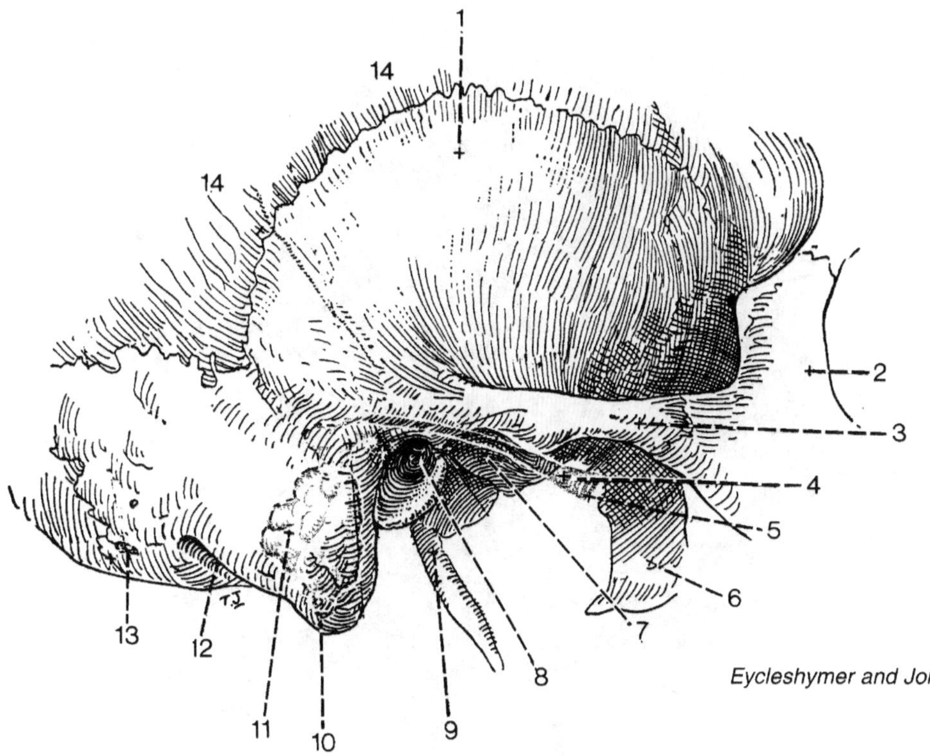

Eycleshymer and Jones

Color and label

1 Squamous part (scale-like, flat, and thin; *squama*, Latin, scale)
2 Zygomatic bone
3 Zygomatic process of temporal bone
4 Auditory tube (eustachian tube, cartilaginous part; this tube connects the middle ear with the nasopharynx; when temporarily opened it equalizes air pressure in the middle ear with the ambient air pressure)
5 Pharyngeal ostium (mouth) of auditory tube
6 Lateral pterygoid plate
7 Mandibular fossa (articulates with head of mandible; forms temporomandibular joint)
8 External acoustic meatus (bony part of ear canal)
9 Styloid process
10 Mastoid (breast-like, *mastos*, Greek, breast)
11 Mastoid air cells inside mastoid process (before antibiotics, infection of these air sinuses could be treated only by surgically scraping out most of the mastoid process air cells.
12 Mastoid notch (posterior belly of digastric muscle attaches to ridge; occipital artery lies in groove)
13 Mastoid foramen (through which passes an emissary vein)
14 Parietal bone

H&N-24 Temporal bone

Right bone. Viewed from the inside

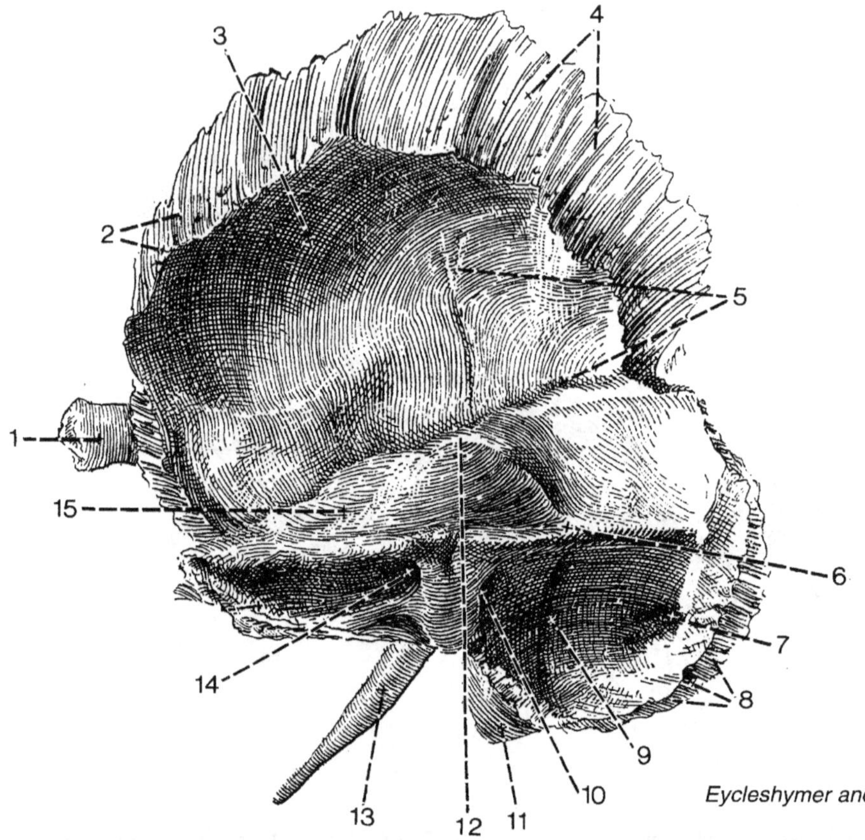

Eycleshymer and Jones

Color and label

1 Zygomatic process
2 Sphenoidal margin
3 Cerebral surface of squamous part
4 Parietal margin
5 Grooves for parietal branches of middle meningeal artery and accompanying veins
6 Groove for superior petrosal sinus
7 Mastoid foramen
8 Occipital margin
9 Sulcus for sigmoid sinus
10 Opening of vestibular aqueduct (contains endolymphatic duct, which forms endolymphatic sac at its end next to the dura mater)
11 Mastoid process
12 Arcuate eminence (marks position of anterior semicircular canal)
13 Styloid process
14 Internal acoustic opening (into which pass the facial nerve, vestibulocochlear nerve, and internal auditory artery)

H&N-25 Superficial muscles of the neck

The platysma has been removed.

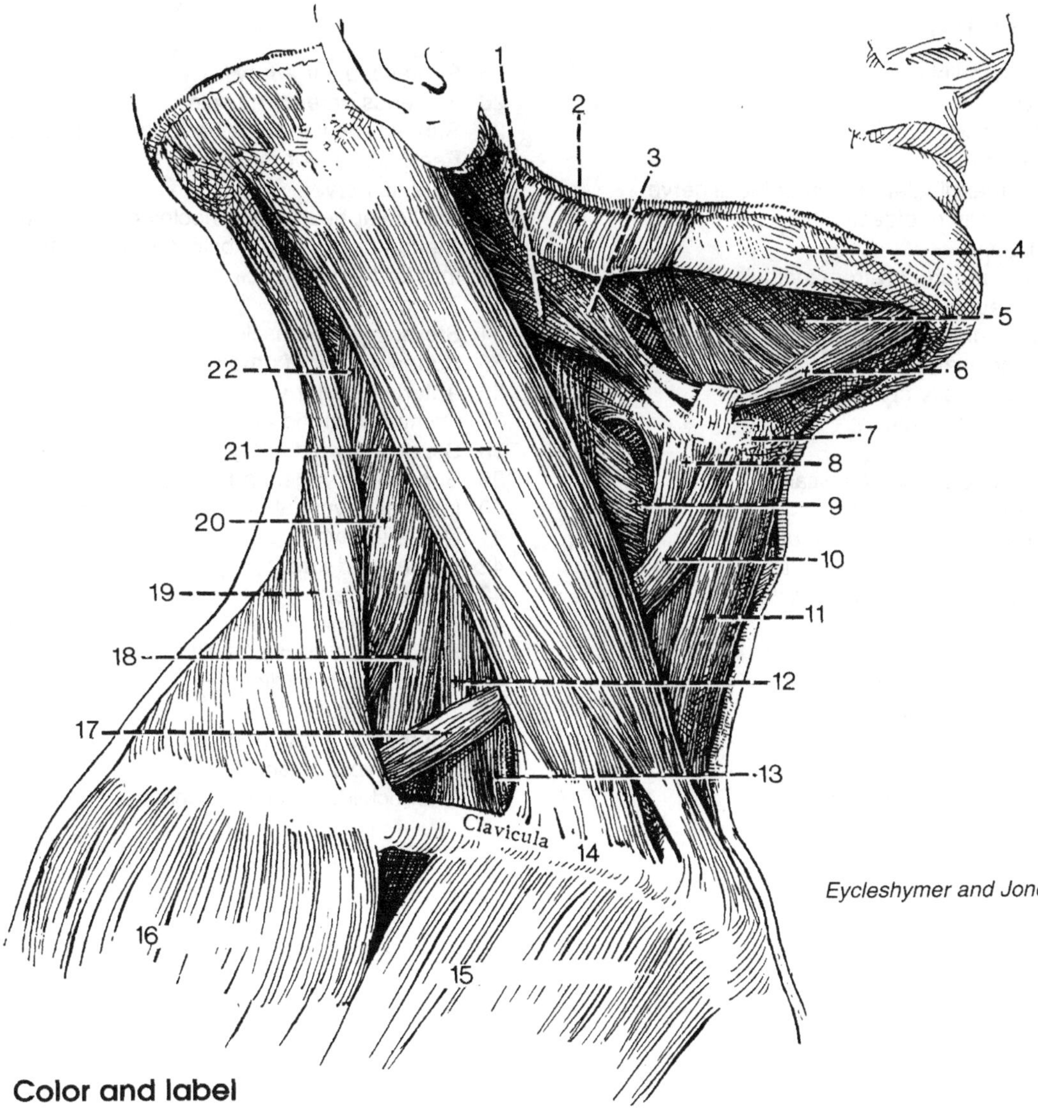

Eycleshymer and Jones

Color and label

1 Posterior belly of digastric
2 Masseter
3 Stylohyoid
4 Mandible
5 Mylohyoid
6 Anterior belly of digastric
7 Hyoid bone
8 Thyrohyoid
9 Inferior pharyngeal constrictor
10 Superior belly of omohyoid
11 Sternohyoid
12 Scalenus medius
13 Scalenus anterior
14 Clavicle
15 Pectoralis major
16 Deltoid
17 Inferior belly of omohyoid
18 Scalenus posterior
19 Trapezius
20 Levator scapulae
21 Sternocleidomastoid
22 Splenius capitis

H&N-26 Left side of neck I

Platysma and deep cervical fascia have been removed

(opposite page)

Color and label

1 Body of mandible
2 Facial vein
3 Buccal fat pad
4 Facial artery
5 Marginal mandibular branch of facial nerve
6 Posterior belly of digastric muscle
7 Parotid gland
8 Posterior branch of retromandibular vein
9 Posterior auricular vein
10 Great auricular nerve
11 Lesser occipital nerve
12 Jugulodigastric lymph nodes
13 External jugular vein
14 Facial vein
15 Superior root of ansa cervicalis on internal carotid artery
16 Transverse cervical nerve (cut)
17 Accessory nerve (N XI) supplies trapezius and sternocleidomastoid muscles
18 Cervical nerves to trapezius
19 Trapezius muscle
20 Superficial cervical vein
21 Upper trunk of brachial plexus
22 Superficial cervical artery
23 Suprascapular nerve
24 Inferior belly of omohyoid muscle
25 Suprascapular artery
26 Scalenus anterior muscle
27 Supraclavicular nerves and their branches
28 Pectoralis major muscle
29 Phrenic nerve
30 Clavicular head of sternocleidomastoid muscle
31 Sternal head of sternocleidomastoid muscle
32 Inferior thyroid vein
33 Thyroid gland
34 Sternothyroid muscle
35 Superior belly of omohyoid muscle
36 Anterior jugular vein
37 Common carotid artery
38 Superior thyroid artery and external laryngeal nerve
39 Superior laryngeal artery
40 Internal laryngeal nerve
41 Nerve to thyrohyoid
42 Suprahyoid artery
43 Lingual artery
44 Body of hyoid bone
45 Hypoglossal nerve (N XII)
46 Anterior belly of digastric
47 Submandibular gland
48 Submental artery and vein
49 Sternohyoid muscle
50 Sternocleidomastoid muscle

H&N-26 Left side of neck I

From the left and front

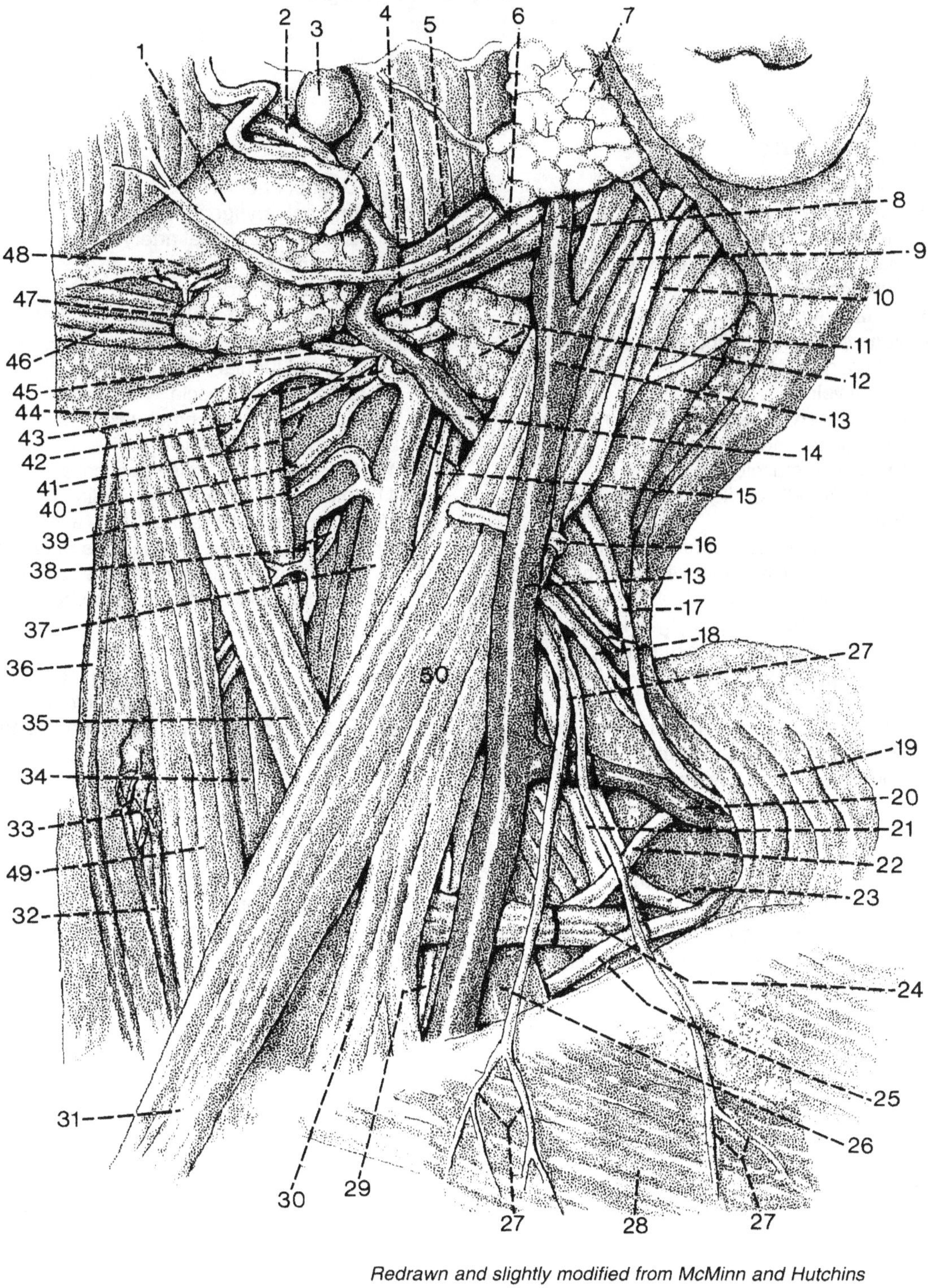

Redrawn and slightly modified from McMinn and Hutchins

H&N-27 Left side of neck II

Deep dissection. Most of the sternocleidomastoid and submandibular gland have been removed.

(opposite page)

Color and label

1 Hyoid bone
2 Anterior belly of digastric muscle
3 Suprahyoid artery
4 Marginal mandibular branch of facial nerve (N VII)
5 Submental artery
6 Facial artery
7 Vena comitans (Latin, vein running with) of hypoglossal nerve
8 Facial vein
9 Facial artery (arising from external carotid artery)
10 Hypoglossal nerve (N XII)
11 Stylohyoid muscle
12 Posterior belly of digastric muscle
13 Parotid gland
14 Sternocleidomastoid muscle (cut)
15 Second cervical nerve ventral ramus
16 Great auricular nerve
17 Carotid sinus at beginning of internal carotid artery (a baroreceptor or pressure receptor; the internal carotid gives off no branches in the neck)
18 Lesser occipital nerve
19 Third cervical nerve ventral ramus
20 Communicating ramus between nerves C3 and C4
21 Fourth cervical nerve ventral ramus
22 Fifth cervical nerve ventral ramus
23 Accessory nerve (N XI)
24 Scalenus medius muscle
25 Upper trunk of brachial plexus
26 Dorsal scapular nerve
27 Trapezius muscle (motor innervation: accessory nerve; sensory: cervical plexus)
28 Thyrohyoid muscle
29 Lingual artery
30 Internal laryngeal nerve
31 Superior laryngeal artery
32 External carotid artery
33 Superior thyroid artery
34 External laryngeal nerve
35 Common carotid artery
36 Internal jugular vein
37 Sternohyoid muscle
38 Superior belly of omohyoid
39 Sternothyroid muscle
40 Superior root of ansa cervicalis
41 Inferior root of ansa cervicalis
42 Ansa cervicalis (*ansa*, Latin, a loop or handle, probably related to a goose's neck, *anser*, goose)
43 Ramus of the ansa cervicalis to the infrahyoid muscles (also called strap muscles)
44 Omohyoid tendon
45 Inferior thyroid artery
46 Thyrocervical trunk (splitting into three arteries)
47 Clavicular head of sternocleidomastoid (cut)
48 Thoracic duct (emptying lymph into the subclavian vein)
49 Subclavian vein
50 Phrenic nerve (motor nerve to the diaphragm; arises mainly from cervical nerve C4)
51 Scalenus anterior muscle
52 Superficial cervical artery
53 Suprascapular artery
54 Suprascapular nerve
55 Inferior belly of omohyoid
56 Scalenus medius muscle

H&N-27 Left side of neck II

Deep dissection

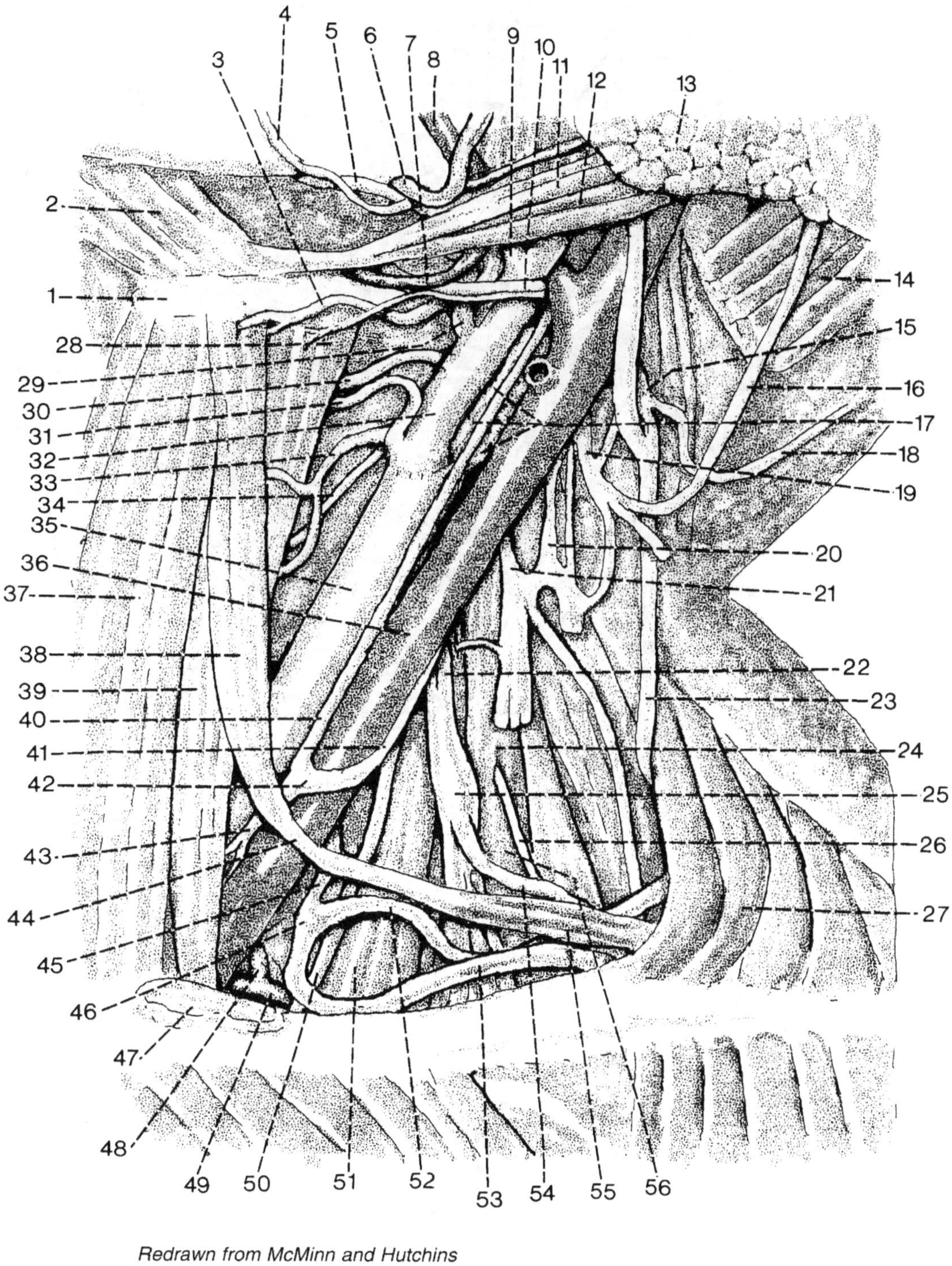

Redrawn from McMinn and Hutchins

H&N-28 Mandibular nerve and maxillary artery I

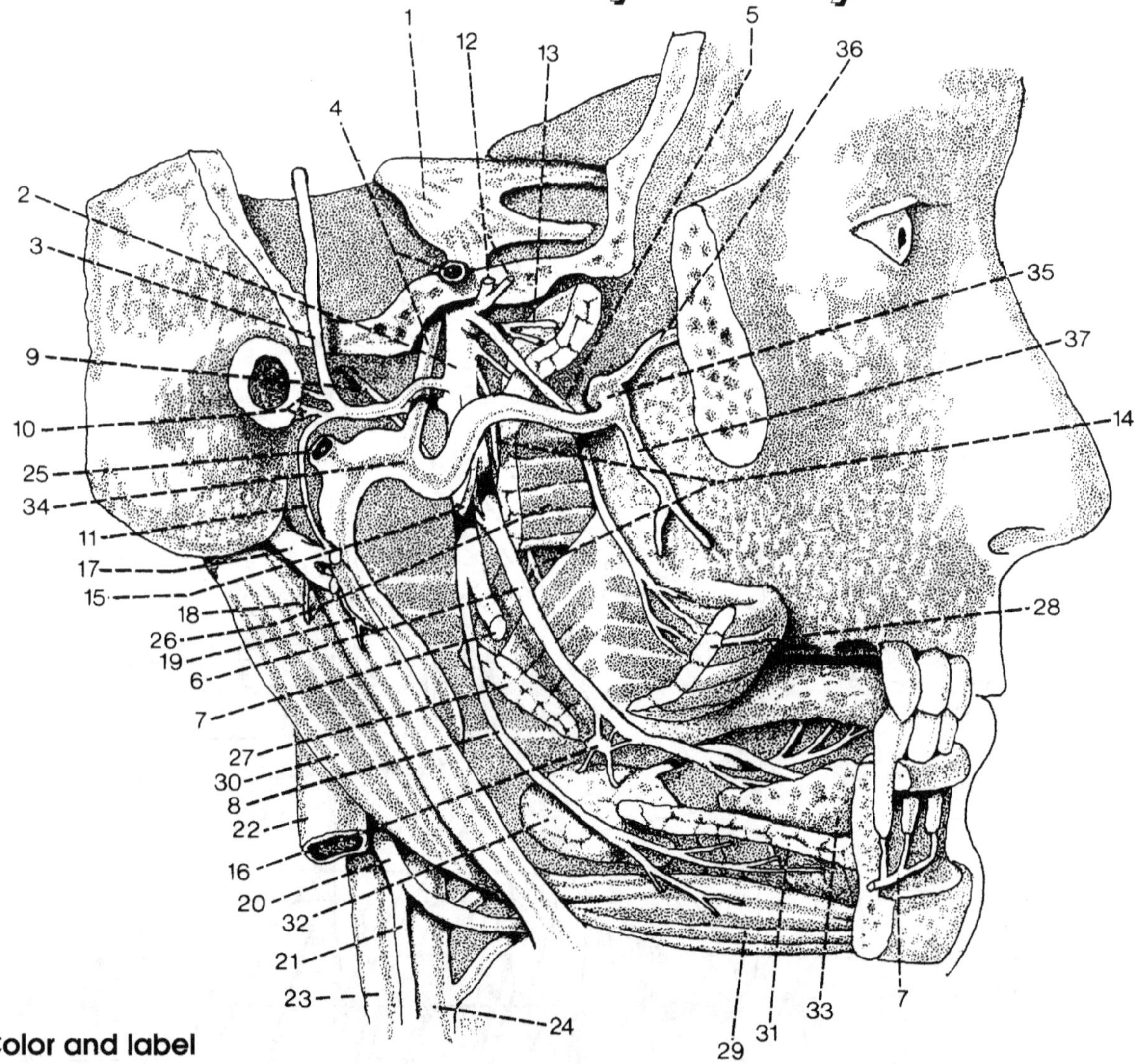

Color and label

1 Trigeminal ganglion
2 Mandibular nerve
3 Auriculotemporal nerve (notice its two roots surrounding the middle meningeal artery)
4 Middle meningeal artery
5 Buccal nerve (sensory to mucous membrane and skin of cheek)
6 Lingual nerve (supplies general sensation to anterior two-thirds of tongue)
7 Inferior alveolar nerve (cut)
8 Mylohyoid nerve (motor to mylohyoid muscle and anterior belly of digastric muscle)
9 Chorda tympani (branch of facial nerve carrying taste fibers and parasympathetic fibers to lingual nerve; exits skull through petrotympanic fissure)
10 External acoustic meatus nerves
11 Communicating branch with facial nerve
12 Deep temporal nerves (motor to temporalis muscle)
13 Lateral pterygoid nerve
14 Medial pterygoid nerve
15 Masseteric nerve
16 Submandibular ganglion
17 Facial nerve
18 Digastric branch of facial nerve (motor to posterior belly of digastric muscle)
19 Stylohyoid branch of facial nerve
20 Hypoglossal nerve
21 Superior root of ansa cervicalis
22 Internal jugular vein
23 Internal carotid artery
24 External carotid artery
25 Superficial temporal artery
26 Lateral pterygoid muscle (cut)
27 Medial pterygoid muscle (cut)
28 Buccinator muscle (cut and reflected)
29 Anterior belly of digastric muscle
30 Posterior belly of digastric muscle
31 Mylohyoid muscle (cut)
32 Sublingual gland (notice its duct crossing the lingual nerve)
33 Sublingual gland
34 Maxillary artery (most of its branches are not shown)
35 Sphenopalatine artery entering nasal cavity through sphenopalatine foramen
36 Infraorbital artery
37 Posterior superior alveolar artery

H&N-29 Mandibular nerve and maxillary artery, II

Color and label

1 Right carotid artery
2 Maxillary artery
3 Superficial temporal artery (cut)
4 Middle meningeal artery (entering skull through foramen spinosum)
5 Posterior superior alveolar arteries
6 Infraorbital artery
7 Sphenopalatine artery
8 Pterygopalatine fossa
9 Sphenopalatine foramen
10 Mandibular nerve (exiting foramen ovale)
11 Deep temporal nerves (to temporal muscle)
12 Buccal nerve (sensory to cheek mucous membrane)
13 Lingual nerve (sensory to anterior two-thrids of tongue)
14 Inferior alveolar nerve (cut; sensory to teeth of lower jaw)
15 Mylohyoid nerve (to mylohyoid muscle and anterior belly of digastric)
16 Chorda tympani nerve (branch of facial nerve carrying taste from anterior two-thirds of tongue and parasympathetic fibers to sublingual and submandibular glands)
17 Auriculotemporal nerve (sensory to skin in front of ear and side of head)
18 Facial nerve (cut)
19 Posterior superior alveolar nerve (branch of maxillary nerve; sensory to upper posterior teeth)
20 Carotid canal
21 Jugular foramen
22 Styloid process (right and left)
23 Occipital condyle (right)
24 Hamulus of medial pterygoid plates (right and left)
25 Foramen magnum
26 Petrotympanic fissure
27 Stylomastoid foramen (facial nerve exits skull here)

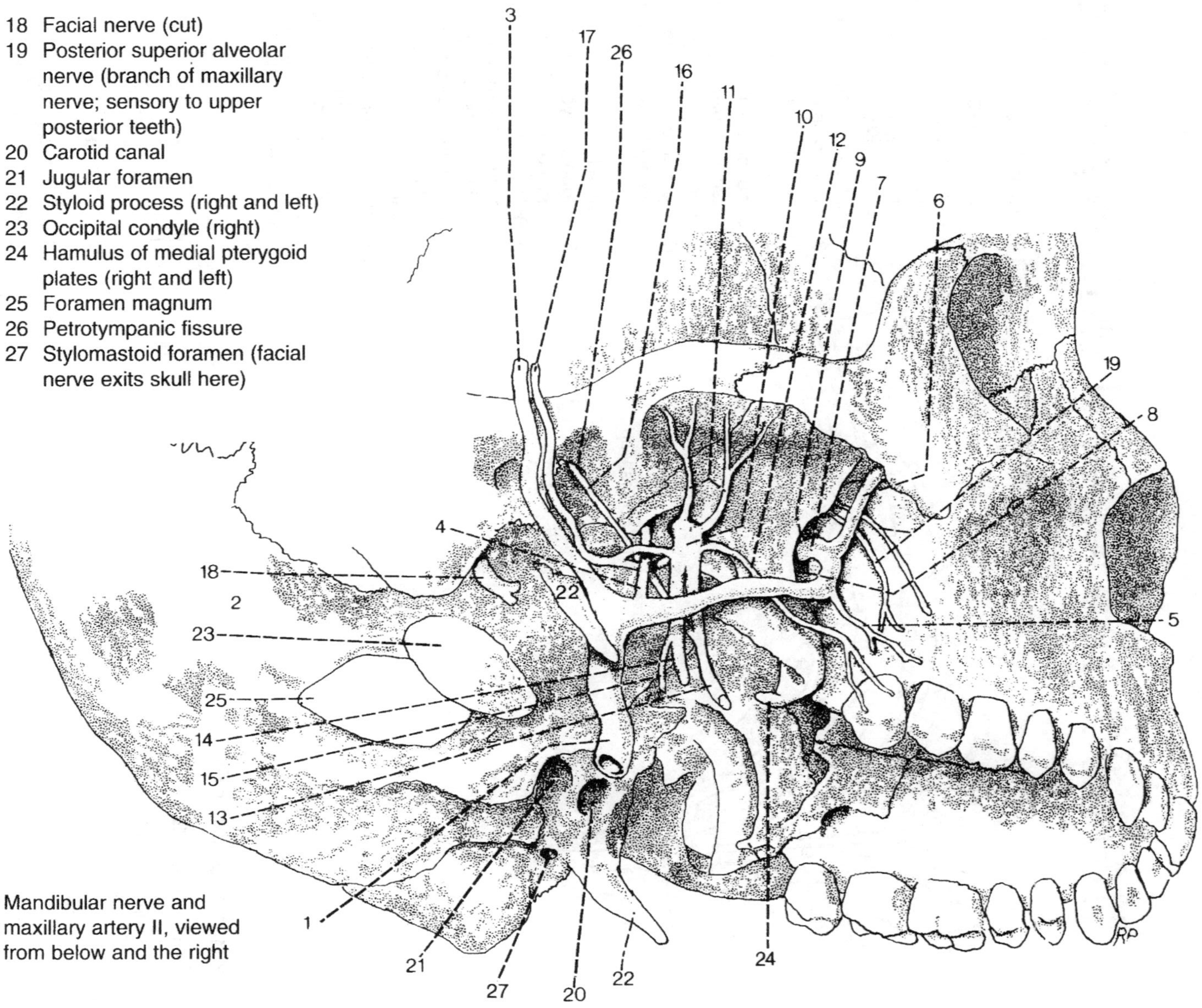

Mandibular nerve and maxillary artery II, viewed from below and the right

H&N-30 The eyelid and eye in orbit

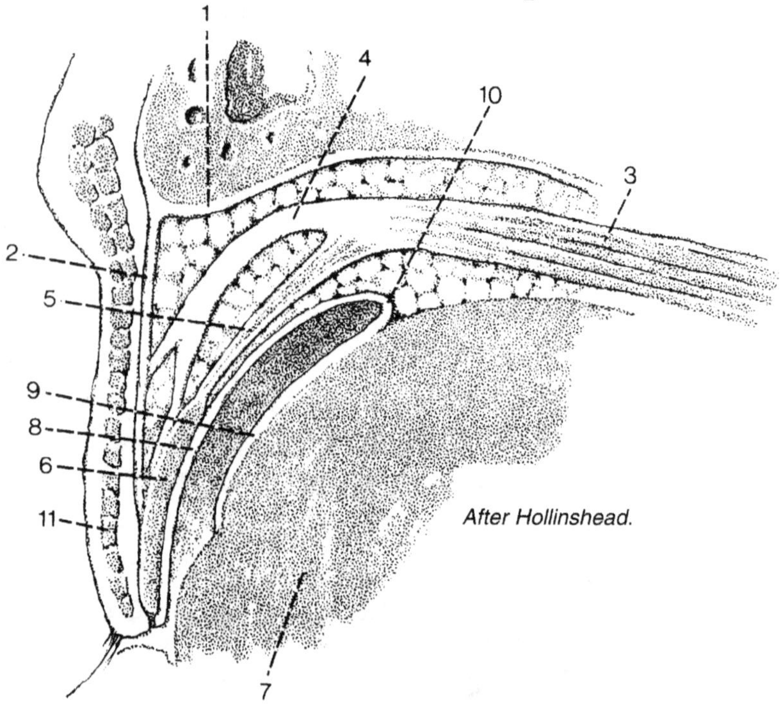

After Hollinshead.

Upper eyelid

Color and label

1 Periorbita (periosteum of the orbit)
2 Orbital septum (dense connective tissue sheet within eyelid, continuous with periorbita)
3 Levator palpebrae muscle (raiser of the upper lid)
4 Levator aponeurosis
5 Superior tarsal muscle (a smooth muscle supplied by sympathetic fibers)
6 Superior tarsus (a dense, curved plate of cartilage-like connective tissue)
7 Eyeball
8 Palpebral (eyelid) conjunctiva (a mucous membrane)
9 Bulbar (eyeball) conjunctiva (space between two layers of conjunctiva is exaggerated here; two layers slide against each other lubricated only by a thin layer of tears)
10 Superior conjunctival fornix (Latin, an arch)
11 Orbicularis oculi muscle (note muscle is within the upper lid as well as on the bony orbit)

Right eye and orbit

Color and label

1 Superior tarsus
2 Inferior tarsus
3 Tendon of levator palpebrae superior
4 Orbital septum
5 Lacrimal gland (orbital and palpebral parts)
6 Lateral palpebral ligament
7 Medial palpebral ligament (cut and relfected)
8 Superior lacrimal canaliculus
9 Inferior lacrimal canaliculus
10 Lacrimal sac
11 Nasolacrimal duct
12 Maxillary bone (cut open to show nasolacrimal duct)

After Wolf-Heidegger

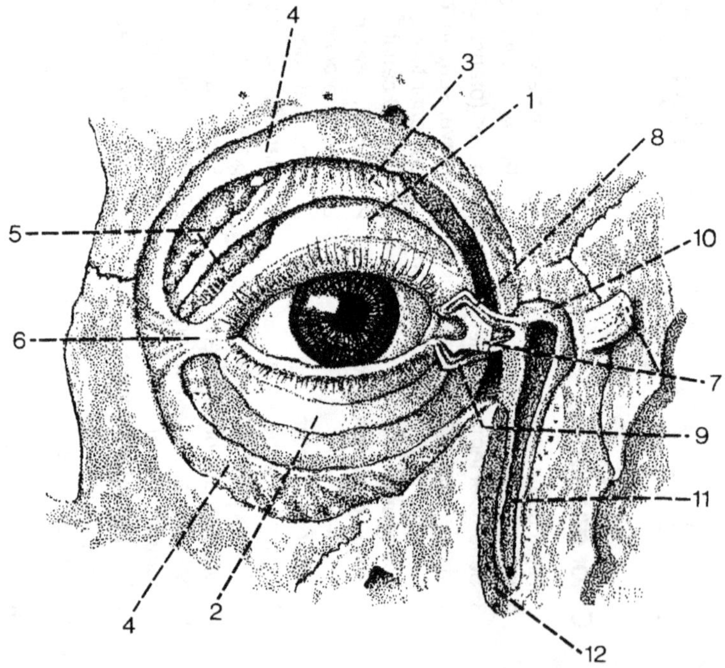

H&N-31 Extraocular muscles

Lateral view of right eye with lateral wall removed

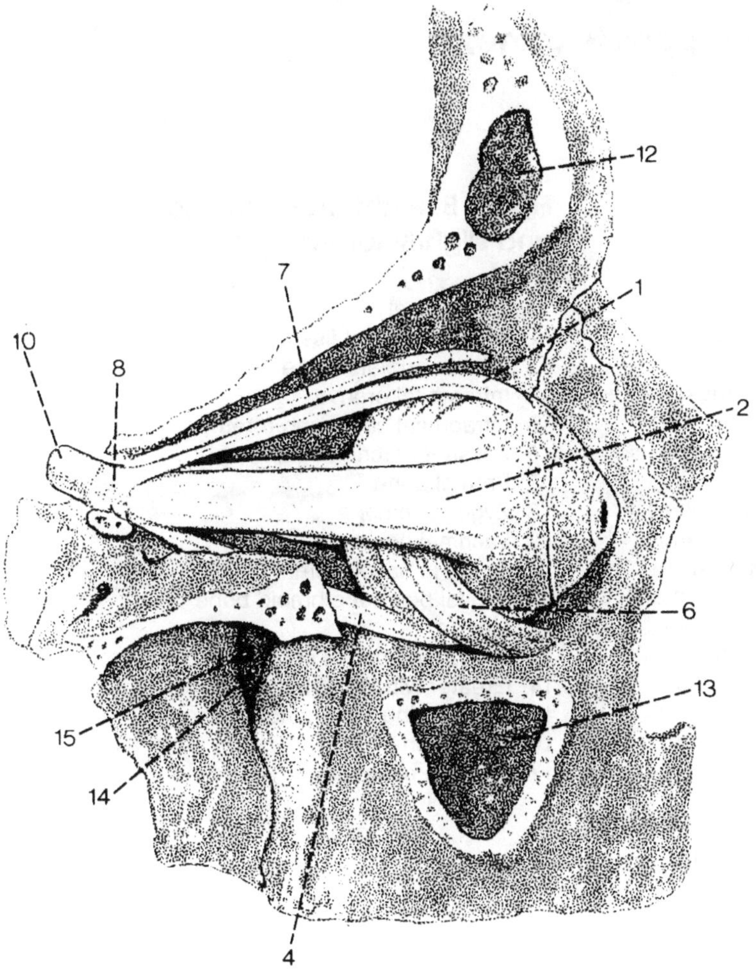

Color and label

1 Superior rectus muscle
2 Lateral rectus muscle
3 Medial rectus muscle
4 Inferior rectus muscle
5 Superior oblique muscle
6 Inferior rectus muscle
7 Levator palpebrae muscle (also levator muscle of upper lid)
8 Anulus tendineus communis (also common tendinous ring)
9 Trochlea (Latin, pulley)
10 Optic nerve (cranial nerve II)
11 Bulbar conjunctiva (cut edge)
12 Frontal sinus
13 Maxillary sinus
14 Pterygopalatine fossa
15 Sphenopalatine foramen

After Wolf-Heidegger

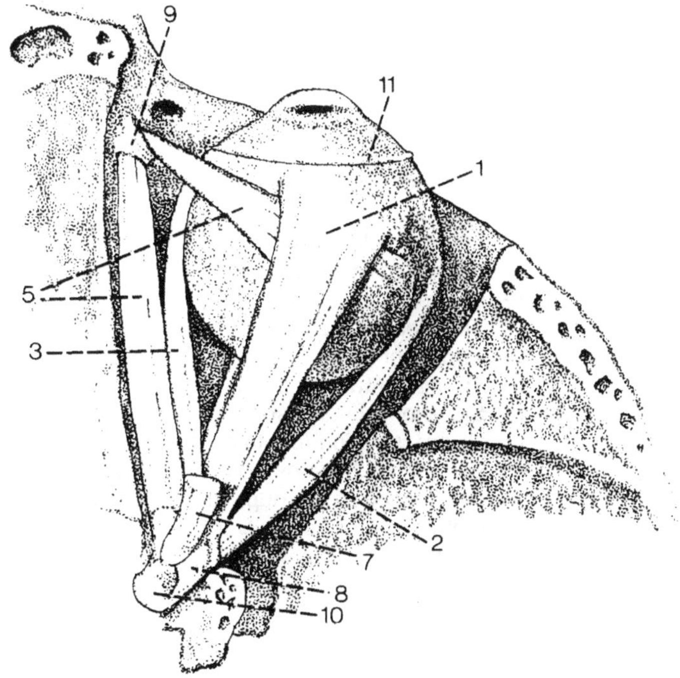

Superior view of right eye with roof of orbit removed

H&N-32 Eye and orbit

(opposite page)

Color and label

Figure A. Right eye

1 Pupil (central opening of iris, through which light enters)
2 Iris (pigmented; responsible for color of eye; blue, green, brown, etc.; regulates size of its central aperature, the pupil, by its circular sphincter muscle, which constricts the pupil, and its radial dilator muscle, which enlarges the pupil)
3 Reflection on cornea (the transparent cornea possesses a greater curvature than the eyeball itself; the curvature of the cornea is greatest in youth and least in old age; distortion of corneal curvature gives rise to astigmatism; more refraction of light occurs at the anterior surface of the cornea than in any other refractive media in the eye. In man the refractive power of the cornea is more than twice that of the lens)
4 Bulbar conjunctiva overlying sclera (sclera is white fibrous coat of eye)
5 Upper lid (palpebra superior)
6 Lower lid (palpebra inferior)
7 Cilia (eyelashes projecting from margin of eyelid)
8 Lacrimal caruncle (Latin, *lacrima*, a tear)

Figure B. Right orbit: anterior and slightly lateral view

1 Optic canal
2 Superior orbital fissure
3 Inferior orbital fissure
4 Infraorbital groove
5 Infraorbital canal and foramen
6 Fossa for lacrimal gland
7 Frontal bone
8 Zygomatic bone
9 Lacrimal bone
10 Probe in nasolacrimal duct
11 Orbital plate of ethmoid bone
12 Maxilla
13 Posterior lacrimal crest
14 Greater wing of sphenoid bone
15 Lesser wing of sphenoid bone
16 Nasal bone
17 Palatine bone

Figure C. Common tendinous ring (anulus tendineus communis)

1 Common tendinous ring (notice that it encircles the optic canal, including the optic nerve and ophthalmic artery, and also encircles part of the superior orbital fissure with the abducent nerve and oculomotor nerve)
2 Optic nerve emerging from the optic canal
3 Ophthalmic artery
4 Superior ramus of oculomotor nerve (innervates superior rectus and levator palpebrae muscles)
5 Inferior ramus of oculomotor nerve (innervates medial rectus, inferior rectus, and inferior oblique muscles)
6 Levator palpebrae muscle
7 Superior rectus muscle
8 Superior oblique muscle
9 Medial rectus muscle
10 Inferior rectus muscle
11 Inferior oblique muscle
12 Lateral rectus muscle
13 Trochlear nerve
14 Abducent nerve
15 Trochlea (Latin, a pulley)
16 Superior orbital fissure
17 Ciliary ganglion (contains postganglionic parasympathetic nerve cell bodies that cause constriction of the pupil and greater curvature of the lens for near vision)
18 Supraorbital notch

H&N-32 Eye and orbit

Anterior aspect

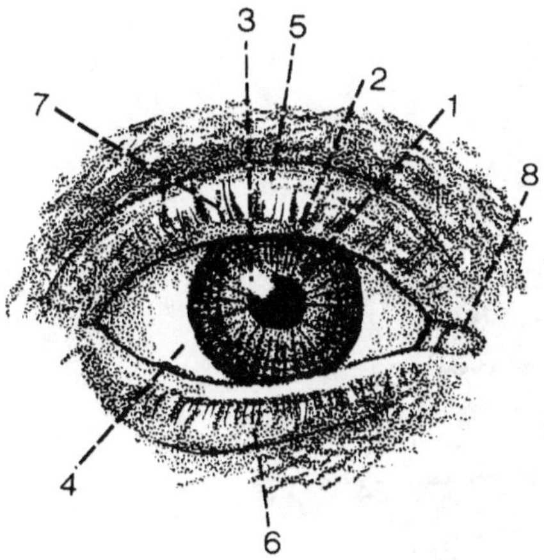

A

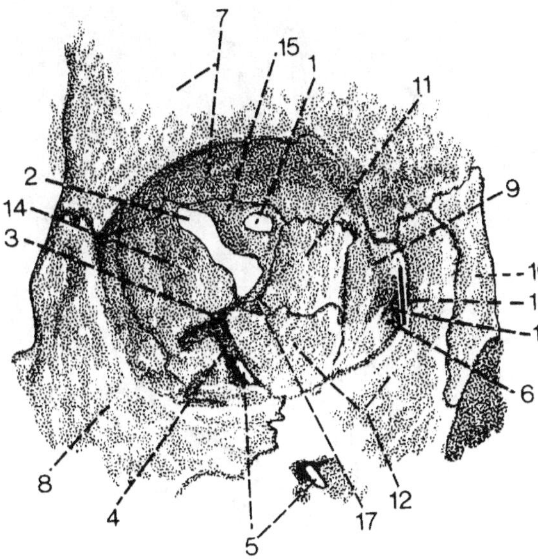

B

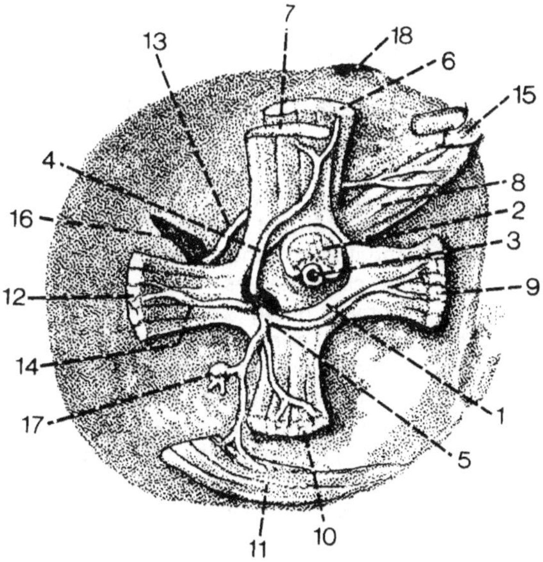

C

H&N-33 Nerves of the orbit

Superior aspect

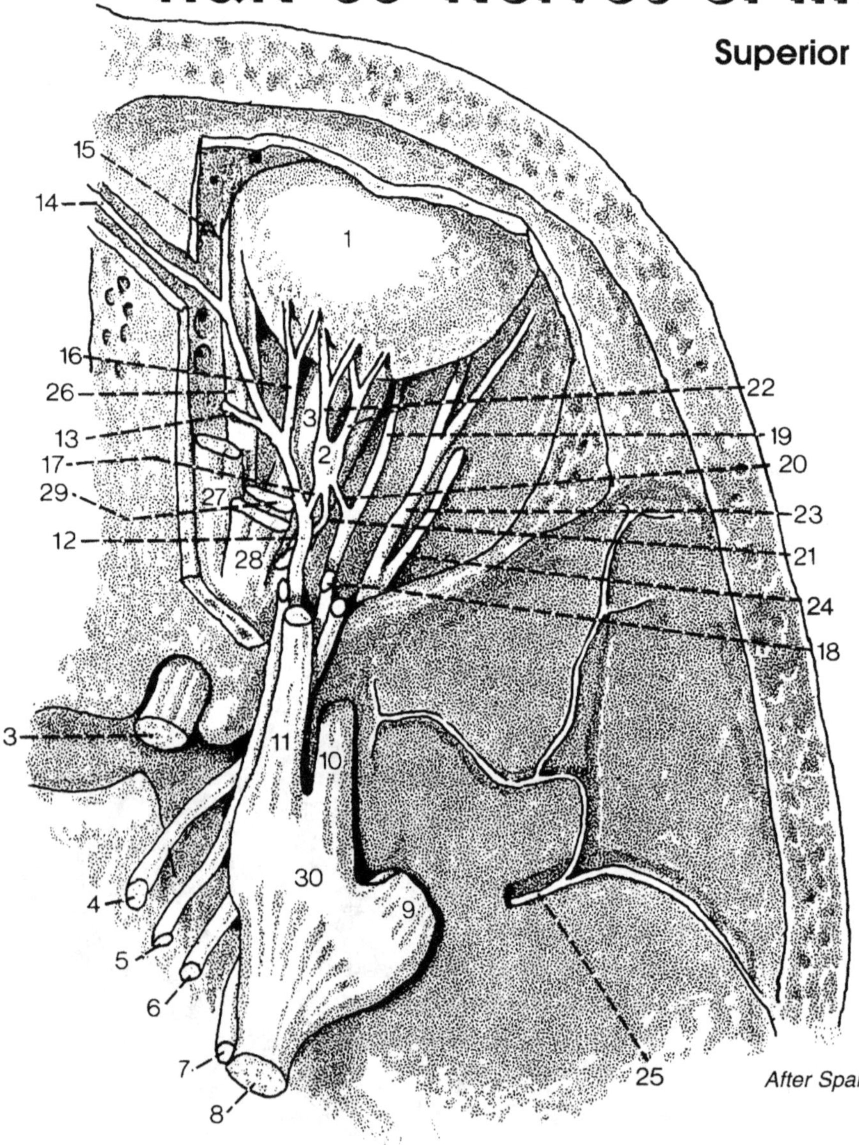

After Spalteholz and Spanner

Color and label

1 Eyeball
2 Ciliary ganglion (parasympathetic)
3 Optic nerve (II)
4 Oculomotor nerve (III)
5 Trochlear nerve (IV)
6 Abducent nerve (VI)
7 Motor root (portio minor) of trigeminal nerve (V)
8 Sensory root (portio major) of trigeminal nerve (V)
9 Mandibular nerve (major branch of trigeminal nerve)
10 Maxillary nerve (major branch of trigeminal nerve)
11 Ophthalmic nerve (major branch of trigeminal nerve; cut)
12 Nasociliary nerve (branch of ophthalmic nerve)
13 Posterior ethmoidal nerve
14 Anterior ethmoidal nerve
15 Infratrochlear
16 Long ciliary nerves
17 Communicating branch of nasociliary nerve with ciliary ganglion
18 Oculomotor nerve superior branch (cut)
19 Oculomotor nerve inferior branch
20 Oculomotor root of ciliary ganglion
21 Sympathetic branch to ciliary ganglion
22 Short ciliary nerves
23 Zygomatic nerve
24 Infraorbital nerve
25 Meningeal branch of mandibular nerve
26 Medial rectus muscle
27 Superior oblique muscle (cut)
28 Levator palpebrae superior muscle (cut)
29 Superior rectus muscle (cut)
30 Trigeminal ganglion

H&N-34 Nerves of the orbit

Lateral aspect

The bones of the right orbit and part of the right maxilla are removed, showing roots of the teeth and their innervation.

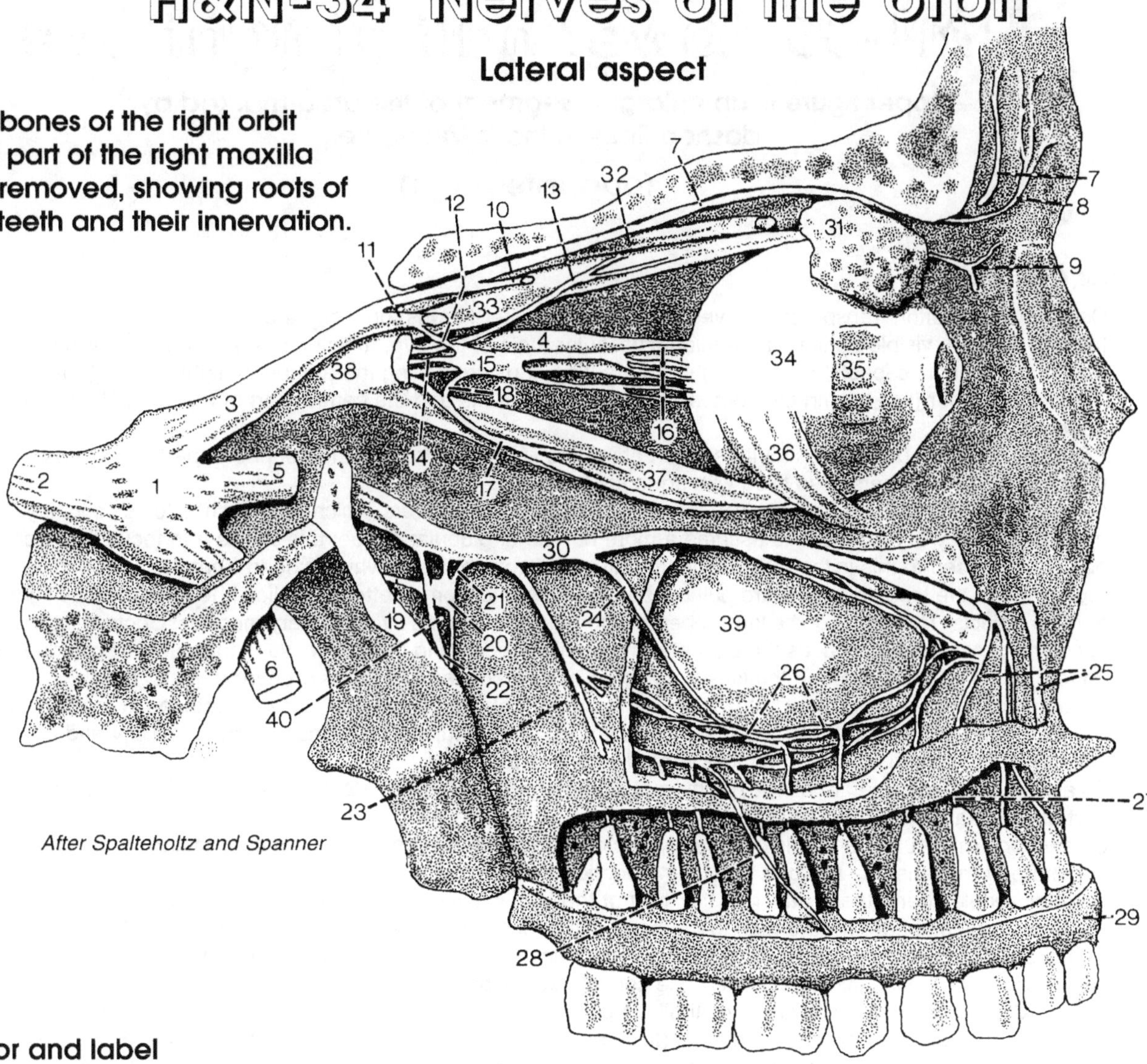

After Spalteholtz and Spanner

Color and label

1 Trigeminal (semilunar) ganglion
2 Sensory root of trigeminal nerve
3 Ophthalmic nerve (V_1)
4 Optic nerve
5 Maxillary nerve (V_2)
6 Mandibular nerve (V_3) (cut)
7 Supraorbital nerve
8 Supraorbital nerve (medial branch)
9 Supratrochlear nerve
10 Lacrimal nerve (cut)
11 Nasociliary nerve (cut)
12 Branch from nasociliary nerve to ciliary ganglion
13 Superior branch of oculomotor nerve
14 Sympathetic branch to ciliary ganglion
15 Ciliary ganglion
16 Short ciliary nerves
17 Inferior branch of oculomotor nerve
18 Oculomotor root to ciliary ganglion
19 Nerve of pterygoid canal
20 Pterygopalatine ganglion
21 Pterygopalatine nerves
22 Palatine nerves
23 Posterior superior alveolar branches
24 Middle superior alveolar branches
25 Anterior superior alveolar branches
26 Superior dental plexus
27 Superior dental branches
28 Gingival branch
29 Gingiva (Latin, *gingiva*, the gum)
30 Infraorbital nerve
31 Lacrimal gland
32 Levator palpebrae superior muscle
33 Superior rectus muscle
34 Eyeball
35 Lateral rectus muscle (cut)
36 Inferior oblique muscle
37 Inferior rectus muscle
38 Common tendinous ring
39 Mucous membrane of maxillary sinus
40 Pterygopalatine fossa

H&N-35 Lower half of right eye

Upper figure is an enlarged segment of the area marked by dashed lines in the lower figure.

(opposite page)

Color and label

1 Cornea (the anterior, transparent, curved portion of the outer fibrous tunic of the eyeball)
2 Iris (the colored, visible portion of the middle vascular tunic of the eye; functions as a diaphragm with the central opening, the pupil, capable of enlarging or contracting, thus controlling the amount of light entering the eye)
3 Anterior chamber (lies behind the cornea and in front of the iris and the central part of the lens; filled with aqueous humor)
4 Posterior chamber (a narrow circular space behind the iris and in front of the peripheral part of the lens and the anterior zonule fibers; also filled with aqueous humor)
5 Lens. The biconvex lens is held in place by the surrounding zonule fibers, which are attached to its periphery. The natural tendency of the lens is to assume a more curved or globular shape; this allows it to focus light from near objects. Apposed to this is the radial outward pull of the zonule fibers, which extend from the surrounding ciliary processes to the lens; their outward pull causes the lens to become flatter and allow the lens to focus light from far objects. The shape of the lens depends upon the surrounding circular ciliary muscles. Contraction of the circular ciliary muscles reduces the diameter of the ciliary body and thereby lessens the outward pull on the edge of the lens, thus allowing the lens to become more biconvex and focus on near objects; this is accommodation. Presbyopia, or "old vision," is the loss of ability to focus on close objects, as in reading, due to the thickening of the lens, which occurs with advanced age, resulting in the loss of lens elasticity and an inability of the lens to assume the more curved biconvex form.
6 Ciliary processes (these are about 70 tiny radially-arranged, wrinkled folds; they lie in the pars plica or folded part of the ciliary body; also called ciliary crown)
7 Ciliary body (muscular part); this completely encircles the lens and consists of smooth muscle that controls the curvature of the lens; the muscles of accommodation
8 Anterior zonule fibers (these attach to the front of the lens where they fuse with the lens capsule)
9 Posterior zonule fibers (these attach to the back of the lens where they fuse with the lens capule)
10 Trabecular meshwork (this is an irregular network of tiny beams or trabeculae at the periphery of the anterior chamber where the iris joins the cornea; the convoluted passages between the trabeclae contain aqueous humor which slowly flows outward eventually to be absorbed by the scleral venous sinus or canal of Schlemm)
11 Scleral venous sinus or canal of Schlemm (this vein encircles the inner part of the corneoscleral junction; it drains the aqueous humor from the anterior chamber of the eye; **glaucoma** is an increase in intraocular pressure sufficient to damage the function or structure of the eye; caused by the blockage of drainage and buildup of aqueous humor in the anterior chamber; *glaukoma,* Greek, gleaming, bluish green, gray)
12 Limbus (the corneoscleral junction)
13 Conjunctiva (bulbar conjunctiva is the transparent mucous membrane on the sclera; it is also reflected onto the inner surface of both upper and lower lids as palpebral conjunctiva)
14 Sclera (the white, fibrous, outer coat of the eyeball)
15 Choroid (the middle, vascular tunic of the eyeball)
16 Retina (the inner, nervous, light-sensitive tunic of the eye)
17 Fovea centralis (the central part of the retina responsible for maximum visual acuity; contains only tightly-packed cones)
18 Outer dural sheath of optic nerve
19 Central artery and vein of the retina
20 Optic nerve
21 Ciliary body (pars plana or smooth part; covered by the non-nervous part of the retina)

H&N-35 Lower half of right eye

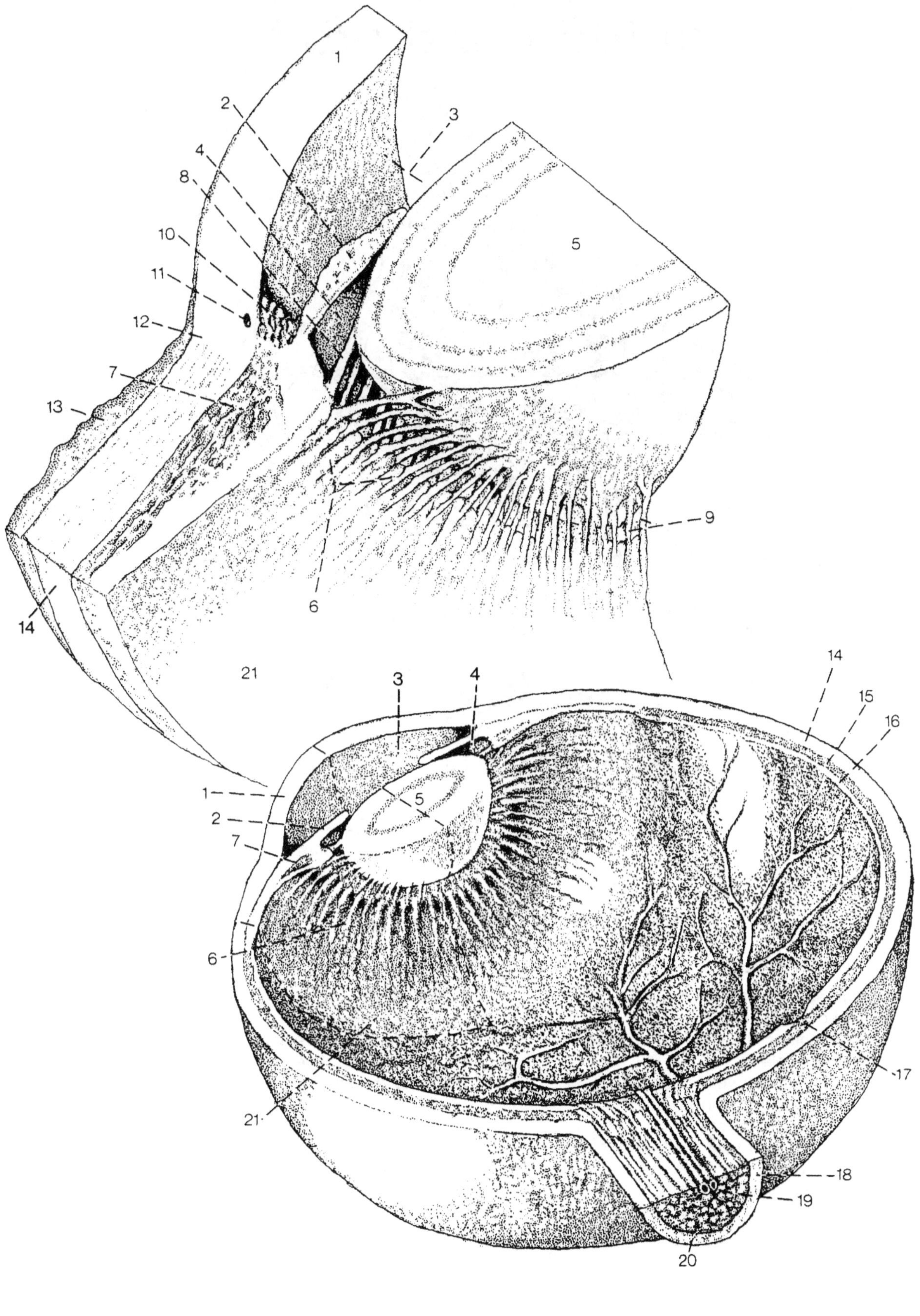

H&N-36 Principal veins of face and orbit

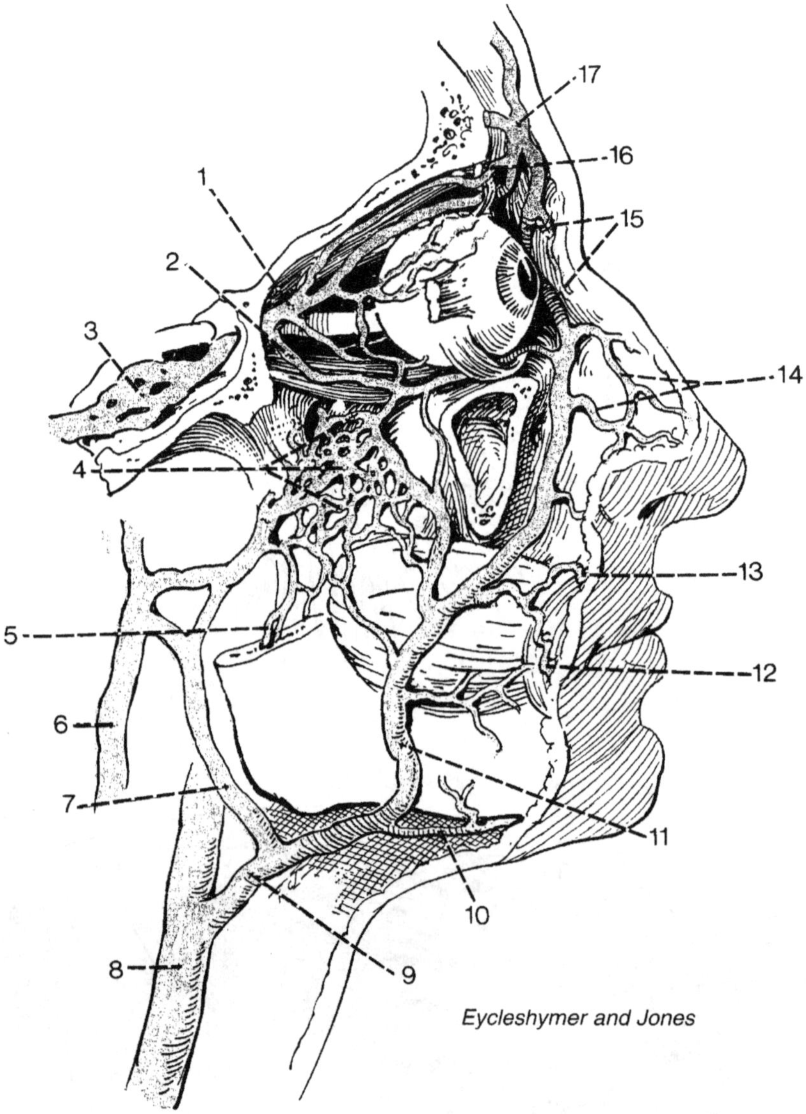

Eycleshymer and Jones

Color and label

1 Superior ophthalmic vein
2 Inferior ophthalmic vein
3 Cavernous sinus
4 Pterygoid plexus
5 Inferior alveolar vein (doubled)
6 External jugular vein
7 Retromandibular vein
8 Internal jugular vein
9 Facial vein
10 Submental vein
11 Facial vein
12 Inferior labial vein
13 Superior labial vein
14 External nasal veins
15 Angular vein
16 Supraorbital vein
17 Anastomosis of angular vein with supraorbital and supratrochlear veins

H&N-37 The lacrimal apparatus

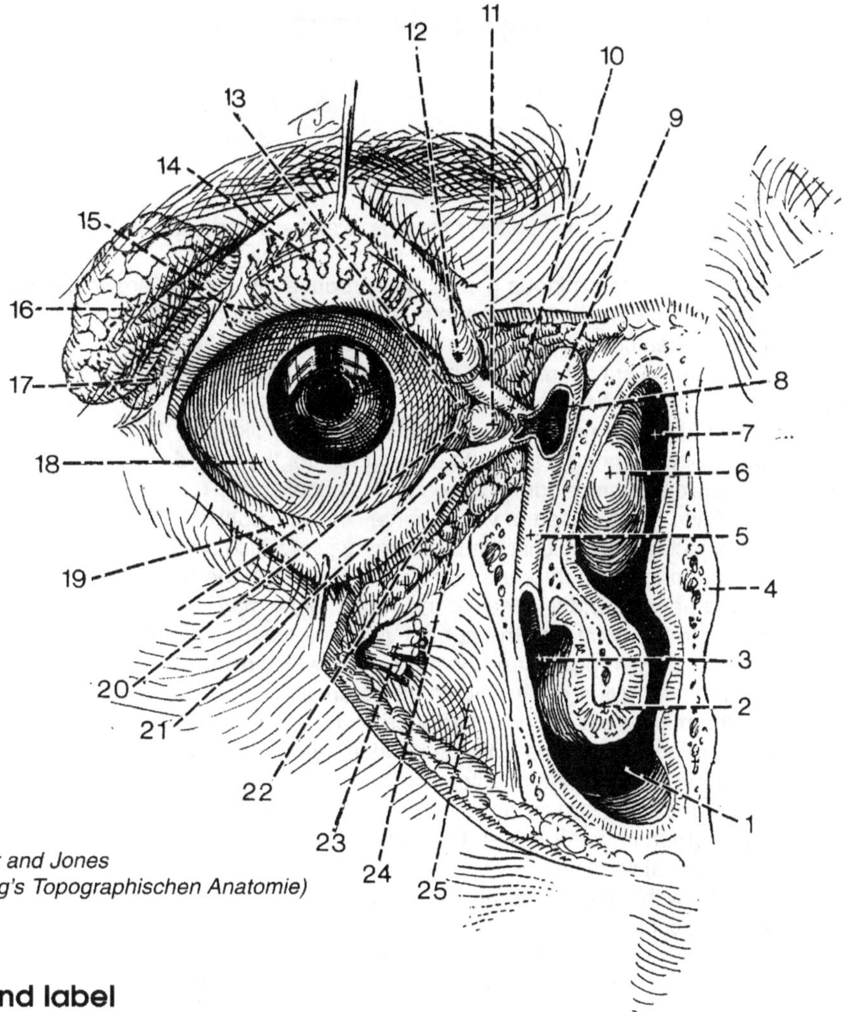

Eycleshymer and Jones
(after Corning's Topographischen Anatomie)

Color and label

1 Nasal cavity
2 Inferior nasal concha (a separate bone)
3 Inferior nasal meatus
4 Nasal septum
5 Nasolacrimal duct
6 Middle nasal concha
7 Nasal cavity
8 Lacrimal sac
9 Fornix of lacrimal sac
10 Lacrimal canaliculus
11 Conjunctival caruncle (a small rounded fleshy body in the medial angle of the eye)
12 Lacrimal punctum (Latin, a tiny hole; opening of lacrimal canaliculus; *pl.* puncta)
13 Semilunar plica (or semilunar fold; covered by lake of tears or lacrimal lake)
14 Tarsal glands
15 Openings of lacrimal ducts
16 Lacrimal gland (orbital part)
17 Lacrimal gland, palpebral part
18 Bulbar conjunctiva
19 Palpebral conjunctiva (lines inside of upper and lower lids)
20 Lakus lacrimalis (thin layer of tears overlying plica semilunaris)
21 Lacrimal papilla with lacrimal punctum
22 Ampulla of lacrimal canaliculus (this actually occurs at the "elbow" or bend in the lacrimal canaliculus)
23 Infraorbital nerve
24 Orbital fat
25 Maxilla

H&N-38 Dissection of ear and cast of bony labyrinth

(opposite page)

Color and label

Figure A

1 Pinna (also called auricle)
2 Cartilaginous walls of external acoustic (or auditory) meatus; walls are cartilage externally and bone internally
3 External acoustic meatus; contains ceruminous glands that produce the orange-brown ear wax, or cerumen, which, when accumulated in excess amounts, may impair hearing
4 Bony wall of external auditory meatus; this canal is about 2.5 cm long and acts as a resonator for sound waves in the critical range of human speech (2000 to 4000 cycles per second), thus amplifying these sounds.
5 Umbo of the ear drum; the ear drum (or tympanic membrane) is shaped like a blunt cone, with the deepest point externally called the umbo (Latin for the raised ornament on a shield); the outside of the ear drum is skin and is supplied by sensory fibers from nerves V and X; because the vagus nerve (X) also supplies the pharynx and larynx, an object lodged against the ear drum may produce a cough.
6 Middle ear cavity; lined with a mucous membrane that covers the walls, the 3 ossicles, their ligaments, and nerves; under certain conditions mucus may accumulate in the middle ear to the point that the normal vibratory movements of the ear drum and 3 ear ossicles are impeded and hearing is impaired; **otitis media** is a general term for inflammation of the middle ear; cranial nerve IX supplies sensory fibers to the middle ear and inner surface of the ear drum; the middle ear is filled with air and communicates with the nasopharynx by way of the auditory tune.
7 Internal jugular vein (note its proximity to the middle ear)
8 Round window (fenestra cochleae); closed by a membrane that acts as a pressure release for waves in the perilymph in the cochlea; it bulges out when the foot plate of the stapes pushes in at the oval window.
9 Vestibule; the fluid-filled cavity within the temporal bone containing the membranous utricle and the saccule.
10 Auditory tube; old name, eustachian tube; this connects the middle ear with the nasopharynx; normally closed, when dilated, as in yawning, it allows air in the middle ear to equalize with the ambient air pressure.
11 Nasopharynx
12 Malleus (Latin, hammer); note that the end of the malleus handle is attached to the inside of the ear drum at the umbo.
13 Incus (Latin, anvil)
14 Lateral semicircular canal; each semicircular canal contains a thinner semicircular duct.
15 Posterior semicircular canal
16 Anterior semicircular canal
17 Facial nerve (N VII; cut)
18 Internal acoustic meatus
19 Vestibulocochlear nerve (VIII)
20 Cochlea (Latin, a snail); the snail-like tubular spiral divided into 3 scalae or compartments: (1) the tympani, (2) the scala media or cochlea duct, and (3) the scala vestibuli.
21 Footplate (or base) of stapes (Latin, stirrup); it covers the oval window; sound-induced vibrations of the footplate send pressure waves into the endolymph of the vestibule which are simultaneously carried into the cochlea.

Figure B

The bony labyrinth is a series of cavities and canals within the petrous portion of the temporal bone. The thinner membranous labyrinth lies within the bony labyrinth. The membranous labyrinth contains endolymph. The outer bony labyrinth contains perilymph, which surrounds and bathes the membranous labyrinth.

H&N-38 Dissection of ear and cast of bony labyrinth

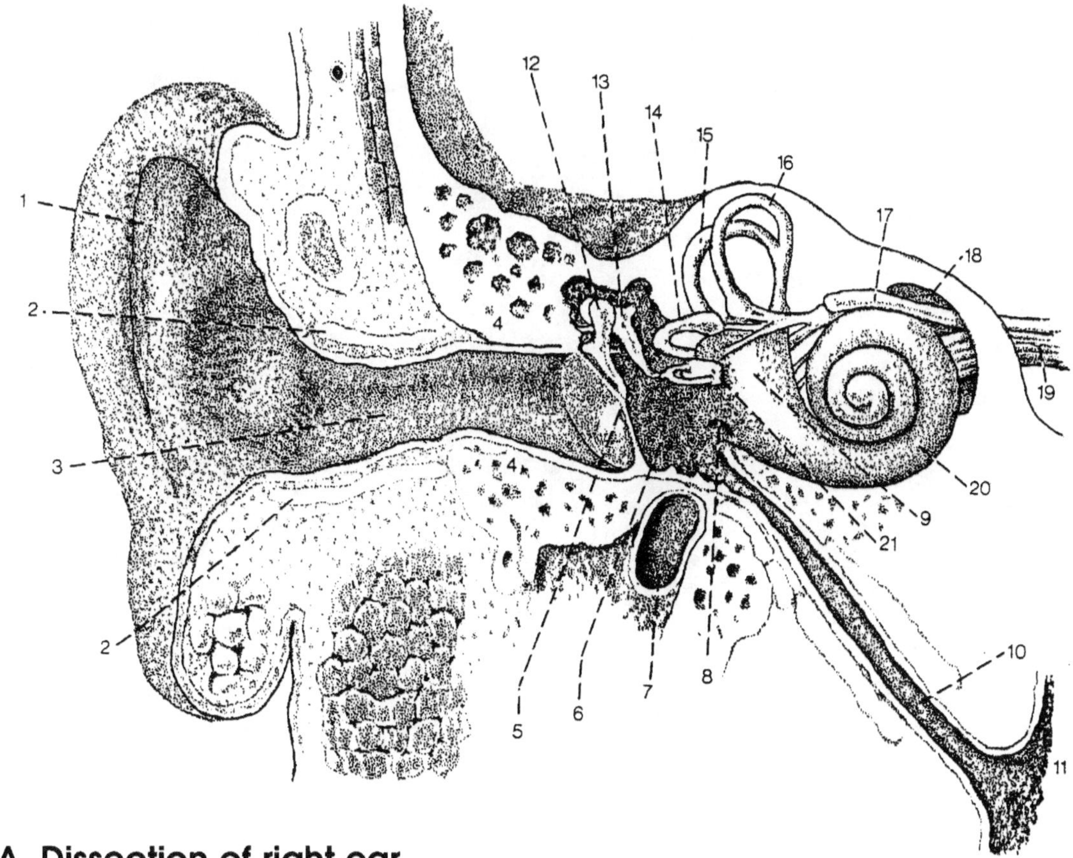

Figure A. Dissection of right ear

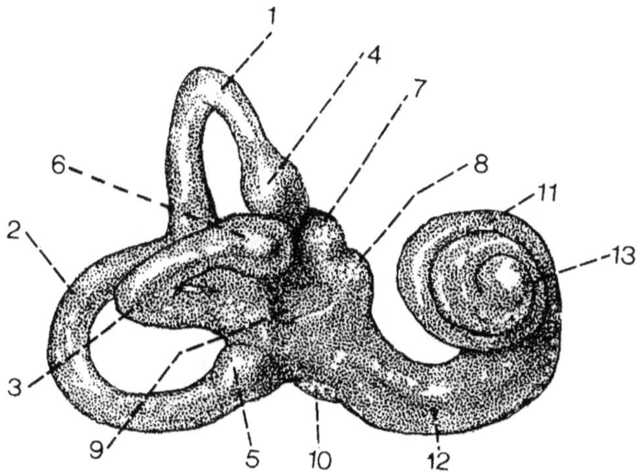

Figure B. Bony labyrinth

Right bony labyrinth (from a cast)

Color and label

1 Anterior semicircular canal
2 Posterior semicircular canal
3 Lateral semicircular canal
4 Anterior bony ampulla
5 Posterior bony ampulla
6 Lateral bony ampulla
7 Elliptical recess
8 Spherical recess
9 Fenestra vestibuli (former name: oval window)
10 Fenestra cochleae (former name: round window)
11 Cochlea
12 Base of cochlea
13 Cupula of cochlea

Based on Spalteholz and Spanner

H&N-39 Dissection of ear

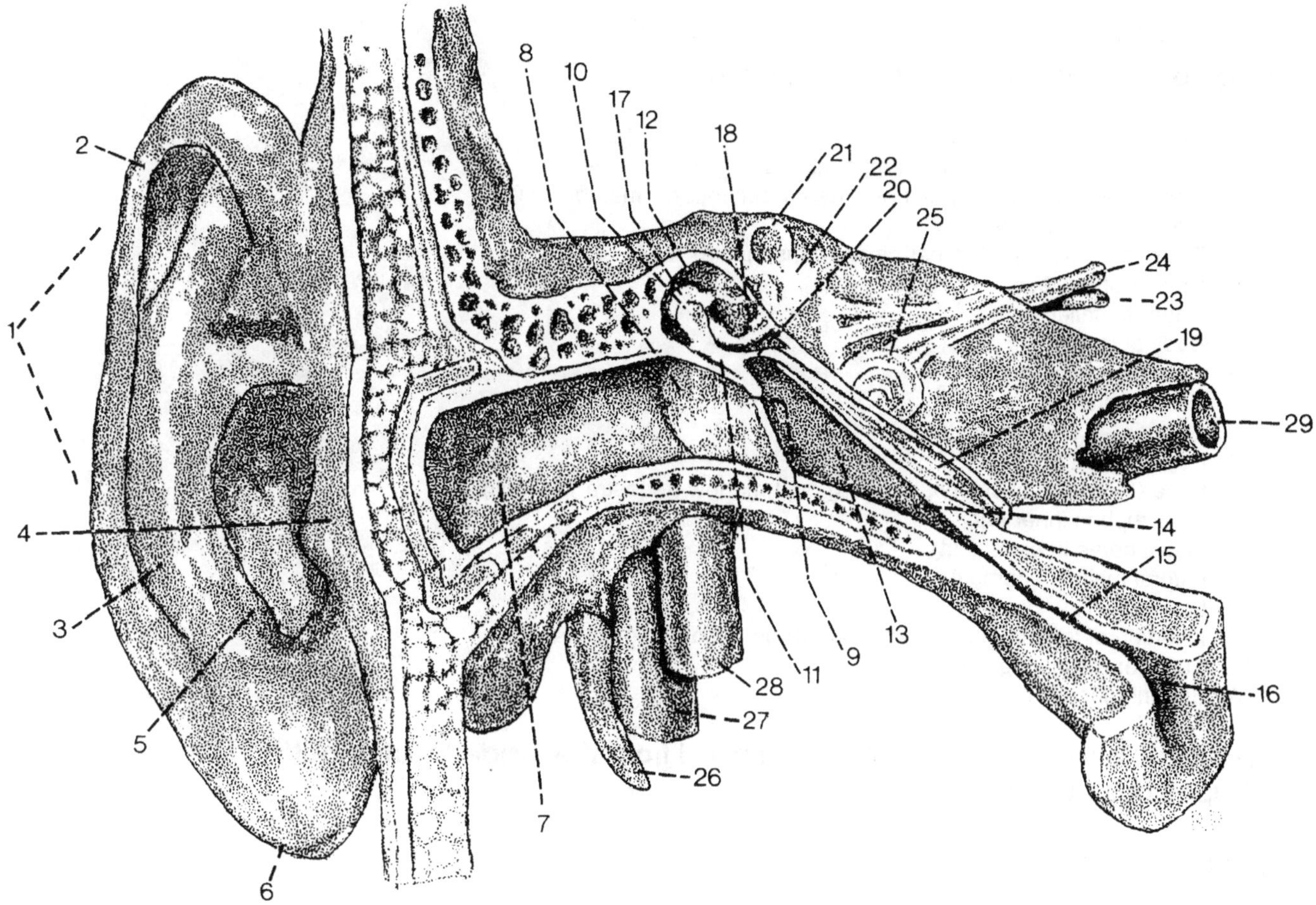

Color and label

1 Auricle (pinna)
2 Helix
3 Antihelix
4 Tragus
5 Antitragus
6 Lobule of auricle
7 External acoustic meatus
8 Tympanic membrane (eardrum)
9 Umbo of tympanic membrane
10 Head of malleus
11 Handle of malleus (attached at umbo)
12 Epitympanic recess
13 Middle ear (tympanic cavity)
14 Auditory tube (bony part)
15 Auditory tube (cartilaginous part)
16 Pharyngeal opening of auditory tube in nasal pharynx
17 Incus
18 Stapes
19 Tensor tympani muscle
20 Tendon of tensor tympani inserting on malleus
21 Superior semicircular canal (within petrous part of temporal bone)
22 Vestibule (cavity containing both utricle and saccule)
23 Vestibular nerve (of vestibulocochlear nerve)
24 Cochlear nerve (of vestibulocochlear nerve)
25 Cochlea
26 Styloid process
27 Internal jugular vein
28 Internal carotid artery (entering carotid canal)
29 Internal carotid artery (emerging from carotid canal)

H&N-40 Middle ear and ear ossicles

(opposite page)

Color and label

Figure A. Right middle ear, anterior view

1 External acoustic meatus
2 Tympanic membrane (ear drum; cut in half)
3 Umbo (central deepest point on exterior of tympanic membrane)
4 Fibrocartilaginous ring
5 Tympanic cavity (middle ear cavity, auris media)
6 Handle of malleus
7 Head of malleus
8 Body of incus
9 Long leg of incus
10 Head of stapes
11 Anterior leg of stapes
12 Posterior leg of stapes
13 Base (footplate) of stapes; covering oval window (fenestra vestibuli)
14 Perilymph in inner ear
15 Facial nerve in canal (cut)
16 Lateral mallear ligament
17 Lateral mallear process
18 Insertion of tensor tympani tendon (cut) on handle of malleus
19 Superior mallear ligament
20 Superior incudial ligament

Figures B and C. Right middle ear viewed from the inside looking out. Stapes has been removed.

Color and label

1 Tympanic membrane
2 Handle of malleus (attached to inside of ear drum at umbo)
3 Insertion of tensor tympani tendon on handle of malleus
4 Chorda tympani nerve (a branch of facial nerve)
5 Head of malleus
6 Body of incus
7 Short leg of incus
8 Long leg of incus
9 Lenticular process of incus (shaped like a small lentil bean)
10 Auditory tube (formerly, eustachian tube)
11 Canal for tensor tympani muscle (muscle has been removed)
12 Superior mallear ligament
13 Superior incudial ligament
14 Posterior incudial ligament
15 Anterior mallear fold
16 Posterior mallear fold
17 Fibrocartilaginous ring of tympanic membrane
18 Facial nerve
19 Anterior tympanic recess
20 Posterior tympanic recess

H&N-40 Middle ear and ear ossicles

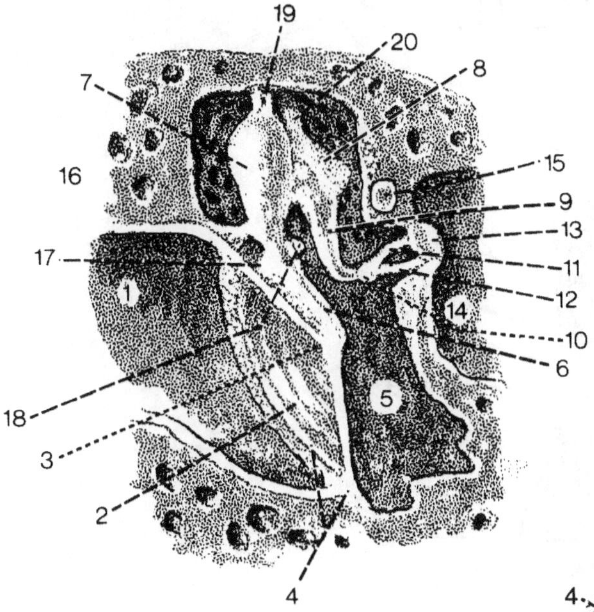

Tympanic membrane and ear ossicles

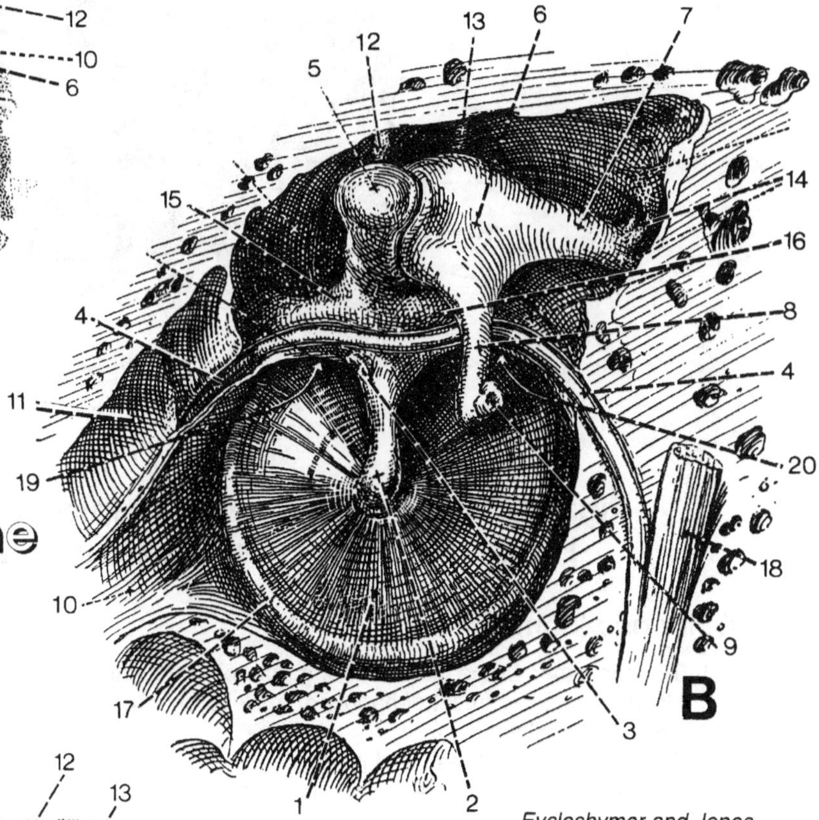

Eycleshymer and Jones

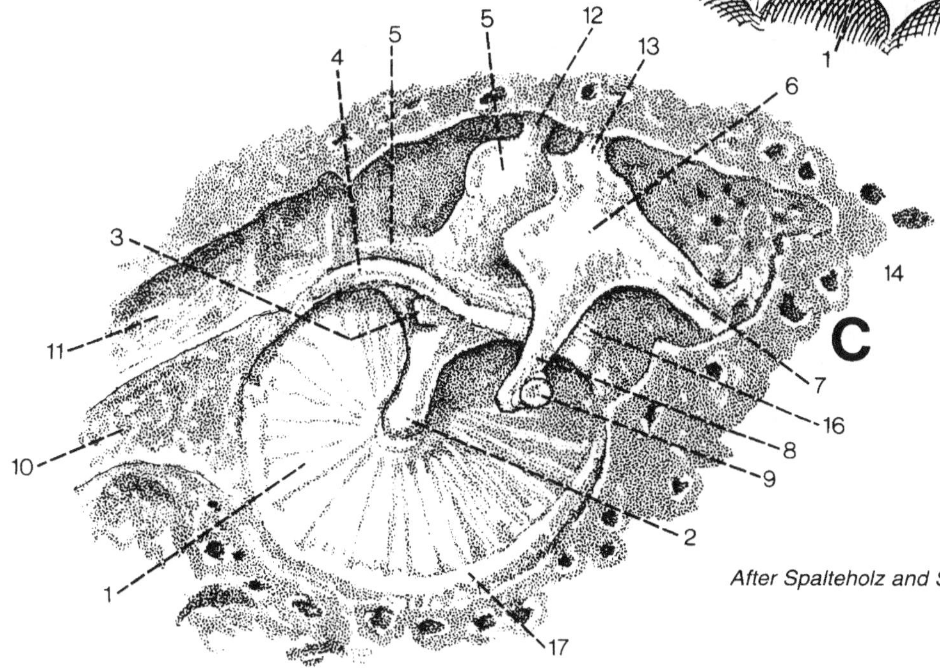

After Spalteholz and Spanner

H&N-41 Ear ossicles and part of eardrum

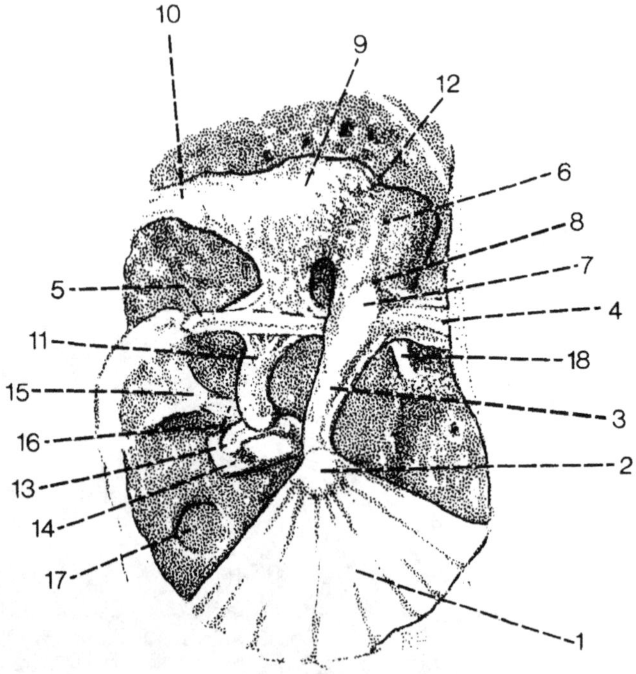

Right middle ear with eardrum largely removed. Looking in from external acoustic meatus.

Color and label

1 Tympanic membrane (eardrum; one quarter intact, three-quarters removed)
2 Umbo (note attachment of handle of malleus on inner surface of eardrum at umbo)
3 Handle of malleus
4 Anterior mallear process and ligament
5 Chorda tympani nerve (so named because of its passing adjacent to the tympanic membrane)
6 Head of malleus
7 Lateral mallear process
8 Neck of malleus
9 Body of incus
10 Short limb of incus
11 Long limb of incus
12 Incudomalleal joint
13 Stapes posterior limb
14 Footplate of stapes on oval window (fenestra vestibuli)
15 Pyramidal eminence containing stapedius muscle
16 Tendon of stapedius muscle
17 Fenestra cochleae (round window; acts as a pressure release for fluid waves in cochlea)
18 Tendon of tensor tympani muscle (acts as a damper on loud, sound-induced vibrations)

H&N-42 Middle ear ossicles

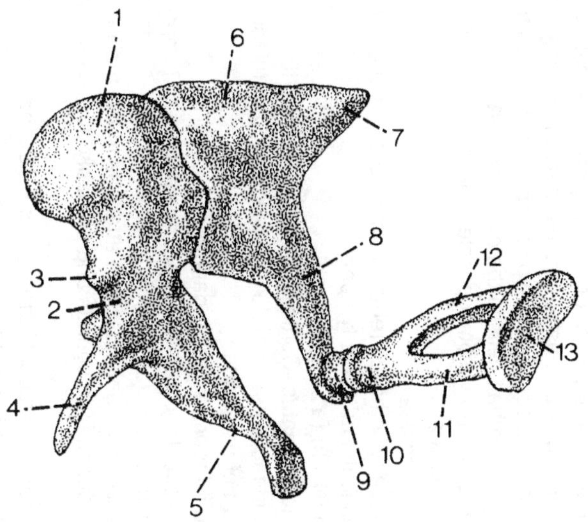

Color and label

1 Head of malleus
2 Neck of malleus
3 Lateral mallear process
4 Anterior mallear process
5 Handle of malleus
6 Body of incus
7 Short process of incus
8 Long process of incus
9 Lenticular process of incus
10 Head of stapes
11 Anterior limb (crus) of stapes
12 Posterior limb (crus) of stales
13 Footplate of stapes
14 Articular surface of malleus (with incus)
15 Articular surface of incus (with malleus)

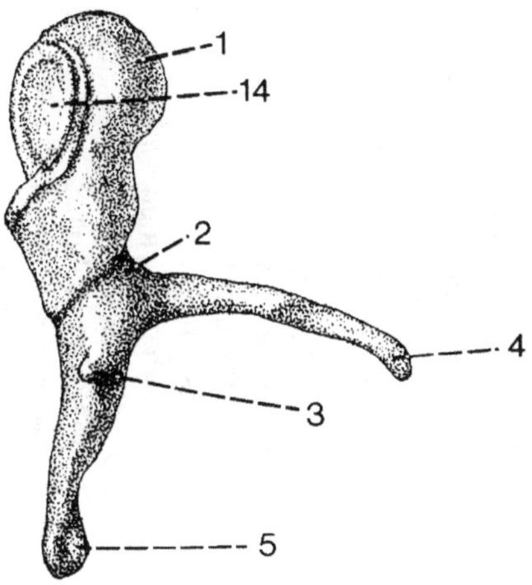

Right malleus lateral view

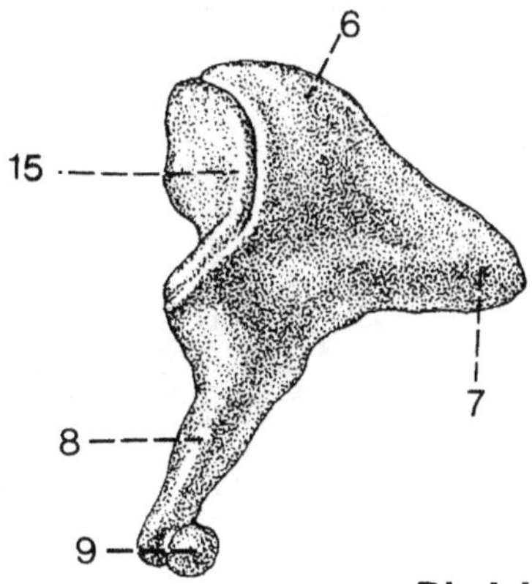

Right incus medial view

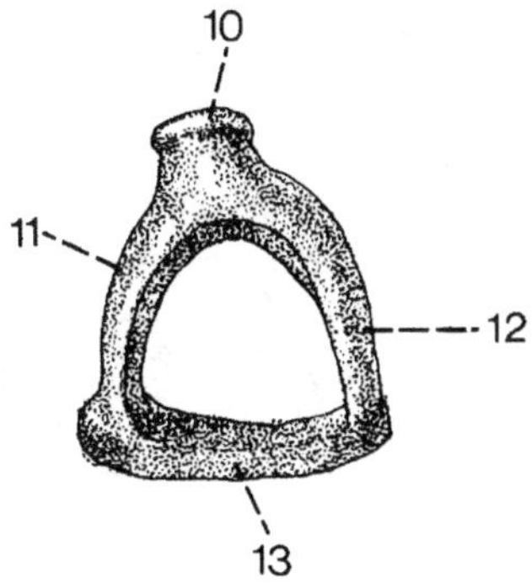

Right stapes superior view

After Wolf-Heidegger

H&N-43 Dissection of right ear showing middle ear and cochlea

(opposite page)

Color and label

1 External auditory (acoustic) meatus
2 Tympanic membrane (eardrum)
3 Middle ear cavity. This is filled with air that can enter and leave only through the eustachian tube; the middle ear cavity is lined with a mucous membrane that covers its walls as well as the ear ossicles, plus that portion of the chorda tympani nerve passing through the middle ear
4 Malleus (note its handle attached to the eardrum at the umbo; sound-induced vibrations are carried across the middle ear cavity and increased in force by the three ear ossicles)
5 Incus (the three ear ossicles are joined by two synovial joints; however, the malleus and incus vibrate as a single unit; the longer length of the malleus in relation to the incus gives a leverage advantage; the end of the malleus handle moves more, whereas the shorter lenticular process end of the incus moves less but with greater force)
6 Base (footplate) of stapes on oval window (fenestra vestibuli). The eardrum is about 15 times greater in area than the footplate of the stapes. This difference in area plus the leverage advantages bestowed by the ossicles' configuration results in an increase in pressure at the oval window that is about 15 times greater than that at the eardrum.
7 Opening of vestibule into scala vestibuli. Sound-induced pressure waves from the vibrating footplate of the stapes set off fluid pressure waves in the perilymph of the vestibule which enter the scala vestibuli where they cause the membranous walls of the duct to be deflected.
8 Scala vestibuli. The snail-like conchlea is divided into three spiral compartments or scalae (Latin, staircase or ladder). The scala vestibuli and scala tympani are filled with perilymph, which has a high sodium content. The scala media, or cochlear duct, is filled with endolymph, which has a high potassium content. Arrows pointing **UP**, that is, towards the apex, indicate the course of pressure waves in the scala vestibuli.
9 Scala tympani. Arrows pointing **DOWN** indicate the course of pressure waves in the scala tympani. In cross-section the three scala each occupy the following amount of cross-section in the cochlea: scala vestibuli, about 150°; the cochlear duct, about 30°; the scala tympani, about 180°
10 Round window (now called fenestra tympani). This is covered by a membrane that moves directly opposite to the movements of the footplate of the stapes. When the footplate moves in against the perilymph in the vestibule, the membrane on the round window moves out, and vice versa. This allows the sound-induced fluid pressure waves to travel up the cochlea. Because the fluid (endolymph and perilymph) is essentially incompressible, and the cells and membrane are mainly fluid, plus the fact that the fluid-filled inner ear is encased in unyielding bone, it is essential that the membrane across the round window acts as a pressure release.
11 Cochlear duct. Filled with endolymph, it contains the organ of Corti. It is here that vibrations in the form of traveling waves in basilar membrane of the cochlear duct are transformed into nerve impulses.
12 Spiral ganglion. This consists of bipolar nerve cell bodies that supply sensory fibers to the hair cells in the organ of Corti.
13 Cochlear portion of the vestibulocochlear nerve
14 Basal turn of cochlea
15 Second turn of cochlea
16 Apex of cochlea witih helicotrema, which is a small opening between the scala vestibuli and scala tympani
17 Facial nerve (N VII) (a small portion)
18 Internal auditory meatus. Contains nerves VII and VIII.
19 Facial nerve in facial canal. Note its proximity to the middle ear cavity.
20 Vestibular part of nerve VIII
21 Superior and inferior vestibular ganglia
22 Superior semicircular canal within petrous portion of temporal bone
23 Tensor tympani muscle (a portion)
24 Tendon of tensor tympani muscle. It attaches to the malleus and dampens its vibrations during loud sounds and probably during chewing and speaking.
25 Auditory (eustachian) tube. Normally it is collapsed so that air does not pass freely between the middle ear and nasopharynx. Chewing and yawning usually open the tube enough to allow air pressure in the middle ear to equalize with that of the outside air.
26 Superior petrosal sinus. A vein enclosed by dura mater
27 Temporal bone

H&N-43 Dissection of right ear showing middle ear and cochlea

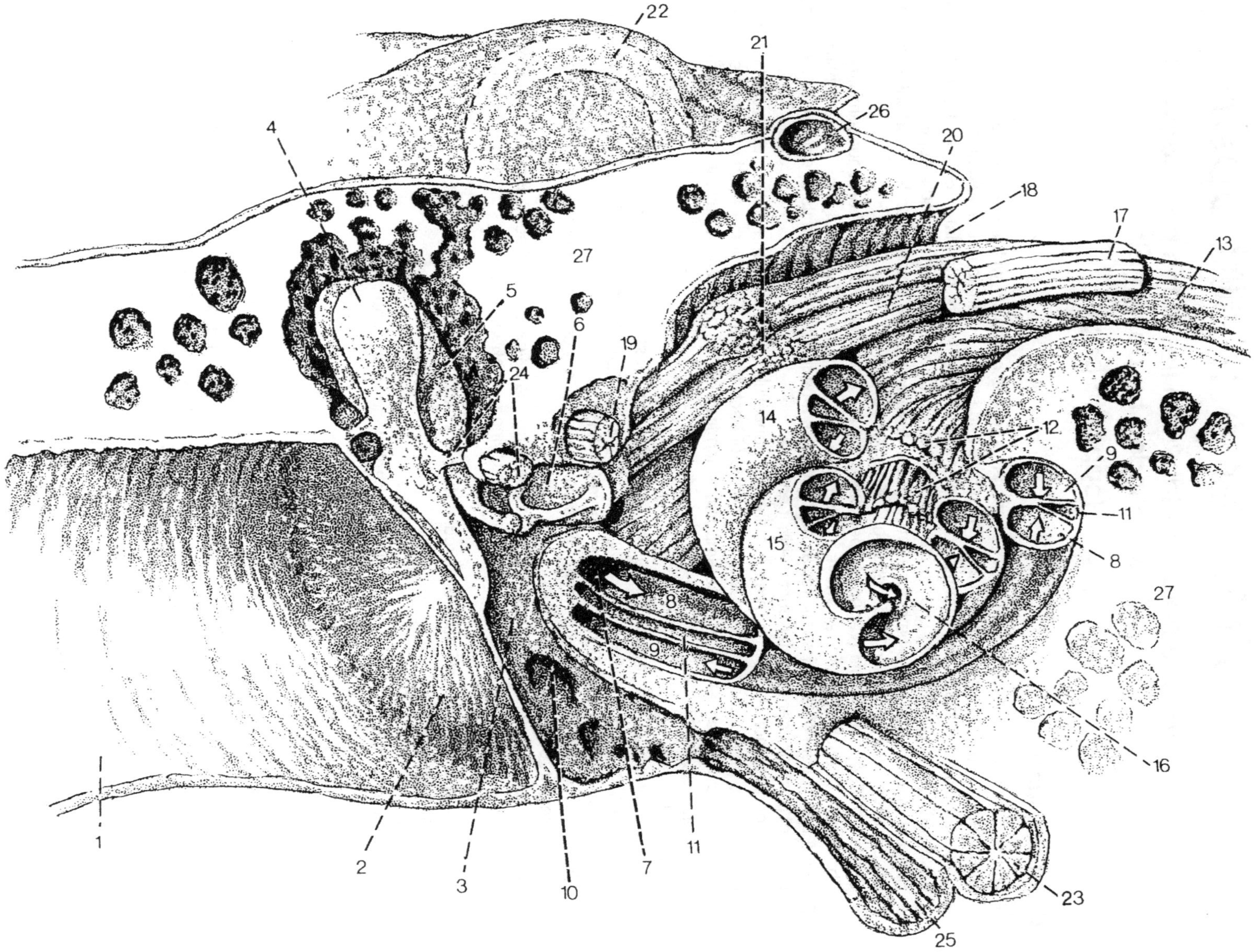

H&N-44 Membranous labyrinth of left inner ear cut open

The membranous labyrinth lies in the bony labyrinth surrounded by perilymph.

(opposite page)

Color and label

1 Utricle (a position and motion sensor); cut open to show its continuity with each of the 3 semicircular ducts
2 Saccule. Cut open to reveal its macula. The utricle and saccule both lie in the vestibule.
3 Utricular macula. It lies mainly in a horizontal plane. Its hair cells are stimulated both by tilting the head and by accelerating and decelerating in a horizontal direction, such as speeding up and stopping suddenly in a car.
4 Saccular macula (*macula* is Latin for spot). It lies in a vertical plane and responds to vertical acceleration and deceleration, such a starting and stopping in a fast elevator.
5 Crista (L. ridge) and cupula (L. cup-shaped object) in the ampulla (L. flask) of anterior semicircular duct. The cupula in each semicircular sways in response to movement of the endolymph in the semicircular ducts.
6 Crista and cupula of lateral semicircular duct within its ampulla seen through its opening into the utricle.
7 Crista of posterior semicircular duct within it ampulla
8 Cupula on posterior crista. The three cupulae are noncellular gelatinous masses on each crista. Hair cells in the three cristae project their processes into the base of each cupula. Turning the head causes the endolymph to deflect the cupula either towards the ampulla, which fires off the hair cells, or away from the ampulla, which hyperpolarizes the air cells.
9 Utricle cut open.
10 Vestibular end of cochlear duct. This abuts on the fenestra vestibuli (round window).
11 Spiral ganglion. Its peripheral processes end in the spiral organ of Corti and its central processes form the cochlear portion of the vestibulocochlear nerve (N VIII)
12 Afferent (incoming, to the brain) nerve fibers from the bipolar neurons in the spiral ganglion. There are also some efferent (outgoing) nerve fibers.
13 Cochlear duct. Shown here without the accompanying scala vestibuli and scala tympani. The cochlear duct, or scala media, is pie-shaped in cross-section, occupying only about 30 degress of the cross-section of the cochlea.
14 Anterior semicircular duct. Each semicircular duct lies within a semicircular canal.
15 Lateral semicircular duct
16 Posterior semicircular duct
17 Endolymphatic duct. Its enlarged end lies adjacent to the dura mater.
18 Nerve to posterior crista ampullaris
19 Upper division of vestibular nerve
20 Lower division of vestibular nerve
21 Cochlear nerve

Vertigo (Latin, *vertere,* to turn): a feeling of whirling or turning around, a giddiness, a dizziness. An hallucination of movement, expecially of rotation, independent of any actual movement. Vestibular vertigo, such as occurs in Meniere's disease, is due to disease within the vestibular labyrinth, which includes the three semicircular ducts, the utricle, and the saccule.

H&N-44 Membranous labyrinth of left inner ear cut open

Removed from bony labyrinth and partially dissected

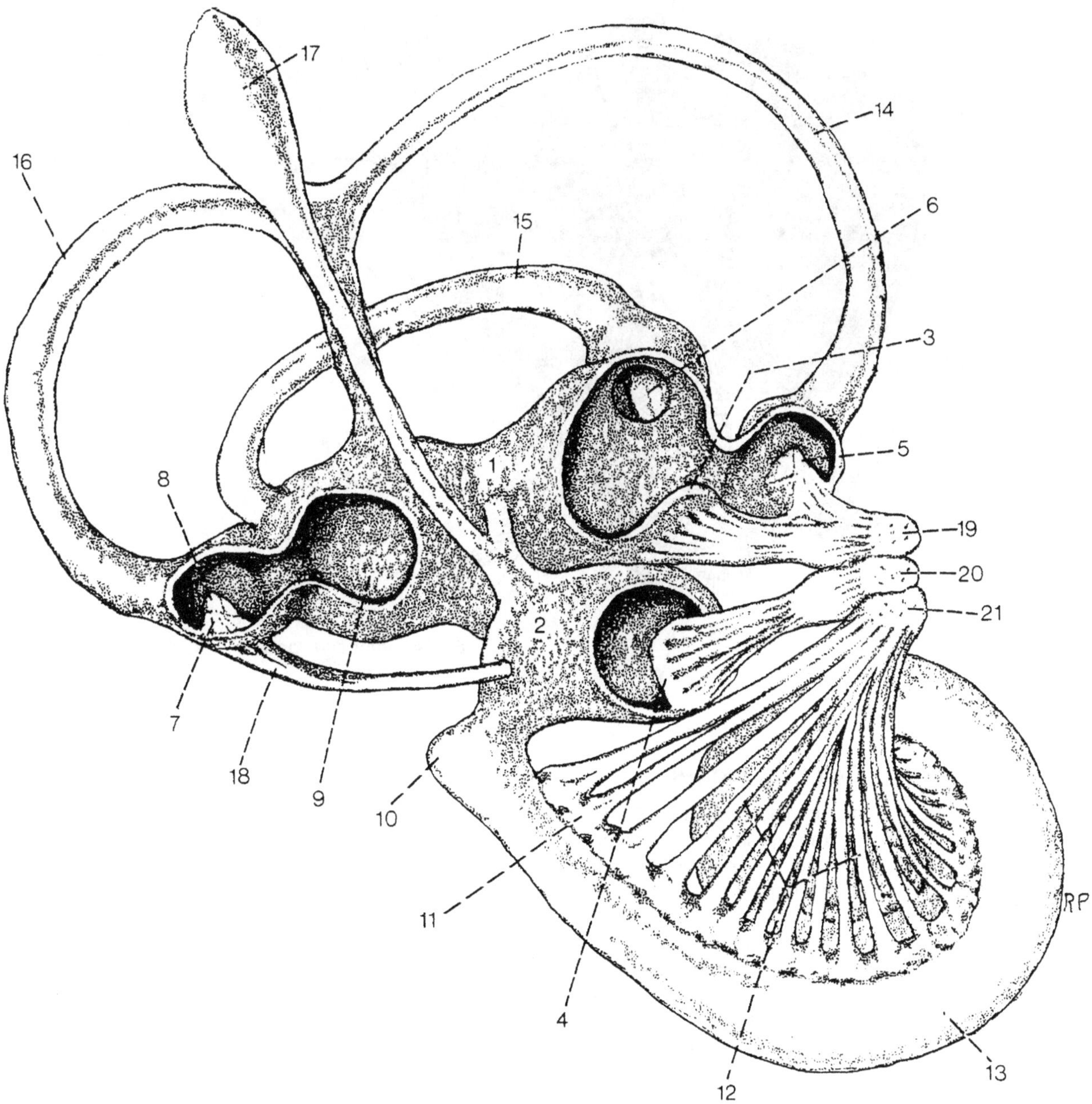

H&N-45 Dissection of right temporal bone showing sigmoid sinus and facial canal

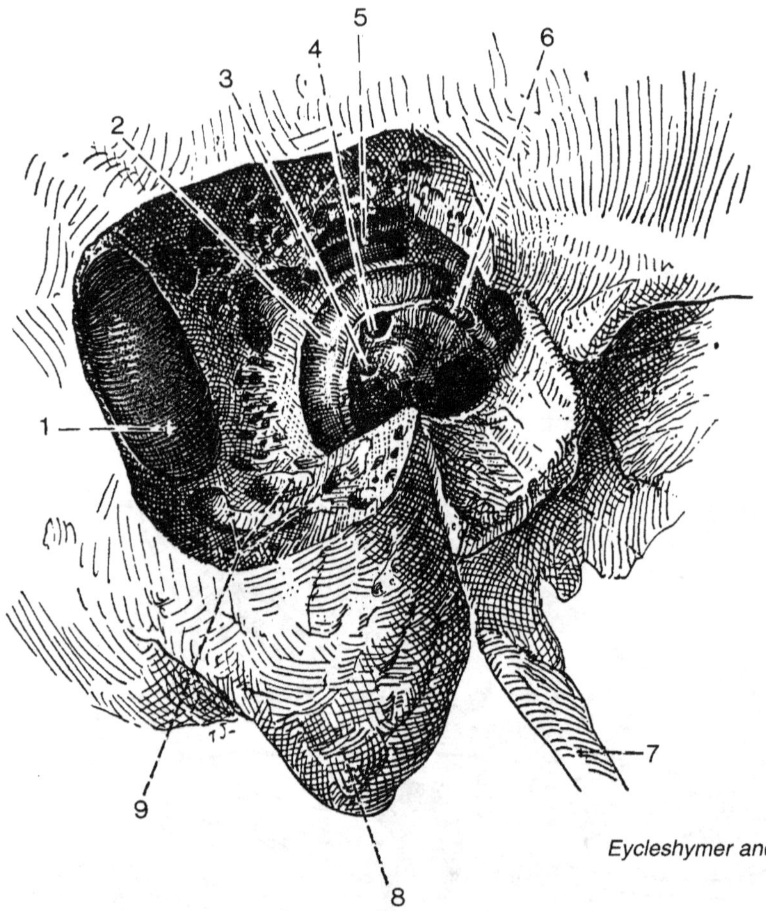

Eycleshymer and Jones

Color and label

1 Sigmoid sinus; directly continuous with transverse sinus; becomes the internal jugular vein upon leaving the skull via the jugular foramen
2 Facial canal
3 Round window
4 Oval window; covered by footplate of stapes
5 Lateral semicircular canal
6 Canal for tensor tympani muscle
7 Styloid process
8 Mastoid process (breast-like, *mastos*, Greek, breast)
9 Mastoid air cells

H&N-46 Section through external ear, middle ear, and inner ear

Somewhat diagrammatic

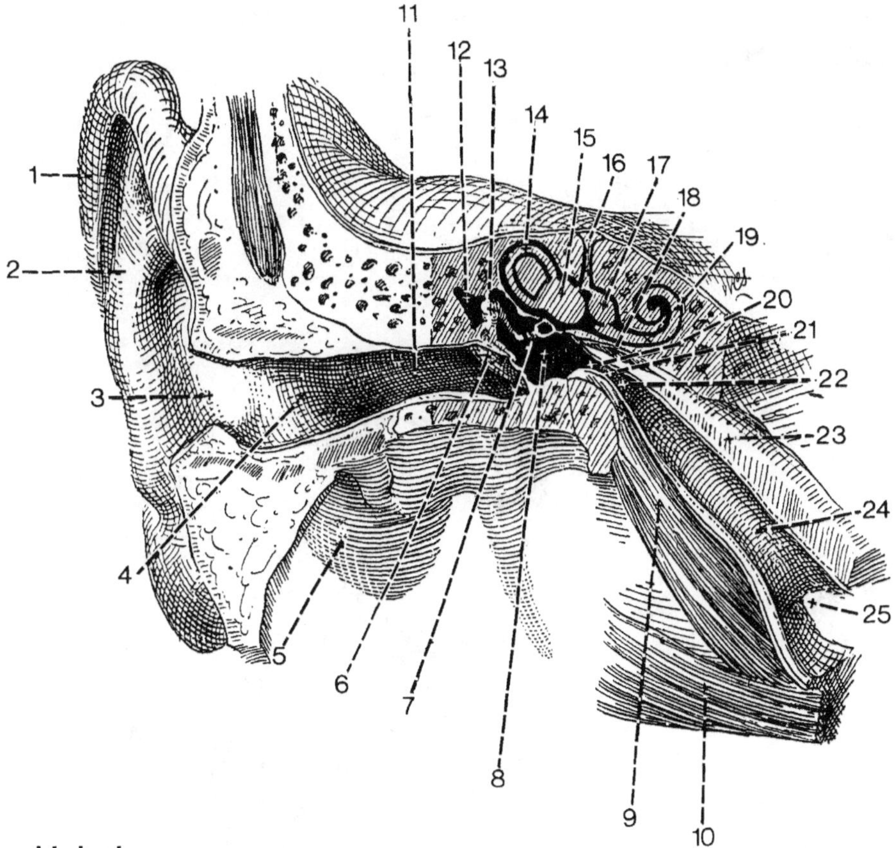

Color and label

1 Helix of auricle (external ear)*
2 Antihelix of auricle*
3 Concha of auricle*
4 External acoustic (auditory) meatus (cartilaginous part)
5 Mastoid process
6 Ear drum (tympanic membrane)
7 Head of stapes
8 Tympanic cavity (cavity of middle ear)
9 Levator veli palatini muscle
10 Superior pharyngeal constrictor muscle
11 External auditory meatus (bony part)
12 Epitympanic recess
13 Head of malleus
14 Anterior semicircular duct (within anterior semicircular canal)
15 Utricle
16 Endolymphatic duct
17 Sacculus; both the saccule and the utricle occupy the vestibule, a small cavity in the temporal bone
18 Tensor tympani muscle
19 Cochlear duct
20 Tympanic opening of the auditory tube (old name, Eustachean tube)
21 Bony part of auditory tube
22 Isthmus of auditory tube
23 Cartilage of auditory tube
24 Cartilaginous part of auditory tube
25 Pharyngeal opening of auditory tube

Eycleshymer and Jones with slight modification

*The Terminologia Anatomica lists 29 anatomical parts of the auricle of the ear, only three of which are identified here.

Tragus
Etymological cartoon

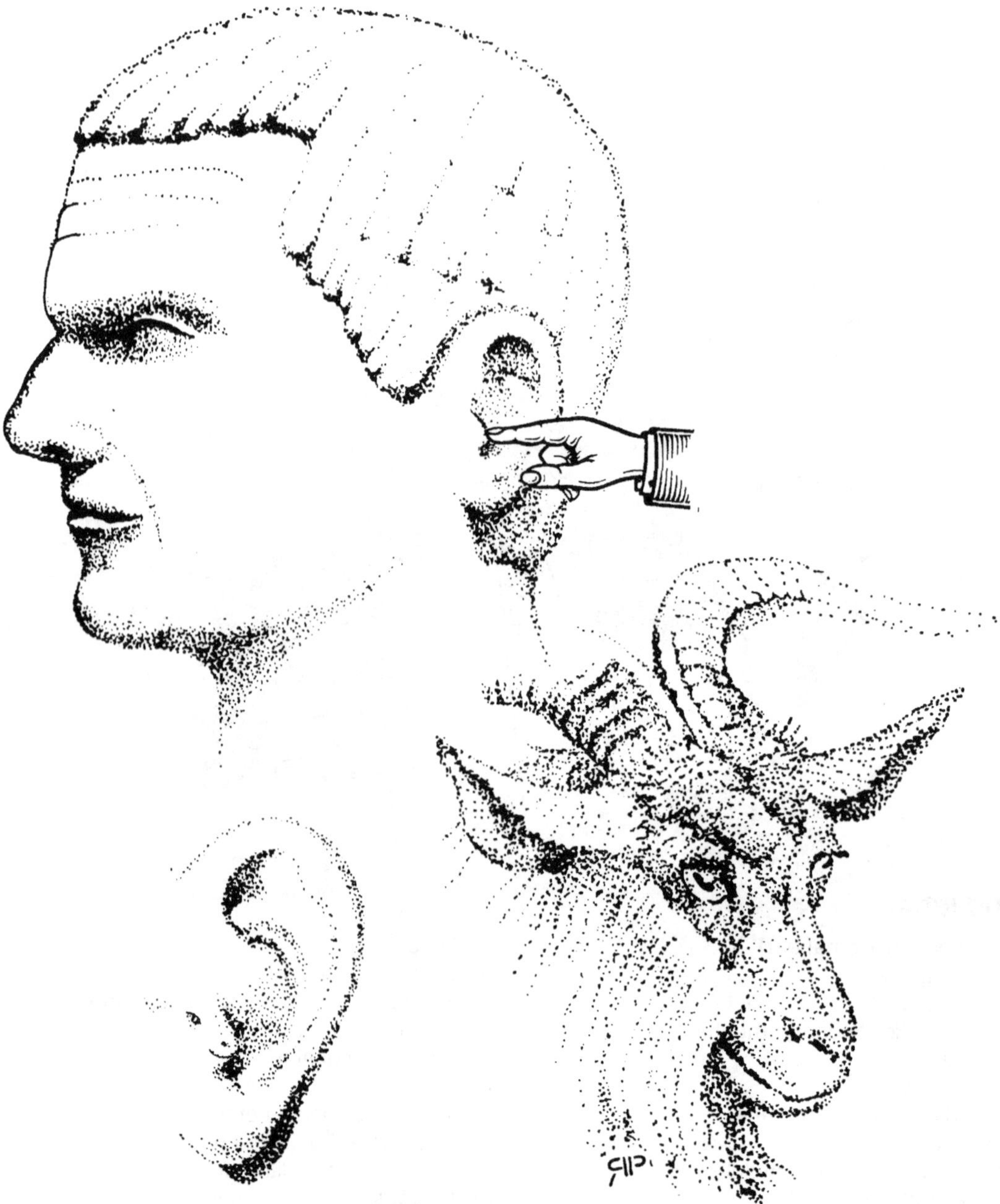

Latin, billy goat

The tragus of the ear was so named because in some old men it grows a little tuft of hair that reminded the ancient anatomists of a billy goat's beard. Tragos is Greek for billy goat and tragus is the Latin. Tragedy originally meant "goat's song."

H&N-47 Cartilages of the nose

Color and label

1 Greater alar cartilage
2 Lateral crus of greater alar cartilage
3 Medial crus of greater alar cartilage
4 Lateral nasal cartilage
5 Accessory nasal cartilage
6 Minor alar cartilage
7 Nasal septal cartilage
8 Nasal bone
9 Maxillary bone

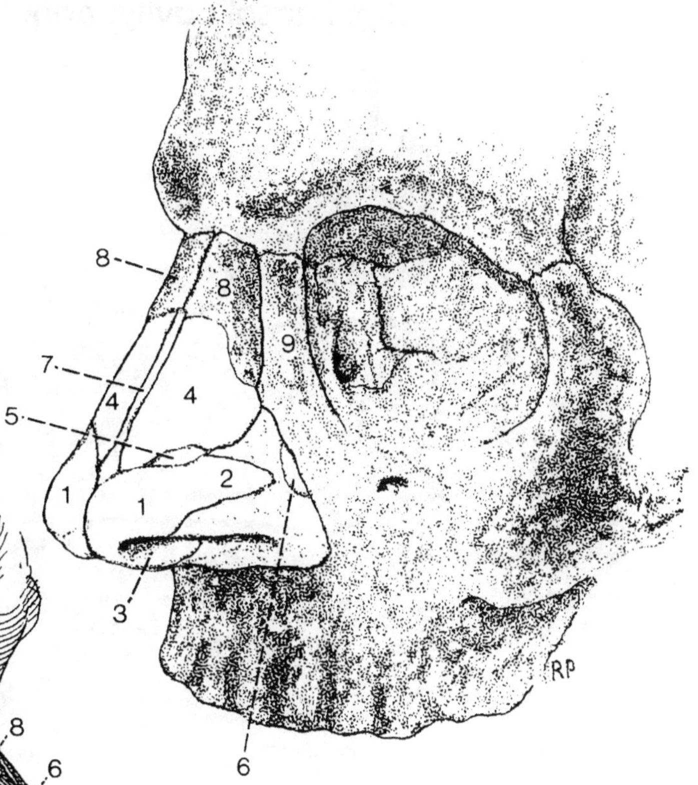

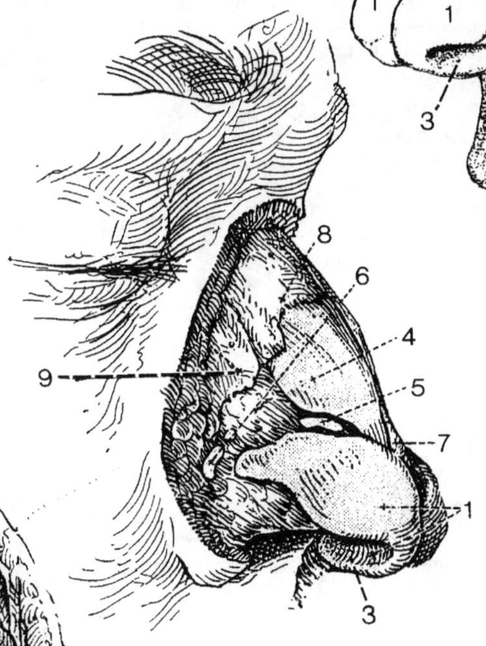

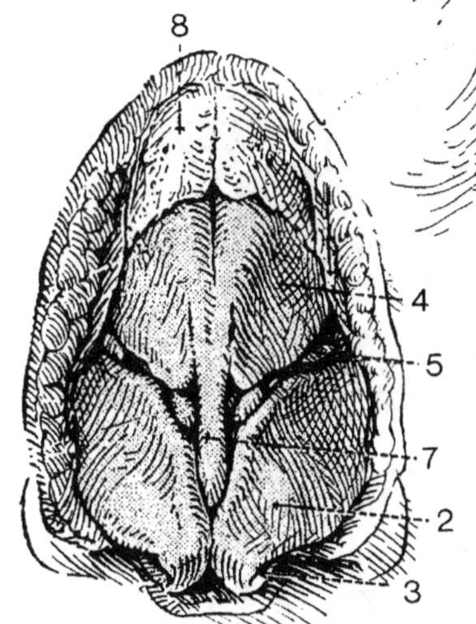

Eycleshymer and Jones

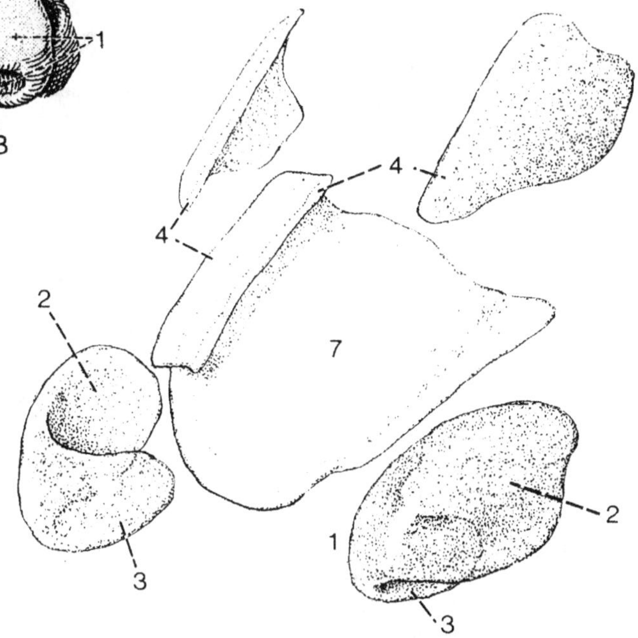

H&N-48 Nasal cavity, lateral wall

Right nasal cavity: conchae cut* in lower figure

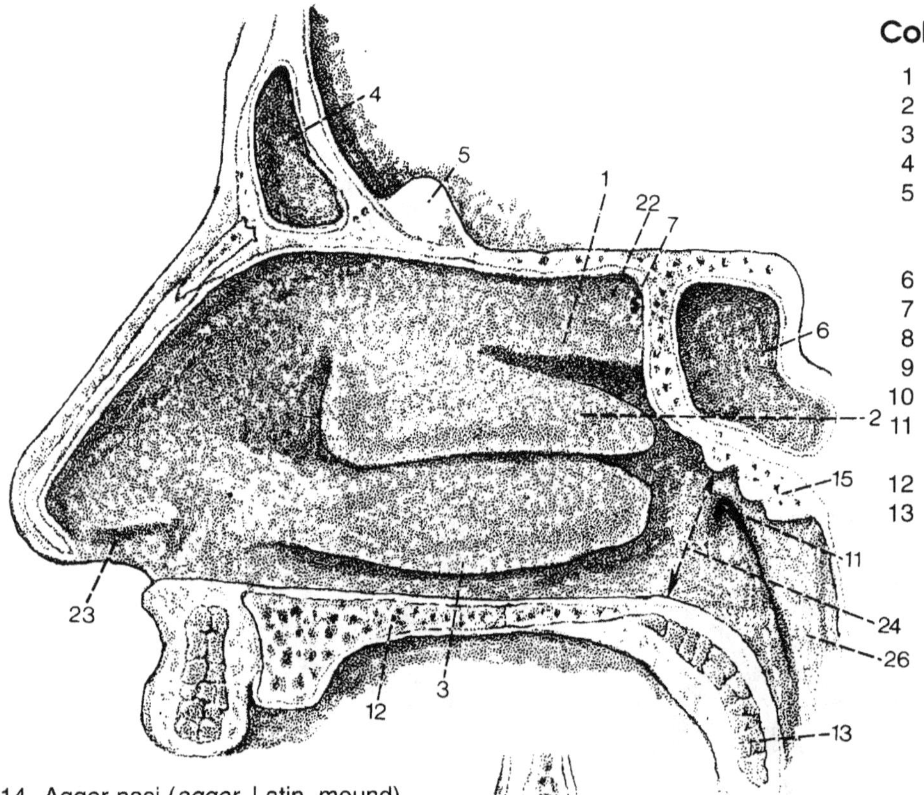

Color and label

1 Superior nasal concha*
2 Middle nasal concha*
3 Inferior nasal concha*
4 Frontal sinus
5 Crista galli (not to be confused with Crystal Gale; *crista galli* is Latin for rooster's comb)*
6 Sphenoidal sinus
7 Opening of sphenoidal sinus
8 Superior nasal meatus
9 Middle nasal meatus
10 Inferior nasal meatus
11 Opening of auditory tube in nasal pharynx
12 Hard palate
13 Soft palate

*Crystal Gale is a country blues singer. Although crista galli and Cristal Gale sound alike, they don't at all look alike.

14 Agger nasi (*agger*, Latin, mound)
15 Pharyngeal tonsil (called adenoids when inflamed)
16 Ethmoidal bulla (Latin, swelling)
17 Openings of ethmoidal air cells
18 Hiatus semilunaris
19 Opening of frontal sinus into hiatus semilunaris
20 Opening of nasolacrimal duct into inferior nasal meatus

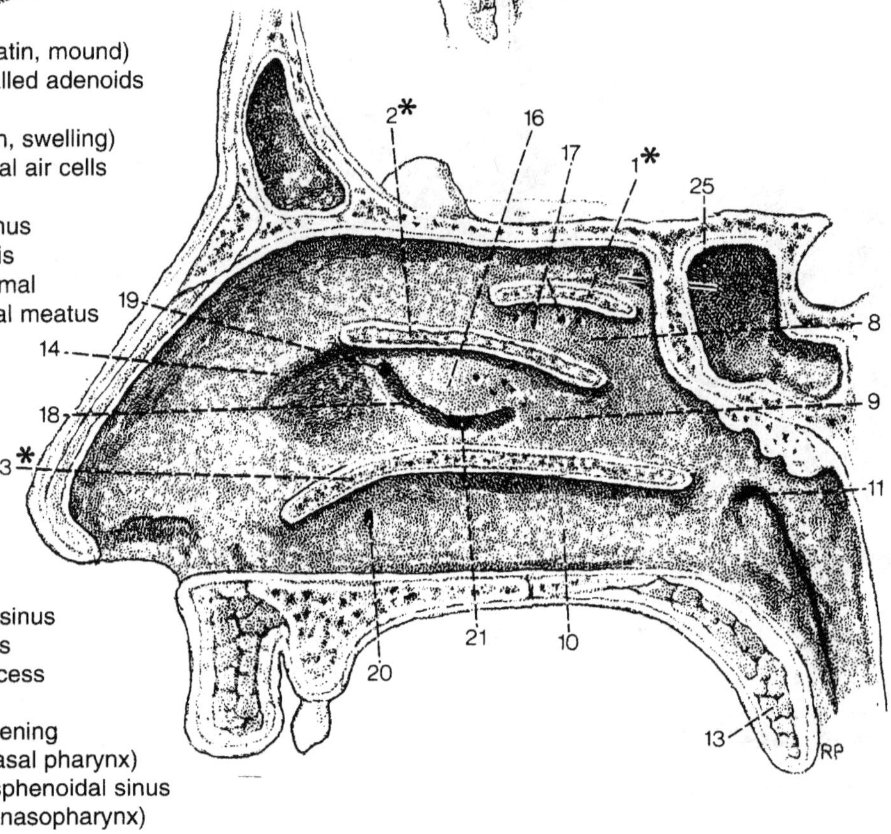

21 Opening of maxillary sinus into hiatus semilunaris
22 Spheno-ethmoidal recess
23 Nasal vestibule
24 Choana (posterior opening of nasal cavity into nasal pharynx)
25 Probe in opening of sphenoidal sinus
26 Nasal pharynx (also, nasopharynx)

H&N-49 Nasal cavity, bones and cartilages

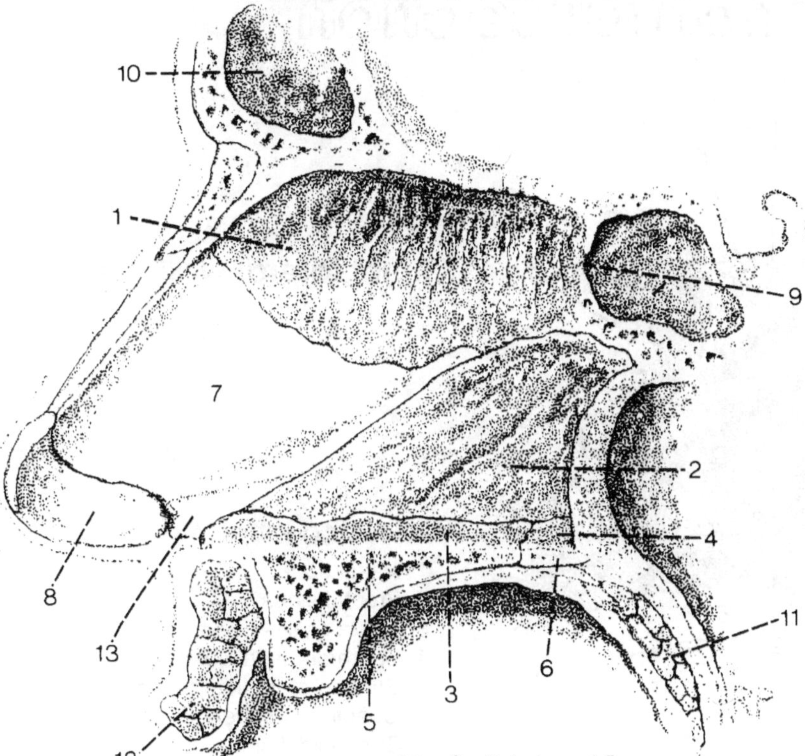

After Spalteholz and Spanner

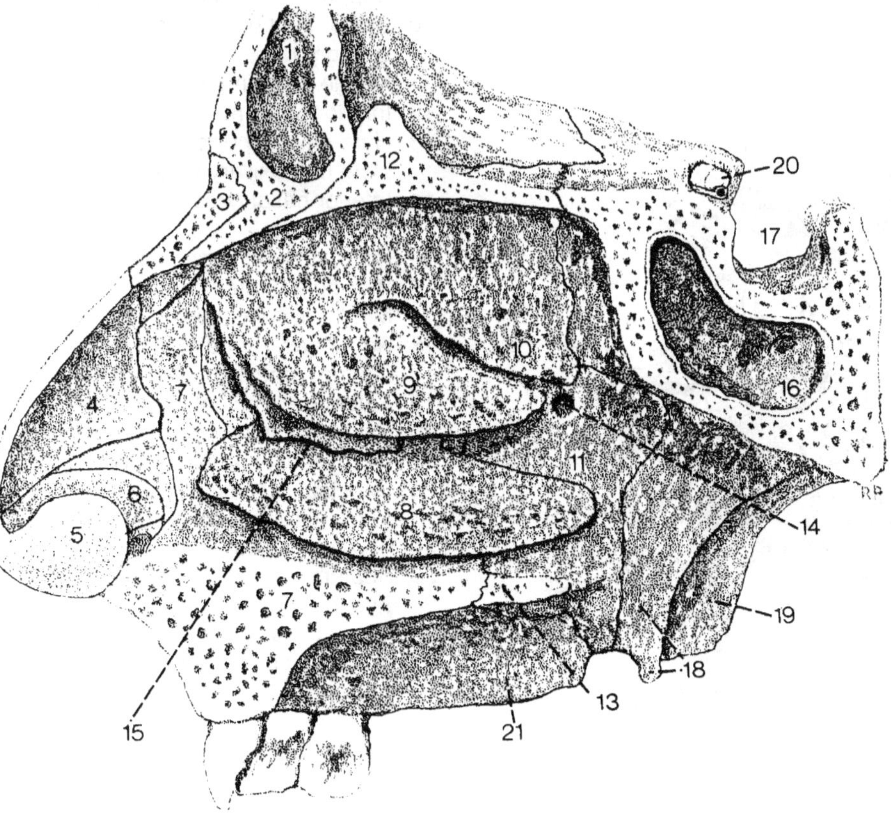

Color and label

1 Perpendicular plate of ethmoid bone
2 Vomer (Latin, plowshare)
3 Nasal spine of maxillary bone
4 Nasal spine of palatine bone
5 Palatine process of maxilla
6 Horizontal plate of palatine bone
7 Nasal septal cartilage
8 Left greater alar cartilage (medial crus) (cut; with lateral crus removed)
9 Sphenoidal sinus and opening
10 Frontal sinus
11 Soft palate
12 Upper lip
13 Vomeronasal cartilage

Right side of nasal cavity

1 Frontal sinus
2 Frontal bone
3 Nasal bone
4 Lateral nasal cartilage
5 Greater alar cartilage (medial crus)
6 Greater alar cartilage (lateral crus)
7 Maxillary bone
8 Inferior nasal concha (a separate bone)
9 Middle nasal concha (part of the ethmoid bone)
10 Superior nasal concha (part of ethmoid bone)
11 Palatine bone (vertical part)
12 Crista galli (part of ethmoid)
13 Palatine bone (horizontal part)
14 Sphenopalatine foramen
15 Uncinate process (part of ethmoid)
16 Sphenoidal sinus
17 Hypophyseal fossa
18 Medial pterygoid plate (part of sphenoid bone)
19 Lateral pterygoid plate (part of sphenoid bone)
20 Optic nerve and ophthalmic artery
21 Alveolar process of maxillary bone

H&N-50 Nasal cavity, lateral wall and frontal section

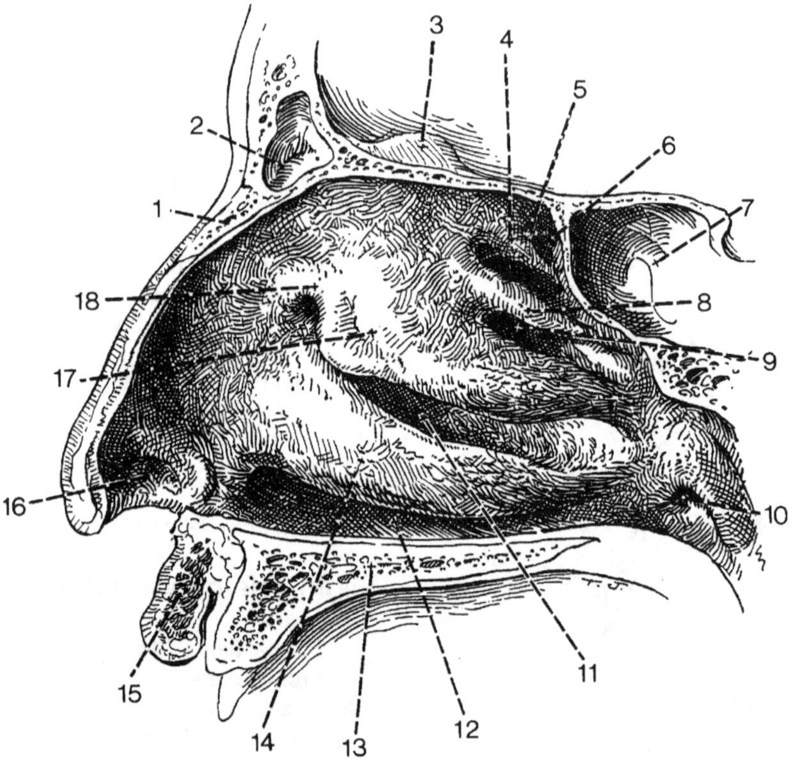

Right lateral wall

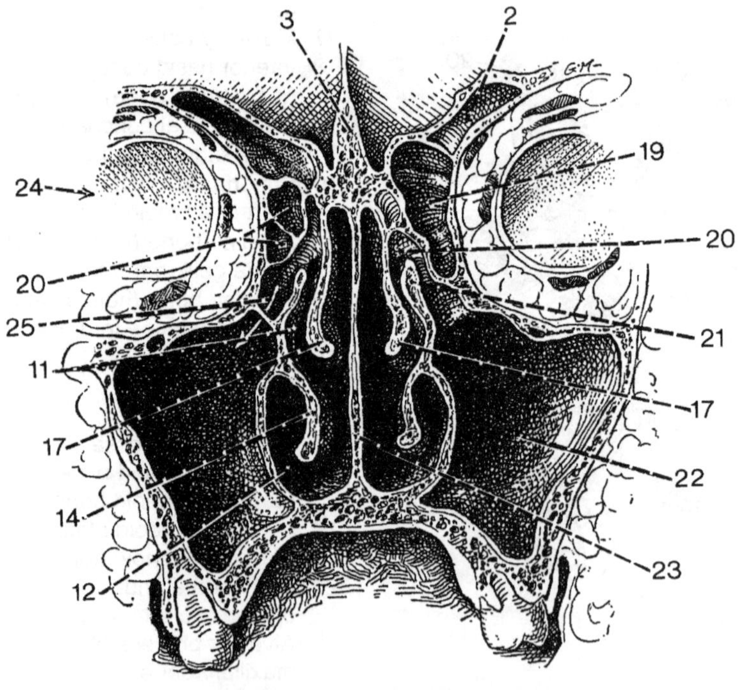

Frontal section

Color and label

1 Nasal bone
2 Frontal sinus
3 Crista galli
4 Supreme nasal concha
5 Spheno-ethmoidal recess
6 Opening of sphenoidal sinus
7 Sphenoidal sinus
8 Superior nasal concha
9 Superior nasal meatus
10 Pharyngeal opening of auditory tube
11 Middle nasal meatus
12 Inferior nasal meatus
13 Hard palate (horizontal plate of maxillary bone)
14 Inferior nasal concha
15 Superior lip (Latin, *labium superius*)
16 Vestibule of the nose
17 Middle nasal concha
18 Agger nasi (*agger*, Latin, heap, mound, rampart)
19 Anterior ethmoidal air cell
20 Ethmoidal bulla (bulla, Latin, a bubble-like protuberance)
21 Uncinate process (uncinate, hook-shaped)
22 Maxillary sinus
23 Septum of nose
24 Eye in orbit
25 Arrow passing through maxillary sinus opening

Eycleshymer and Jones

H&N-51 Pterygopalatine ganglion

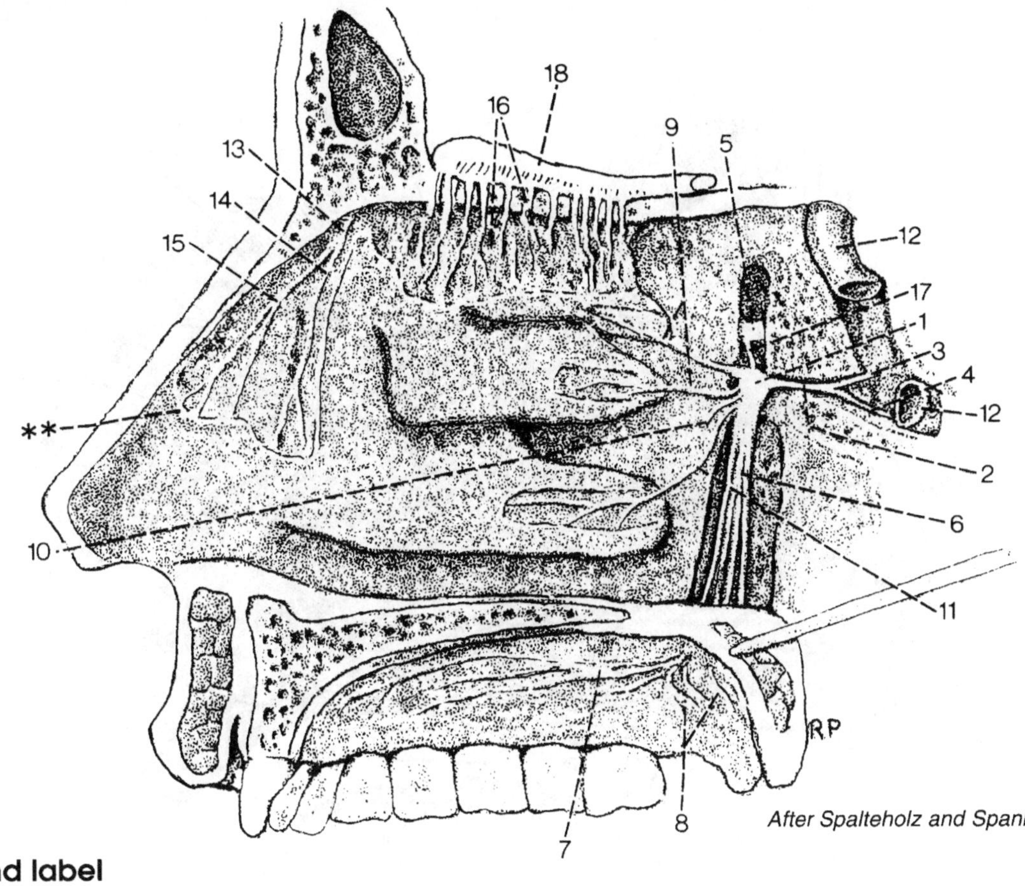

After Spalteholz and Spanner

Color and label

1 Pterygopalatine ganglion*; contains postganglionic parasympathetic neurons with secretomotor axons destined for the posterior nasal glands and lacrimal gland; only pregangionic parasympathetic axons synapse within this ganglion, other fibers bypass it.
2 Nerve of the pterygoid canal; made up of the greater petrosal (taste and parasympatheic fibers from the facial nerve) and the deep petrosal nerve (sympathetic fibers from cell bodies in the superior cervical ganglion).
3 Greater petrosal nerve
4 Deep petrosal nerve
5 Maxillary in the pterygopalatine fossa*
6 Palatine nerves; descending in palatine canal*
7 Greater palatine nerves
8 Lesser palatine nerves
9 Lateral superior posterior nasal branches of maxillary nerve and pterygopalatine ganglion
10 Medial superior posterior nasal branches to nasal septum from maxillary nerve and pterygopalatine ganglion (cut)
11 Lateral inferior posterior nasal branches of maxillary nerve and pterygopalatine ganglion
12 Internal carotid artery (cut both entering [bottom], and leaving [top] the cavernous sinus)
13 Internal nasal branches of anterior ethmoidal nerve of ophthalmic nerve
14 Lateral nasal branches
15 External nasal branches
16 Olfactory nerves (cranial nerve I; note axons ending in olfactory bulb after passing through cribriform [sieve-like, full of holes] plate of ethmoid bone)
17 Pterygopalatine nerves
18 Olfactory bulb

*Pterygopalatine fossa and palatine canal opened from medial aspect

**Mucous membrane removed to display nerves

H&N-52 Olfactory nerves and arterial supply of nasal cavity

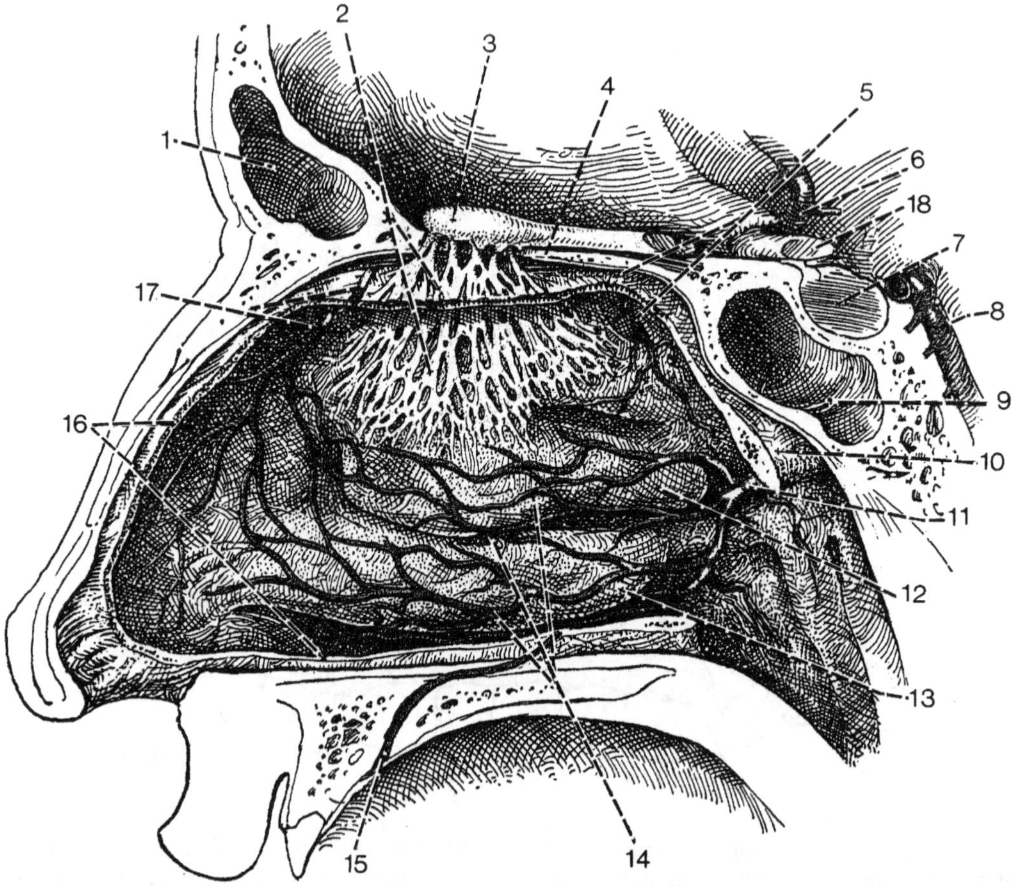

Color and label

1 Frontal sinus
2 Olfactory nerves (cranial nerve I); note their passing through the cribriform plate; note also olfactory nerves on the nasal septum (where both septum and nerves are cut)
3 Olfactory bulb; compared to mammals such as dogs, humans have relatively small olfactory bulbs and rely largely on vision, rather than olfaction, for perceiving our surroundings. (Macrosmatic means having a well-developed olfactory sense; microsmatic means having a poorly developed olfactory sense; *osme*, Greek, smell)
4 Cribriform plate of ethmoid bone
5 Posterior ethmoidal artery; including cut branch on nasal septum (also cut)
6 Internal carotid artery
7 Hypophysis (pituitary gland)
8 Basilar artery
9 Sphenoid sinus
10 Nasal septum (posterior part; cut)
11 Sphenopalatine artery
12 Middle nasal concha
13 Inferior nasal concha
14 Lateral posterior nasal arteries
15 Artery in incisive canal (anastomosis between septal nasal artery and greater palatine artery)
16 Nasal septum (cut)
17 Anterior ethmoidal artery
18 Optic nerve (cranial nerve II; cut)

Eycleshymer and Jones

H&N-53 Right wall of nasal cavity and ethmoidal air cells

The middle and superior conchae have been removed.

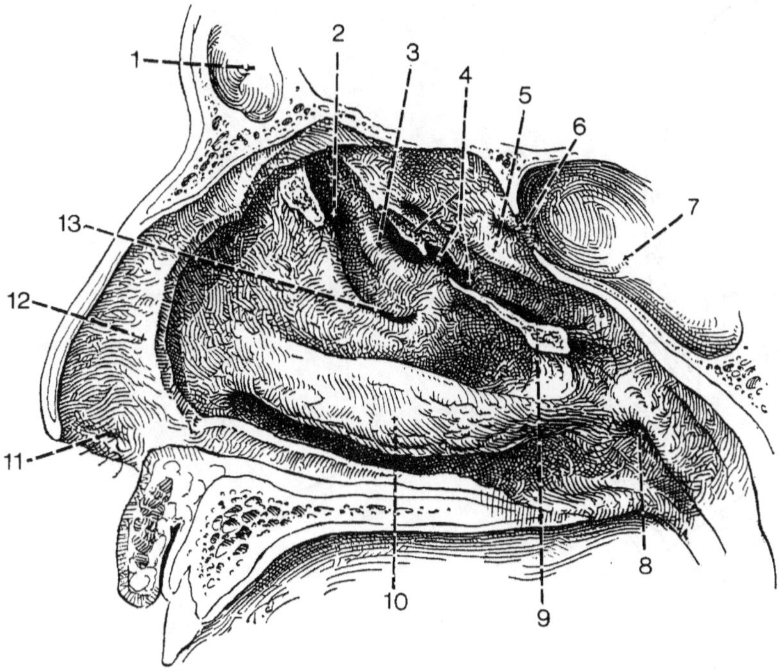

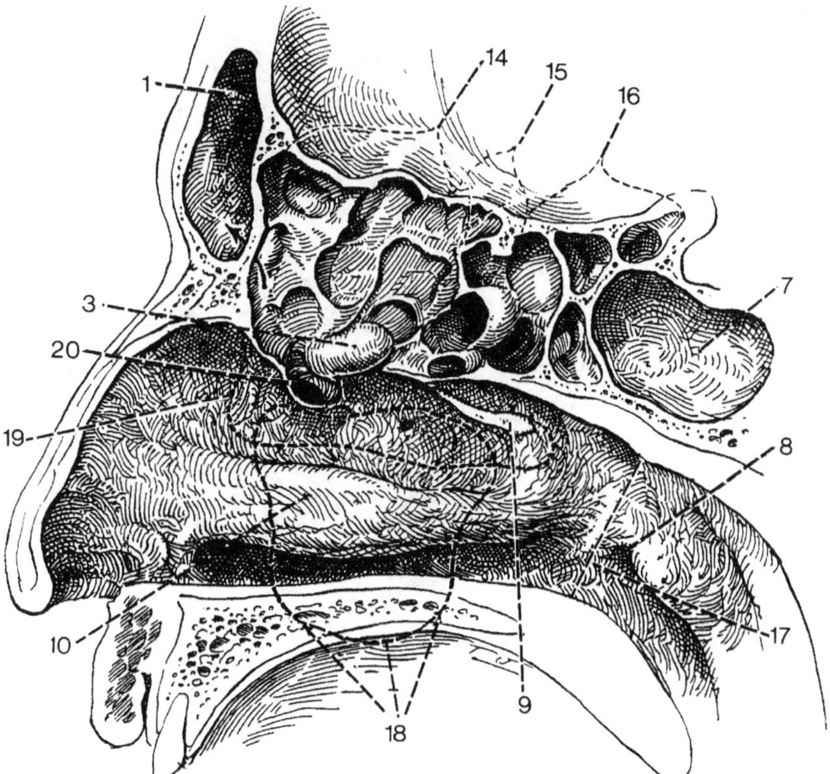

Color and label

1 Frontal sinus
2 Ethmoidal infundibulum
3 Ethmoidal bulla
4 Superior nasal concha (cut and removed) and superior nasal meatus
5 Highest (supreme) nasal concha
6 Opening of sphenoidal sinus
7 Sphenoidal sinus; note the variation in both size and shape in the frontal and sphenoidal sinuses in the two figures.
8 Pharyngeal opening of the auditory tube
9 Middle nasal concha (cut and removed)
10 Inferior nasal concha
11 Nasal vestibule
12 Nasal septum (cut and largely removed)
13 Hiatus semilunaris
14 Anterior ethmoidal (air) cells
15 Middle ethmoidal (air) cells
16 Posterior ethmoidal (air) cells
17 Posterior nasal aperature (or choana)
18 Projected outline of maxillary sinus
19 Outline of middle nasal concha (cut and removed)
20 Opening into maxillary sinus

Eycleshymer and Jones with modification

H&N-54 Projection of paranasal sinuses on front and side of face

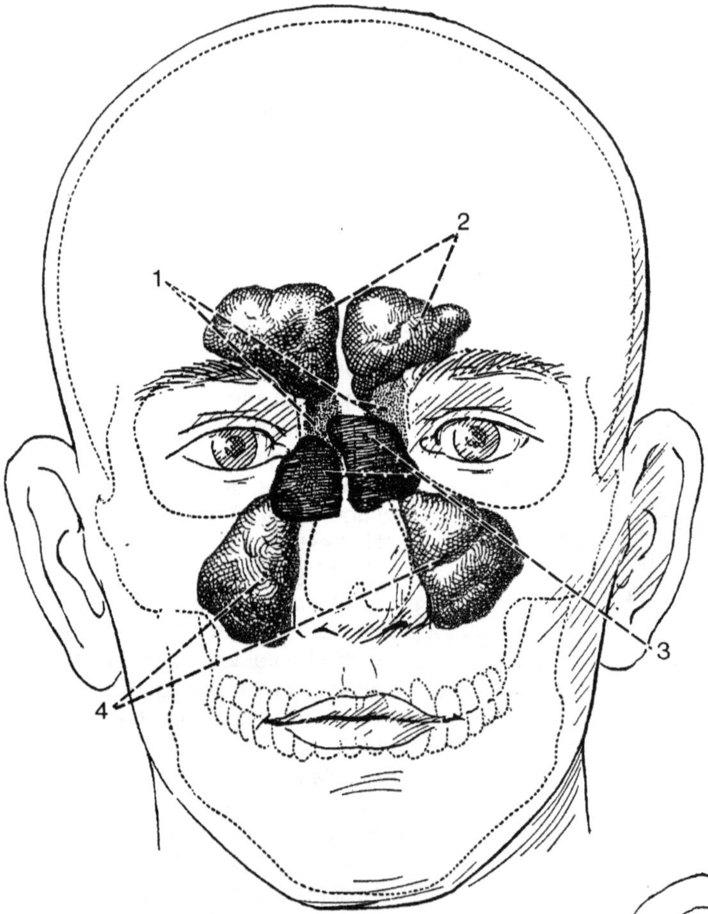

Eycleshymer and Jones

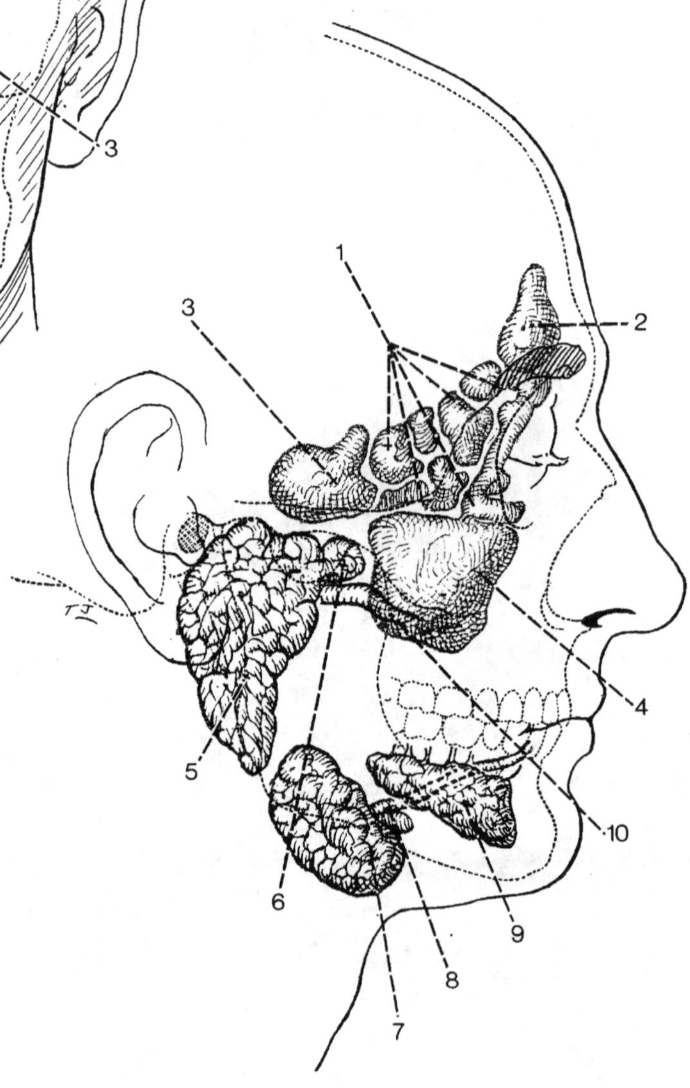

Salivary glands are also projected in lower figure

Color and label

1 Ethmoidal (air) cells*
2 Frontal sinsuses
3 Sphenoidal sinsuses
4 Maxillary sinsuses
5 Parotid gland
6 Accessory parotid gland
7 Submaxillary gland
8 Submaxillary duct
9 Sublingual gland
10 Parotid duct

*The official anatomical name for the small air filled cavities in the upper sides of the nasal cavity is **ethmoidal cells**. To avoid any confusion with the word **cells,** the author has inserted the word **air**.

H&N-55 Oral and nasal cavities in sagittal section

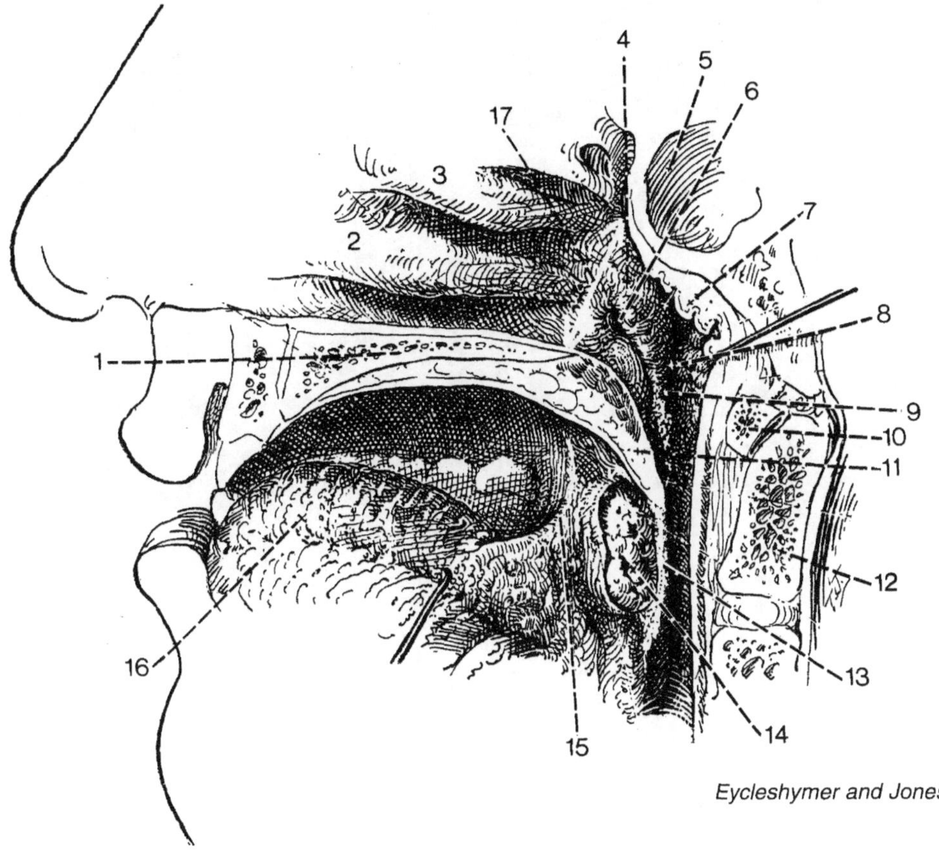

Eycleshymer and Jones

Color and label

1 Hard palate
2 Inferior nasal concha
3 Middle nasal concha
4 Torus tubularis (tubal prominence; *torus*, Latin, raised ridge, bulge); the protuberance of the base of cartilaginous part of the auditory tube in the lateral wall of the nasopharynx behind the orifice of the auditory tube.
5 Sphenoidal sinus
6 Pharyngeal orifice (opening) of auditory tube
7 Pharyngeal tonsil; usually absent in adults (the term *adenoids* denotes hypertrophy of this tonsil)
8 Pharyngeal recess
9 Salpingopharyngeal fold
10 Anterior arch of first cervical vertebra (atlas)
11 Soft palate
12 Second cervical vertebra (axis)
13 Palatopharyngeal arch
14 Palatine tonsil
15 Palatoglossal arch
16 Dorsum of tongue
17 White arrow indicates right choana (posterior nasal aperature; *choana*, Latin, a funnel); the two choanae are oval openings connecting each nasal cavity with the nasal pharynx.

H&N-56 Skull, coronal section

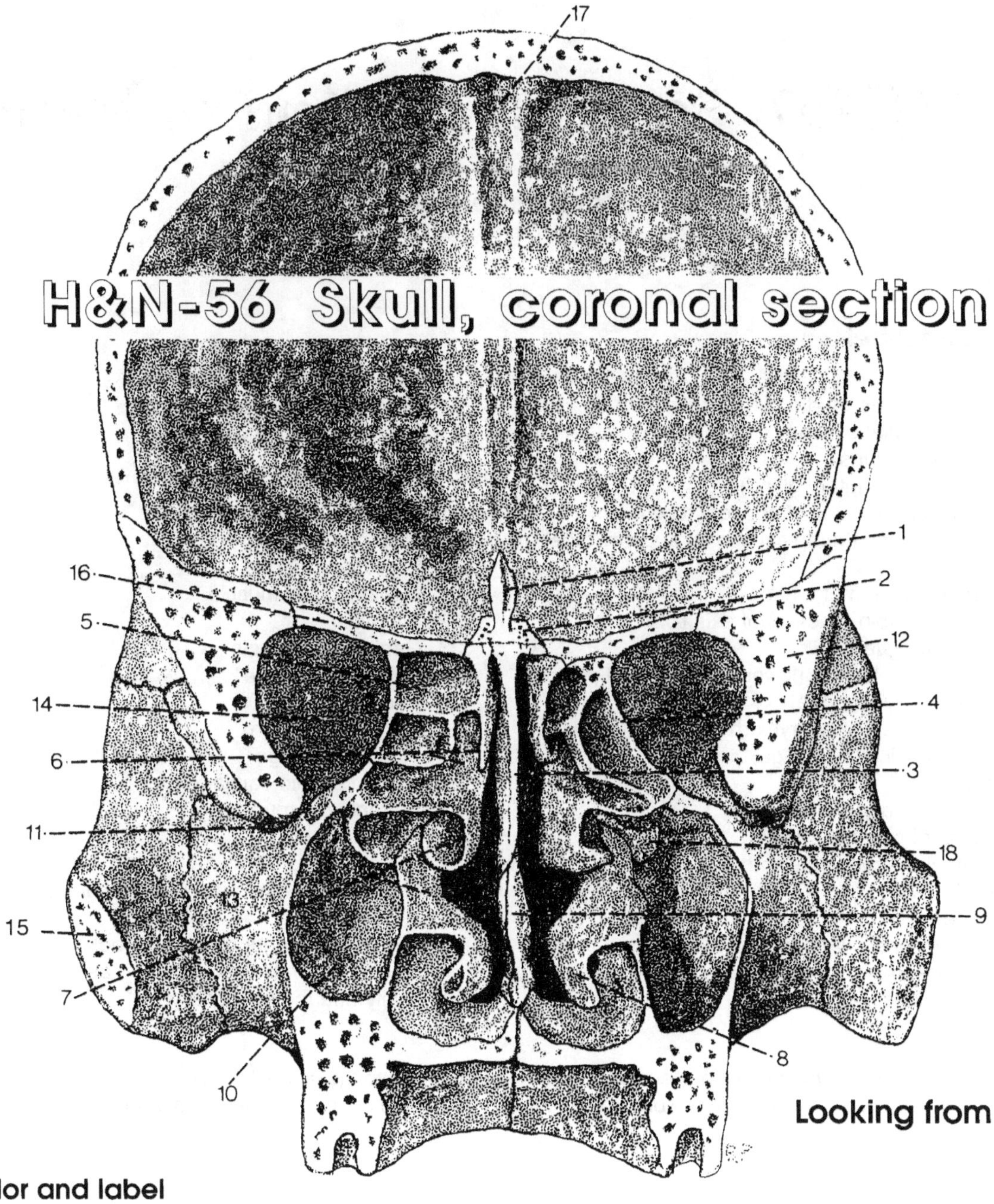

Looking from behind

Color and label

1 Crista galli (Latin, rooster's crest; part of ethmoid)
2 Cribriform (Latin, sieve-like) plate of ethmoid (contains foramina for olfactory nerves)
3 Perpendicular plate of ethmoid
4 Orbital plate of ethmoid (formerly called *lamina papyraceus* because to the ancient anatomists it was as thin as papyrus paper)
5 Ethmoidal air cells (these number 3-18 on each side)
6 Superior nasal concha (Latin, seashell; part of ethmoid) and superior nasal meatus (the passage immediately below it)
7 Middle nasal concha (part of ethmoid) and middle nasal meatus
8 Inferior nasal concha (a separate bone) and inferior nasal meatus
9 Vomer (Latin, plowshare)
10 Maxillary sinus
11 Inferior orbital fissure
12 Greater wing of sphenoid bone
13 Maxillary bone (or maxilla)
14 Orbit
15 Zygomatic bone (zygomatic arch cut)
16 Orbital part of frontal bone
17 Groove for superior sagittal sinus
18 Uncinate (Latin, hook-like) process of ethmoid

After Spalteholz and Spanner

H&N-57 Sagittal section of head

(opposite page)

Color and label

1 Crista galli
2 Cribriform plate of ethmoid bone
3 Superior nasal concha
4 Sphenoidal sinus
5 Hypophysis (pitutary gland)
6 Pharnygeal opening of auditory tube
7 Torus tubularis (bump caused by auditory tube)
8 Soft palate
9 Foramen cecum of tongue
10 Dens (odontoid process) of axis (C2)
11 Root of tongue
12 Oral part of pharynx (lower border of soft palate to level of hyoid bone)
13 Laryngeal part of pharynx (hyoid bone to lower border of cricoid cartilage)*
14 Epiglottis
15 Transverse arytenoid muscle
16 Lamina of cricoid cartilage
17 Vocal folds (true vocal cords)
18 Esophagus
19 Trachea
20 Brachiocephalic vein (old name, innominate vein)
21 Brachiocephalic artery (old name, innominate artery)
22 Frontal sinus
23 Nasal bone
24 Middle nasal concha
25 Inferior nasal concha
26 Hard palate
27 Upper lip
28 Body of tongue
29 Lower lip
30 Septum of tongue
31 Genioglossus muscle
32 Mandible
33 Geniohyoid muscle
34 Mylohyoid muscle
35 Hyoid bone
36 Vestibule of larynx
37 Thyroid cartilage
38 Arch of cricoid cartilage
39 Sternohyoid muscle
40 Thyroid gland
41 Sternothyroid gland
42 Manubrium of sternum (*manubrium*, Latin, handle)

White arrow: right choana (Greek, afunnel): the paired openings between the nasal cavity and the nasopharynx

*The nasal part of the pharynx lies posterior to the nasal cavities above the soft palate. Unlike the oral and laryngeal parts, which temporarily close during swollowing, the nasal part of the pharynx (or nasopharynx) always remains open.

H&N-57 Sagittal section of head

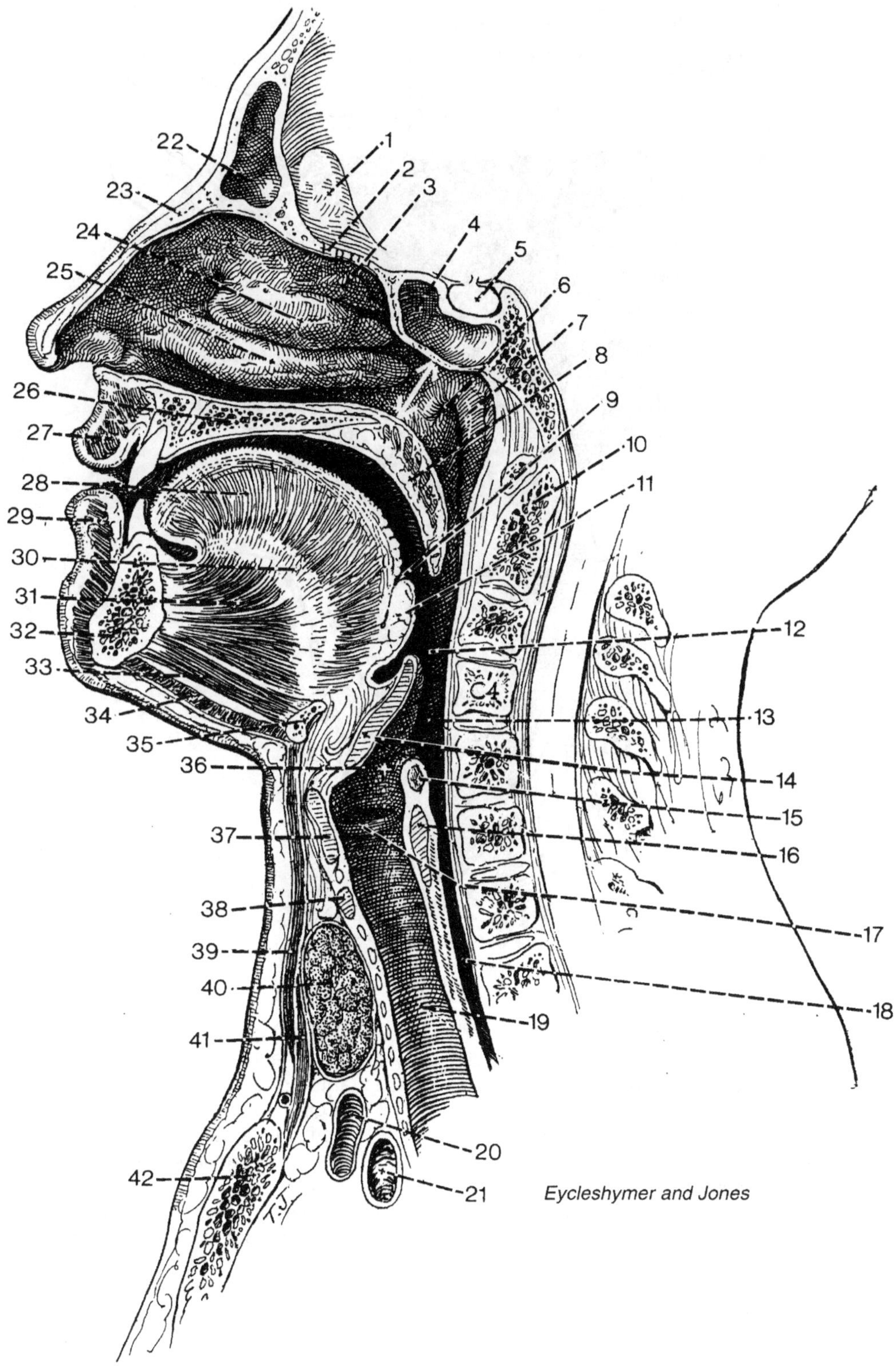

H&N-58 Pharynx

Viewed from behind. Posterior wall has been cut and retracted.

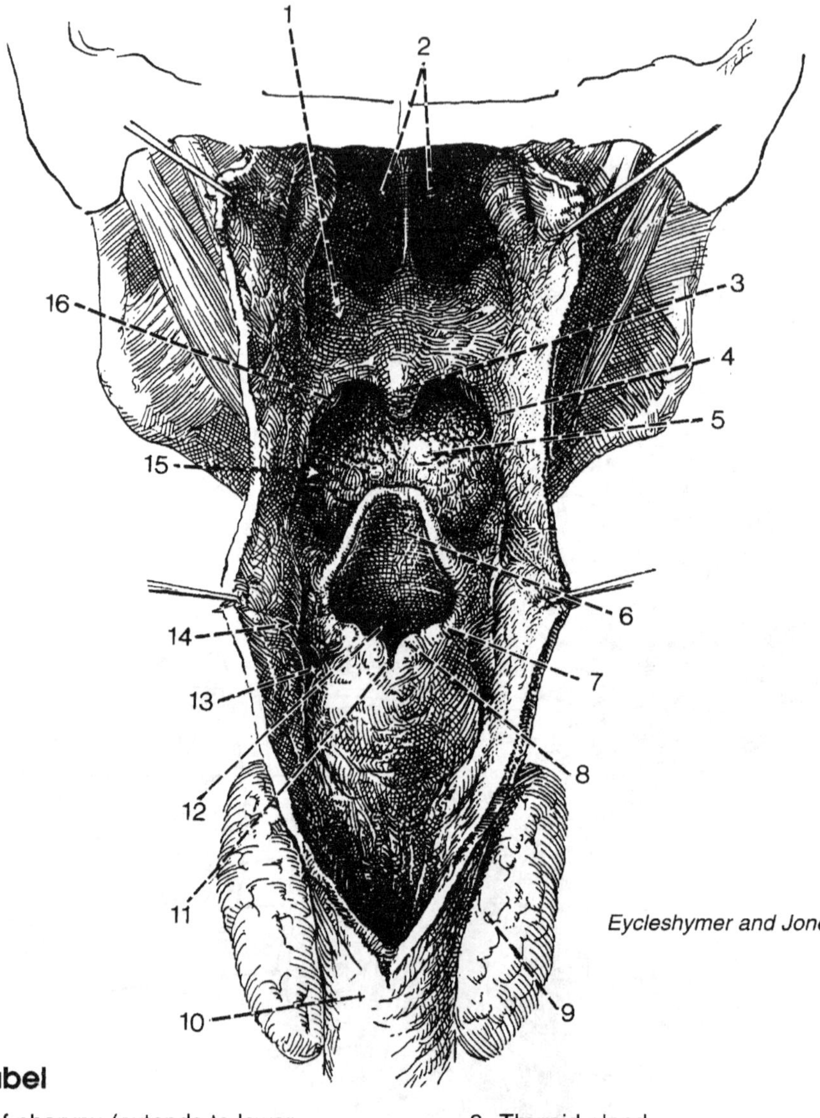

Eycleshymer and Jones

Color and label

1 Nasal part of pharynx (extends to lower edge of soft palate)
2 Choanae (two posterior openings of nasal cavity into nasal pharynx)
3 Uvula (Latin, little grape) of the soft palate
4 Palatopharyngeal arch
5 Root of tongue (pain, touch, temperature, and taste supplied by glossopharyngeal nerve)
6 Epiglottis; this covers the opening to the larynx when swollowing.
7 Cuneiform tubercle (caused by the underlying cuneiform cartilage)
8 Corniculate tubercle (caused by the underlying corniculate cartilage)
9 Thyroid gland
10 Esophagus
11 Interarytenoid incisure (*incisura*, Latin, a cut, a groove); a small notch between the two corniculate cartilages and the apices of the arytenoid cartilages on the posterior aditus of the larynx.
12 Aditus (opening) to the larynx
13 Piriform recess; a site where foreign bodies may lodge and abscesses may develope.
14 Laryngeal part of pharynx; extends from level of hyoid bone to lower border of cricoid cartilage.
15 Oral part of pharynx; extends from lower border of soft palate to level of hyoid bone.
16 Palatine tonsil

H&N-59 Muscles of the tongue, pharynx, and larynx

Right side

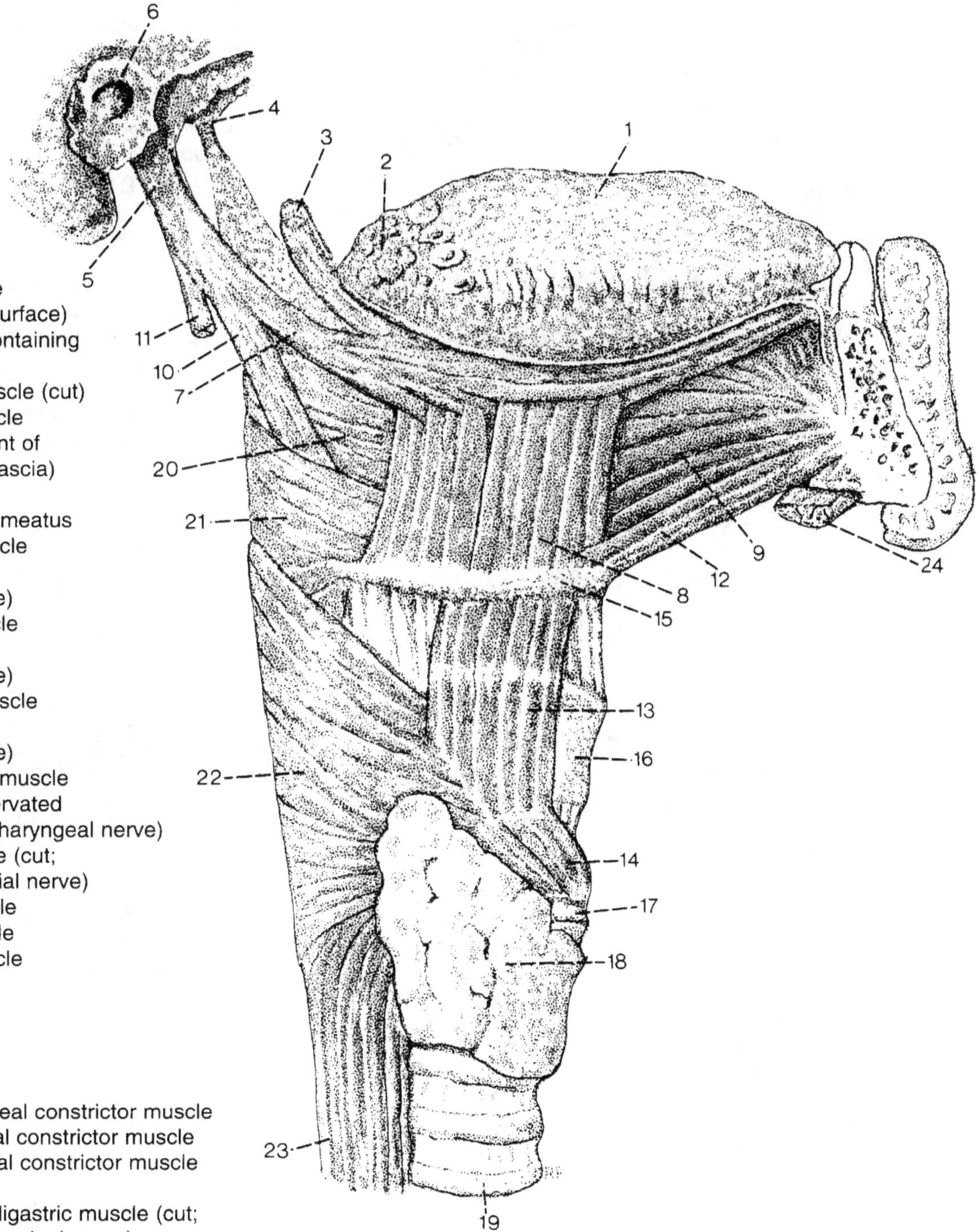

Color and label

1 Dorsum of tongue (superior visible surface)
2 Root of tongue containing lingual follicles
3 Palatoglossal muscle (cut)
4 Pharyngeal tubercle (cranial attachment of pharyngobasilar fascia)
5 Styloid process
6 External auditory meatus
7 Styloglossus muscle (innervated by hypoglossal nerve)
8 Hyoglossus muscle (innervated by hypoglossal nerve)
9 Genioglossus muscle (innervated by hypoglossal nerve)
10 Stylopharyngeus muscle (only muscle innervated solely by glossopharyngeal nerve)
11 Stylohyoid muscle (cut; innervated by facial nerve)
12 Geniohyoid muscle
13 Thyrohyoid muscle
14 Cricothyroid muscle
15 Hyoid bone
16 Thyroid cartilage
17 Cricoid cartilage
18 Thyroid gland
19 Trachea
20 Superior pharyngeal constrictor muscle
21 Middle pharyngeal constrictor muscle
22 Inferior pharyngeal constrictor muscle
23 Esophagus
24 Anterior belly of digastric muscle (cut; innervated by trigeminal nerve)

After Wolf-Heidegger

H&N-60 Oral cavity

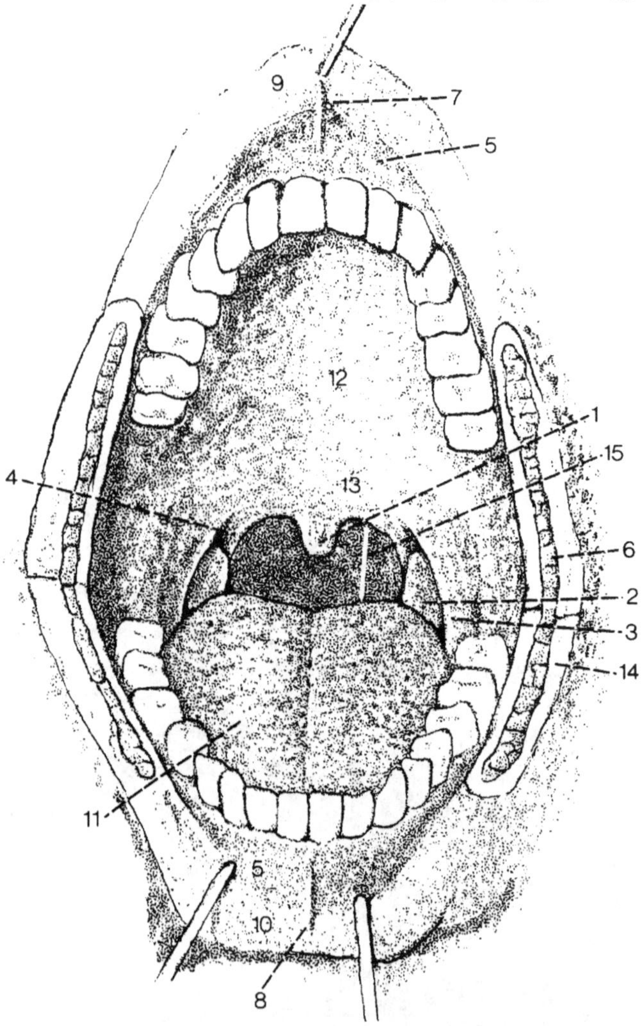

Color and label

1 Uvula (Latin, little grape)
2 Palatine tonsil
3 Palatoglossal arch*
4 Palatopharyngeal arch*
5 Gingiva (Latin, gum)
6 Buccinator muscle (Latin, trumpeter)
7 Frenulum of upper lip (Latin, a small bridle)
8 Frenulum of lower lip
9 Upper lip (Latin, labium superius)
10 Lower lip (Latin, labium inferius)
11 Dorsum of tongue
12 Hard palate
13 Soft palate
14 Cheek (bucca, Latin) (cut)
15 Isthmus of fauces (posterior opening of mouth into pharynx; vertical white line)

*These two arches were also called the pillars of the fauces (Latin, throat).

Palatine glands exposed on right side. Glands removed on left side to show greater and lesser palatine nerves.

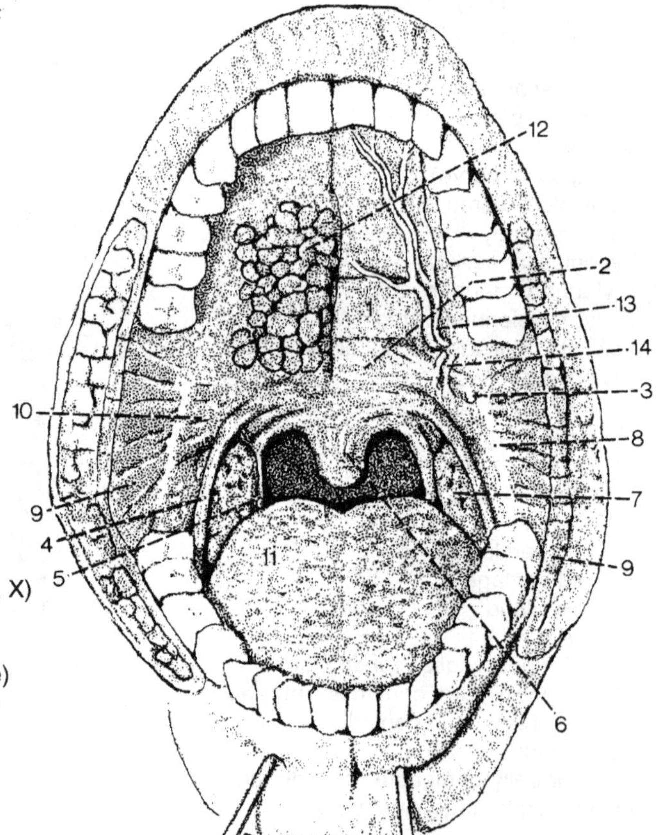

Color and label

1 Hard palate
2 Soft palate
3 Hamulus (Latin, little hook) of medial pterygoid plate
4 Palatoglossal muscle
5 Palatopharyngeal muscle (both muscles 4 and 5 are innervated by the pharyngeal plexus: nerves IX, X)
6 Muscle of the uvula (musculus uvulae)
7 Palatine tonsil
8 Pterygomandibular raphe (Latin, a seam or suture)
9 Buccinator muscle
10 Superior pharyngeal constrictor muscle
11 Dorsum of tongue
12 Palatine glands
13 Greater palatine vessels and nerve (run forward)
14 Lesser palatine vessels and nerve (run backward)

Redrawn from Spalteholz and Spanner

H&N-61 Tongue

Inferior surface of tongue and related structures

Color and label

1 Frenulum of tongue
2 Plica fimbriata (Latin, fimbriated fold)
3 Sublingual fold (plica subligualis) (contains openings of sublingual gland ducts)
4 Sublingual caruncle (opening of submandibular duct and main sublingual duct)

After Spalteholz and Spanner

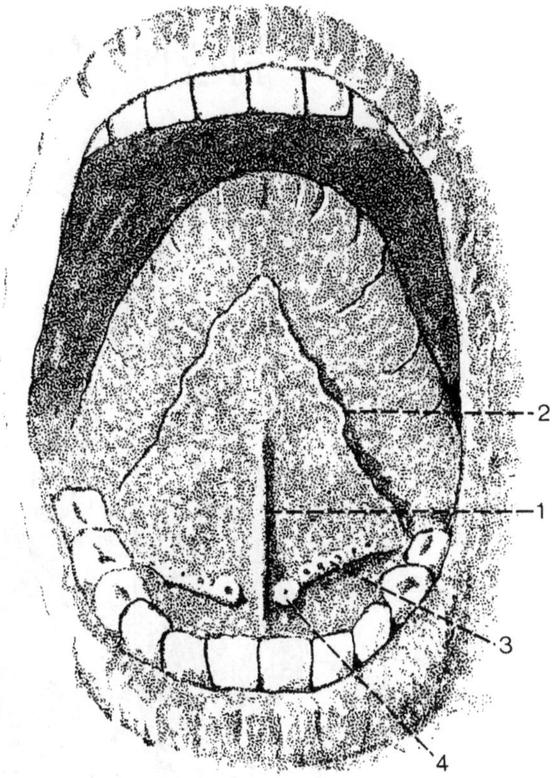

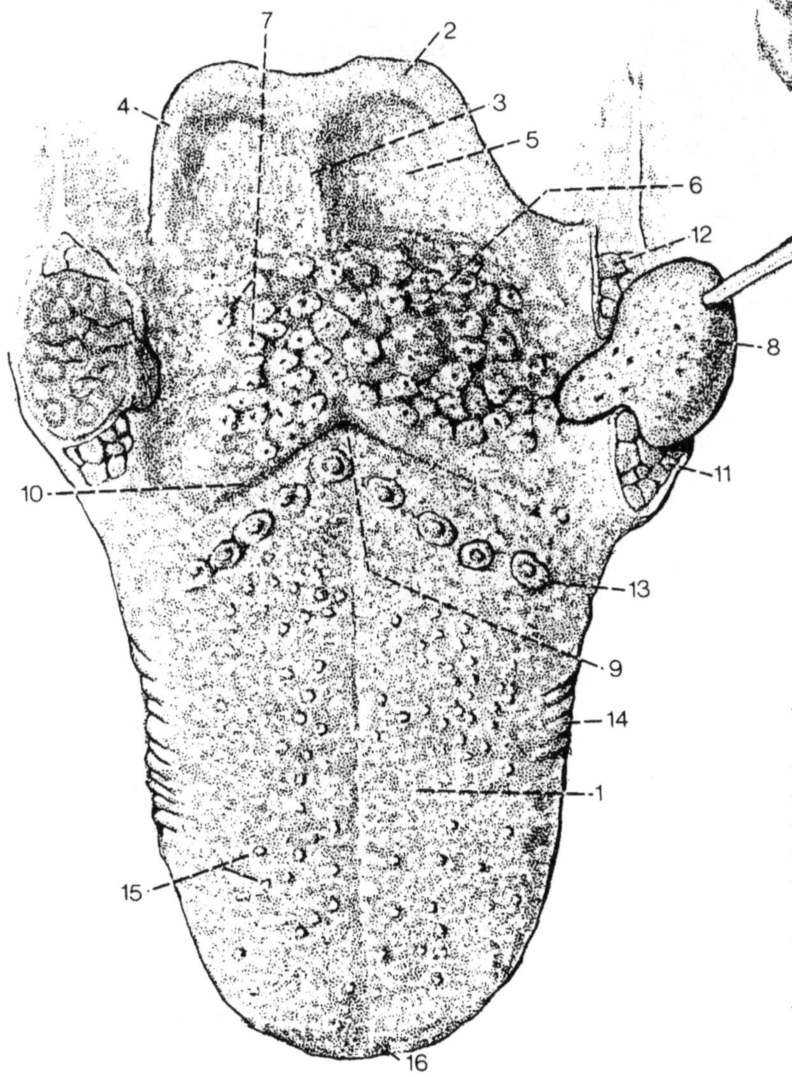

Superior aspect of the tongue and related structures

Color and label

1 Dorsum of tongue
2 Epiglottis
3 Median glosso-epiglottic fold
4 Lateral glosso-epiglottic fold
5 Vallecula (Latin, little valley) epiglottica
6 Lingual tonsil (lymph nodules)
7 Openings of lingual tonsillar crypts
8 Palatine tonsil (often inflamed and removed in childhood)
9 Foramen cecum linguae (blind hole of the tongue)
10 Sulcus terminalis (*sulcus*, akin to the Greek, *holkos*, a furrow)
11 Palatoglossal arch and muscle (cut)
12 Palatopharyngeal arch and muscle (cut)
13 Vallate papilla
14 Foliate papilla (Latin, *folium*, a leaf)
15 Fungiform papilla (Latin, *fungus*, a mushroom)
16 Apex of tongue

After Spalteholz and Spanner

H&N-62 Tongue II

Upper figure
Inferior surface of tongue
Right side dissected

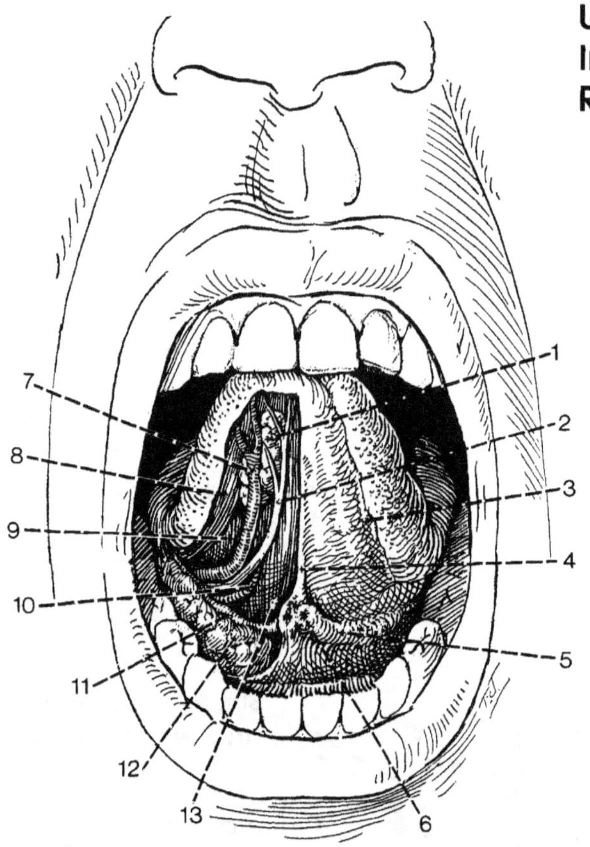

Color and label

1 Anterior lingual gland
2 Lingual nerve
3 Fimbriated plica (or fold)
4 Frenulum of tongue
5 Sublingual plica (or fold)
6 Sublingual caruncle
7 Lingual vein
8 Styloglossus muscle
9 Inferior longitudinal muscle of tongue
10 Deep lingual artery
11 Submandibular duct
12 Sublingual gland
13 Genioglossus muscle

Lower figure median section of tongue

Color and label

1 Mandible
2 Hyoid bone
3 Genioglossus muscle
4 Mylohyoid muscle
5 Geniohyoid muscle
6 Superior longitudinal muscle
7 Transverse lingual muscle
8 Foramen cecum of tongue
9 Lingual tonsil(s)
10 Epiglottis
11 Lower lip
12 Vestibule of larynx
13 Vestibular fold (false vocal cord)
14 Vocal fold (vocal cord, true vocal cord)

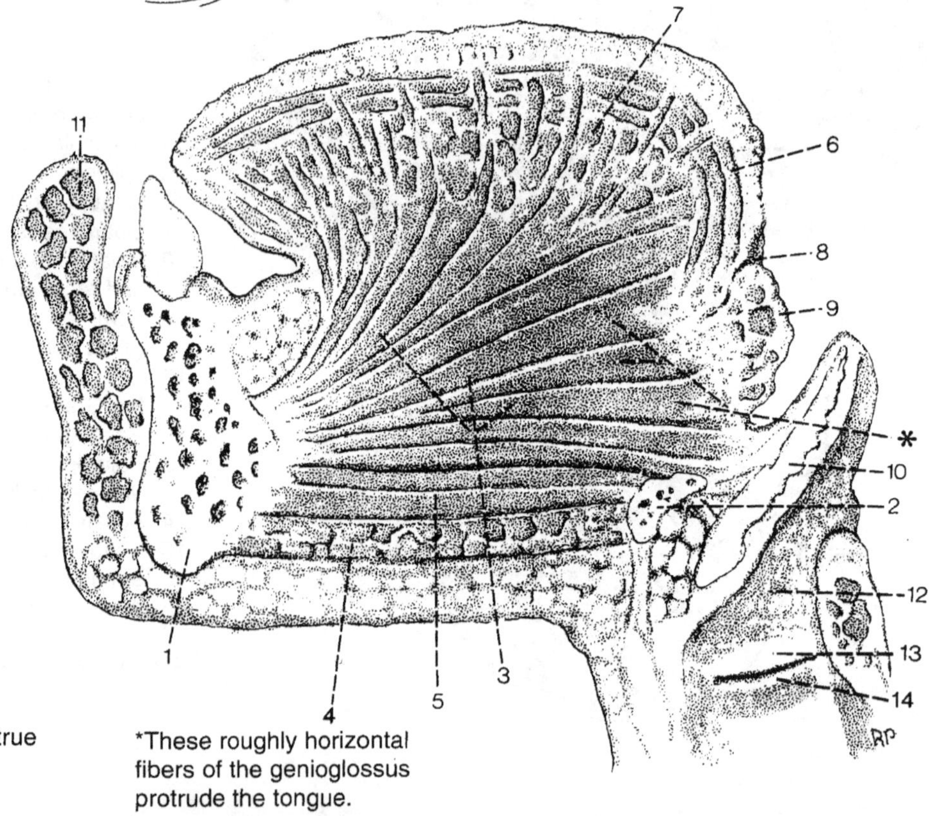

*These roughly horizontal fibers of the genioglossus protrude the tongue.

H&N-63 Tongue and related structures, in coronal section

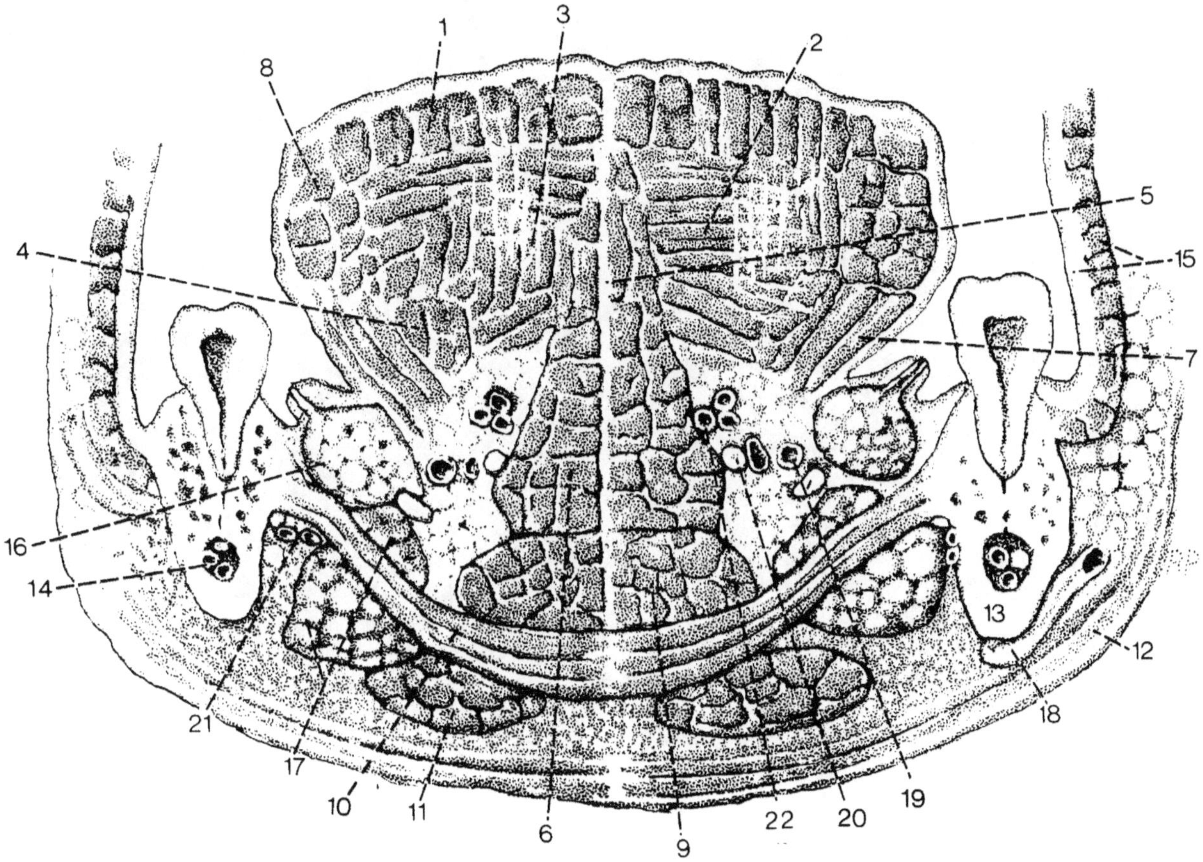

Color and label

1 Superior longitudinal muscle*
2 Transverse lingual muscle*
3 Vertical lingual muscle*
4 Inferior longitudinal muscle*
5 Lingual septum
6 Genioglossus muscle**
7 Hyoglossus muscle**
8 Styloglossus muscle**
9 Geniohyoid muscle
10 Mylohyoid (*myle*, Greek, mill, millstone) muscle
11 Digastric (two-bellied) muscle
12 Platysma muscle
13 Mandible
14 Inferior alveolar nerve, artery, and vein in mandibular canal
15 Buccinator muscle and buccal mucosa (space between tongue and cheek is exaggerated)
16 Sublingual gland and duct opening at sublingual fold
17 Submandibular gland (notice that the gland lies both above and below the mylohyoid muscle)
18 Facial artery
19 Submandibular duct (above) and lingual nerve (below)
20 Hypoglossal nerve and vein
21 Mylohyoid nerve, artery, and vein
22 Deep lingual artery and vein

*Intrinsic muscles of the tongue. They arise and insert within the tongue
**Extrinisic tongue muscles these arise outside the tongue and insert into the tongue.

H&N-64 Temporomandibular joint

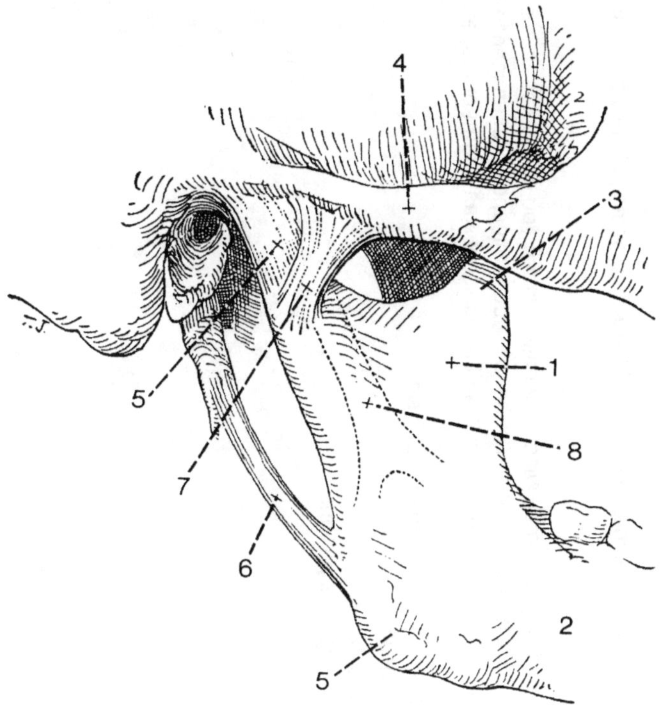

Color and label

1 Ramus of mandible
2 Body of mandible
3 Coronoid process of mandible
4 Zygomatic arch
5 Angle of mandible
6 Stylomandibular ligament
7 Temporomandibular ligament (lateral ligament; medial ligament on inside)
8 Sphenomandibular ligament (on inside of ramus)
9 Head of mandible (partially removed)
10 Articular tubercle
11 Articular disk
12 Mandibular fossa
13 External acoustic meatus
14 Mastoid process
15 Styloid process

Eycleshymer and Jones

Right temporomandibular joint
Lateral view

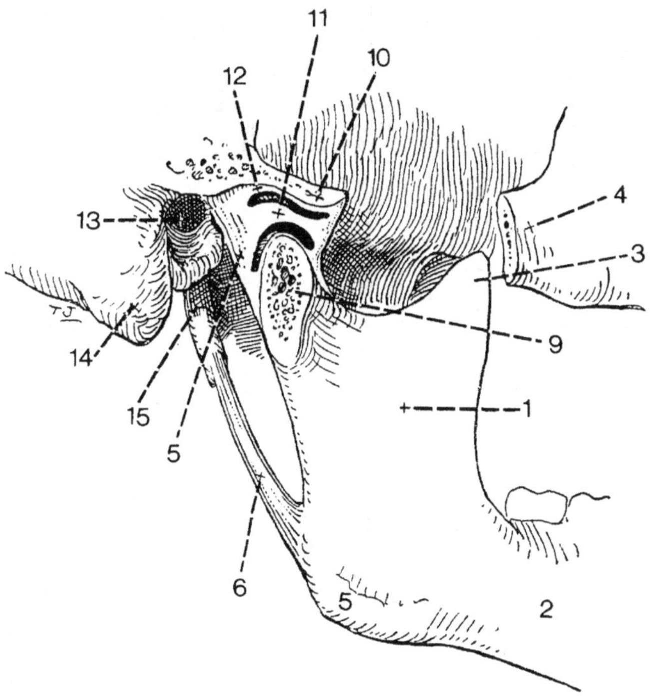

Etymological cartoon: Latin words used to describe parts of the nervous system

1 *Locus ceruleus*, blue place. This mass of nerve cells in the brain derives its name from its blue color.

2 *Tectum*, roof. The former name was *lamina quadrigemina*, the plate with the four bodies–that is, the four colliculi ("little hills").

3 *Vitrum*, glass. *In vitro* means "in glass" (that is, in a test tube or petri dish).

4 *Fenestra*, window. the ear has two small *fenestrae*, the oval window and the round window. Fenestrated capillaries have tiny holes in their walls.

5 *Lithos*, stone (Greek). Otoliths, or ear stones, are found in the inner ear.

6 *Lemniscus*, ribbon. This term describes a flat bundle of axons.

7 *Brachia conjunctiva*, the arms that come together. This was the old name for the superior cerebellar peduncles because the two peduncles would come together and decussate.

8 *Macula*, spot. In ancient Rome instead of calling "here Spot, here Spot" (that is, if you had a dog with a big spot), you would call, "veni macula, veni macula." Immaculate means spotless.

9 *Substantia gelatinosa*, jelly-like substance. This layer of the spinal cord gray matter, now designated layer II of Rexed, appears jelly-like because of the absence of myelinated fibers.

10 *Ampulla*, a swelling or a flask.

11 *Genu*, knee. Geniculate means bent, as in geniculate ganglion or lateral geniculate body. You may wish to genuflect when you encounter an important person, such as an anatomy professor, especially before an exam. You might also wish to address him or her as "your eminence." An eminence is something that rises above its surroundings. In anatomy an eminence means a bump, and in the church or in the palace it was a term of respect for a very important person who rose above his contemporaries.

12 *Peduncle*, little foot or stalk. The cerebellum is attached to the brain stem by six peduncles (three on each side).

13 *Operculum*, a cover or lid. The operculum of the cerebral hemisphere covers the insula.

14 *Amygdala*, almond. This mass of neurons in the temporal lobe has an almond shape.

15 *Putamen*, a shell or husk. This shell-shaped mass of neurons partially envelops the globus pallidus.

16 *Uncus*, hook. The uncinate gyrus on the temporal lobe suggests a hook.

17 *Decussate*, to intersect or to cut in the form of an X.

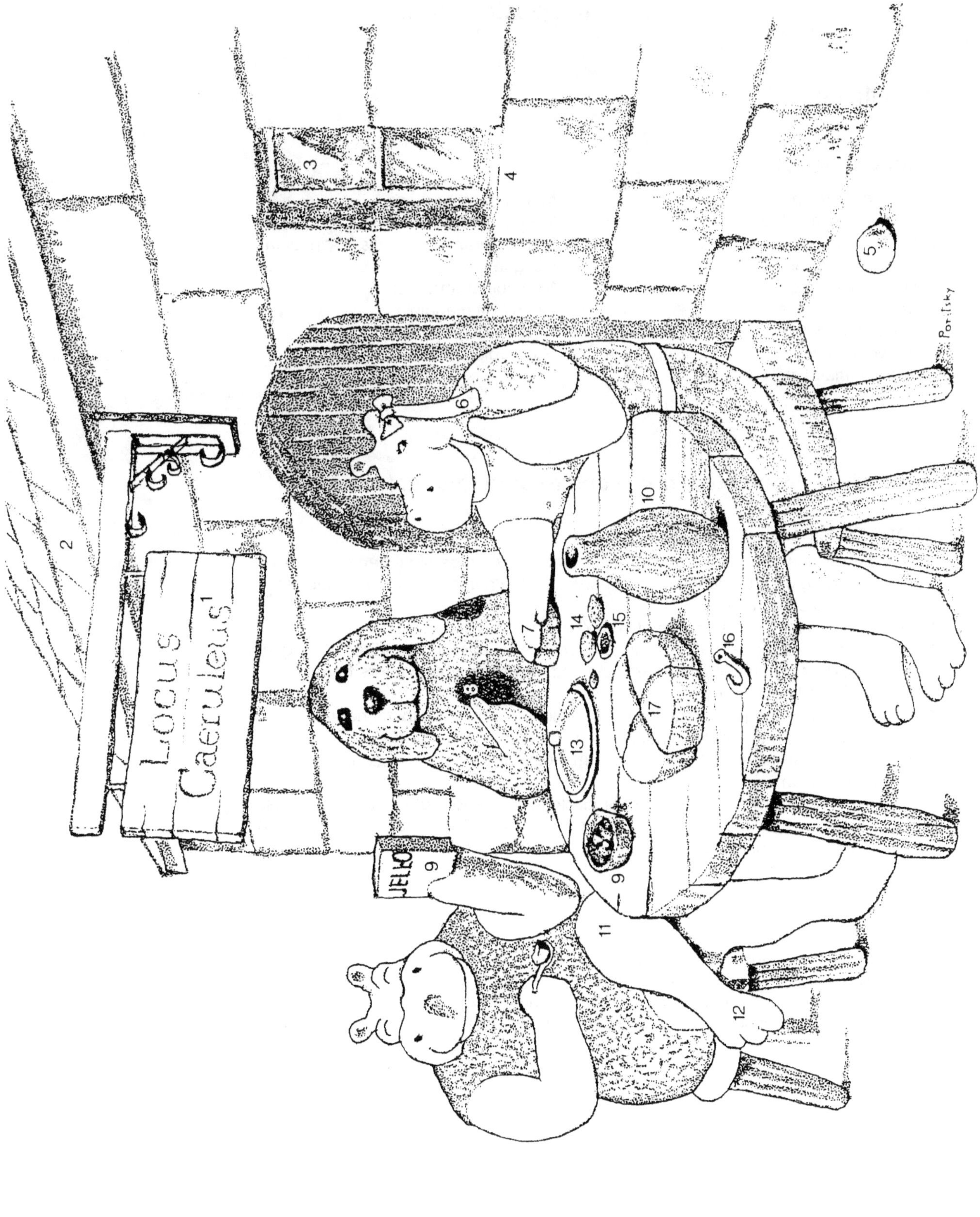
Locus Caeruleus[1]
JELLO

H&N-65 Mandible

(opposite page)

Upper figure

Color and label

1 Body of mandible
2 Ramus of mandible
3 Angle of mandible
4 Coronoid process
5 Mandibular notch
6 Condylar process
7 Neck of mandible
8 Pterygoid fovea
9 Head of mandible
10 Mental protuberance
11 Mental tubercle
12 Mental foramen (*mentis*, Latin, chin)
13 Oblique line
14 Mandibular foramen
15 Lingula of mandible
16 Mylohyoid grove
17 Mylohyoid line

Lower figure: Mandibular nerve and related structures

Color and label

1 Mandibular nerve; cut, third and largest branch of the trigeminal nerve (nerve V); note its giving off 4 branches: buccal nerve, lingual nerve, inferior alveolar nerve, and auriculotemporal nerve.
2 Buccal nerve (sensory to inside of cheek)
3 Lingual nerve (supplies pain, touch, temperature to anterior two-thirds of tongue)
4 Chorda tympani nerve; cut, carries taste and parasympathetic fibers from facial nerve (VII) to lingual nerve.
5 Submandibular ganglion (contains postganglionic parasympathetic neurons which send fibers to submandibular gland and sublingual gland)
6 Inferior alveolar nerve (note its entering mandibular foramen and canal; sensory to teeth and gums)
7 Mylohyoid nerve (motor to mylohyoid muscle and anterior belly of digastric muscle)
8 Auriculotemporal nerve (notice its origin from the mandibular nerve by two roots)
9 Otic ganglion (supplies postganglionic fibers to the parotid gland)
10 Origin of genioglossus muscle (cut)
11 Geniohyoid muscle (*genion*, Greek, chin)
12 Mylohyoid muscle
13 Hyoid bone
14 Submandibular gland
15 Submandibular duct (note its crossing **over** the lingual nerve)
16 Sublingual gland (notice its several ducts which open at the sublingual fold)
17 Digastric muscle posterior belly (cut) and sling restraining intermediate tendon

H&N-65 Mandible

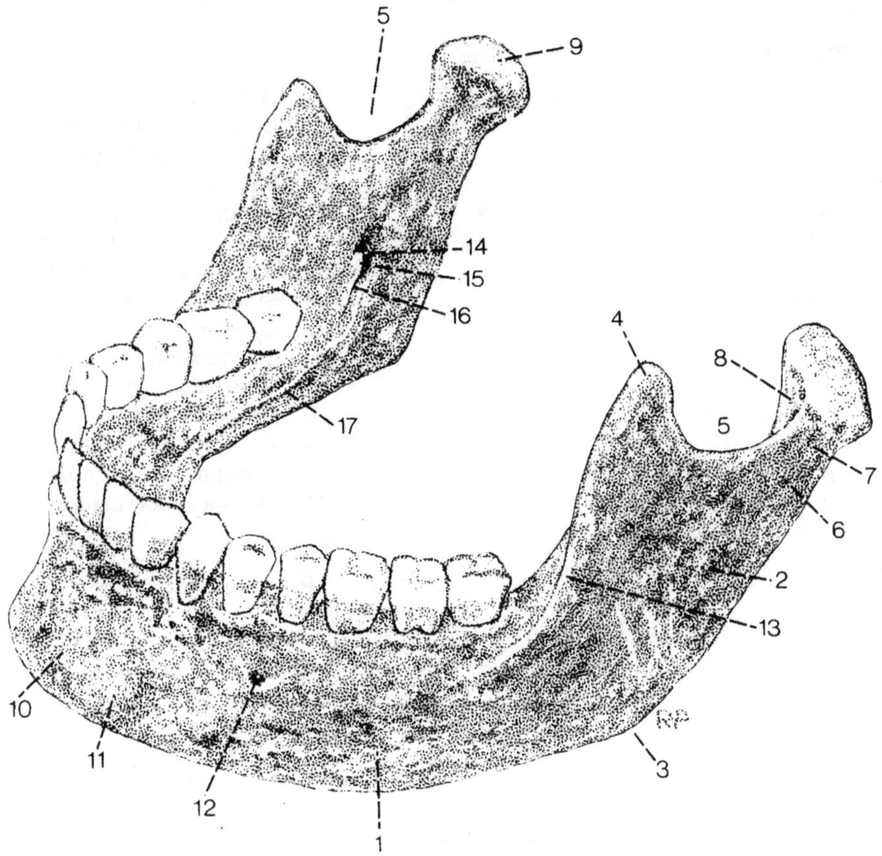

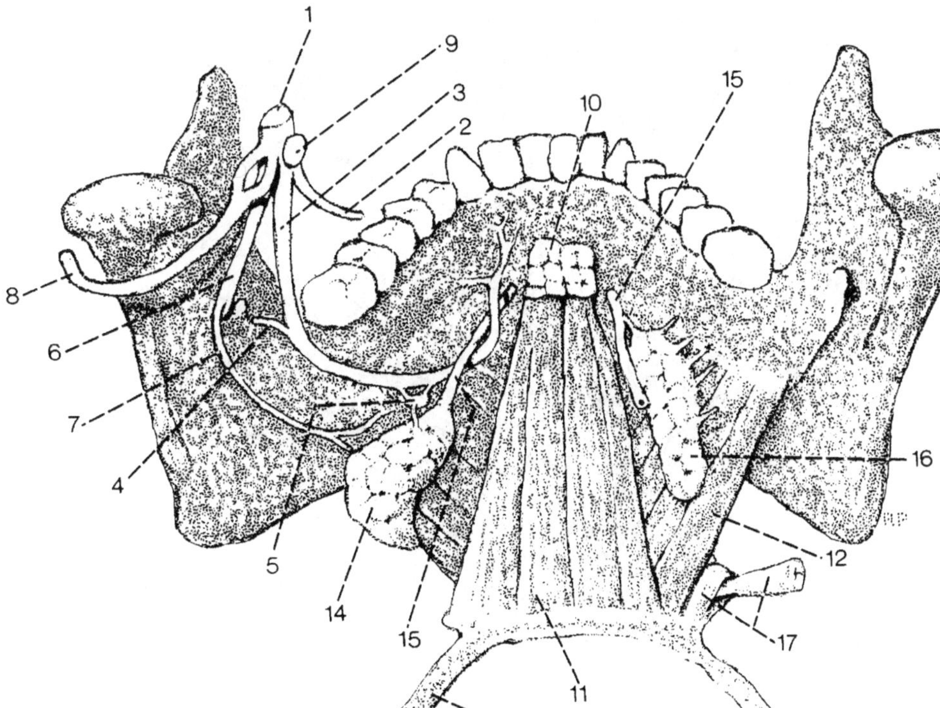

H&N-66 Salivary glands

Color and label

1 Superficial temporal artery and vein
2 Parotid gland
3 Temporal fascia
4 Buccinator muscle
5 Orbicularis oculi muscle
6 Zygomaticus major muscle
7 Accessory parotid gland
8 Parotid duct
9 Labial glands
10 Gingiva
11 Probe in parotid duct
12 Sublingual caruncle
13 Major sublingual duct
14 Minor sublingual ducts
15 Sublingual gland
16 Lingual nerve
17 Geniohyoid muscle
18 Submandibular duct
19 Hypoglossal nerve
20 Mylohyoid muscle (cut)
21 Hyoglossus muscle
22 Anterior belly of digastric muscle (cut)
23 Submandibular gland
24 Sternohyoid muscle
25 Omohyoid muscle (anterior belly; cut)
26 Sternocleidomastoid muscle
27 Internal jugular vein
28 Greater auricular nerve
29 Posterior belly of digastric muscle
30 Submandibular ganglion
31 Sternocleidomastoid muscle

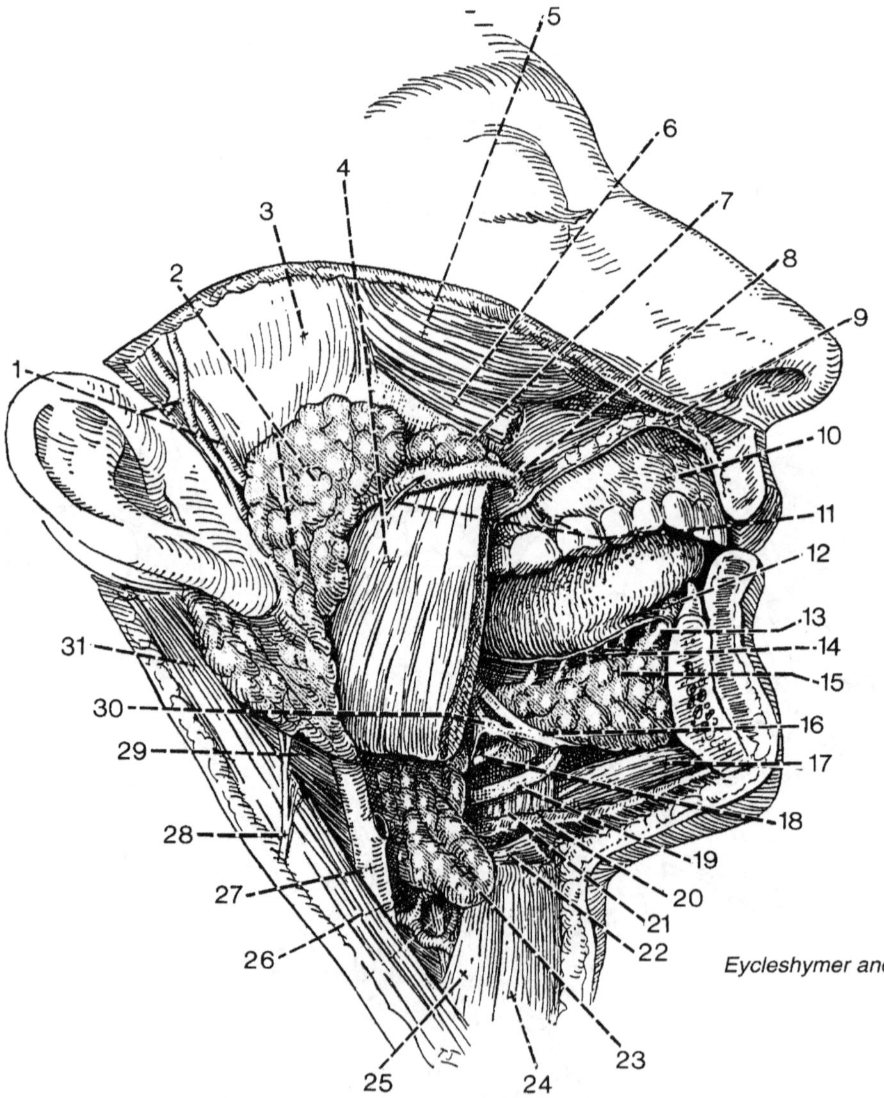

Eycleshymer and Jones

H&N-67 Oral cavity from inside

Tongue and pharyngeal mucosa and wall removed

Color and label

1 Hard palate
2 Soft palate (cut and removed)
3 Oral mucosa
4 Sublingual papilla
5 Submandibular duct
6 Submandibular gland
7 Sublingual gland and ducts
8 Lingual nerve
9 Hypoglossal nerve (cut)
10 Deep lingual artery (cut)
11 Chorda tympani nerve
12 Inferior alveolar nerve
13 Medial pterygoid muscle (cut)
14 Genioglossus muscle origin on mandible
15 Geniohyoid muscle
16 Mylohyoid muscle
17 Anterior belly of digastric muscle
18 Posterior belly of digastric muscle
19 External carotid artery
20 Internal carotid artery
21 Vagus nerve
22 Ascending pharyngeal artery
23 Facial artery
24 Lingual artery
25 Glossopharyngeal nerve (N IX)
26 Stylohyoid ligament
27 Styloglossus muscle (cut)
28 Hyoglossus muscle (cut)
29 Middle pharyngeal constrictor muscle
30 Hyoid bone
31 Inferior nasal concha

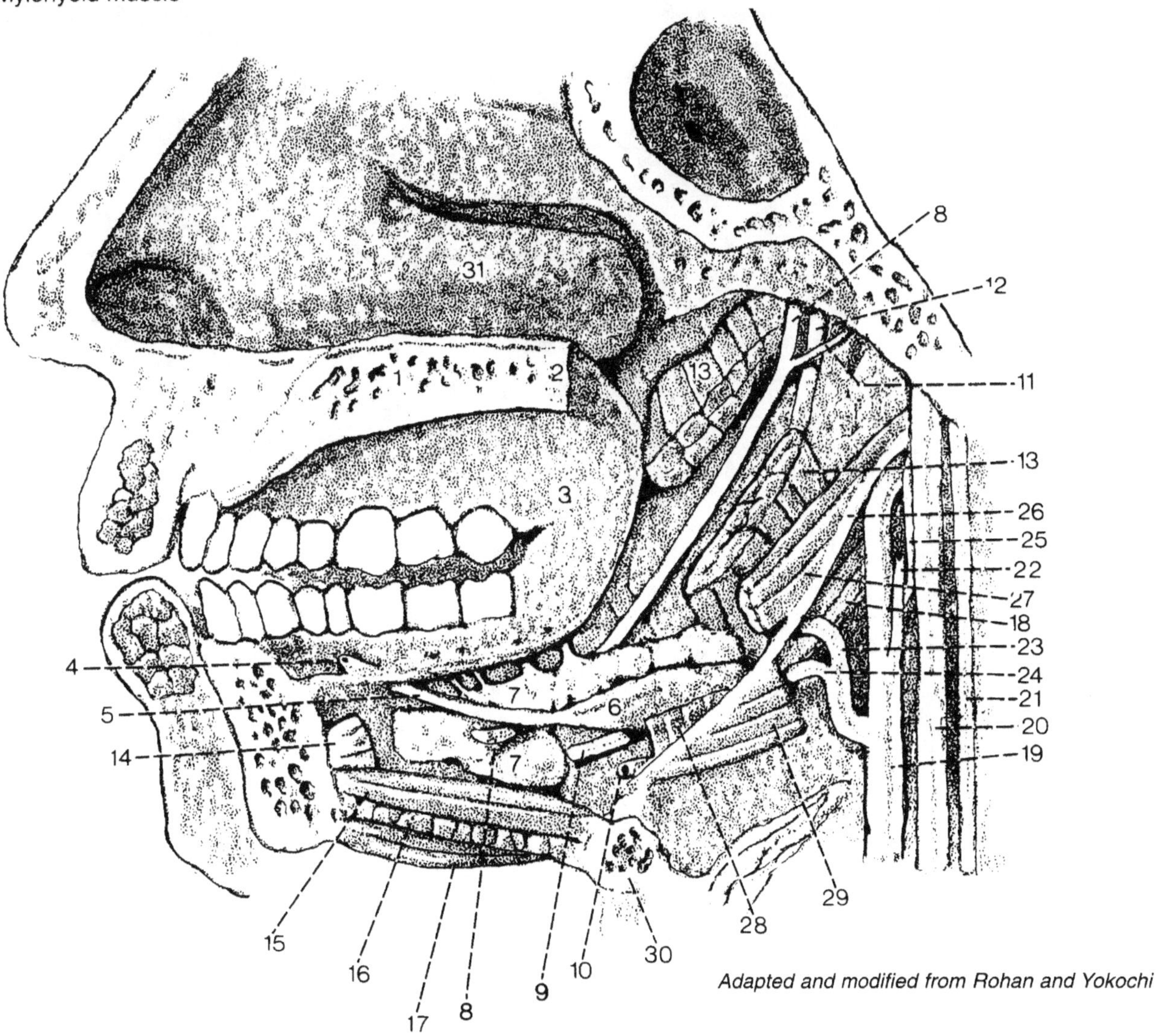

Adapted and modified from Rohan and Yokochi

H&N-68 Infratemporal fossa

Color and label

1 Facial nerve
2 Retromandibular vein
3 External jugular vein
4 Superficial temporal vein
5 External carotid artery
6 Maxillary artery
7 Superficial temporal vein
8 Middle meningeal artery
9 Masseteric artery
10 Inferior alveolar artery
11 Deep temporal arteries
12 Buccal artery
13 Pterygoid branch
14 Buccal nerve
15 Inferior alveolar nerve
16 Lingual nerve
17 Sphenomandibular ligament
18 Auriculotemporal nerve
19 Facial nerve
20 Ramus of mandible (cut)
21 Neck of mandible (cut)
22 External pterygoid muscle
23 Medial pterygoid muscle
24 Masseter muscle (cut)
25 Buccinator muscle (partially cut)
26 Sternocleidomastoid muscle

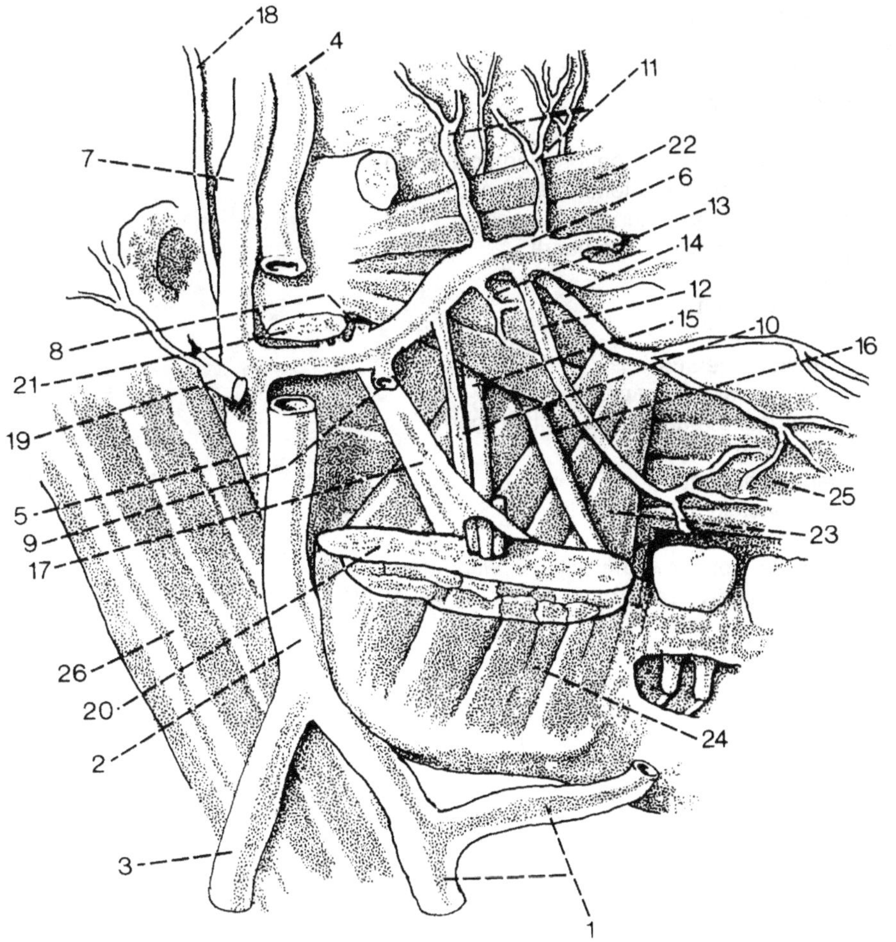

H&N-69 Maxillary artery

(opposite page)

Color and label

1 External carotid artery
2 Maxillary artery
3 Superficial temporal artery
4 Masseteric artery (to masseter muscle)
5 Inferior alveolar artery (supplies teeth in lower jaw; with inferior alveolar vein and nerve; both not shown)
6 Pterygoid branches (supplies pterygoid muscles)
7 Buccal artery (supplies buccinator and cheek)
8 Anterior deep temporal artery (supplies temporalis muscle)
9 Posterior deep temporal artery (supplies temporalis muscle)
10 Posterior superior alveolar artery (supplies upper back teeth)
11 Infraorbital artery (entering orbit)
12 Sphenopalatine artery (entering nose through sphenopalatine foramen)
13 Descending palatine artery
14 Deep auricular artery
15 Anterior tympanic artery
16 Mental artery
17 Lateral pterygoid muscle (superior superficial head)
18 Lateral pterygoid muscle (inferior deep head)
19 Medial pterygoid muscle (superficial head)
20 Medial pterygoid muscle (deep head)
21 Buccinator muscle
22 Masseter muscle (cut)
23 Zygomatic arch (cut)
24 External auditory meatus
25 Temporomandibular joint capsule
26 Ramus of mandible (partially cut, with coronoid process removed)
27 Middle meningeal artery
28 Sternocleidomastoid muscle

Keep in mind: veins, not shown here, travel with arteries and are often doubled; that is, two veins often accompany a single artery.

H&N-69 Maxillary artery

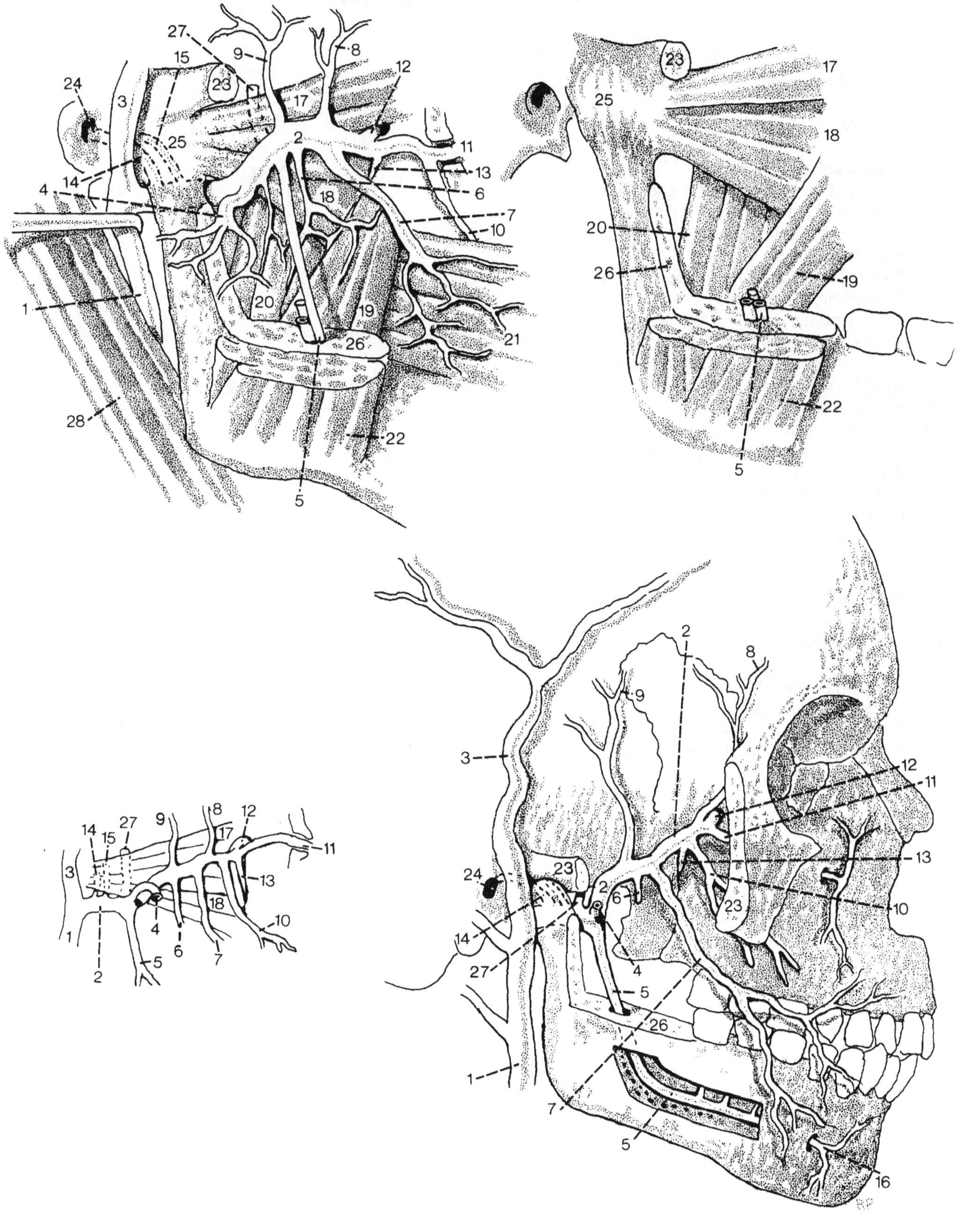

H&N-70 Muscles of the pharynx

Right side (opposite page)

Color and label

1 Auditory tube (cartilaginous)
2 Tensor veli palatini muscle
3 Levator veli palatini muscle
4 Tendon of tensor veli palatini and palatine aponeurosis
5 Hamulus of medial pterygoid plate
6 Pterygomandibular raphe
7 Buccinator muscle
8 Superior pharyngeal constrictor muscle
9 Palatopharyngeus muscle
10 Salpingopharyngeus muscle
11 Glossopharyngeus muscle (part of superior constrictor)
12 Middle pharyngeal constrictor muscle
13 Styloglossus muscle
14 Hyoglossus muscle
15 Stylohyoid ligament
16 Inferior pharyngeal constrictor muscle
17 Mylohyoid muscle
18 Geniohyoid muscle
19 Thyrohyoid membrane
20 Stylopharyngeus muscle
21 Fibers to pharyngo-epiglottic fold
22 Longitudinal muscle of pharynx
23 Internal branch of superior laryngeal nerve
24 Thyroid cartilage
25 Cricoid cartilage
26 Trachea
27 Arytenoid cartilage
28 Corniculate cartilage
29 Pharyngeal aponeurosis
30 Cricopharyngeus muscle (part of inferior constrictor)
31 Esophageal circular muscle
32 Esophageal longitudinal muscle
33 Pharyngobasilar fascia
34 Hyoid bone

H&N-70 Muscles of the pharynx

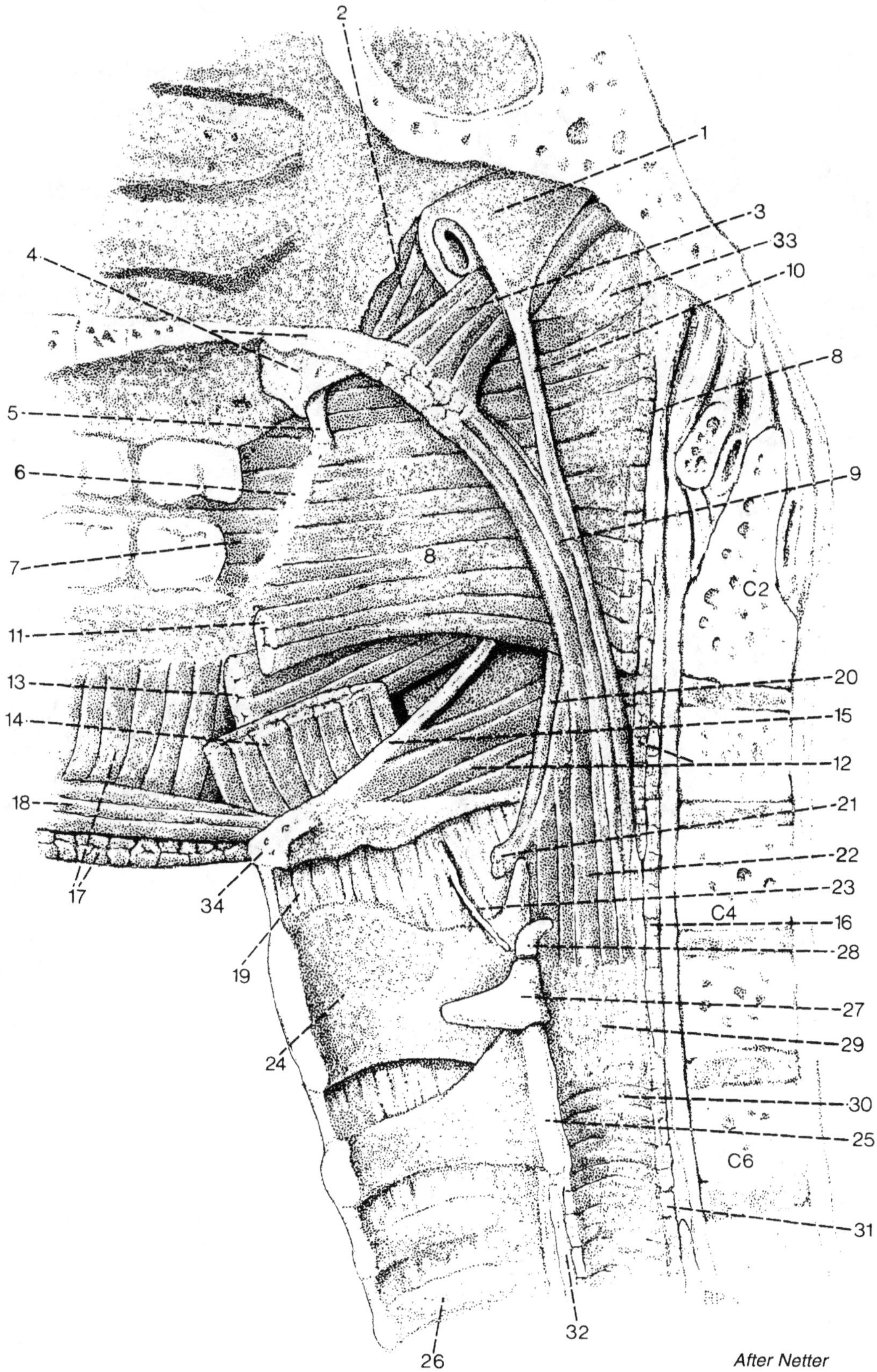

After Netter

H&N-71 Arytenoid and cricoid cartilages

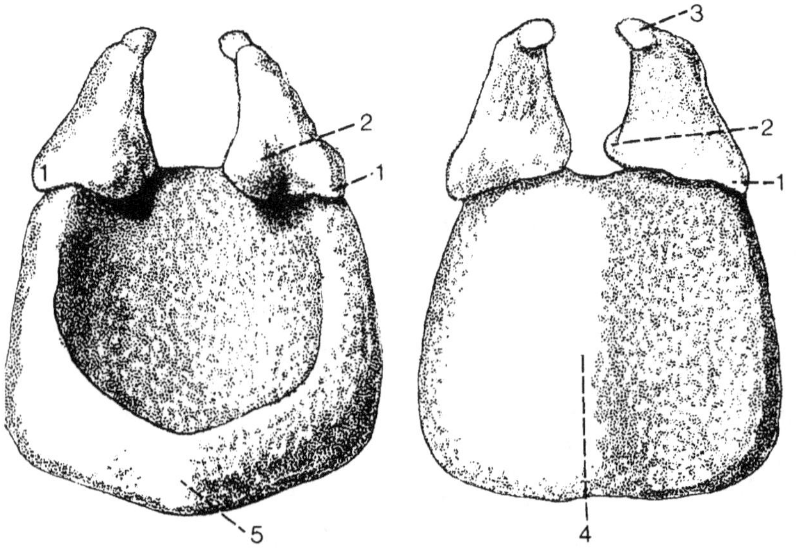

Anterior Posterior

Left, anterior view;
Right, posterior view

Color and label

1 Muscular process of arytenoid cartilage
2 Vocal process of arytenoid cartilage
3 Corniculate cartilage
4 Lamina of cricoid cartilage
5 Arch of cricoid cartilage

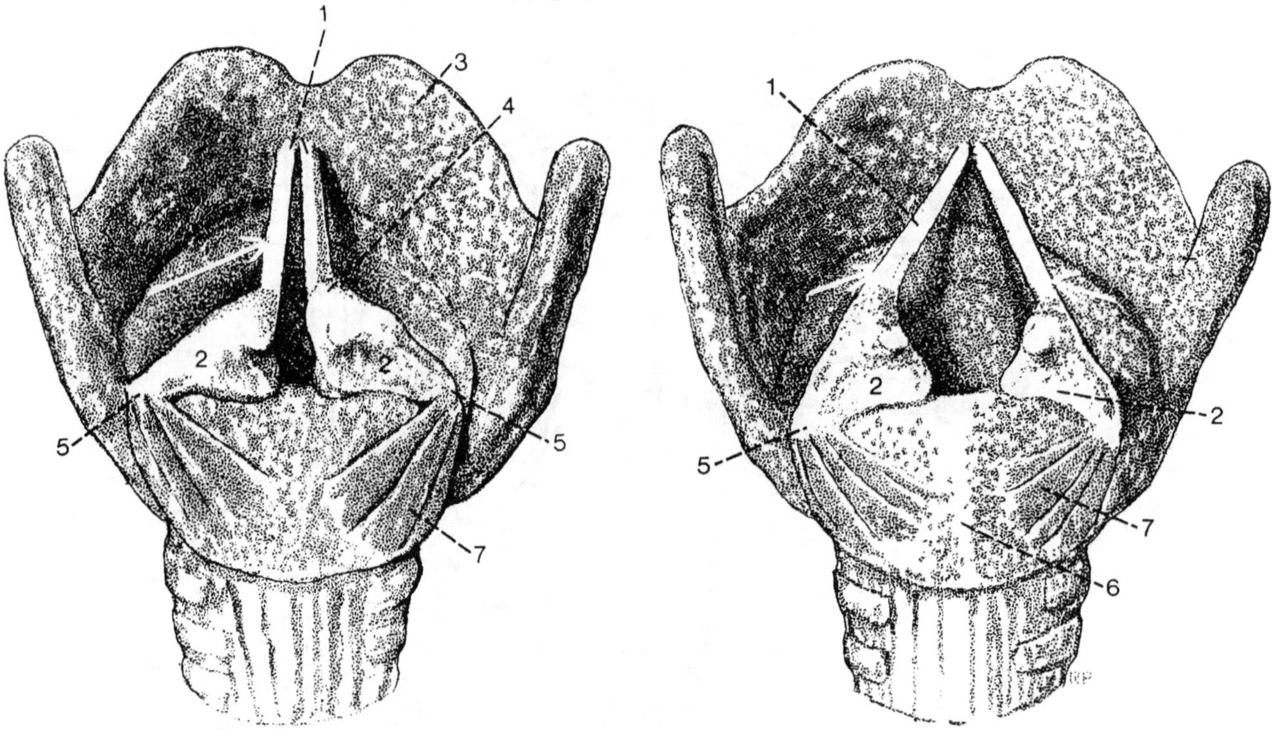

Adduction **Vocal ligaments in** Abduction

Color and label

1 Vocal ligaments
2 Arytenoid cartilages
3 Thyroid cartilage
4 Vocal process of arytenoid cartilage
5 Muscular process of arytenoid cartilage
6 Lamina of cricoid cartilage
7 Posterior cricoarytenoid muscles; these two muscles are the sole abductors (pull apart) of the vocal ligaments, thus opening the space between the vocal cords (the rima glottidis).
8 White arrows indicate the conus elasticus (not shown here, see next page); these extend from the cricoid cartilage to the vocal ligaments.

H&N-72 Vocal ligaments and muscles

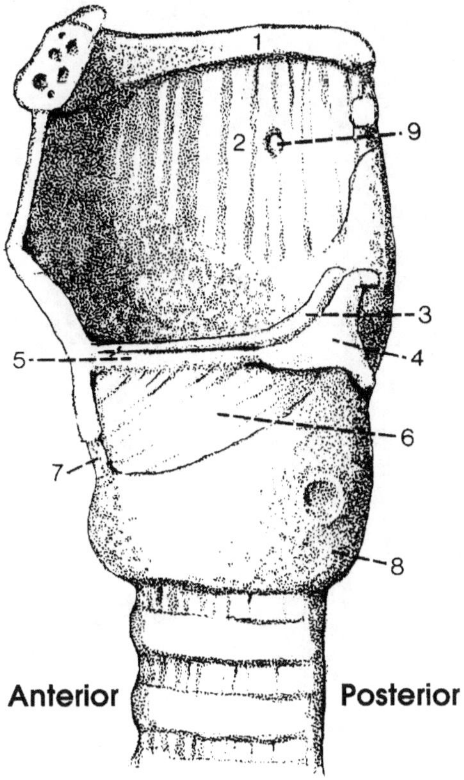

Larynx partially bisected

Left half of hyoid bone and thryroid cartilage removed

Color and label

1 Right half of hyoid bone
2 Right thyrohyoid membrane
3 Right arytenoid cartilage
4 Left arytenoid cartilage
5 Vocal ligaments
6 Conus elasticus
7 Cricothyroid ligament
8 Cricoid cartilage
9 Foramen for passage of internal branch of superior laryngeal nerve and artery

Muscles of right side of larynx

Right side of thyroid cartilage removed

Color and label

1 Aryepiglottis muscle
2 Thyroarytenoid muscle
3 Arytenoid muscle muscle
4 Lateral cricoarytenoid muscle
5 Cricothyroid muscle
6 Posterior cricoarytenoid muscle

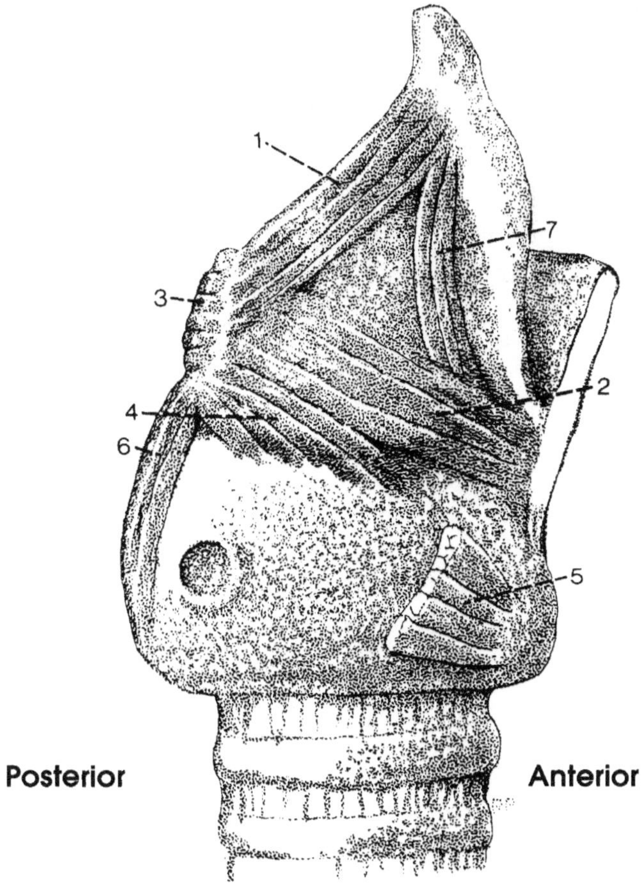

H&N-73 Larynx, cartilages

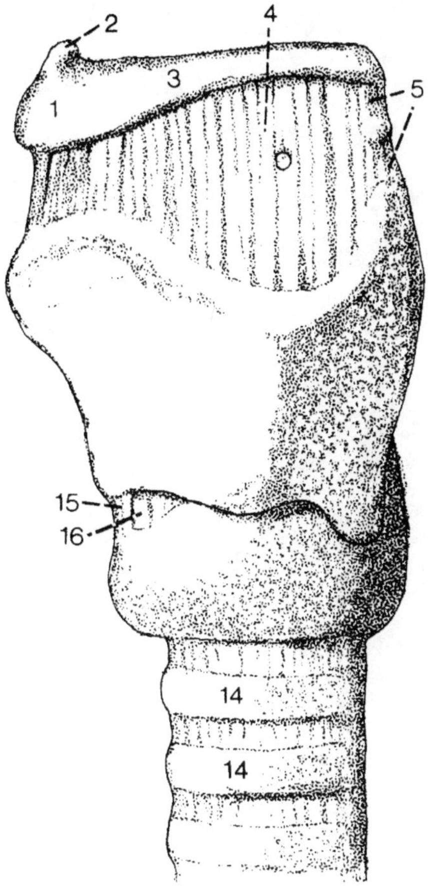

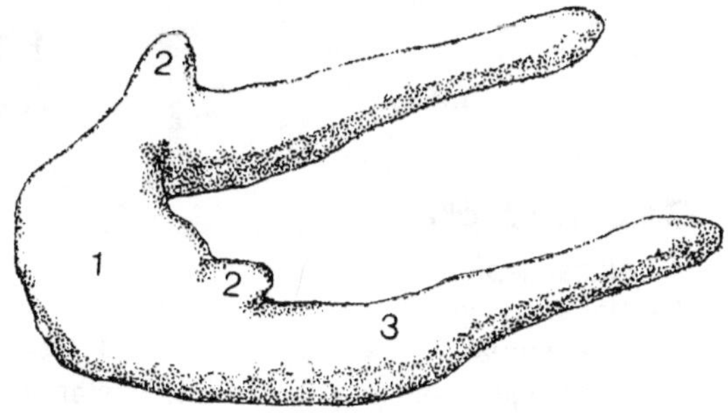

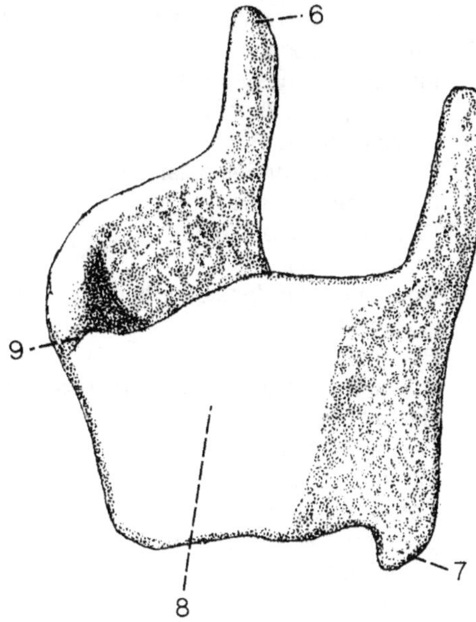

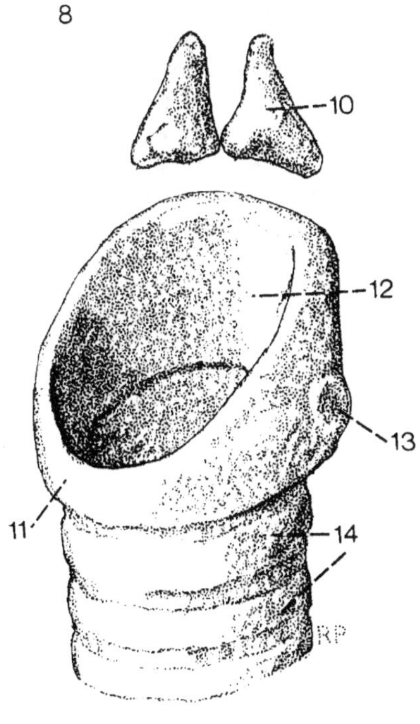

Larynx (above)

Hyoid bone and cartilages of the larynx (right)

Color and label

1 Body of hyoid bone
2 Lesser horn (cornu) of hyoid bone
3 Greater horn (cornu) of hyoid bone
4 Thyrohyoid membrane
5 Lateral thyrohyoid ligament
6 Superior horn of thyroid cartilage
7 Inferior horn of thyroid cartilage
8 Lamina of thyroid cartilage
9 Superior thyroid notch
10 Arytenoid (Greek, *arytaina*, pitcher, ladle) cartilage
11 Arch of cricoid cartilage
12 Lamina of cricoid cartilage
13 Facet for inferior horn of thyroid cartilage
14 Tracheal rings
15 Cricothyroid ligament
16 Conus elasticus (extends from cricoid cartilage to vocal ligament

H&N-74 Pharynx

Posterior aspect (opposite page)

Color and label

1 Nasal septum
2 Nasal conchae
3 Pharyngeal
4 Pharyngeal wall (cut open along posterior raphe)
5 Nasal pharynx (nasopharynx)
6 Oral pharynx (oropharynx)
7 Laryngeal pharynx (laryngopharynx)
8 Soft palate and uvula
9 Dorsum sellae and clivus (Latin, slope) of occipital bone
10 Petrous portion of temporal bone
11 Facial canal and its termination at the stylomastoid foramen
12 Styloid process
13 Mastoid process and mastoid air cells
14 Opening of auditory tube
15 Torus tubularis
16 Torus of levator veli palatini muscle
17 Pharyngeal recess
18 Palatopharyngeal fold
19 Palatine tonsil
20 Root of tongue (posterior third) with lingual lymph follicles (tonsil)
21 Epiglottis
22 Piriform recess
23 Superior laryngeal nerve and vessel under mucous membrane
24 Hyoid bone (greater horn)
25 Thyroid cartilage (superior horn)
26 Interarytenoid notch
27 Corniculate tubercle (covering corniculate cartilage)
28 Cuneiform tubercle (covering cuneiform cartilage)
29 Aryepiglottic fold
30 Esophagus
31 Thyroid gland and vessels
32 Parathyroid gland
33 Mucous membrane overlying posterior cricoarytenoid and lamina of cricoid cartilage
34 Aditus (Latin, entrance) to larynx
35 Vallate papillae
36 Posterior belly of digastric muscle
37 Parotid gland
38 Submandibular gland

H&N-74 Pharynx

Posterior aspect

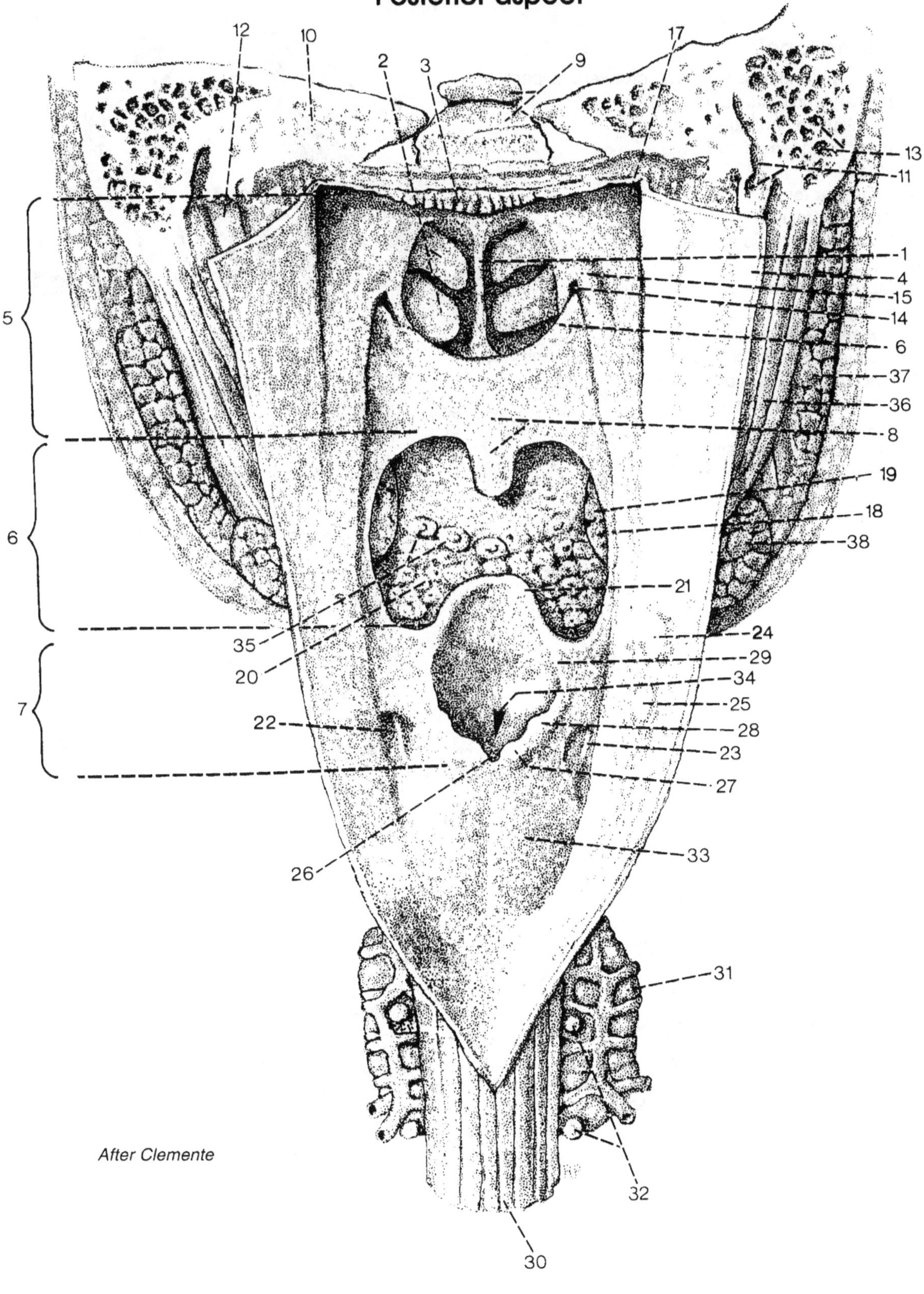

After Clemente

H&N-75 Arytenoid cartilages

Color and label

1 Right arytenoid cartilage (anterolateral aspect)
2 Left arytenoid cartilage
3 Corniculate cartilage
4 Apex of arytenoid cartilage
5 Neck
6 Triangilar fossa
7 Arcuate crest
8 Base of arytenoid cartilage
9 Oblong fossa
10 Muscular process
11 Vocal process
12 Vocal ligaments (cut)
13 Conus elasticus (cut) (cricovocal membrane)
14 Cricoid cartilage (cut)
15 Vestibular ligament (cut)
16 Vocalis muscle (cut)
17 Thyroarytenoid muscle (cut)
18 Lateral cricoarytenoid muscle (cut)

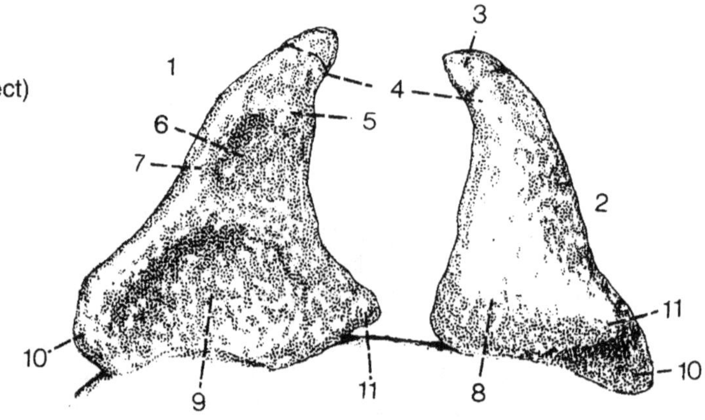

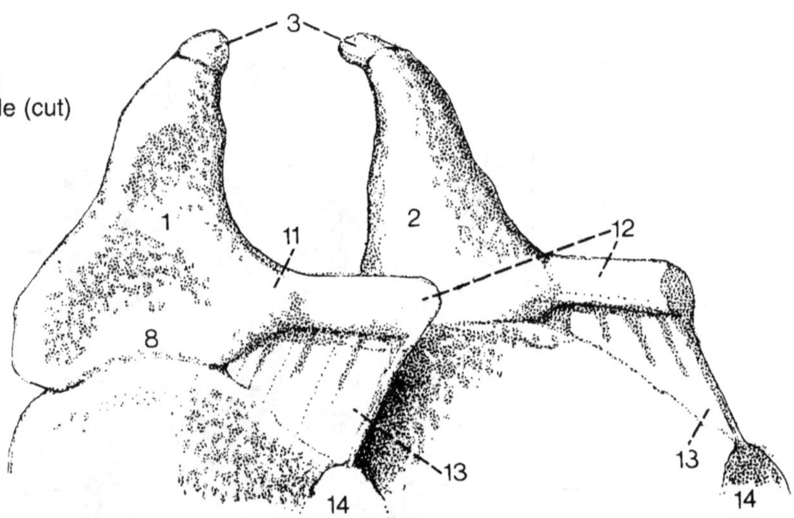

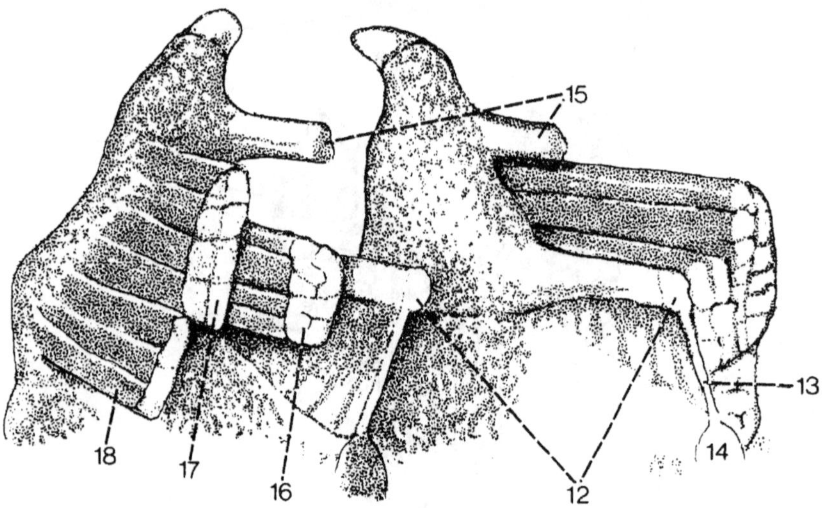

H&N-76 Larynx, cartilages

Posterior aspect

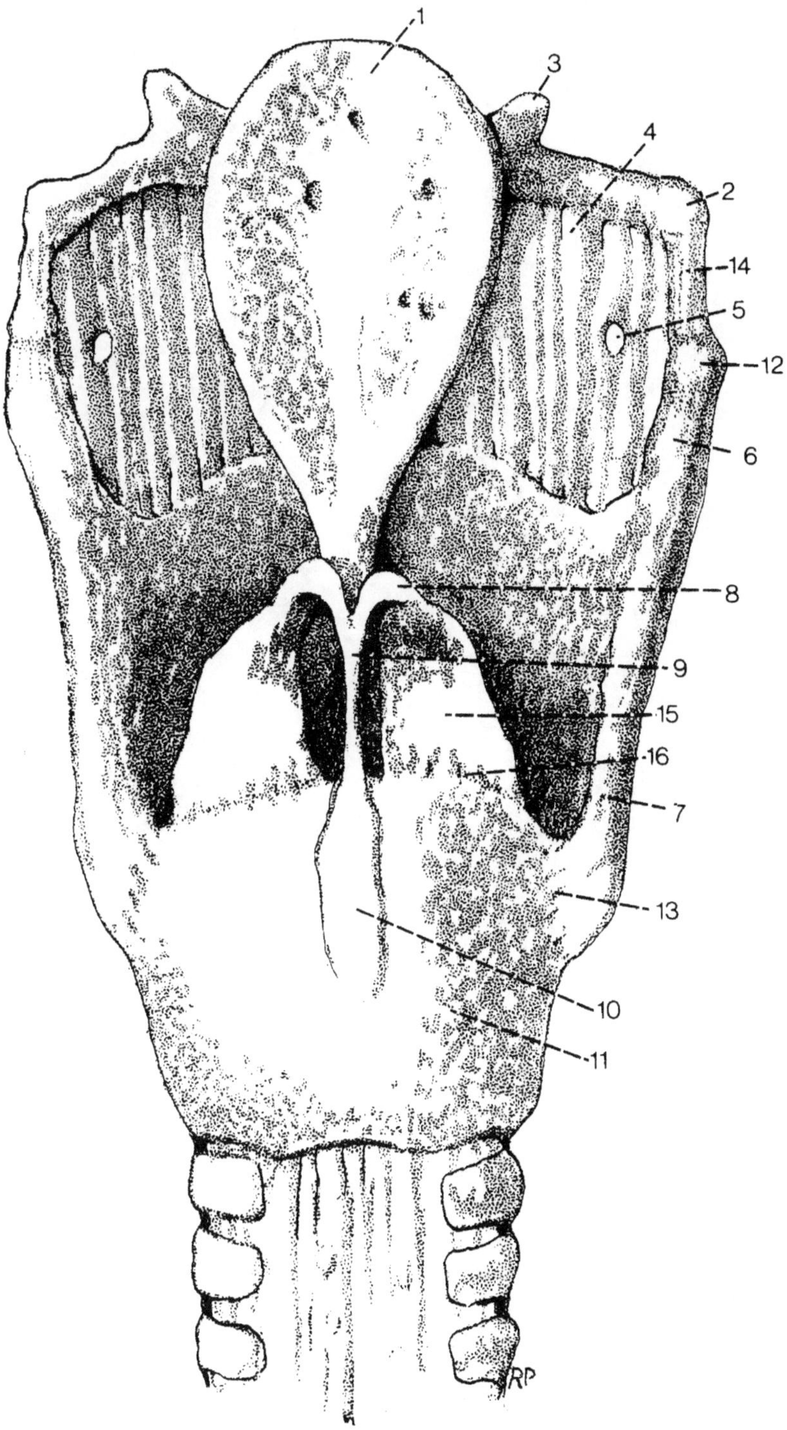

Color and label

1 Epiglottis
2 Hyoid bone greater horn
3 Hyoid bone lesser horn
4 Thyrohyoid membrane
5 Foramen for internal branch of superior laryngeal nerve and superior laryngeal artery
6 Superior horn of thyroid cartilage
7 Inferior horn of thyroid cartilage
8 Corniculate cartilage
9 Corniculopharyngeal ligament
10 Cricopharyngeal ligament
11 Lamina of cricoid cartilage
12 Triticeal cartilage
13 Cricothyroid joint and ligament
14 Lateral thyrohyoid ligament
15 Arytenoid cartilage
16 Cricoarytenoid joint and ligament

H&N-77 Larynx, nerves and muscles

Posterior view

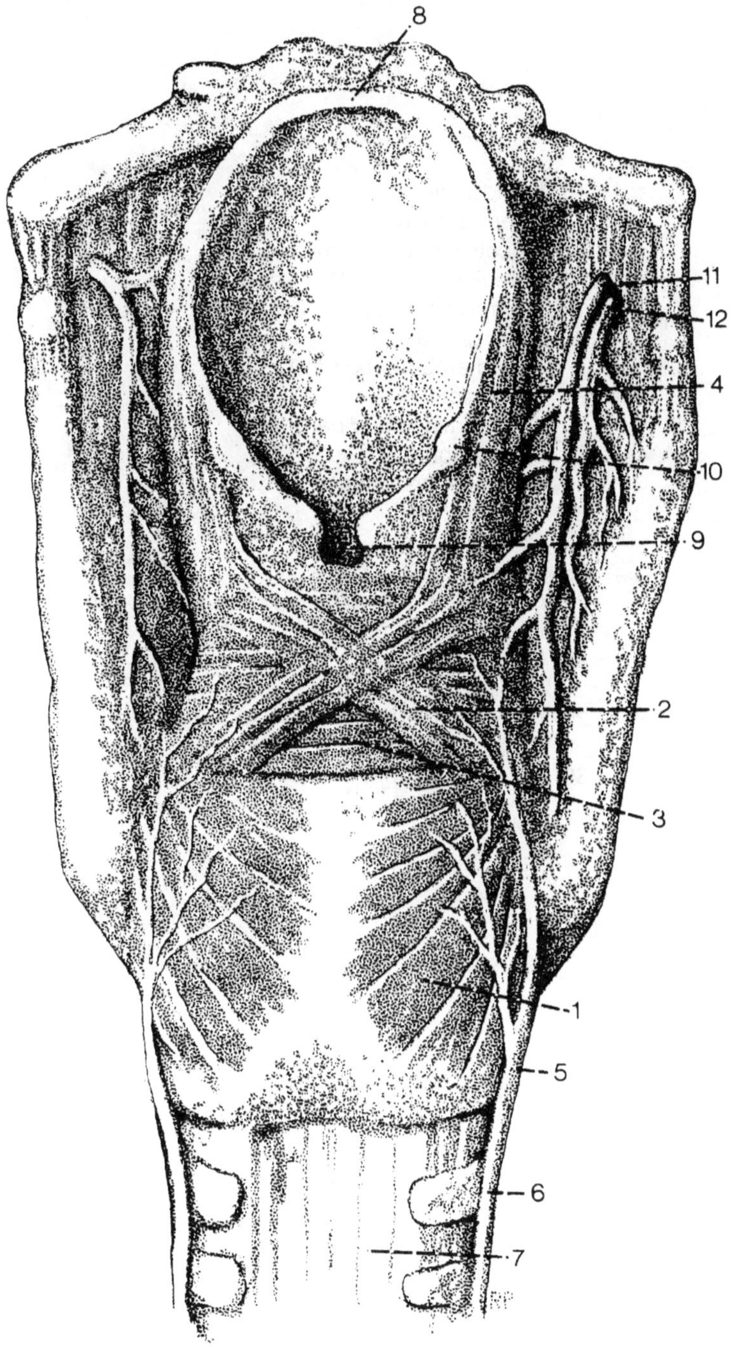

Color and label

1 Posterior cricoarytenoid muscle (only abductor of the vocal folds)
2 Oblique arytenoid muscle
3 Transverse arytenoid muscle
4 Aryepiglottic muscle (also considered part of oblique arytenoid)
5 Inferior laryngeal nerve
6 Recurrent laryngeal nerve
7 Membranous tracheal wall and glands
8 Epiglottis
9 Interarytenoid notch
10 Cuneiform cartilage and tubercle
11 Internal branch of superior laryngeal nerve
12 Superior laryngeal artery

H&N-78 Larynx, coronal section

Viewed from behind

(opposite page)

Figure A and B

Color and label

1 Vestibular fold (false vocal cord)
2 Vestibular ligament
3 Ventricle of larynx
4 Vocal ligament
5 Vocal fold (true vocal cord)
6 Vocalis muscle
7 Thyroarytenoid muscle
8 Lateral cricoarytenoid muscle
9 Rima glottidis (space between vocal folds); divided into: intermembranous part, intercartilaginous part, interarytenoid fold
10 Cricothyroid muscle
11 Arch of cricoid cartilage
12 Tracheal rings
13 Epiglottis
14 Vestibule of larynx (laryngeal space above vestibular folds)
15 Infraglottic space (laryngeal space below vocal folds)
16 Hyoid bone
17 Conus elasticus (cricovocal membrane)
18 Aryepiglottic muscle
19 Thyrohyoid muscle
20 Rima glottidis (intermembranous part)
21 Rima glottidis (intercartilaginous part)
22 Root of tongue (posterior one-third)
23 Palatine tonsil
24 Piriform recess
25 Cuneiform tubercle
26 Corniculate tubercle
27 Interarytenoid notch
28 Laryngeal pharynx leading to esophagus
29 Epiglottic depression (vallecula epiglottica)
30 Aryepiglottic fold

H&N-78 Larynx, coronal section

Larynx and surrounding structures

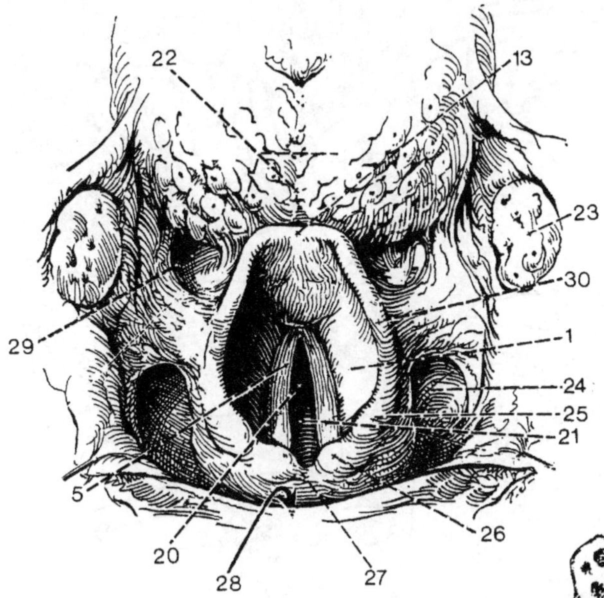

Figure B (viewed from above)

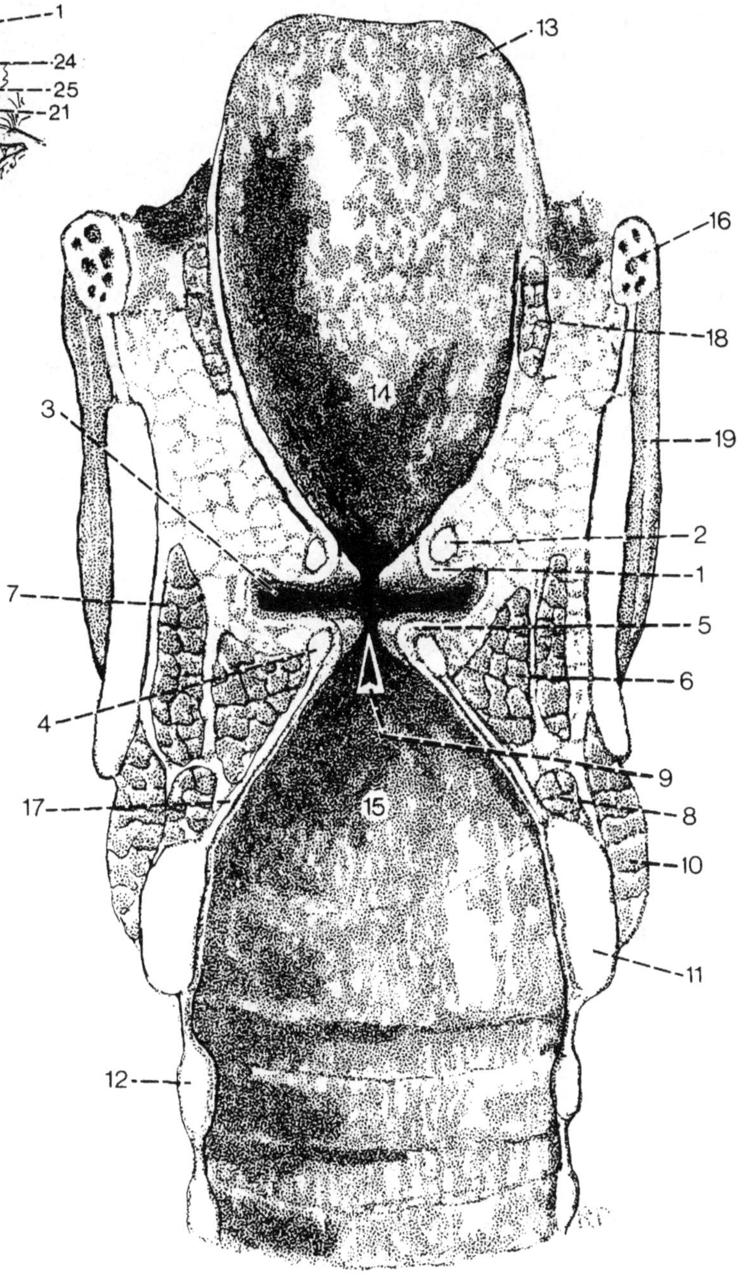

Figure A
(viewed from behind)

H&N-79 Muscle origins and insertions on side of skull

Color the origins (O) RED and the insertions (I) BLUE

1 Temporalis (O)
2 Temporalis (I)
3 Masseter (O)
4 Masseter (I)
5 Buccinator (O)*
6 Zygomatic major (O)
7 Orbicularis oculi (orbital part) (O)
8 Corrugator supercilii (O)
9 Orbicularis oculi (lacrimal part) (O)
10 Levator labii superioris alaeque nasi (O)
11 Orbicularis oculi (orbital part) (O)
12 Zygomatic minor (O)
13 Levator labii superioris (O)
14 Compressor naris (O)
15 Levator anguli oris (O)
16 Orbicularis oris (O)
17 Mentalis (O)
18 Orbicularis oris (O)
19 Depressor labii inferioris (O)
20 Depressor anguli oris (O)
21 Sternocleidomastoid (I)
22 Occipitalis (O)
23 Trapezius (O)
24 Semispinalis capitis (I)
25 Obliquus capitis superior (I)
26 Rectus capitis posterior major (I)
27 Rectus capitis posterior minor (I)
28 Splenius capitis (I)
29 Digastric (O)
30 Longissimus capitis (I)
31 Stylohyoid (O)
32 Styloglossus (O)
33 Platysma (O)

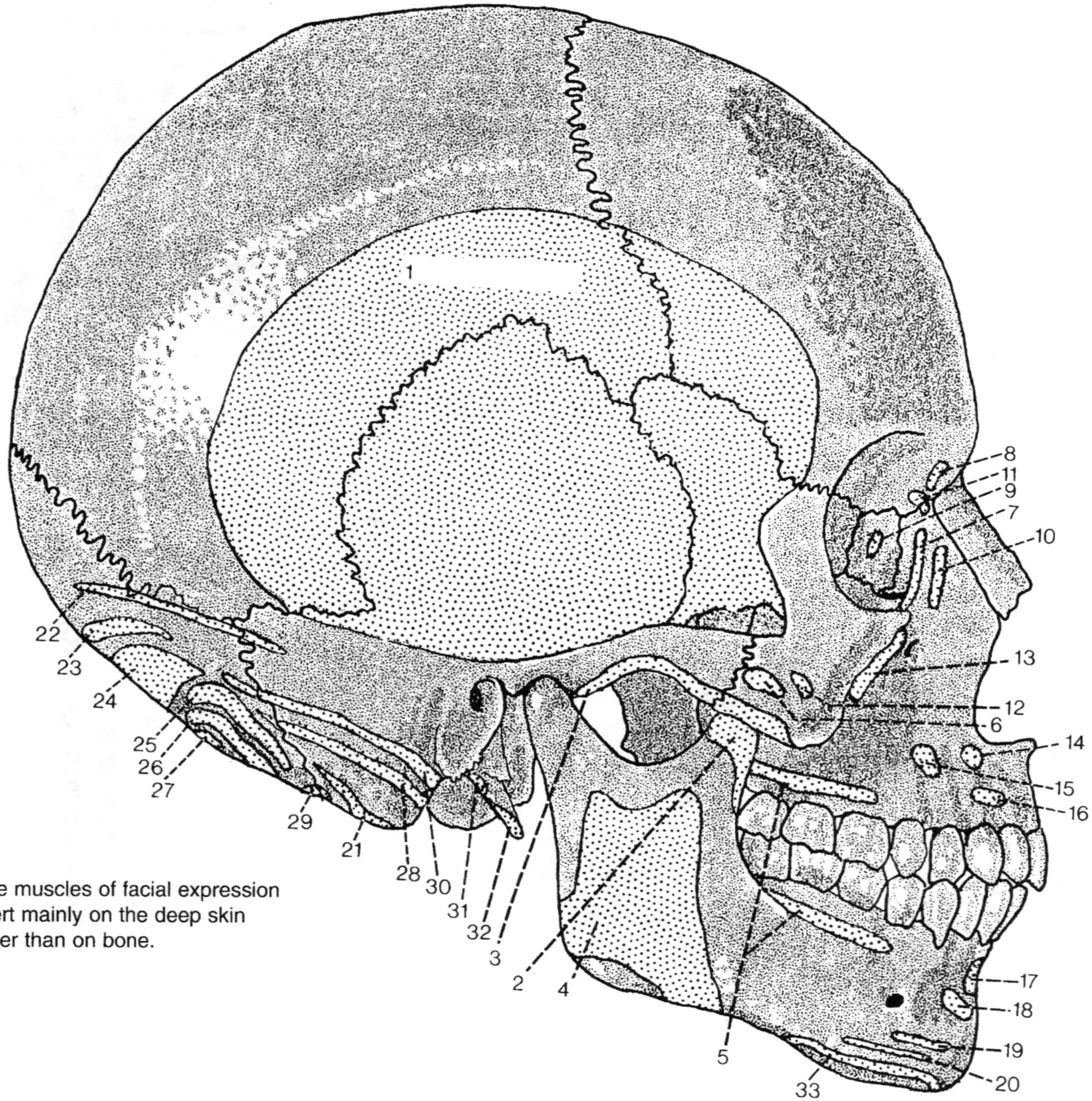

*The muscles of facial expression insert mainly on the deep skin rather than on bone.

H&N-80 Skull

Inferior aspect

Color each bone a different color

Temporal (T)
Sphenoid (S)
Occipital (O)
Zygomatic (Z)
Maxillary (M)
Palatine (Pal)
Vomer (V)

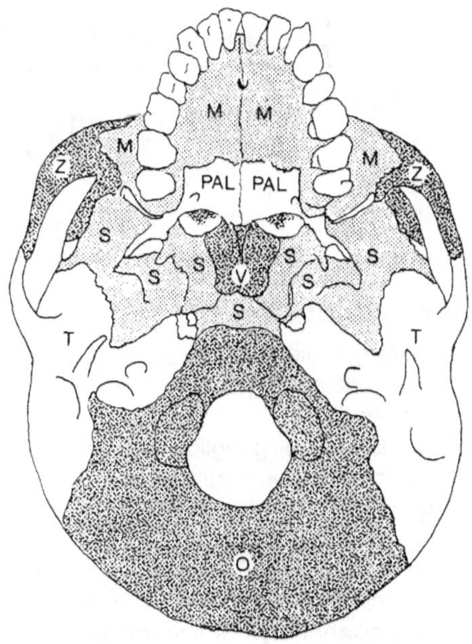

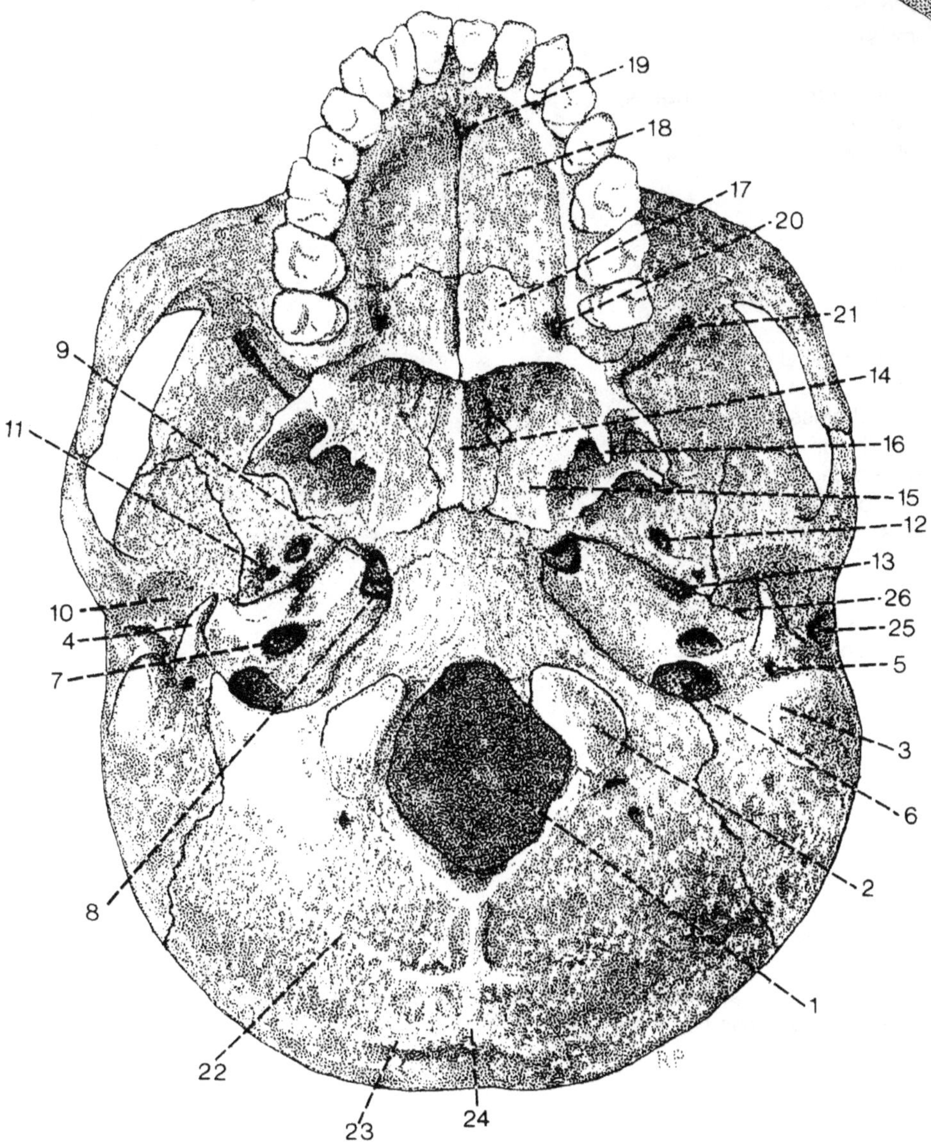

...and label

1 Foramen magnum
2 Occipital condyle
3 Mastoid foramen
4 Styloid process
5 Stylomastoid foramen
6 Jugular foramen
7 Carotid canal external aperature
8 Carotid canal internal aperature
9 Foramen lacerum (plugged up with cartilage in life)
10 Mandibular fossa
11 Foramen spinosum
12 Foramen ovale
13 Auditory tube sulcus
14 Vomer
15 Medial and lateral pterygoid plates
16 Pterygoid hamulus
17 Horizontal plate of palatine bone
18 Palatine process of maxillary bone
19 Incisive foramen
20 Major palatine foramen
21 Inferior orbital fissure
22 Inferior nuchal line
23 Superior nuchal line
24 External occipital protuberance (inion)
25 External auditory meatus
26 Petrotympanic fissure

H&N-81 Autonomic outflow in the head I

(opposite page)

Color and label

1 Ciliary ganglion*
2 Pterygopalatine ganglion*
3 Otic ganglion*
4 Submandibular ganglion*
5 Trigeminal nerve sensory root
6 Trigeminal nerve motor root
7 Trigeminal ganglion
8 Nasociliary branch of ophthalmic nerve
9 Long ciliary nerve (sensory to eye)
10 Short ciliary nerve (autonomics)
11 Oculomotor nerve (N III)
12 Oculomotor root to ciliary ganglion (parasympathetics)
13 Sympathetic root to ciliary ganglion
14 Internal carotid artery and plexus
15 Maxillary nerve
16 Pterygopalatine nerves
17 Palatine nerves
18 Posterior lateral nasal nerves
19 Nerve of the pterygoid canal (Vidian nerve)
20 Facial nerve
21 Greater petrosal nerve (branch of facial nerve, N VII)
22 Deep petrosal nerve (sympathetics)
23 Lesser petrosal nerve (branch of glossopharyngeal nerve, N IX)
24 Lingual nerve (branch of mandibular nerve)
25 Chorda tympani nerve (branch of facial nerve)
26 Inferior alveolar nerve (branch of mandibular nerve)
27 Glossopharyngeal nerve (N IX)
28 Vagus nerve (N X)
29 Superior laryngeal branch of vagus nerve
30 Superior cardiac branch of vagus nerve
31 Superior cervical sympathetic ganglion
32 Carotid nerve
33 Middle meningeal artery and plexus
34 Maxillary artery and plexus
35 External carotid artery and plexus
36 Carotid sinus nerve (branch of glossopharyngeal nerve)
37 Carotid sinus
38 Common carotid artery
39 Pharyngeal plexus (nerves X and IX)
40 Superior cervical sympathetic cardiac nerve
41 Auriculotemporal nerve

*These four parasympathetic ganglia contain postganglionic parasympathetic nerve cell bodies upon which preganglionic parasympathetic fibers synapse.

H&N-81 Autonomic outflow in the head, I

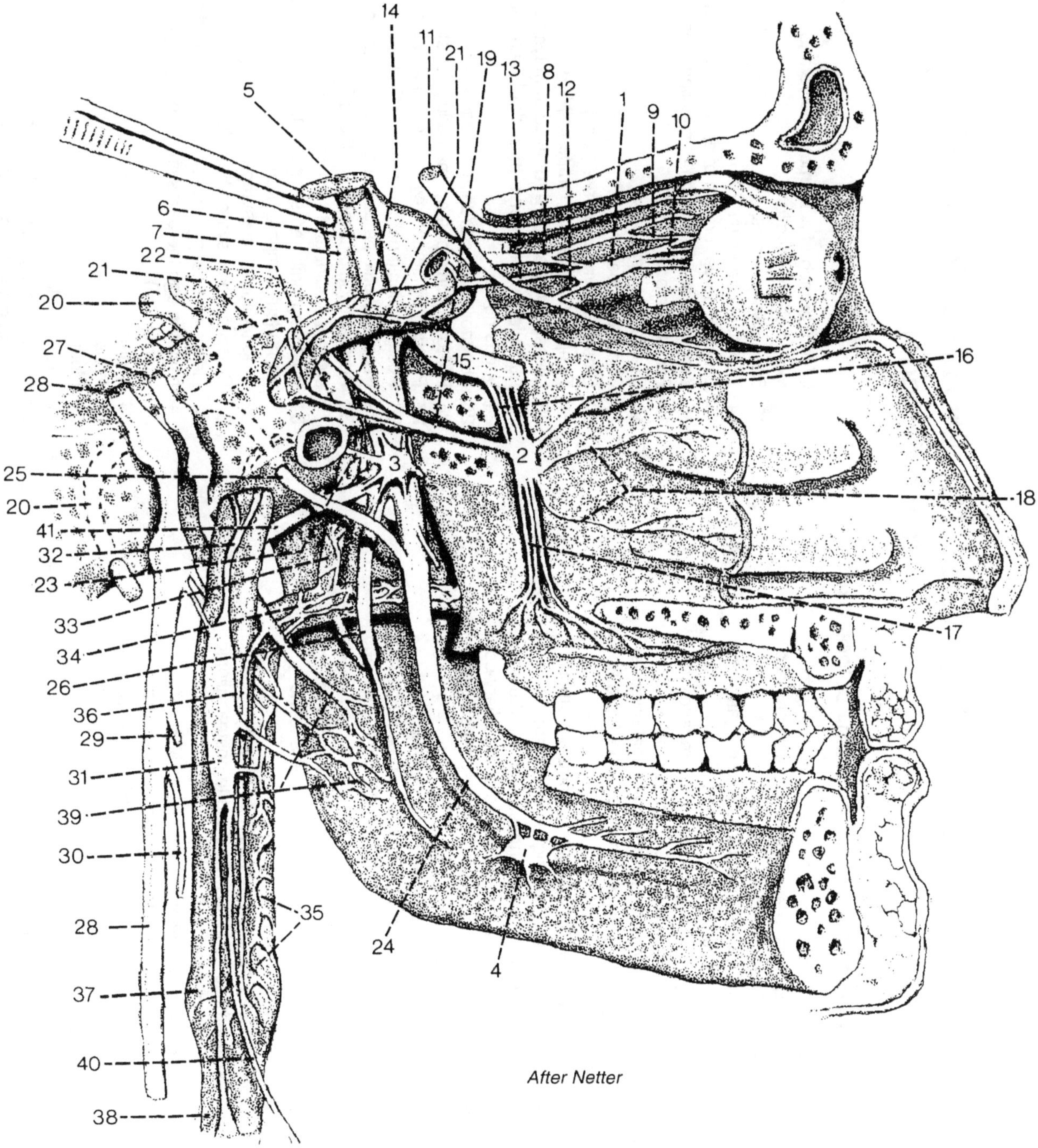

After Netter

H&N-82 Autonomic outflow in the head II

(opposite page)

Color the neurons and trace the paths of their axons

1 Accessory oculomotor nucleus (old name: Edinger-Westfall nucleus) with preganglionic parasympathetic neurons* and fibers (axons)
2 Superior (rostral) salivatory nucleus with preganglionic parasympathetic neurons* and fibers (axons)
3 Inferior (caudal) salivatory nucleus with preganglionic parasympathetic neurons* and fibers (axons)
4 Dorsal nucleus of vagus nerve (dorsal vagal nucleus) with preganglionic parasympathetic neurons* and fibers (axons)
5 Ciliary ganglion with postganglionic parasympathetic neurons giving rise to postganglionic fibers to the constrictor muscles of the iris (these diminish the size of the pupil) and to the circular muscles of the ciliary body (these allow the lens to become more spherical and focus on near objects)
6 Pterygopalatine ganglion with postganglionic parasympathetic neurons giving rise to postganglionic fibers to the lacrimal gland and glands of the nose and palate
7 Otic ganglion with postganglionic parasympathetic neurons giving rise to postganglionic fibers to the parotid gland
8 Submandibular ganglion with postganglionic parasympathetic neurons giving rise to postganglionic fibers to the submandibular and sublingual gland
9 Preganglionic sympathetic nerve cell body in interomediolateral column of thoracic spinal cord
10 Postganglionic sympathetic nerve cell body in superior cervical ganglion
11 Oculomotor nerve (N III)

*Each of the greatly enlarged neurons (or nerve cells) shown here represent hundreds or thousands of microscopic neurons.

12 Inferior branch of oculomotor nerve and oculomotor root to ciliary ganglion
13 Short ciliary nerves
14 Trigeminal nerve (N V)
15 Lacrimal nerve (branch of ophthalmic nerve)
16 Zygomaticofacial branch of maxillary nerve
17 Facial nerve (N VII)
18 Greater petrosal nerve
19 Chorda tympani nerve
20 Glossopharyngeal nerve (N IV)
21 Tympanic nerve and tympanic plexus
22 Lesser petrosal nerve (derived from tympanic plexus)
23 Auriculotemporal nerve (branch of mandibular nerve)
24 Vagus nerve
25 Superior cardiac branch of vagus nerve
26 Postganglionic parasympathetic fiber(s) to eye
27 Postganglionic parasympathetic fiber(s) to lacrimal gland
28 Postganglionic parasympathetic fibers to nasal glands
29 Postganglionic parasympathetic fiber(s) to palatine glands
30 Postganglionic parasympathetic fibers to submandibular and sublingual glands
31 Postganglionic parasympathetic fiber(s) to parotid gland via auriculotemporal nerve
32 Preganglionic parasympathetic fiber(s) to heart
33 Postganglionic sympathetic fiber(s) to nose via carotid plexus and deep petrosal nerve; (sympathetic fibers pass through the parasympathetic ganglion with no interruption)
34 Midbrain
35 Pons
36 Medulla
37 Lacrimal gland
38 Nasal glands and nasal conchae
39 Parotid gland (a small portion)
40 Sublingual gland
41 Submandibular gland

H&N-82 Autonomic outflow in the head II

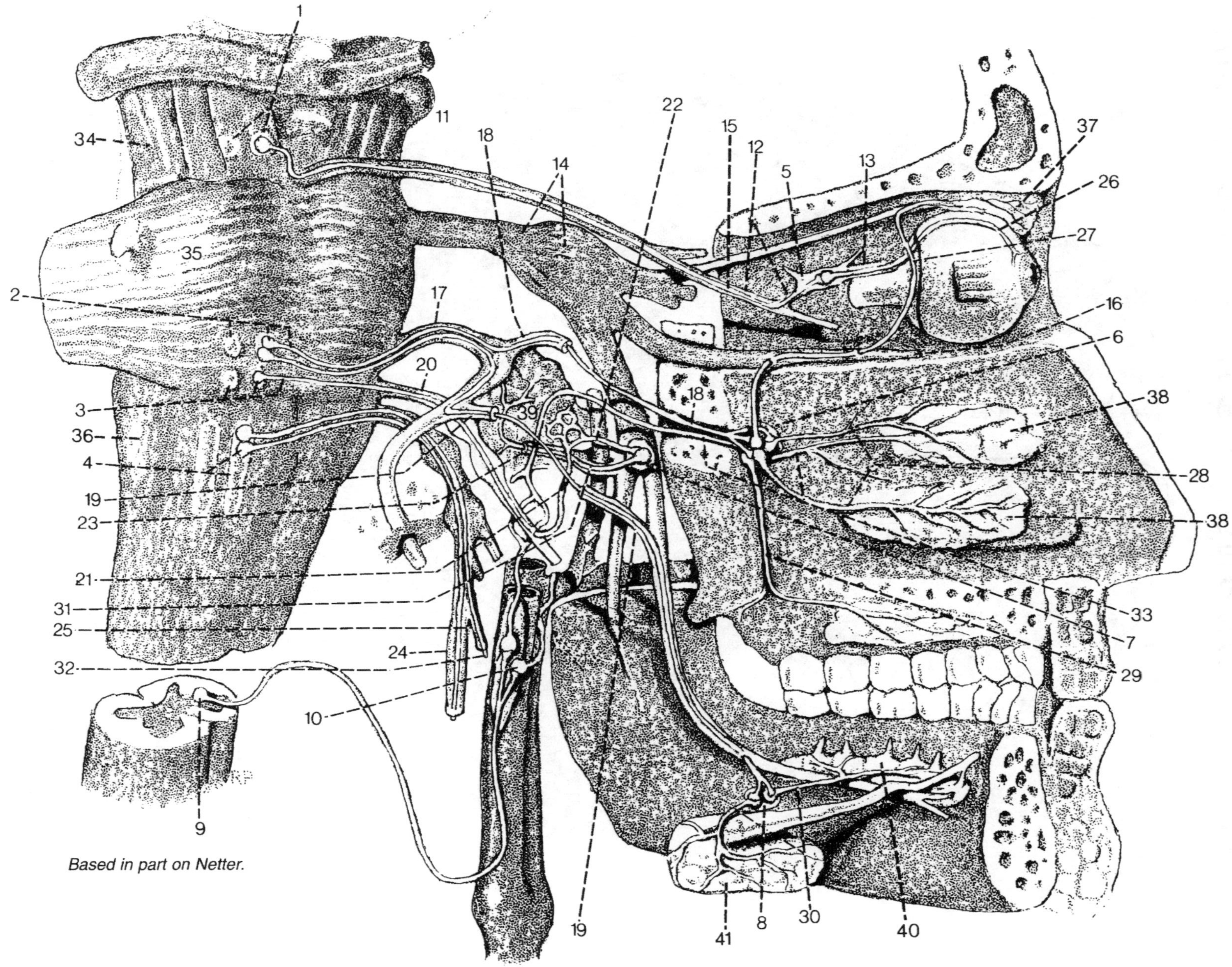

Based in part on Netter.

H&N-83 Inferior view of the brain

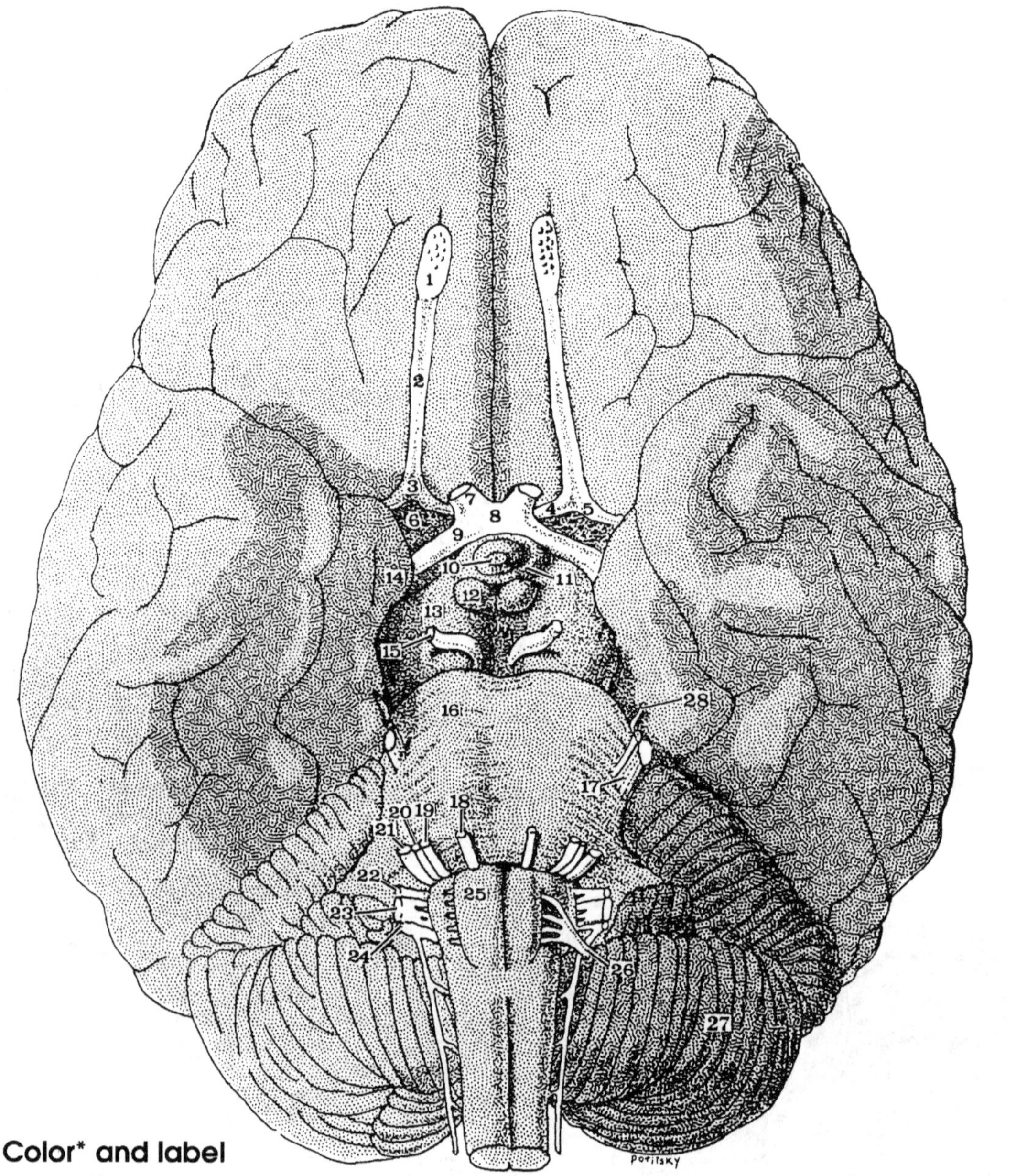

Color* and label

1 Olfactory bulb*
2 Olfactory tract*
3 Olfactory trigone*
4 Medial olfactory stria*
5 Lateral olfactory stria*
6 Anterior perforated substance
7 Optic nerve (cranial nerve II)
8 Optic chiasma*
9 Optic tract*
10 Infundibulum
11 Tuber cinereum
12 Mamillary body
13 Cerebral peduncle
14 Uncus
15 Oculomotor nerve (cranial nerve III)*
16 Pons
17 Trigeminal nerve (cranial nerve V)*
18 Abducent nerve (cranial nerve VI)*
19 Facial nerve (cranial nerve VII) (motor part)*
20 Nervus intermedius (part of facial nerve)*
21 Vestibulocochlear nerve (cranial nerve VIII)*
22 Glossopharyngeal nerve (cranial nerve IX)*
23 Vagus nerve (cranial nerve X)*
24 Accessory nerve (cranial nerve XI)*
25 Pyramids
26 Hypoglossal nerve (cranial nerve XII)*
27 Cerebellum (hemisphere)
28 Trochlear nerve (cranial nerve IV)*

H&N-84 Medial view of right half of brain

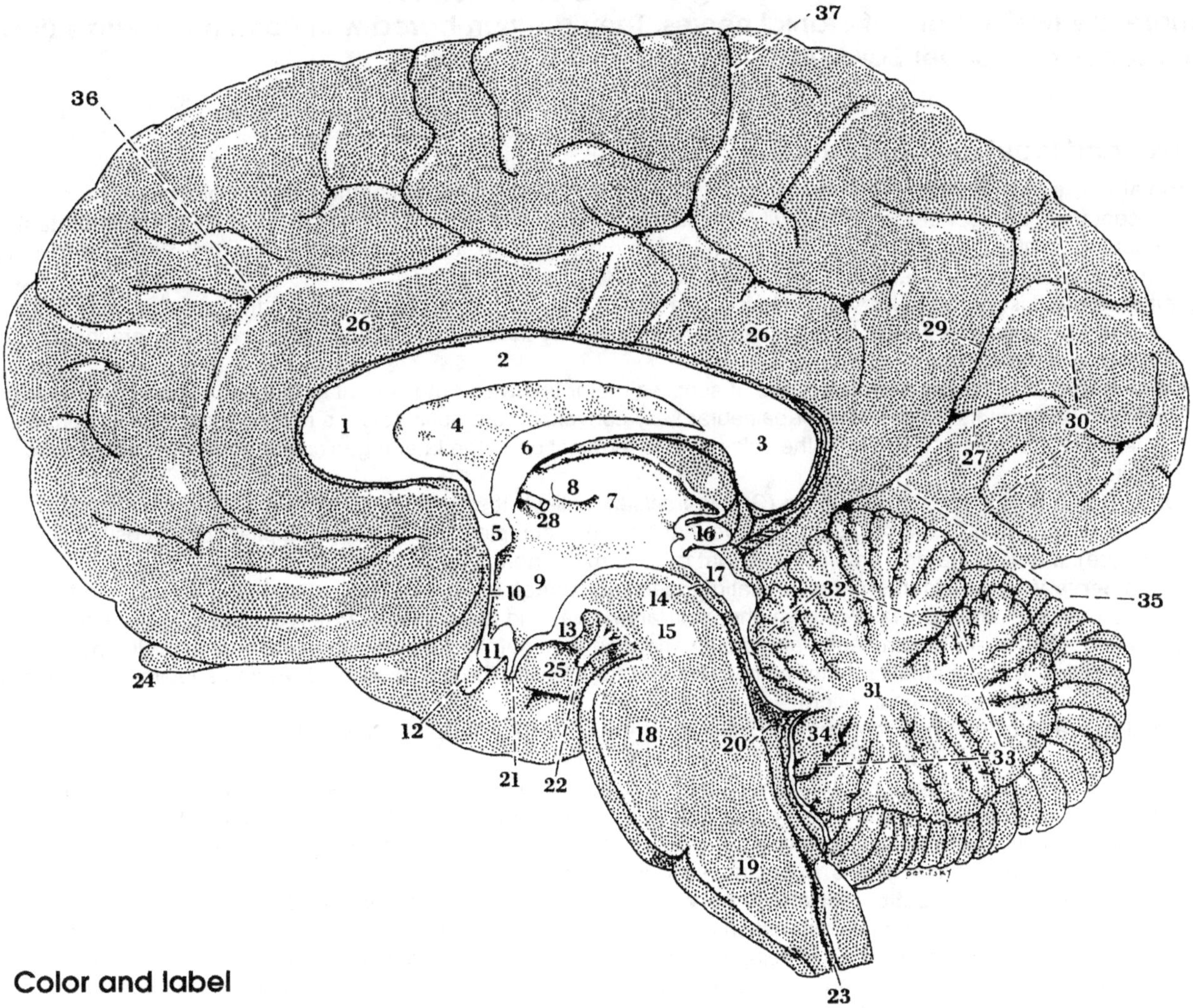

Color and label

1 Genu of corpus callosum
2 Body of corpus callosum
3 Splenium of corpus callosum
4 Septum pellucidum
5 Anterior commissure
6 Fornix
7 Thalamus
8 Interthalamic adhesion
9 Hypothalamus
10 Lamina terminalis
11 Optic chiasm
12 Optic nerve
13 Mamillary body
14 Cerebral aqueduct
15 Decussation of superior cerebellar peduncles
16 Pineal body
17 Mesencephalic tectum (formerly lamina quadrigemina)
18 Pons
19 Medulla
20 Fourth ventricle
21 Infundibulum
22 Oculomotor nerve
23 Central canal of spinal cord
24 Olfactory bulb
25 Uncus of temporal lobe
26 Cingulate gyrus
27 Calcarine sulcus
28 Probe in interventricular foramen
29 Parieto-occipital sulcus
30 Occipital lobe
31 White matter of vermis
32 Anterior lobe of cerebellum
33 Posterior lobe of cerebellum
34 Nodulus of cerebellum
35 Common stem of parieto-occipital sulcus and calcarine sulcus
36 Cingulate sulcus
37 Marginal part of cingulate sulcus

H&N-85 The cranial nerves

Ventral aspect of brain stem showing exit of cranial nerves.
There are twelve pairs of cranial nerves. They are numbered with Roman numerals (just like the successive Super Bowls!).

Color and label (unlabelled side)

Cranial nerve I is the **olfactory nerve** (Latin, *olfacia*, to smell). It is made up of the axons of bipolar olfactory receptors in the roof of the nasal cavity. These axons group into about 20 bundles called fila that penetrate the cribriform plate of the ethmoid bone and end in the olfactory bulb. The axons of the olfactory nerve are thin and unmyelinated and are easily broken should the olfactory bulb be raised.

Cranial nerve II is the **optic nerve**. It consists of about one million axons that arise from the ganglion cells in the retina. The optic nerve is the only nerve that is enclosed by the three meninges, the dura mater, arachnoid mater, and the pia mater.

Cranial nerve III is the **oculomotor nerve**. It supplies motor fibers and movement to four extrabulbar eye muscles and the raiser of the eyelid (levator palpebrae). By convention the optic nerve is named "optic nerve" from the eyeball to the optic chiasm; from the chiasm to its termination in the lateral geniculate body it is called "optic tract."

Cranial nerve IV is the **trochlear nerve** (Greek, *trochlea*, pulley). It supplies only one extrabulbar muscle, the superior oblique. It is the only cranial nerve that becomes completely crossed (it supplies the opposite superior oblique). It also is the only cranial nerve that exits from the dorsal aspect of the brain stem.

Cranial nerve V is the **trigeminal nerve** (Latin, *trigeminus*, threefold). It is mainly sensory and divides into three large branches, the ophthalmic nerve, the maxillary nerve, and the mandibular nerve. These three nerves supply the face, eye, nose, mouth, teeth, and the anterior two-thirds of the tongue with pain, touch, and temperature sensibilities. It has a smaller motor component that travels with the mandibular nerve and supplies the muscles of the jaw (muscles of mastication).

Cranial nerve VI is the **abducent nerve** (Latin, *abducere*, to lead away). It supplies only one extrabulbar eye muscle, the lateral rectus which turns the eye lateral.

Cranial nerve VII is the **facial nerve**. It arises by two roots. The larger motor root supplies the muscles of facial expression. Immediate lateral to the motor root is the smaller root, the **nervus intermedius**. The nervus intermedius contains taste fibers from the anterior two-thirds of the tongue and parasympathetic fibers that supply the lacrimal gland, nasal glands, submandibular gland, and sublingual gland.

Cranial nerve VIII is the **vestibulocochlear nerve**. It carries two distinct sensory modalities from the inner ear. The older vestibular portion carries information about the position and movement of the head. The vestibular part of the inner ear responds to the head being turned, tilted, or accelerated in a straight line. The newer cochlear portion of the vestibulocochlear carries hearing sensibility from the cochlea to the medial geniculate body.

Cranial nerve IX is the **glossopharyngeal nerve** (Greek, literally "tongue-throat"). It is mainly sensory to the upper pharynx and soft palate. It supplies pain, touch, temperature, and taste to the posterior one-third of the tongue. It supplies motor fibers that join with those of the vagus nerve to form the pharyngeal plexus, which innervates the soft palate and upper pharynx. Parasympathetic fibers in the glossopharyngeal nerve supply the parotid gland.

Cranial nerve X is the **vagus nerve**. It contains five different kinds of fibers. These include preganglionic parasympathetic fibers that innervate the esophagus, heart, lungs, stomach, and intestines. Numerous visceral afferent (incoming) fibers function in cardiac and pulmonary reflexes. The vagus supplies motor control of the pharynx and larynx. Taste fibers from taste buds on the epiglottis travel within the vagus nerve, as do a few afferent fibers from the skin of the ear.

Cranial nerve XI is the **accessory nerve** (old name, spinal accessory nerve). It arises by two roots, a cranial one from the medulla and a spinal one from the cervical spinal cord. It supplies only two muscles, the trapezius and the sternocleidomastoid.

Cranial nerve XII is the **hypoglossal nerve**. It supplies all the homolateral tongue muscles (on the same side).

H&N-85 The cranial nerves

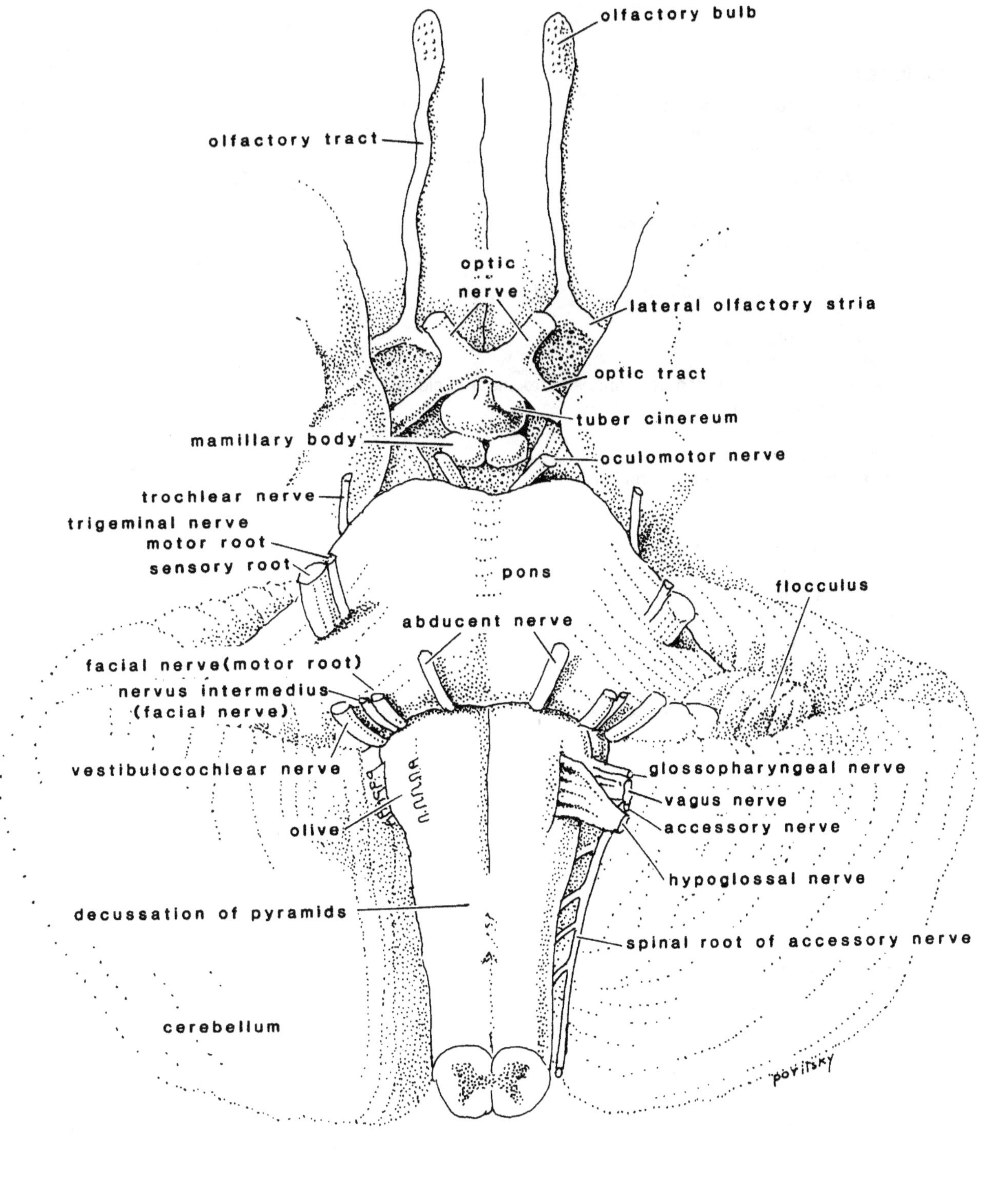

H&N-86 Brain stem

Dorsal aspect
(opposite page)

Color and label

1 Cavity of septum pellucidum
2 Corpus callosum (a small section)
3 Septum pellucidum
4 Internal capsule
5 Putamen
6 Stria terminalis and thalamostriate vein
7 Tail of caudate nucleus
8 Ventricle III
9 Choroid membrane (tela choroidea) of third ventricle
10 Pineal gland
11 Brachium of inferior colliculus
12 Inferior colliculus
13 Trochlear nerve (originated from opposite trochlear nucleus)
14 Superior cerebellar peduncle
15 Facial colliculus
16 Vestibular area
17 Lateral aperature of fourth ventricle (IV)
18 Hypoglossal trigone
19 Vagal trigone
20 Obex (caudal angle of ventricle IV)
21 Fasciculus gracilis
22 Fasciculus cuneatus
23 Posterior intermediate sulcus
24 Posterior median sulcus
25 Tubercle of nucleus cuneatus
26 Tubercle of nucleus gracilis
27 Tenia of ventricle IV (line of attachment of choroid membrane to rim of ventricle IV)
28 Accessory nerve (N XI)
29 Vagus nerve (N X)
30 Glossopharyngeal nerve (N IX)
31 Stria medularis of ventricle IV
32 Inferior cerebellar peduncle (old name, restiform body)
33 Middle cerebellum peduncle (old name, brachium pontis)
34 Superior medullary velum
35 Trigeminal nerve (N V)
36 Superior colliculus
37 Medial geniculate body
38 Lateral geniculate body
39 Habenular triangle
40 Internal capsule (sublenticular part)
41 Thalamus
42 Fornix (body; cut)
43 Caudate nucleus (body)
44 Lateral ventricle (left)
45 Caudate nucleus (head)

H&N-86 Brain stem

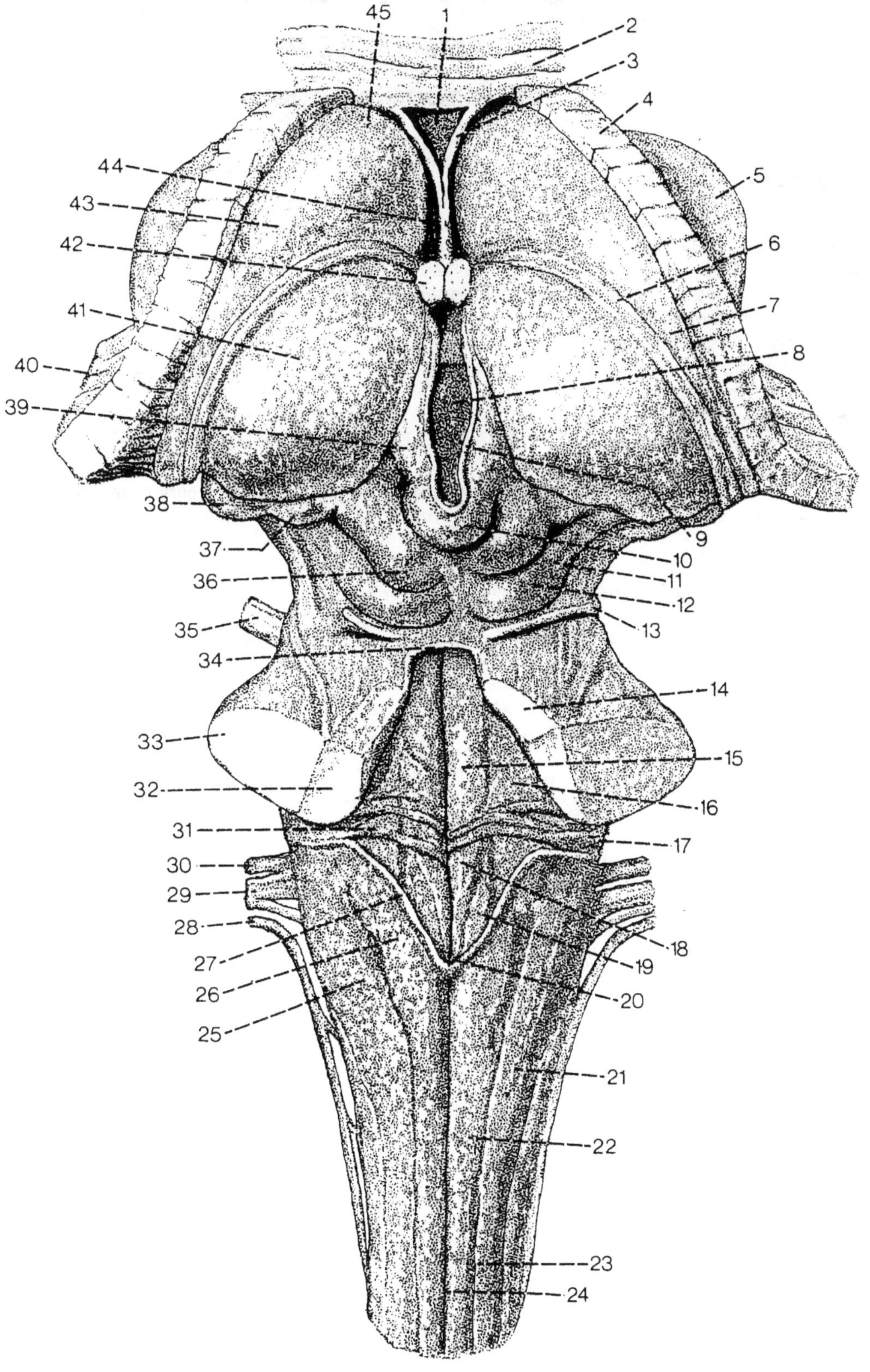

H&N-87 Arterial supply at base of brain

Anterior aspect

(opposite page)

(opposite page)

Color and label

1 Vertebral arteries (right and left)*
2 Internal carotid arteries (right and left)*
3 Anterior spinal artery
4 Basilar artery (formed by the union of the two vertebral arteries)
5 Posterior inferior cerebellar artery
6 Anterior inferior cerebellar artery
7 Labyrinthine artery
8 Superior cerebellar artery
9 Posterior cerebral artery
10 Posterior communicating artery
11 Middle cerebral artery
12 Anterior cerebral artery (note its course in the longitudinal cerebral fissure as it curves around the genu of the corpus callosum)
13 Anterior communicating artery (prone to aneurysms)
14 Branch of the posterior cerebral artery
15 Pontine branches off basilar artery

*These four arteries, the right and left vertebral arteries and the right and left internal carotid arteries, are the sole supply of arterial blood to the brain.

H&N-87 Arterial supply at base of brain

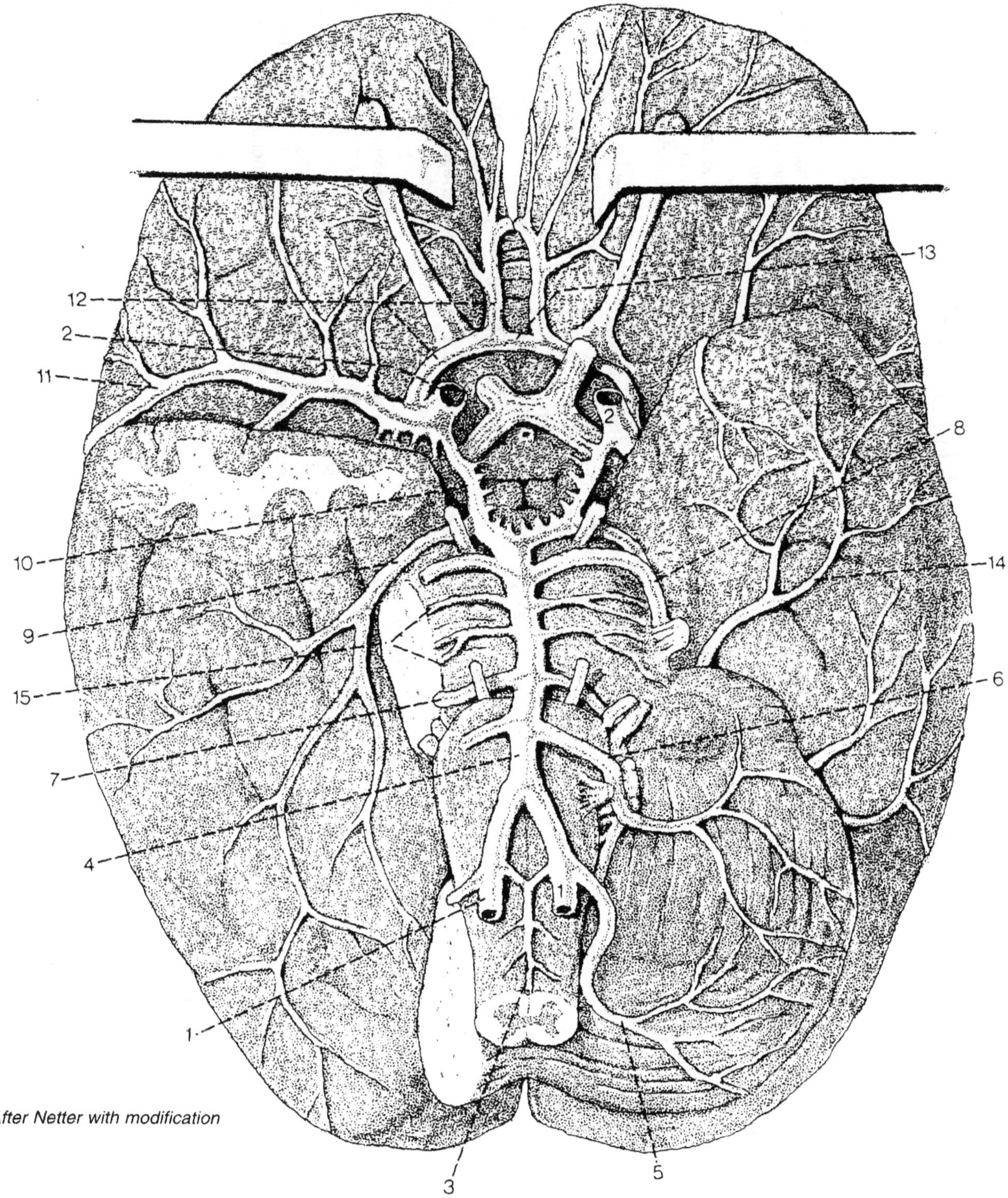

After Netter with modification

Thalamus means bedroom
Etymological cartoon

Thalamus meant bedroom or inner chamber in both Latin and Greek. Why the thalamus, which is a solid mass of neurons, should be named a room or chamber is something of a mystery. It probably goes back to the ancients' belief that hollow chambers in the brain stored particles of sensation conveyed to the brain by hollow nerves. The optic nerve supposedly carried particles of vision to its chamber, the optic thalamus. A careful examination of the brain would have revealed to the ancients that the lateral geniculate body, which is that part of the thalamus where the optic nerve ends, is not hollow but rather solid; nor is any other part of the thalamus hollow. Unfortunately the ancients' knowledge of brain anatomy was founded more on doctrine than on actual dissection and examination. For a long time the term **optic thalamus** was used for the thalamus, even after it was shown that it was solid, not hollow. Eventually "optic" was discarded and the name was shortened to simply thalamus.

Pituitary gland. At one time the pituitary gland was believed to secrete phlegm. Its name is derived from the Latin *pituita*, which means phlegm. Pituita itself is an onomatope, which means it is imitative of the sound associated with it, which in this case is the sound of spitting, much like our expression "ptooey." The ancients thought that the brain extracted phlegm from the blood. The phlegm was then funneled into the pituitary gland. In fact, the name of the pituitary stalk, **infundibulum,** means funnel in Latin. From the pituitary gland the phlegm was supposedly conveyed to the roof of the nose, where it migrated through tiny holes in the cribriform plate into the nose.

Ostium (Latin) meant door. It is now used in anatomy for a small opening of a vessel. It is derived from *os* (mouth).

Tectum (Latin) was either a celing or a roof. The tectum is that part of the midbrain dorsal to the cerebral aqueduct. The former name for the tectum was **lamina quadrigemina**, the "plate with the quadruplets," that is, the four colliculi.

Colliculus (Latin) meant little hill, from *collis*, hill.

Folia (Latin) meant leaves. One leaf was a **folium**. The transverse folds of the cerebellar cortex are called folia.

Ramus (Latin) meant branch.

Arbor (Latin) meant tree. The **arbor vitae**, "tree of life," was the old name for the white matter in the cerebellum.

Dendrite is derived from the Greek **dendron** (tree) and means little tree or tree-like.

Radix (Latin) meant root. **Radicular** relates to a root. **Radiculitis** means inflammation of a nerve root. A **radical** change is a change so drastic that it gets down to the roots, and may even pull out the roots!

Funiculus (Latin) is derived from **funis** (rope) and meant little rope or string. The white matter of the spinal cord is divided into three funiculi.

Pulivinus (Latin) meant a cushion. **Pulivinar** meant couch. The pulivinar of the thalamus resembles a cushion.

Kline was a bed in ancient Greece. Words such as **clinic**, **recline**, **incline** all come from this root. A **clinician** was originally one who visited and treated patients at the bedside.

Murus (Latin) was a wall. **Intramural** ganglia are groups of nerve cells within the walls of the heart, the intestines, and other viscera. **Intramural** sports are held within the walls of the school or college.

Clinoid process means bed post, being derived from kline (bed). The four **clinoid processes** are found in the skull, where they make up part of the **sella turcica,** or "Turkish saddle," which holds the pituitary gland.

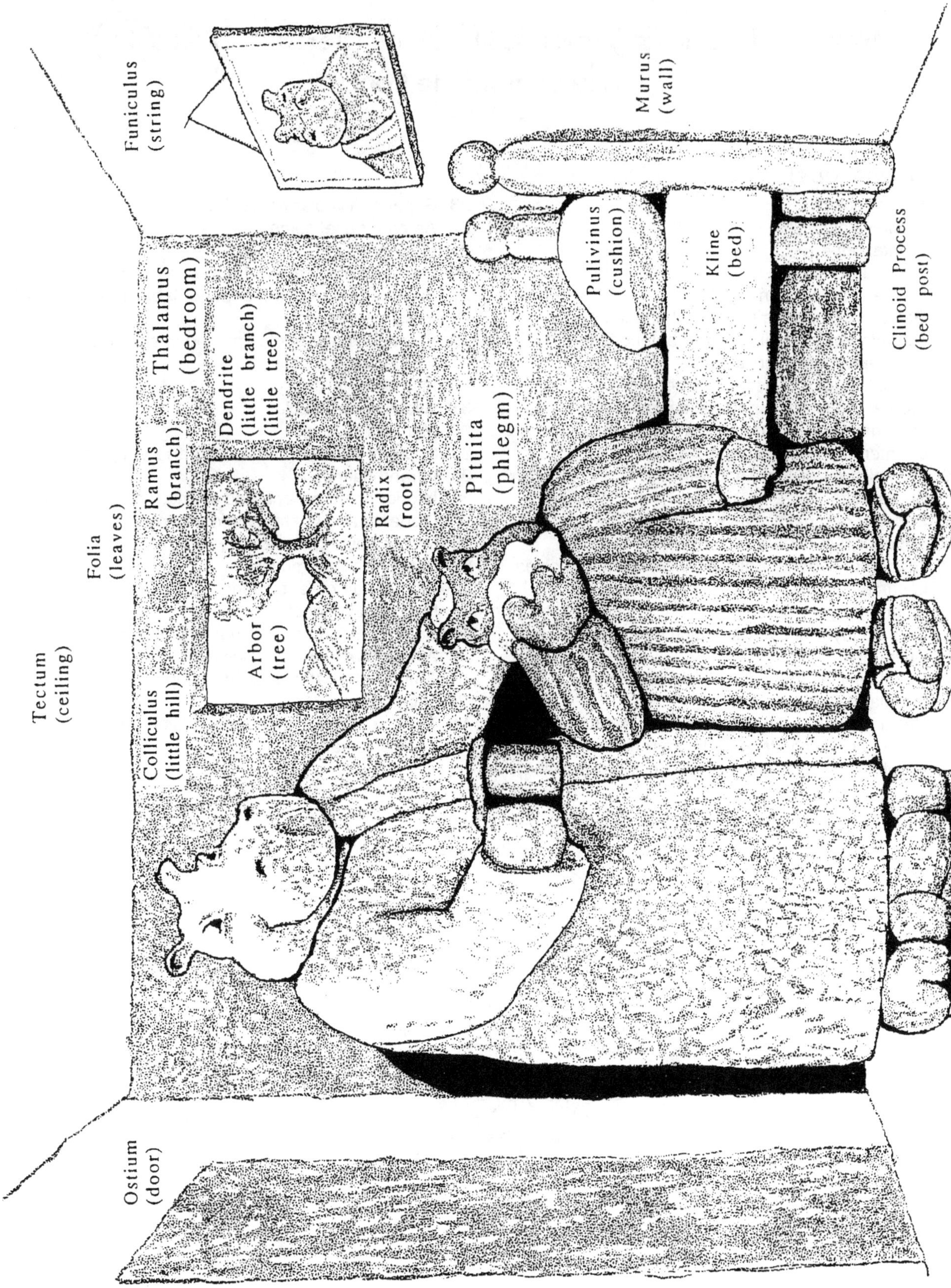
Ostium
(door)
Tectum
(ceiling)
Colliculus
(little hill)
Folia
(leaves)
Arbor
(tree)
Ramus
(branch)
Radix
(root)
Thalamus
(bedroom)
Dendrite
(little branch)
(little tree)
Pituita
(phlegm)
Funiculus
(string)
Pulivinus
(cushion)
Kline
(bed)
Murus
(wall)
Clinoid Process
(bed post)

H&N-88 Head frontal section; level of eyes and nasal cavity

Viewed from the front

Color and label

1 Skin of scalp
2 Frontal diploic vein
3 Frontal bone
4 Bone of frontal crest
5 Frontal lobe of brain
6 Galea aponeurotica (epicranial aponeurosis); extends from frontalis muscle anteriorly to occipitalis muscle posteriorly
7 Loose connective tissue layer of scalp
8 Frontal branch of superficial temporal vein
9 Terminal branch of frontopolar artery (branch of anterior cerebral artery)
10 Frontal sinuses (right and left)
11 Supraorbital nerve
12 Superior ophthalmic vein
13 Superior rectus muscle (tendon)
14 Tendon of superior oblique muscle within trochlea
15 Lacrimal gland
16 Sclera of eye
17 Choroid layer of eye (dark pigmented layer)
18 Crista galli
19 Nasal cavities and left middle nasal concha
20 Maxillary sinus
21 Nasal septum (perpendicular plate of ethmoid above, septal cartilage and vomer below)
22 Levator labii superioris muscle (facial expression)
23 Superior alveolar nerve (left)
24 Anterior nasal spine
25 Maxilla
26 Root and pulp cavity of upper left canine in maxilla
27 Facial artery (above), superior labial artery (below)
28 Buccinator muscle
29 Submandibular ducts opening in sublingual papillae (caruncles)
30 Inferior labial artery
31 Hyoglossus muscle
32 Mentalis muscle
33 Superior alveolar nerves and artery (right)
34 Infraorbital nerve
35 Inferior nasal concha and inferior nasal meatus (beneath and lateral to inferior nasal concha)
36 Middle nasal concha
37 Inferior oblique muscle
38 Ethmoid air cells (sinuses)
39 Nasolacrimal duct
40 Superficial temporal vein and artery (frontal branch)
41 Anterior temporal diploic veins
42 Tendon of levator palpebrae superioris muscle
43 Orbital fat
44 Terminal branch of sphenopalatine artery in incisive canal

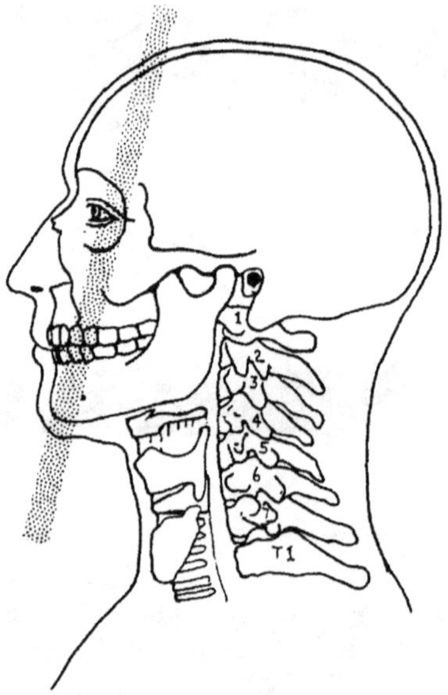

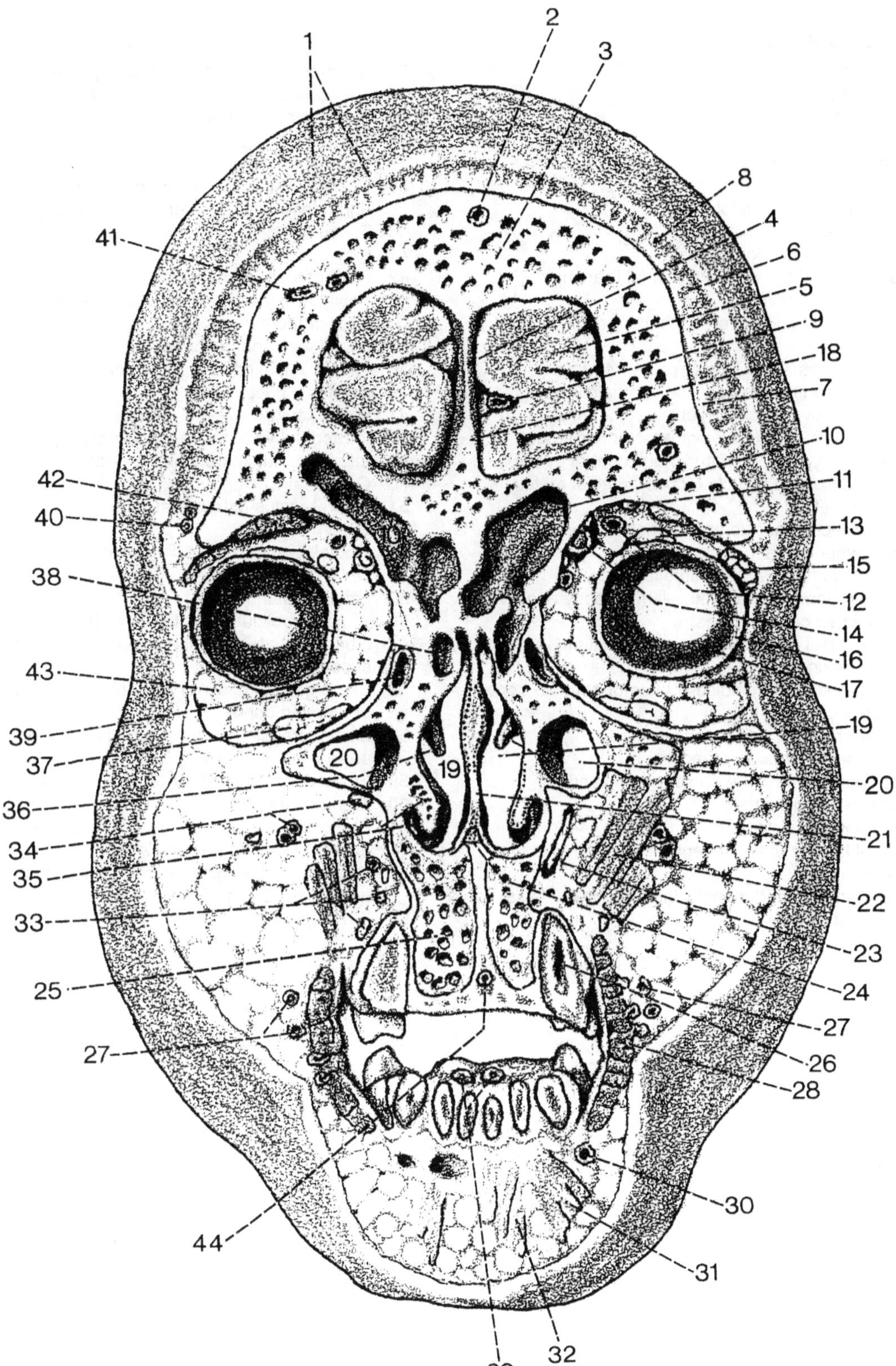
1
2
3
8
41
4
6
5
9
18
7
10
42
11
40
13
15
38
12
14
16
43
17
39
19
37
20
19
20
36
21
34
35
22
33
23
25
24
27
27
26
28
44
30
31
32
29

H&N-89 Eye muscles, sinuses level

Color and label

1 Falx cerebri
2 Superior sagittal sinus
3 Dura mater
4 Diploic veins
5 Superior frontal gyrus
6 Middle frontal gyrus
7 Anterior temporal diploic vein
8 Inferior frontal gyrus
9 Gyrus rectus (straight gyrus)
10 Superficial temporal artery (frontal branch)
11 Supraorbital nerve and artery
12 Superficial temporal vein (frontal branch)
13 Lacrimal nerve
14 Superior rectus and levator palpebrae muscles
15 Superior ophthalmic vein and ophthalmic artery
16 Fundus of eye (back portion)—retina (inner gray) and choroid layer (dark pigmented middle coat)
17 Sclera of eye (outer white fibrous coat of eyeball)
18 Superior oblique muscle (above), medial rectus muscle (below)
19 Inferior rectus muscle and inferior division of oculomotor nerve
20 Infraorbital nerve and infraorbital artery
21 Ethmoid bone (orbital plate—lamina papyracea)
22 Ethmoid air cells (sinuses)
23 Middle nasal concha and middle nasal meatus (space)
24 Maxillary sinus
25 Nasal septum (perpindicular plate of ethmoid bone above and vomer below)
26 Greater palatine artery and nerve
27 Facial nerve—buccal branches
28 Hard palate (maxillary portion) and glands in mucosa of hard palate
29 Buccinator muscle
30 Buccal branch of facial nerve
31 Facial artery
32 Labial arteries and mandibular branches of facial nerve
33 Platysma muscle
34 Submandibular duct and sublingual gland
35 Inferior alveolar nerve in mandible
36 Genioglossus muscle
37 Mandible
38 Submental veins
39 Sublingual vein (in sublingual gland) and inferior alveolar nerve in mandibular canal
40 Tongue
41 Oral cavity
42 Root of tooth in mandible
43 Facial artery and buccal branches of facial nerve
44 Root of tooth in maxilla
45 Facial vein and buccal branches of facial nerve
46 Inferior nasal concha (turbinate) and inferior nasal meatus (space)
47 Nasal cavity
48 Infraorbital vein, nerve, and artery
49 Inferior rectus extraocular muscle
50 Orbital fat
51 Lateral rectus extraocular muscle
52 Zygomatic bone
53 Medial rectus extraocular muscle
54 Optic nerve
55 Lacrimal gland
56 Superior oblique muscle (medial), superior rectus muscle, levator palpebrae muscle (directly above superior rectus)
57 Crista galli (in midline) and cribriform plate (both part of ethmoid bone)
58 Medial orbitofrontal artery (branch of anterior cerebral artery)
59 Frontopolar artery (branch of anterior cerebral artery)
60 Frontal bone
61 Branches of ascending frontal artery (candelabra artery) of middle cerebral artery
62 Cerebral cortex (gray matter)—contains 6 layers of nerve cell bodies
63 White matter (largely myelinated axons)

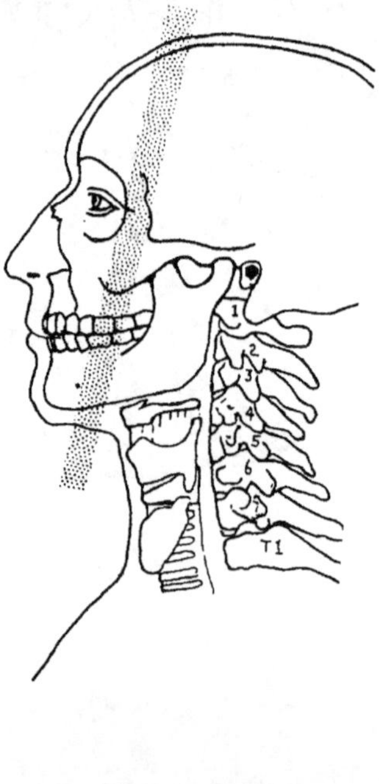

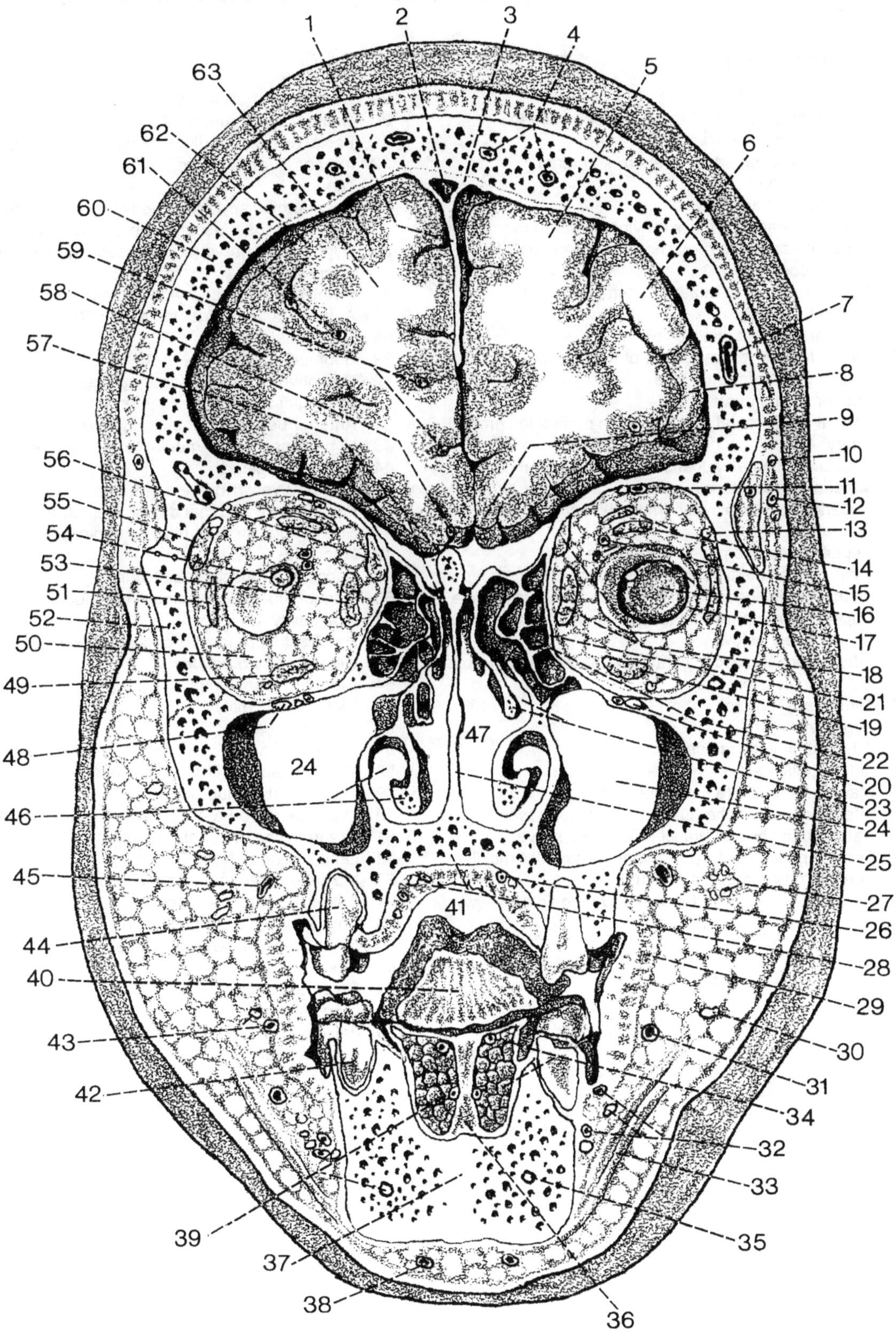
1
2
3
4
5
6
7
8
9
10
11
12
13
14
15
16
17
18
19
20
21
22
23
24
25
26
27
28
29
30
31
32
33
34
35
36
37
38
39
40
41
42
43
44
45
46
47
48
49
50
51
52
53
54
55
56
57
58
59
60
61
62
63

H&N-90 Maxillary sinuses level

Color and label

1 Superior sagittal sinus
2 Longitudinal cerebral fissure (space between cerebral hemispherres)
3 Callosomarginal artery (branch of anterior cerebral artery)
4 Superior frontal gyrus
5 Anterior cerebral arteries curving upwards in front genu of corpus callosum (become pericallosal arteries)
6 Frontal bone
7 Frontal tributary of superficial temporal vein
8 Middle frontal gyrus
9 Anterior temporal diploic vein
10 Straight gyrus (gyrus rectus) of frontal lobe
11 Orbital gyrus of frontal lobe
12 Inferior frontal gyrus
13 Lateral orbitofrontal artery (branch of middle cerebral artery)
14 Levator palpebrae superioris muscle, frontal nerve, superior rectus muscle
15 Superior ophthalmic vein (medial), lacrimal nerve (lateral)
16 Superficial temporal vein and artery
17 Optic nerve in optic canal, ophthalmic artery (immediately above the nerve), lateral rectus muscle
18 Superior oblique muscle (above), medial rectus muscle (immediately below)
19 Inferior rectus muscle, infraorbital nerve (in infraorbital groove in floor of orbit)
20 Temporalis muscle
21 Zygomatic arch
22 Ethmoid air cells (sinuses)
23 Left maxillary sinus
24 Masseter muscle (a small portion)
25 Inferior nasal concha (turbinate), inferior nasal meatus
26 Parotid duct, buccal branches of facial nerve
27 Greater palatine artery and nerve (branch of maxillary nerve in mucosa of hard palate)
28 Molar teeth in maxilla (above) and mandible (below)
29 Buccinator muscle, facial vein
30 Septum of tongue, dorsal lingual vein
31 Facial artery, mandibular branches of facial nerve
32 Inferior alveolar nerve, vein, and artery in mandibular canal
33 Submandibular duct immediately above lingual nerve
34 Genioglossus muscle, deep lingual vein
35 Hypoglossal nerve (above), sublingual branch of lingual artery (below)
36 Mylohyoid muscle, mylohyoid nerve
37 Anterior belly of digastric muscle (left)
38 Sublingual gland
39 Submental vein
40 Geniohyoid muscles (right and left)
41 Genioglossus muscle (right side)
42 Anterior belly of right digastric muscle
43 Hypoglossal nerve medial to lingual artery
44 Sublingual gland
45 Inferior alveolar nerve, vein, artery in mandibular canal
46 Facial artery and mandibular branch(es) of facial nerve
47 Submandibular duct (lingual nerve just below)
48 Mandible
49 Buccinator muscle, facial vein
50 Lingual mucosa on dorsum of tongue
51 Oral cavity
52 Parotid duct (buccal branches of facial nerve)
53 Glands of hard palate
54 Right maxillary sinus
55 Right nasal cavity
56 Left nasal cavity
57 Zygomatic arch
58 Middle nasal concha, middle nasal meatus
59 Lateral rectus muscle
60 Lacrimal nerve (lateral), frontal nerve (medial)
61 Greater wing of sphenoid bone
62 Orbital plate of frontal bone
63 Medial orbitofrontal artery and olfactory tract
64 Anterior cerebral arteries
65 Anterior temporal diploic vein
66 Frontal lobe of cerebral hemisphere (white matter)
67 Cingulate gyrus
68 Galea aponeurotica (epicranial aponeurosis)
69 Cingulate sulcus
70 Falx cerebri
71 Lingual artery
72 Buccal fat pad

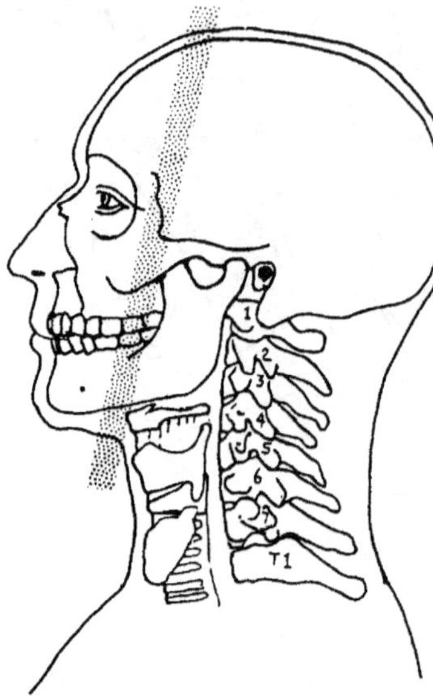

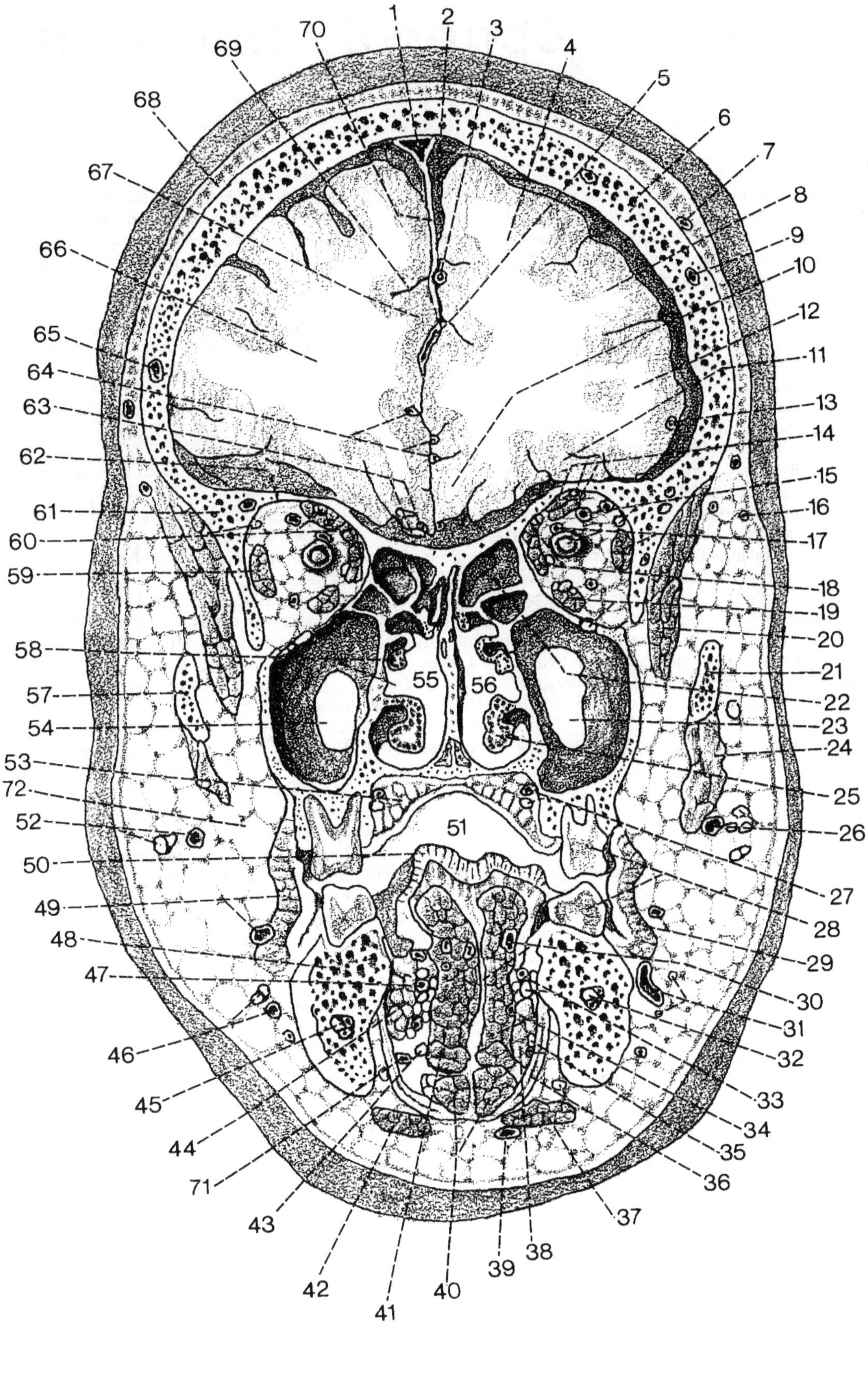
1
2
3
4
5
6
7
8
9
10
11
12
13
14
15
16
17
18
19
20
21
22
23
24
25
26
27
28
29
30
31
32
33
34
35
36
37
38
39
40
41
42
43
44
45
46
47
48
49
50
51
52
53
54
55
56
57
58
59
60
61
62
63
64
65
66
67
68
69
70
71
72

H&N-91 Sphenoid sinuses level

Color and label

1 Superior sagittal sinus
2 Subarachnoid space (contains cerebrospinal fluid, traversed by arachnoid trabeculae)—usually is obliterated after death by arachnoid mater separating from dura mater and collapsing on pia mater
3 Falx cerebri
4 Callosomarginal artery (branch of anterior cerebral)
5 Pericallosal artery (continuation of anterior cerebral artery)
6 Anterior temporal diploic vein
7 Corpus callosum (genu)
8 Lateral ventricle (left)
9 Caudate nucleus (head) abutting lateral ventricle
10 Parietal branch of middle cerebral artery
11 Lateral (Sylvian) fissure
12 Superficial middle cerebral vein
13 Middle cerebral artery
14 Anterior temporal artery (off posterior cerebral artery)
15 Deep temporal arterial branch (off maxillary artery), deep temporal nerve (off motor root of V3), and vein in temporalis muscle
16 Zygomatic arch
17 Greater and lesser palatine nerves descending within palatine canal(s) from pterygopalatine fossa to oral cavity
18 Parotid duct, buccal branch of facial nerve
19 Masseter muscle
20 Facial vein
21 Inferior alveolar nerve, artery, and vein inside mandibular canal

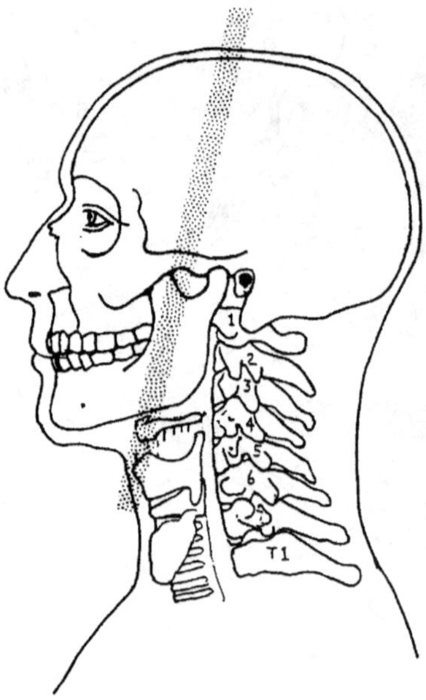

22 Left submandibular duct (superior) and lingual nerve (inferior) within sublingual gland
23 Submental artery and vein, submandibular gland
24 Geniohyoid muscles (right and left), septum of tongue
25 Digastric muscle
26 Mylohyoid muscle
27 Hypoglossal nerve (inferior), lingual artery (superior)
28 Right submandibular duct (superior) and lingual nerve (inferior) within sublingual gland
29 Facial artery
30 Inferior alveolar nerve, artery, and vein inside mandibular canal
31 Facial vein
32 Palatine glands in mucosa of hard palate, greater palatine nerve
33 Inferior alveolar artery, vein, and nerve headed toward mandibular foramen
34 Parotid duct, buccal branches of facial nerve, transverse facial artery
35 Coronoid process of mandible, masseter muscle
36 Inferior nasal concha (turbinate), nasal septum (vomer)
37 Temporalis muscle and maxillary artery in infratemporal fossa
38 Zygomatic arch and tendon of temporalis muscle
39 Maxillary nerve
40 Optic nerve and ophthalmic artery within optic canal
41 Superficial temporal artery and vein (frontal branches)
42 Anterior clinoid process
43 Temporal lobe of brain
44 Middle meningeal artery (frontal branch)
45 Gyrus rectus, olfactory tract
46 Inferior frontal gyrus of cerebral hemisphere
47 Anterior cerebral arteries
48 Middle frontal gyrus of cerebral hemisphere
49 Cingulate gyrus
50 Galea aponeurotica (extends from frontalis muscle)
51 Superior frontal gyrus
52 Arachnoid granulation
53 Lateral venous lacuna (outpouching of superior sagittal sinus)—note the pit in inner surface of the skull caused by arachnoid granulation
54 Body of tongue
55 Oral cavity
56 Nasal cavity (left)
57 Sphenoid sinuses (right and left), septum
58 Cranial nerves III, IV, VI, ophthalmic nerve, and superior ophthalmic vein in cavernous sinus
59 Pterygopalatine ganglion

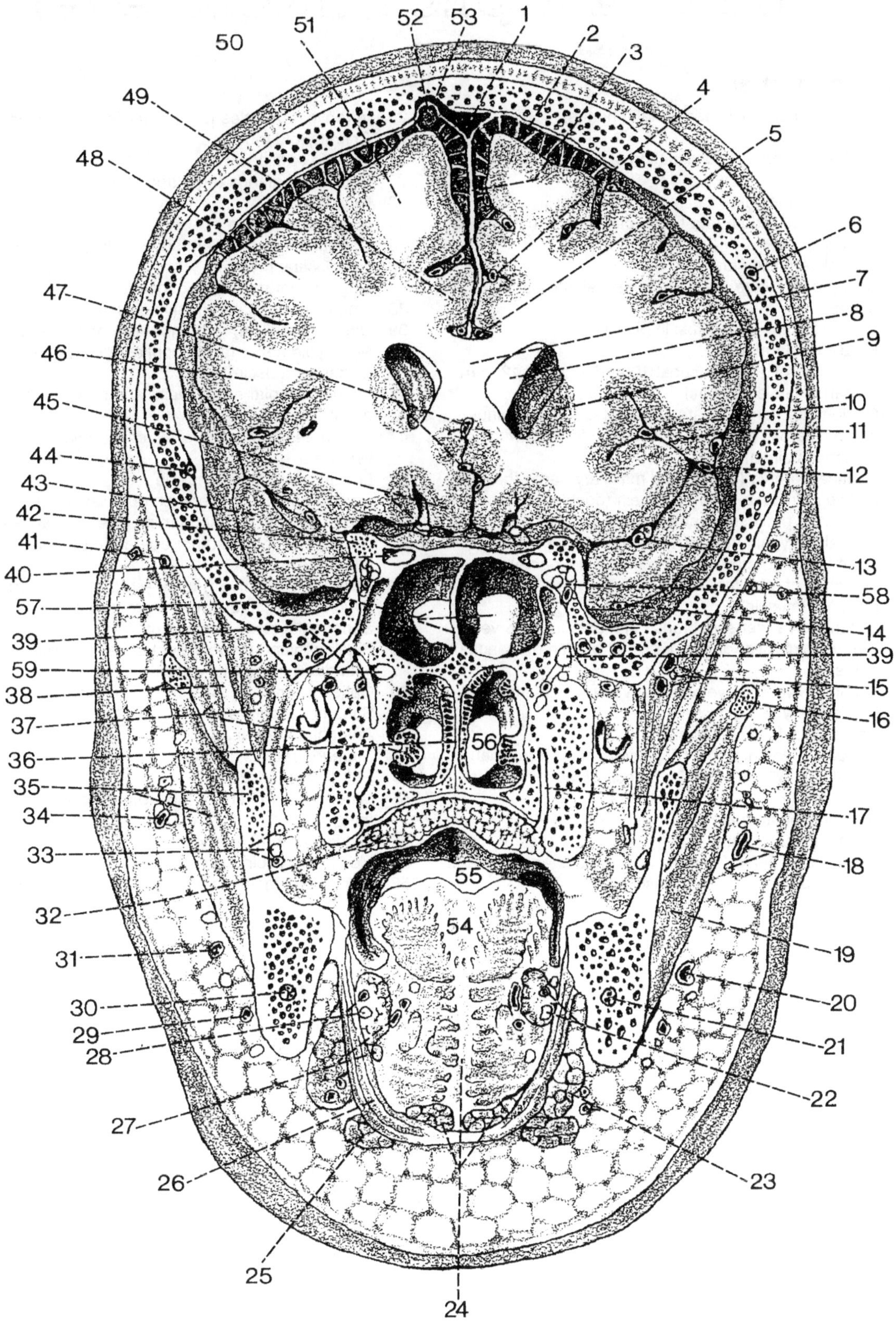

50
51
52
53
1
2
3
4
5
6
7
8
9
10
11
12
13
58
14
39
15
16
17
18
19
20
21
22
23
24
25
26
27
28
29
30
31
32
33
34
35
36
37
38
59
39
57
40
41
42
43
44
45
46
47
48
49
54
55
56

H&N-92 Optic chiasm level

Color and label

1 Sagittal suture (between parietal bones)
2 Falx cerebri
3 Pericallosal artery (continuation of anterior cerebral artery)
4 Corpus callosum
5 Septum pellucidum (the two septa appear to be fused together)
6 Lateral ventricle (left)
7 Squamosal suture (between temporal and parietal bones)
8 Lateral fissure (of Sylvius; in brain)
9 Middle cerebral artery
10 Internal carotid artery (cut at 10 and again at 12, here as part of circle of Willis)
11 Oculomotor nerve (in lateral wall of cavernous sinus)
12 Internal carotid artery (here coursing forward within cavernous sinus)
13 Abducens nerve (above) and maxillary nerve (below)
14 Middle meningeal artery and vein (doubled)
15 Zygomatic process of temporal bone
16 Lateral pterygoid muscle, nerve to lateral pterygoid (from the motor portion of the trigeminal nerve), branches of maxillary artery
17 Masseter muscle
18 Buccal nerve (sensory branch of mandibular nerve)
19 Parotid duct (over or above buccal branch of mandibular nerve)
20 Inferior alveolar nerve and artery in mandibular canal
21 Medial pterygoid muscle
22 Nerve to mylohyoid muscle
23 Lingual nerve (lateral), styloglossus muscle (medial)
24 Facial vein with mandibular branch of facial nerve
25 Facial artery
26 Submandibular duct
27 Submandibular gland
28 Hypoglossal nerve (lateral) and lingual artery (medial), separated by hyoglossus muscle
29 Infrahyoid muscles (strap muscles of the neck)
30 Cricothyroid muscle
31 Thyroid cartilage
32 Sublingual glands (right and left)
33 Hyoid bone
34 Mylohyoid muscle
35 Lingual artery (medial), submandibular gland (lateral)
36 Hyoglossus muscle
37 Lingual septum, intrinsic tongue muscles
38 Lingual nerve (lateral), styloglossus muscle (medial)
39 Uvula (in midline) and underside of soft palate
40 Mylohyoid nerve (also supplies anterior belly of diagastric muscle)
41 Inferior alveolar artery, vein, and nerve in mandibular canal
42 Tensor veli palatini muscle, lesser palatine nerve and vessels
43 Levator veli palatini muscle
44 Parotid duct, buccal branch of facial nerve
45 Posterior wall of nasopharynx (site of pharyngeal tonsil) viewed through posterior aperature of nasal cavity (choanae)
46 Auditory (eustachian) tube—cartilaginous part
47 Zygomatic arch (zygomatic process of temporal bone)
48 Sphenoidal sinus and septum
49 Pituitary gland (hypophysis) in sella turcica, infundibulum (pituitary stalk)
50 Optic chiasm
51 Squamosal suture
52 Anterioir cerebral arteries
53 Superior sagittal sinus
54 Soft palate (sectioned)
55 Middle cerebral artery (above), anterior clinoid process (below)
56 Middle cerebral artery
57 Medial pterygoid plate
58 Lateral pterygoid plate (note how thin they are)

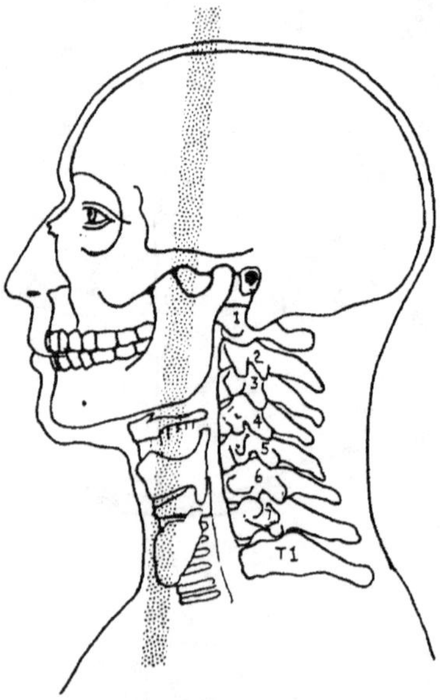

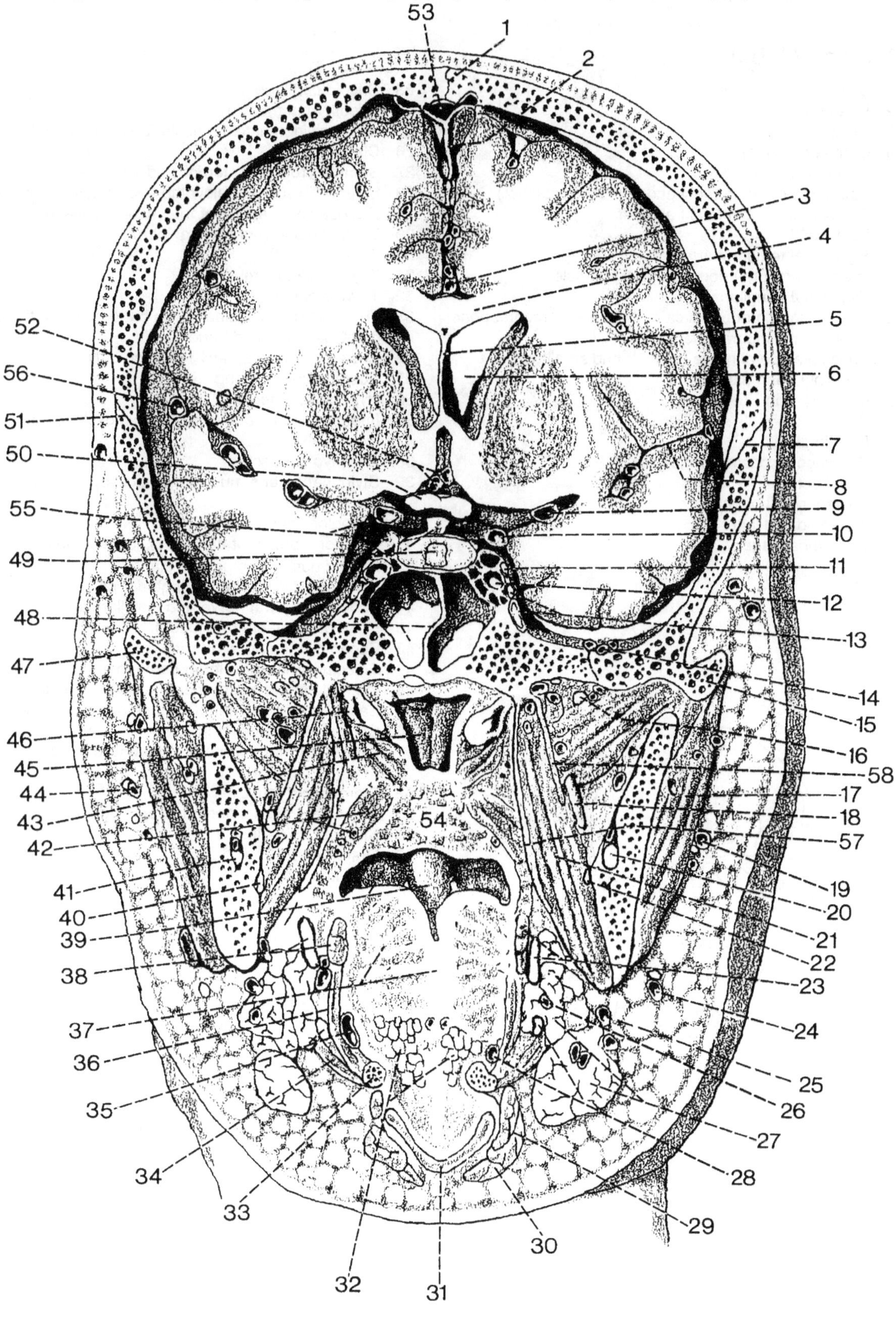
53
1
2
3
4
5
6
7
8
9
10
11
12
13
14
15
16
58
17
18
57
19
20
21
22
23
24
25
26
27
28
29
30
31
32
33
34
35
36
37
38
39
40
41
42
43
44
45
46
47
48
49
55
50
51
56
52
54

H&N-93 Carotid canal level

Color and label

1 Supeior sagittal sinus
2 Falx cerebri
3 Cingulate gyrus
4 Corpus callosum
5 Lateral ventricle
6 Septum pellucidum (right and left fused together)
7 Fornix (body)—both right and left
8 Ventricle III
9 Superficial temporal artery
10 Inferior (temporal) horn of lateral ventricle
11 Trigeminal ganglion
12 Internal carotid artery in carotid canal in temporal bone
13 Superficial temporal artery
14 Auriculotemporal nerve (medial) and small part of mandible head (lateral)
15 Maxillary vein
16 Parotid duct
17 Parotid gland
18 Pharyngeal constrictor muscles
19 Hyoid bone
20 Posterior wall of pharynx
21 Arytenoid cartilage
22 Thyroid cartilage
23 Cricoid cartilage
24 Cricothyroid muscle
25 Sternocleidomastoid muscle (clavicular head)
26 Clavicle (left)
27 Sternothyroid and sternohyoid muscles
28 Infraglottic space (below the vocal folds)—back wall is mucosa-lined lamina of the cricoid cartilage
29 Thyroid gland (right lateral lobe)
30 Clavicle (right)
31 Thyroarytenoid muscle
32 Thyrohyoid muscle
33 Thyrohyoid membrane (white band between thyroid cartilage and hyoid bone)
34 Superior laryngeal nerve (branch of N X)
35 Submandibular gland
36 Hypoglossal nerve (N XII)
37 Intermediate tendon of digastric muscle (connects its two bellies)
38 Stylohyoid muscle
39 Stylopharyngeus muscle and glossopharyngeal nerve (N IX)
40 Styloglossus muscle
41 Anterior tubercle of atlas (C1), longus capitis muscle
42 Parotid duct within parotid gland
43 Body of sphenoid bone (posterior part)
44 Auriculotemporal nerve and maxillary artery
45 Head of mandible (right side)
46 Superficial temporal artery
47 Articular disk inside temporomandibular joint
48 Internal carotid artery (right) in carotid canal
49 Basilar artery on ventral surface of pons of brain stem
50 Oculomotor nerve (N III)
51 Lateral (Sylvian) cerebral fissure with middle cerrebral artery
52 Sternohyoid muscle
53 Branches of facial nerve in parotid gland
54 Sternothyroid muscle
55 First tracheal ring
56 Maxillary artery

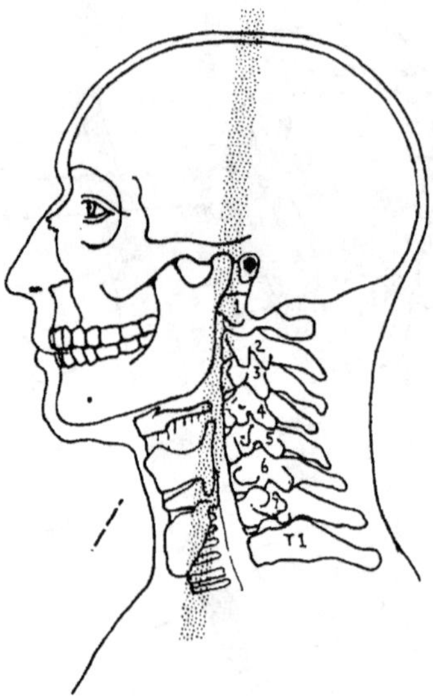

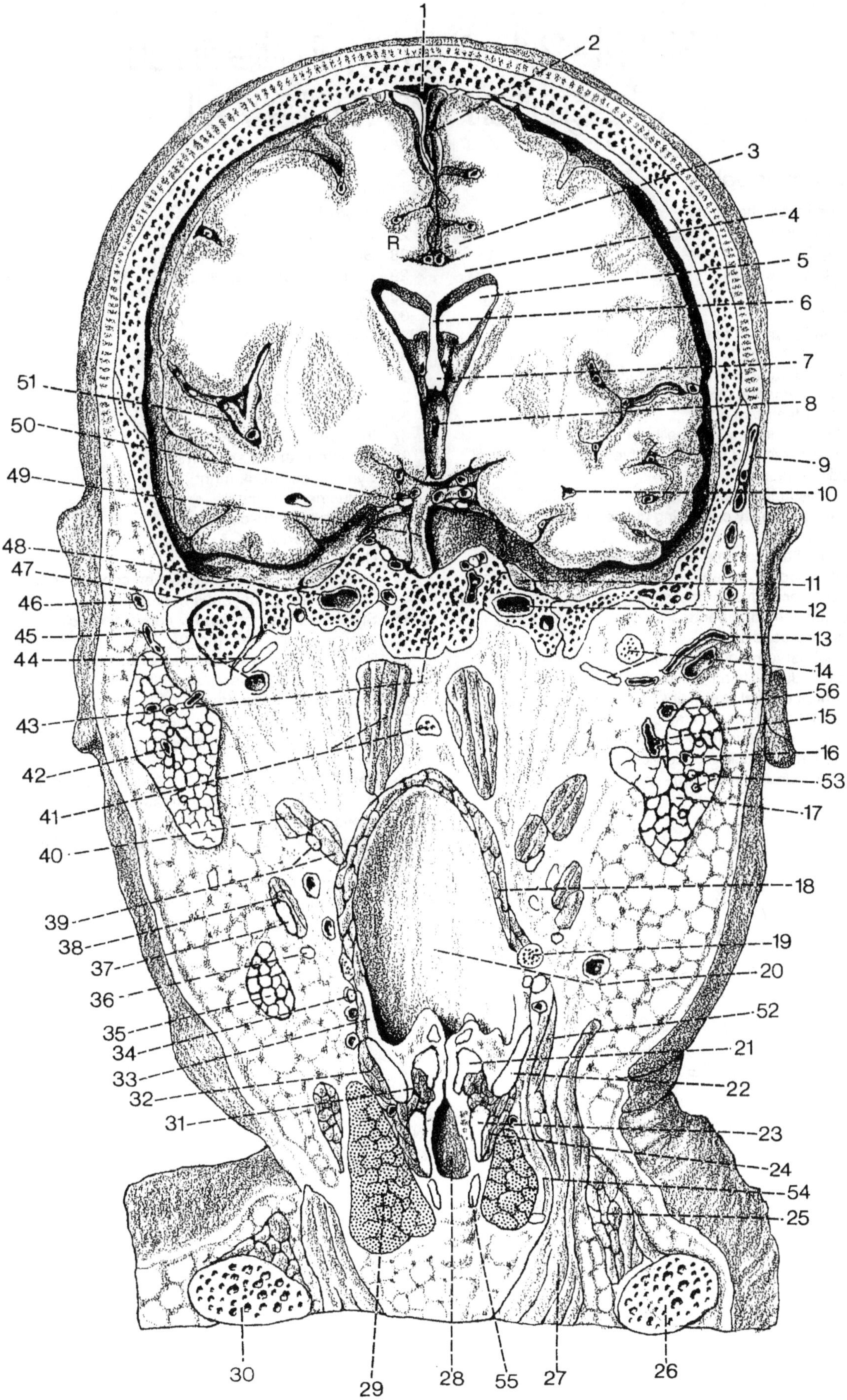
1
2
3
4
5
6
7
8
9
10
11
12
13
14
56
15
16
53
17
18
19
20
52
21
22
23
24
54
25
26
27
55
28
29
30
31
32
33
34
35
36
37
38
39
40
41
42
43
44
45
46
47
48
49
50
51
R

H&N-94 Pons, internal jugular vein level

Color and label

1 Superior sagittal sinus
2 Falx cerebri
3 Cingulate gyrus
4 Corpus callosum
5 Left lateral ventricle
6 Fornix
7 Lateral (Sylvian) fissure
8 Superior temporal gyrus
9 Inferior (temporal) horn of left lateral ventricle
10 Middle temporal gyrus
11 Inferior temporal gyrus
12 Edge of tentorium cerebelli
13 Facial nerve and vestibulocochlear nerve in internal auditory (acoustic) meatus
14 Air cells in temporal bone
15 Vestibule (cavity containing utricle and saccule) of inner ear
16 External auditory meatus (ear canal)
17 Left hypoglossal nerve (N XII) in hypoglossal canal
18 Facial nerve (N VII) descending through facial canal in petrous temporal bone
19 Occipital condyle
20 Facial nerve branches within parotid gland
21 Parotid duct within parotid gland
22 Atlanto-occipital joint (joint between vertebra C1 and occipital condyles at base of skull)
23 Odontoid process (dens) of C2 (axis)
24 Dorsal root ganglion of cervical spinal nerve C2
25 Internal jugular vein (left)—cut in several places

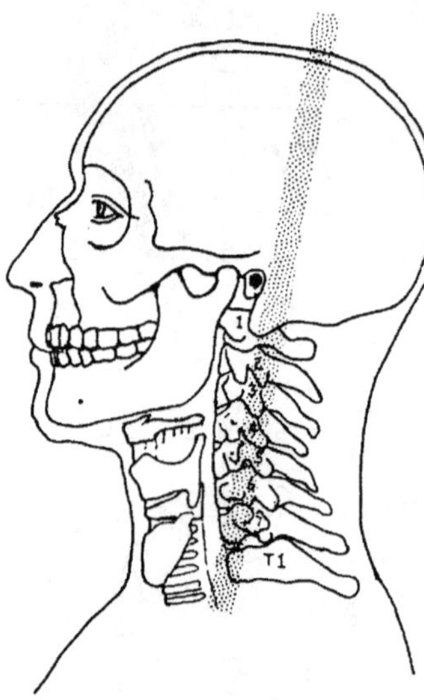

26 Internal carotid artery
27 Maxillary vein
28 Sternocleidomastoid muscle
29 Common carotid artery (left)
30 Thoracic duct
31 Clavicle (left)
32 Subclavian vein
33 Esophagus
34 Lymph glands
35 Thyroid gland
36 Clavicle (right)
37 Internal jugular vein (right)
38 Common carotid artery (right)
39 Sympathetic trunk (right)
40 Vagus nerve (right)
41 Longus colli muscle
42 Cervical vertebra C3
43 Cervical vertebra C2
44 Atlanto-axial joint (joint between cervical vertebrae C1 and C2) and right vagus nerve (N X)
45 Stylohyoid ligament and stylohyoid muscle
46 Internal jugular vein (right)
47 Parotid duct and facial nerve branches in parotid gland
48 Basilar artery on ventral medulla
49 Hypoglossal nerve (right)
50 Facial nerve (right) within facial canal
51 Tympanic cavity (middle ear, lateral) and cochlea (medial)
52 Nerves VII (facial) and VIII (vestibulocochlear, right) entering internal auditory meatus
53 Vestibule of right inner ear
54 Epitympanic recess (upper compartment of middle ear)
55 Pons
56 Middle meningeal artery
57 Hippocampal formation within temporal lobe of brain
58 Substantia nigra of midbrain
59 Ventricle III
60 Jugular foramen

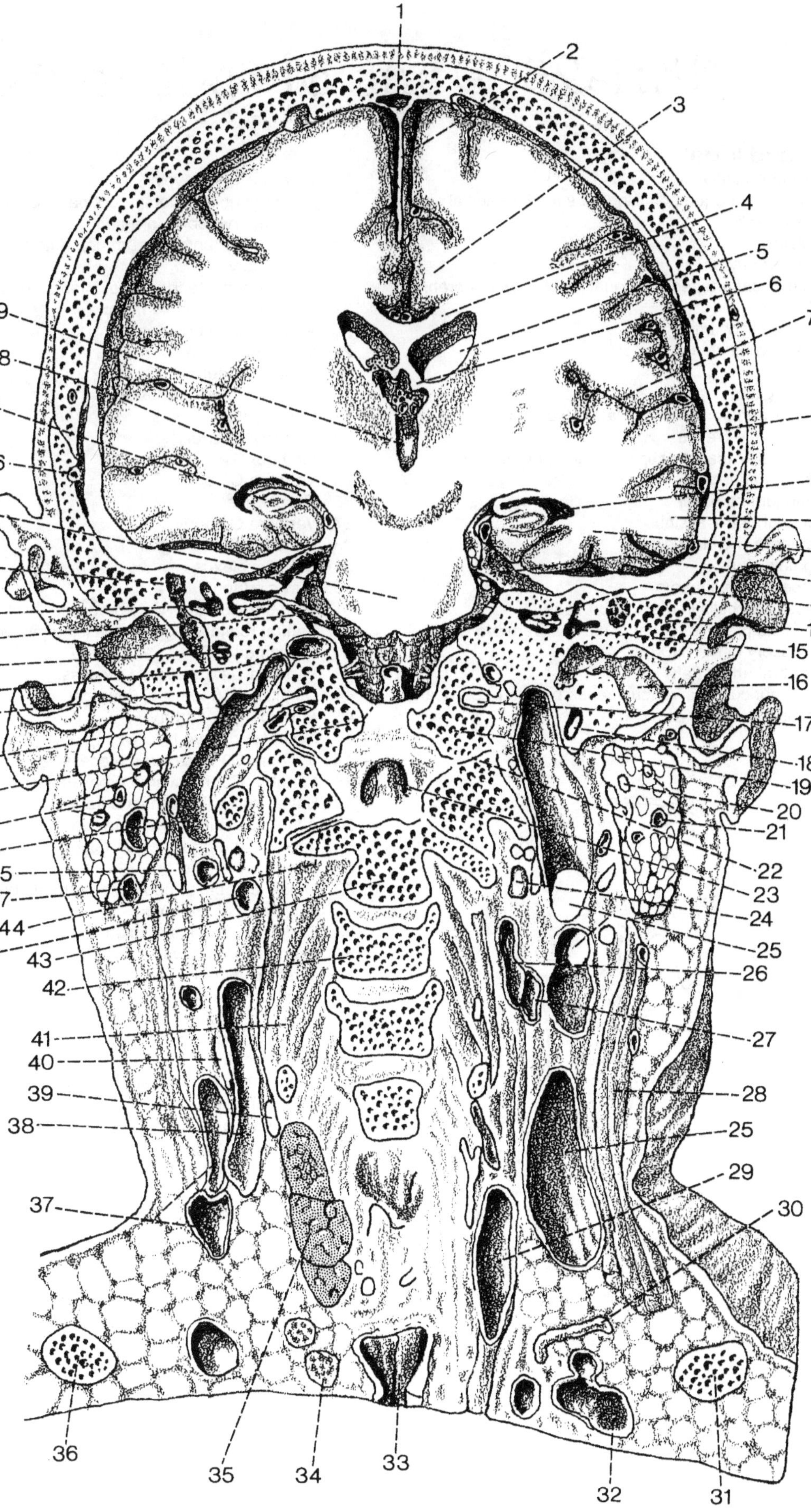
1
2
3
4
5
6
7
8
9
10
11
12
13
14
15
16
17
18
19
20
21
22
23
24
25
26
27
28
25
29
30
59
58
57
56
55
54
53
52
51
60
50
49
48
47
46
45
27
44
26
43
42
41
40
39
38
37
36
35
34
33
32
31

H&N-95 Dens of axis level

Color and label

1 Superior sagittal sinus
2 Lateral lacuna (outpouching) of superior sagittal sinus
3 Falx cerebri
4 Diploic vein
5 Cingulate gyrus
6 Pericallosal arteries (continuation of anterior cerebral arteries)
7 Corpus callosum
8 Lateral ventricle
9 Fornix
10 Pineal gland
11 Inferior (temporal) horn of lateral ventricle and choroid plexus
12 Ventricle IV (narrow superior end approaching cerebral aqueduct)
13 Tentorium cerebelli
14 Superior petrosal sinus
15 Cerebellar hemisphere
16 Sigmoid sinus
17 Lesser occipital nerve
18 Mastoid air cells in mastoid process
19 Odontoid process (dens) of cervical vertebra C2
20 Accessory nerve (N XI)
21 Vertebral artery (left)
22 Great auricular nerve (cutaneous branch of cervical plexus)

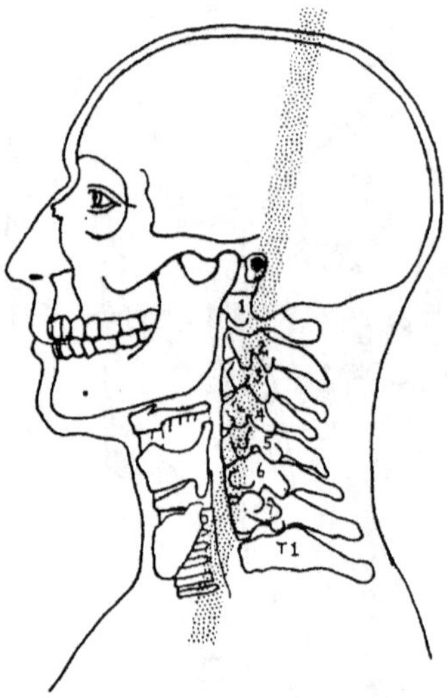

23 External jugular vein
24 Spinal ganglion (dorsal root ganglion) of spinal nerve; C3 in intervetebral foramen
25 Spinal cord (anterior surface); note anterior rootlets of spinal nerves
26 Portion of posterior wall of internal jugular vein
27 Sternocleidomastoid muscle
28 Vertebra C5 body
29 Spinal nerve C6
30 Vertebral artery
31 Scalenus medius muscle
32 Clavicle (left)
33 Subclavian artery
34 First rib
35 Vertebra C6 body
36 Esophagus
37 Vertebra C7 body
38 Vertebral artery (right)
39 Brachial plexus
40 Clavicle (right)
41 Vertebra C5 transverse process
42 Ventral rootlets (right) coalescing into ventral root of spinal nerve C5
43 Vertebra C4 transverse process
44 Denticulate (toothlike) ligament
45 Anterior spinal artery
46 Accessory nerve N XI (right)
47 Vertebra C3 transverse process
48 Vertebra C2 transverse process and right vertebral artery
49 Spinal nerve C2 with its dural sheath
50 Atlanto-occipital joint (between skull and C1 vertebra), transverse process of C1 (atlas)
51 Occipital condyle
52 Middle cerebellar peduncle (formerly brachium pontis Latin, arm of the pons)
53 Superior colliculus of midbrain
54 Internal cerebral veins (join posteriorly to form great cerebral vein of Galen)
55 Splenium of corpus callosum
56 Artifactual space caused by collapse of arachnoid membrane onto pia mater and obliteration of subarachnoid space—normally arachnoid membrane rests directly inside dura mater. A subdural hematoma would form in this potential space.
57 Arachnoid granulation (stretched and distorted)
58 Medulla oblongata
59 Anterior scalene muscle

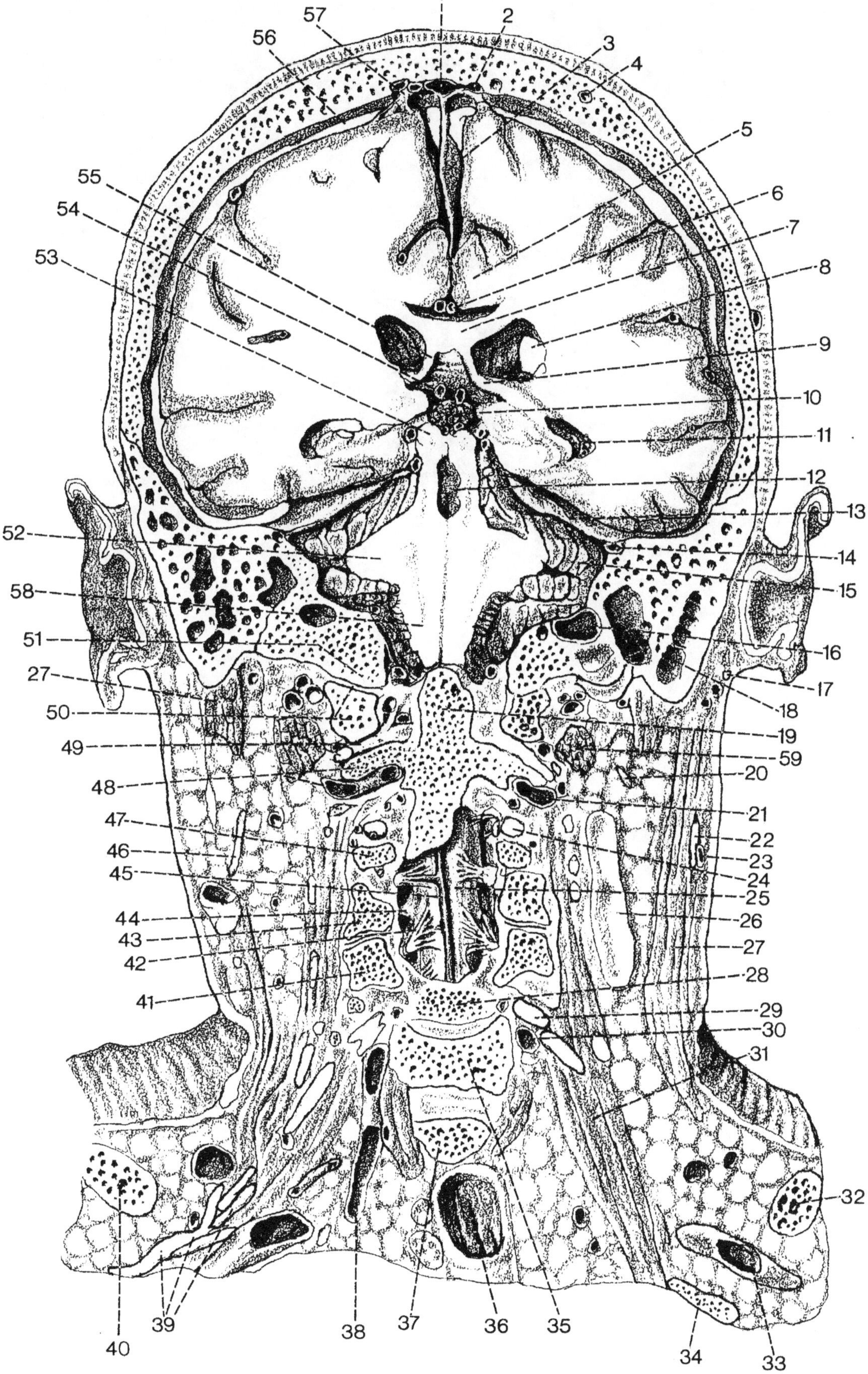
57
2
56
3
4
5
55
6
54
7
53
8
9
10
11
12
13
52
14
58
15
51
16
27
17
18
50
19
49
59
48
20
21
47
22
46
23
45
24
25
44
26
43
27
42
28
41
29
30
31
32
39
38
37
36
35
40
34
33

www.ingramcontent.com/pod-product-compliance
Lightning Source LLC
LaVergne TN
LVHW082012200926
848481LV00010B/2843
9780983578420